Care of the Jaundiced Neonate

Care of the Jaundiced Neonate

David K. Stevenson, MD
Harold K. Faber Professor of Pediatrics
Department of Pediatrics
Division of Neonatal and Developmental Medicine
Stanford University School of Medicine
Stanford, California

M. Jeffrey Maisels, MB BCh, DSc
Physician in Chief, Beaumont Children's Hospital
Professor and Chair
Department of Pediatrics
Oakland University William Beaumont School of Medicine
Royal Oak, Michigan

Jon F. Watchko, MD
Professor of Pediatrics
University of Pittsburgh School of Medicine
Division of Newborn Medicine
Magee-Womens Research Institute
Pittsburgh, Pennsylvania

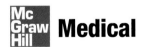

New York   Chicago   San Francisco   Lisbon   London   Madrid   Mexico City
Milan   New Delhi   San Juan   Seoul   Singapore   Sydney   Toronto

The McGraw·Hill Companies

Care of the Jaundiced Neonate

1 2 3 4 5 6 7 8 9 0 CTP/CTP 17 16 15 14 13 12

ISBN 978-0-07-176289-2
MHID 0-07-176289-2

This book was set in Minion by Thomson Digital.
The editors were Alyssa K. Fried and Robert Pancotti.
The production supervisor was Catherine H. Saggese.
The illustration manager was Armen Ovsepyan.
Project management was provided by Charu Bansal, Thomson Digital.
The text designer was Mary McKeon; the cover designer was Elizabeth Pisacreta.
China Translation & Printing Services, Ltd. was printer and binder.

Library of Congress Cataloging-in-Publication Data

Care of the jaundiced neonate / editors, David K. Stevenson, M. Jeffrey Maisels, Jon F. Watchko.
    p. ; cm.
  Includes bibliographical references and index.
  ISBN 978-0-07-176289-2 (hardcover : alk. paper)
  I. Stevenson, David K. (David Kendal), 1949- II. Maisels, M. Jeffrey. III. Watchko, Jon F.
  [DNLM: 1. Jaundice, Neonatal. WS 421]
  618.923'625–dc23
                                    2012007113

To our families and to all others and their babies,
most of whom become jaundiced for a while after birth.

Contents

Contributors

Cristina Bellarosa, PhD
Senior Researcher
Italian Liver Foundation
Trieste, Italy

Vinod K. Bhutani, MD, FAAP
Professor
Department of Pediatrics
Stanford University School of Medicine
Stanford, California

Dag Bratlid, MD, PhD, MHA
Professor of Pediatrics
Department of Laboratory Medicine,
    Children's and Women's Health
Faculty of Medicine, Norwegian
    University of Science and Technology
Trondheim, Norway

Dora Brites, PhD
Senior Researcher and Full Professor
Neuron Glia Biology in Health and Disease
Faculty of Pharmacy, University of Lisbon
Lisbon, Portugal

Maria Alexandra Brito, PharmD, PhD
Professor
Research Institute for Medicines and
    Pharmaceutical Sciences (iMed.UL)
Faculty of Pharmacy, University of Lisbon
Lisbon, Portugal

Jane E. Brumbaugh, MD
Fellow, Neonatal-Perinatal Medicine
Department of Pediatrics
University of Minnesota
Minneapolis, Minnesota

Glenn R. Gourley, MD, AGAF
Professor of Pediatrics
University of Minnesota
Minneapolis, Minnesota

Cathy Hammerman, MD
Department of Neonatology
Shaare Zedek Medical Center
Professor of Pediatrics
Faculty of Medicine of The Hebrew University
Jerusalem, Israel

Thor Willy Ruud Hansen, MD, PhD, MHA, FAAP
Professor of Pediatrics
Women & Children's Division
Oslo University Hospital, Rikshospitalet
Oslo, Norway

Michael Kaplan, MB, ChB
Department of Neonatology
Shaare Zedek Medical Center
Professor of Pediatrics
Faculty of Medicine of The Hebrew University
Jerusalem, Israel

Zhili Lin, MD, PhD
Director
Research and Development
PerkinElmer Genetics, Inc.
Bridgeville, Pennsylvania

M. Jeffrey Maisels, MB BCh, DSc
Physician in Chief, Beaumont Children's Hospital
Professor and Chair
Department of Pediatrics
Oakland University William Beaumont School of Medicine
Royal Oak, Michigan

Antony F. McDonagh, PhD
Department of Medicine and The Liver Center
Division of Gastroenterology
University of California, San Francisco
San Francisco, California
Consulting Professor
Department of Pediatrics
Division of Neonatal and Developmental Medicine
Stanford University School of Medicine
Stanford, California

Lucie Muchova, MD, PhD
Assistant Professor of Medical Chemistry and Biochemistry
4th Department of Internal Medicine & Institute of
   Clinical Biochemistry & Laboratory
Diagnostics 1st Medical Faculty
Charles University of Prague
Prague, Czech Republic

Thomas B. Newman, MD, MPH
Attending Physician, Benioff Children's Hospital
Professor of Epidemiology and Biostatistics and
   Pediatrics and Chief, Division of Clinical Epidemiology
School of Medicine
University of California, San Francisco
San Francisco, California

Bolajoko O. Olusanya, MBBS, FRCPCH, PhD
Developmental Pediatrician & Honorary Lecturer
Community Health & Primary Care
College of Medicine, University of Lagos
Surulere, Lagos, Nigeria

Steven M. Shapiro, MD, MSHA
Professor of Pediatrics
Chief, Section Pediatric Neurology
Children's Mercy Hospital and Clinics and
   University of Missouri-Kansas City
Kansas City, Missouri
Professor of Neurology
Kansas University Medical Center
Kansas City, Kansas

Tina M. Slusher, MD, FAAP
Associate Professor
Pediatrics, Division of Global Pedatrics
University of Minnesota and Hennepin
   County Medical Center
Minneapolis, Minnesota

David K. Stevenson, MD
Harold K. Faber Professor of Pediatrics
Department of Pediatrics
Division of Neonatal and Developmental Medicine
Stanford University School of Medicine
Stanford, California

Claudio Tiribelli, MD, PhD
Professor of Medicine
Medical Sciences
Italian Liver Foundation & University of Trieste
Trieste, Italy

Libor Vitek, MD, PhD, MBA
Professor of Medical Chemistry and Biochemistry
4th Department of Internal Medicine and Institute of
   Clinical Biochemistry and Laboratory Medicine
1st Faculty of Medicine
Charles University of Prague
Prague, Czech Republic

Hendrik J. Vreman, PhD
Senior Research Scientist
Department of Pediatrics
Stanford University School of Medicine
Stanford, California

Jon F. Watchko, MD
Professor of Pediatrics
University of Pittsburgh School of Medicine
Division of Newborn Medicine
Magee-Womens Research Institute
Pittsburgh, Pennsylvania

Ronald J. Wong, BS
Senior Research Scientist
Department of Pediatrics
Stanford University School of Medicine
Stanford, California

Preface

Neonatal jaundice is perhaps the most common of all pediatric problems and hazardous levels of unconjugated bilirubin pose a direct threat of permanent brain damage (kernicterus). Current population-based kernicterus estimates of the prevalence for term neonates in developed countries range from approximately 1:50,000 to 1:200,000. In low- and middle-income countries, although the prevalence is unknown, kernicterus appears to be a much more serious problem. Thus, the prevention of kernicterus remains a concern for neonatal caregivers worldwide.

In addition, it is now increasingly apparent that some neonatal hyperbilirubinemia is the result of complex gene–environment interactions and that the molecular pathogenesis of bilirubin-induced neurotoxicity follows a cascade of events not previously appreciated. This volume was designed to bring together the relevant basic science and clinical information necessary for understanding the genesis of neonatal hyperbilirubinemia and bilirubin-induced brain damage as well as information regarding care of the jaundiced neonate. We are fortunate to have recruited outstanding experts in the field who share their insightful perspectives based on current knowledge and extensive clinical experience, so that this book can serve as an essential reference for both practitioners and investigators.

This volume addresses a broad array of interrelated topics, ranging from the genetics, biochemistry, transport, and metabolism of bilirubin to neonatal hyperbilirubinemia, public policy measures, clinical management, and interventions designed to prevent and treat neonatal hyperbilirubinemia and to reduce the burden of bilirubin encephalopathy in developed and low- and middle-income countries. The pathobiology of bilirubin-induced neurotoxicity, the clinical diagnosis and outcome of kernicterus, and the important contributions of hemolytic disease and glucose-6-phosphate dehydrogenase deficiency to neonatal hyperbilirubinemia are detailed. The book also includes discussion of risk assessment and treatment with phototherapy and other modalities. Collectively the chapters complement each other; they point out gaps in knowledge as well as consensus regarding practice. We hope that this book provides both the clinician and the investigator with a firm basis for future study and the stimulus to move the field forward.

David K. Stevenson, MD
M. Jeffrey Maisels, MB BCh, DSc
Jon F. Watchko, MD

Acknowledgments

This work was supported by the Mary L. Johnson Research Fund, the Christopher Hess Research Fund, the L.H.M. Lui Research Fund, the Clinical and Translational Science Award 1UL1 RR025744 for the Stanford Center for Clinical and Translational Education and Research (Spectrum) from the National Center for Research Resources, National Institutes of Health, the Mario Lemieux Centers for Patient Care and Research of the Mario Lemieux Foundation, and The 25 Club of Magee-Womens Hospital.

Genetics of Neonatal Jaundice

Jon F. Watchko and Zhili Lin

■ INTRODUCTION

Neonatal hyperbilirubinemia and resultant jaundice are common,[1,2] affecting up to ~80% of newborns.[1] Although generally a benign postnatal transitional phenomenon, a select number of infants develop more significant and potentially hazardous levels of total serum bilirubin (TSB) (Table 1-1)[3,4] that may pose a direct threat of brain damage.[3,5,6] Numerous factors contribute to the development of hyperbilirubinemia including genes involved in: (i) the production of bilirubin from heme; (ii) the metabolism of bilirubin; and (iii) heritable conditions that may reduce red blood cell (RBC) life span and predispose to hemolysis, thereby increasing the bilirubin load[7–17] in neonates. The genetics of neonatal hyperbilirubinemia is the focus of this chapter.

In contrast to fully penetrant genetically dominant conditions or those that are mainly environmentally derived, severe neonatal hyperbilirubinemia (TSB >20 mg/dL [342 µmol/L])[3,4] is frequently manifested as a pediatric *complex trait or disorder*. The term *complex* in this context infers the condition is: (i) prevalent (>1% of neonates);[3,4] (ii) multifactorial;[16,17] and (iii) polygenic[16,17] (Figure 1-1).[18] In fact, severe neonatal hyperbilirubinemia is often marked by: (1) etiologic heterogeneity; (2) key environmental influences; and/or (3) the interaction of multiple gene loci, which individually show relatively limited effects, but with each other and nongenetic factors[7–17,19]—a contributing role to hyperbilirubinemia risk.

Characterizing the genetics underlying complex traits is fraught with challenges.[18] Several lines of epidemiologic evidence,[20] however, support the assertion that genetic contributors are clinically relevant modulators of neonatal hyperbilirubinemia. These include: (i) the clinical significance of a positive family history; (ii) twin studies; (iii) the impact of genetic heritage on hyperbilirubinemia risk; and (iv) male/female differences. This information will be briefly reviewed before an analysis of known icterogenic and candidate genes involved in the control of TSB concentration.

■ POSITIVE FAMILY HISTORY

A positive family history can serve as a marker for shared genetic susceptibility.[21] In this regard, several studies, with one recent exception,[22] have identified *a previous sibling with a history of neonatal jaundice* as an important risk factor for neonatal hyperbilirubinemia with adjusted odds ratios (OR) ranging from 2.29 (95% confidence interval [CI]: 1.87–2.81)[23] to 6.0 (1.0–36.0),[24] most reporting a greater than 2-fold higher risk.[23,24] Moreover, there appears to be a direct relationship between the magnitude of peak TSB levels and hyperbilirubinemia risk in subsequent siblings; if a previous sibling had a TSB level >12 mg/dL (205 µmol/L), the risk of a similar TSB in a subsequent sibling was 2.7 times higher than that in controls; if TSB level >15 mg/dL (257 µmol/L), the risk in subsequent siblings increased to 12.5 times greater than that in controls.[25] These findings resonate well with the report of Nielsen et al. of a significant positive correlation between peak TSB levels of siblings.[26] A family history of jaundice in a newborn is also associated with a greater risk of having a TSB >95th percentile on the Bhutani nomogram[16]

■ **TABLE 1-1.** Estimated Occurrence of Neonatal Hyperbilirubinemia Severity

TSB (mg/dL)[a]	Proposed Definition	Estimated Occurrence
≥17.0 (291 μmol/L)	Significant	~1:10
≥20.0 (342 μmol/L)	Severe	~1:70
≥25.0 (428 μmol/L)	Extreme	~1:700
≥30.0 (513 μmol/L)	Hazardous	~1:10,000

[a]TSB, total serum bilirubin.

Adapted from Bhutani VK, Johnson LH, Maisels MJ, et al. Kernicterus: epidemiological strategies for its prevention through systems-based approaches. *J Perinatol.* 2004;24:650–662, with permission from Macmillan Publishers Ltd, copyright 2004.

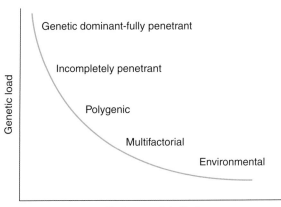

FIGURE 1-1. The relationship between genetic load and environment in the development of disease is shown in this schema.[18] An etiologic continuum from strictly genetic, through polygenic–multifactorial, to largely environmental is observed. Severe neonatal hyperbilirubinemia is characteristically a polygenic–multifactorial trait. (Reproduced from Bomprezzi R, Kovanen PE, Martin R. New approaches to investigating heterogeneity in complex traits. *J Med Genet.* 2003;40:553–559, with permission from BMJ Publishing Group Ltd.)

and a TSB >25 mg/dL (428 μmol/L) in subsequent siblings.[24] This consistent relationship across investigations may reflect in part the heritable risk of hemolytic disease due to ABO or Rh isoimmunization, glucose-6-phosphate dehydrogenase (G6PD) deficiency, and/or exposure to a common environmental factor in addition to a shared genetic background.[23] The sustained excess risk in full siblings of infants with neonatal jaundice independent of known hyperbilirubinemia risk factors (e.g., breastfeeding, prematurity) expected to recur in sibships,[23–25] however, suggests that genetic rather than nongenetic effects are largely responsible.

■ TWIN STUDIES

Twin studies, despite their limitations, have been used for decades to decipher the environmental and genetic backgrounds of complex traits and estimate their heritability.[27] Clinical study comparing monozygotic (identical) with dizygotic (fraternal) twins demonstrate that zygosity, that is, genetic factors, plays an important role in the genesis of neonatal hyperbilirubinemia.[28] Ebbesen and Mortensen, in the only classic twin study of neonatal hyperbilirubinemia reported to date, compared the difference in TSB concentration between monozygotic and dizygotic newborn twins and observed that the median difference between the monozygotic twins was approximately half of that found in dizygotic twins confirming that zygosity, that is, genetic factors, was significant.[28] These findings were controlled for confounders known to modulate neonatal bilirubinemia, including sex, gestational age, postnatal age, maternal smoking, mode of

feeding, postnatal weight loss, and ABO blood-type incompatibility. The high degree of concordance in TSB levels between identical twin pairs in this northern European cohort closely mirrors that reported by Tan in Chinese homozygous twins.[29]

■ GENETIC HERITAGE

Epidemiologic study has revealed significant differences in hyperbilirubinemia incidence (Figure 1-2)[30] and in the risk for more marked hyperbilirubinemia across populations.[24,30,31] Although complex phenotypes vary within and between populations,[32] the study of genetic differentiation across populations can shed insight into the genetic architecture of a given trait.[33] The term population in this context refers to a "geographically and culturally determined collection of individuals who share a common gene pool."[32] Gene flow has been modest between populations in the United States so that despite genetic admixture many populations including African Americans, Asians, and Pacific Islanders still closely represent their indigenous origins from a genetic perspective, and this genetic heritage can impact disease susceptibility.[33] Most notably regarding jaundice, neonates of East

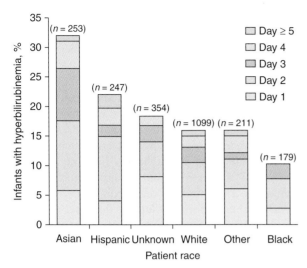

FIGURE 1-2. Incidence of neonatal hyperbilirubinemia as a function of postnatal age in days and mother's race. Hyperbilirubinemia was defined as a TSB ≥5 mg/dL (86 μmol/L) at <24 hours of age, ≥10 mg/dL (171 μmol/L) at 24–48 hours of age, or ≥13 mg/dL (222 μmol/L) thereafter. (Reprinted with permission from Newman TB, Easterling MJ, Goldman ES, Stevenson DK. Laboratory evaluation of jaundice in newborns. *Am J Dis Child*. 1990;144:365, copyright © 1990, American Medical Association. All rights reserved.)

Asian ancestry encompassing the populations of mainland China, Hong Kong, Japan, Macau, Korea, and Taiwan demonstrate a higher incidence of hyperbilirubinemia than other populations[30] and an overall increased risk for a TSB of ≥20 mg/dL (342 μmol/L) (OR: 3.1 [95% CI: 1.5–6.3]).[24] Severe jaundice requiring treatment, rehospitalization for jaundice, or a birth hospitalization stay for greater than 5 days is more likely (relative risk [RR]: 1.7 [95% CI: 1.12–2.58]) in infants of full East Asian parentage.[31] As such, East Asian ancestry is listed as a major risk factor for severe hyperbilirubinemia in the 2004 American Academy of Pediatrics (AAP) clinical practice guideline.[34] Investigators have speculated as to the nature of this phenomenon invoking potential population differences in the incidence of ABO hemolytic disease and G6PD deficiency as well as environmental exposures to Chinese *Materia Medica* among others.[35] Indeed, G6PD deficiency is an important contributor to hyperbilirubinemia risk in East Asian newborns.

Innate variation in hepatic bilirubin clearance[35] also contributes to the biologic basis of hyperbilirubinemia risk in Asian newborns as revealed by genetic

analysis of enzymatic variants that modulate hepatic bilirubin uptake and conjugation. Bilirubin conjugation with glucuronic acid is mediated by the specific hepatic bilirubin uridine diphosphate glucuronosyltransferase isoenzyme *UGT1A1* (OMIM *191740) as detailed in section "*UGT1A1* Polymorphisms." Four different *UGT1A1 coding* sequence variants—G211A (*UGT1A1*6*), C686A (*UGT1A1*27*), C1091T (*UGT1A1*73*), and T1456G (*UGT1A1*7*)—have been described in East Asian populations, each associated with a significant reduction in UGT1A1 enzyme activity and a Gilbert syndrome phenotype.[14,17,36–39] Gilbert syndrome is characterized by mild, chronic or recurrent unconjugated hyperbilirubinemia in the absence of liver disease or overt hemolysis.[40] Of these *UGT1A1* coding sequence variants, the *UGT1A1*6* polymorphism predominates in East Asian populations with an allele frequency ranging from ~13% to 23% increasing to ~30% in East Asian neonates with hyperbilirubinemia ≥15 mg/dL (257 μmol/L).[37] UGT1A1 isoenzyme activity in subjects homozygous for *UGT1A1*6* range between ~14%[37] and ~32% of wild type[38] and this variant is associated with a 2- to 3-fold increased risk for neonatal hyperbilirubinemia[15,37,41–44] as well as prolonged indirect hyperbilirubinemia in breast-fed neonates.[45,46] One recent report from China also suggests an association between *UGT1A1*6* allele frequency and the risk for TSB >20 mg/dL (342 μmol/L) and bilirubin encephalopathy.[47] Hypomorphic *UGT1A1 promoter sequence* polymorphisms, including the TATA box variant *UGT1A1*28* (A[TA]$_6$TAA to A[TA]$_7$TAA) and phenobarbital-responsive enhancer module (PBREM) variant *UGT1A1*60* (−3279T>G), are also observed in East Asian populations,[48] albeit typically at lower allele frequencies than *UGT1A*6*, but their coexpression with *UGT1A1*6* and other *UGT1A1 coding sequence* variants to form compound heterozygous genotypes is observed in 6.9% of Chinese neonates.[44] The coupling of hypomorphic *UGT1A1* promoter and coding sequence variants would be expected to reduce UGT1A1 isoenzyme activity further and thereby enhance neonatal hyperbilirubinemia risk. Coexpression of *UGT1A1* coding sequence and promoter variants merits further study as a contributor to the higher incidence of hyperbilirubinemia in East Asian neonates.[44]

Gene variants of the hepatic solute carrier organic anion transporter 1B1 (*SLCO1B1*) (OMIM *604843), a sinusoidal transmembrane receptor that may facilitate the hepatic uptake of unconjugated bilirubin as detailed in section "*SLCO1B1* Polymorphisms," are also prevalent in East Asian populations.[15,49] Nonsynonymous *SLCO1B1* gene variants that limit the efficacy of hepatic bilirubin uptake could ultimately impair hepatic bilirubin clearance and predispose to hyperbilirubinemia. One putative allele, *SLCO1B1*1b* (A388G), is reported to enhance neonatal hyperbilirubinemia risk in Taiwanese neonates,[15] an effect not seen however in Thai[50] or Malaysian Chinese newborns.[51] Coupling of icterogenic *UGT1A1* and *SLCO1B1* variants is reported to enhance neonatal hyperbilirubinemia risk in Taiwanese newborns,[15] one that is further increased when the infant is also exclusively breastfed.[15]

In contrast to infants of East Asian heritage, African American neonates as a group show a lower overall incidence of clinically significant hyperbilirubinemia[6,22,30,52–57] including less frequent: (i) TSB levels that approach or exceed the 2004 AAP hour-specific phototherapy treatment threshold (OR: 0.43, 95% CI: 0.23–0.80[22]; OR: 0.35, 95% CI: 0.22–0.55[52,53]) and (ii) TSB levels of ≥20 mg/dL (342 μmol/L) (OR: 0.56, 95% CI: 0.41–0.76[6]; OR: 0.36, 95% CI: 0.148–0.885[52]). As such, African American race is listed as a factor associated with decreased risk of significant jaundice in the 2004 AAP clinical practice guideline.[34] The prevalence of peak TSB levels in the 0–12 mg/dL (0–205 μmol/L) "physiologic" range, however, is comparable between African American and white newborns (Table 1-2).[54,57] The mechanisms that underlie the overall

lower prevalence of significant hyperbilirubinemia in African American newborns are not clear.[57] The high allele frequencies of less efficient hypomorphic *UGT1A1* promoter variants (*UGT1A1*28* and *UGT1A1*37* representing seven and eight thymine–adenine [TA] repeats in the promoter TATA box region, respectively, that limit *UGT1A1* transcription as contrasted with the wild-type six repeats denoted as *UGT1A1*1*) and *SLCO1B1* A388G gene polymorphism in African American subjects[16,57,58] would, if anything, impair hepatic bilirubin clearance and uptake, respectively, and predispose to hyperbilirubinemia. These findings suggest other genetic and/or environmental factors account for the lower incidence of marked hyperbilirubinemia in African American neonates. In this regard, the higher formula-feeding prevalence reported among African American mothers[59,60] would likely limit enterohepatic bilirubin circulation and facilitate enteric bilirubin elimination, thereby reducing hepatic bilirubin load and hyperbilirubinemia risk. However, even among formula-fed newborns, neonates identified as African American have lower hyperbilirubinemia risk than their white, Latino, and Asian counterparts.[52] Clarification of this phenomenon must await further investigation.

Although African American neonates have an apparent overall lower risk for significant hyperbilirubinemia, a clinically noteworthy few go on to develop hazardous hyperbilirubinemia.[3,4,57] Indeed, African Americans are

■ TABLE 1-2. Peak Total Serum Bilirubin (TSB) in Black and White Newborns (Birth Weight > 2500 g)

TSB (mg/dL)	White (*n*)	%	Black (*n*)	%	*P*-Value[a]	Odds Ratio[b] (Black/White)
0–7	11,908	69.4	11,734	69.5	.85	1 (0.96–1.05)
8–12	3243	18.9	3309	19.6	.11	1.05 (0.99–1.1)
13–15	531	3.1	412	2.4	<.0003	0.78 (0.69–0.89)
16–19	315	1.8	202	1.2	<.0001	0.64 (0.53–0.76)
≥20	153	0.9	97	0.6	<.0001	0.64 (0.49–0.83)
Total	16,150		15,754			
Unknown	1012		1133			
Grand total	17,162		16,887			

[a]Black versus white, Chi square with Yate's correction.

[b]95% confidence interval. Adapted from Collaborative Perinatal Project; data were collected from 1959 to 1966 prior to introduction of phototherapy.

Reprinted from Watchko JF. Hyperbilirubinemia in African American neonates: clinical issues and current challenges. *Semin Fetal Neonatal Med.* 2010;15:176–182, with permission from Elsevier, copyright 2010.

overrepresented in the US Pilot Kernicterus Registry[3,4,55] accounting for more than 25% of US kernicterus cases,[3,4,57] and black race is an independent risk factor for bilirubin encephalopathy (OR: 19.0; 95% CI: 2.5–144.7) in the United Kingdom and Ireland as well.[61] G6PD deficiency accounts for ~60% of African American newborns with kernicterus[3,4,57] with late-preterm gestation and ABO hemolytic disease being other clinically important clinical contributors to severe hyperbilirubinemia risk in African American neonates.[57] Clinical study designed to enhance the identification of African American newborns predisposed to develop hazardous hyperbilirubinemia is of particular merit including the potential utility of birth hospitalization point of care G6PD screening.[57,62]

Regarding genetic heritage, it is important to recognize that ethnicity does not properly capture or characterize an individual's genotype or even genetic variation among individuals; more accurate assessment will be obtained by genotyping specific disease-associated alleles.[32,33] In the absence of being able to perform genotyping studies routinely, however, population affiliation will continue to be of clinical value in broadly assessing risk.[17,34]

■ MALE SEX

Several reports demonstrate that male neonates have higher TSB levels than female neonates[2,23,63,64] and are overrepresented in: (i) infant cohorts readmitted to the hospital for management of neonatal jaundice[2,64,65] (OR: 2.89 [95% CI: 1.46–5.74])[2]; (ii) the US Pilot Kernicterus Registry, a database of voluntarily reported cases of kernicterus, where there is an ~2-fold greater predominance of males ($n = 84$) than females ($n = 38$)[3]; and (iii) autopsied cases of kernicterus (male:female ratio 127:90).[66] Others have failed to demonstrate sex as a significant risk factor for hyperbilirubinemia (>95th percentile on Bhutani nomogram).[16] In general, however, the current literature suggests both an increased risk for marked hyperbilirubinemia and an increased susceptibility to bilirubin-induced injury in male neonates. Regarding the former, the prevalence of the Gilbert syndrome is reportedly more than 2-fold higher in males (12.4%) than in females (4.8%).[67] The UGT1A1 gene variants that underlie Gilbert syndrome detailed below would be expected to enhance the risk of neonatal hyperbilirubinemia, particularly when coexpressed with other

icterogenic conditions,[12,15,16] including G6PD deficiency which given its X-linked nature is also more prevalent in males. In addition, several clinical studies suggest greater male susceptibility to bilirubin-induced central nervous system (CNS) injury,[68–71] a phenomenon also noted in the Gunn rat model of neonatal hyperbilirubinemia and kernicterus.[72,73] A potential role for sex hormones in this process remains unexplored but merits study as gonadotropin surges during late embryonic and early postnatal life impact CNS development.[74] Innate gender-based neuronal differences independent of circulating sex steroids may also contribute to this sexually dimorphic vulnerability to CNS injury.[75]

■ SPECIFIC GENES AND THEIR VARIANTS THAT MODULATE NEONATAL BILIRUBIN CONCENTRATION

Numerous genes are involved in controlling neonatal bilirubin concentration and can be categorized as those that modulate: (i) heme production (namely, conditions that predispose to hemolysis and/or reduce RBC life span); (ii) the catabolism of heme to bilirubin (heme oxygenase [HO]; biliverdin reductase); (iii) hepatic bilirubin uptake (SLCO1B1); (iv) hepatocyte bilirubin binding (glutathione S-transferase [GST; ligandin]); and (v) hepatic bilirubin clearance (UGT1A1). Specific gene mutations and polymorphisms related to each category are reviewed below in sequence as schematized in Figure 1-3. Regulatory genes, particularly those of the nuclear receptor superfamily that modulate the expression of genes involved in bilirubin metabolism, will also be detailed.[76]

■ HERITABLE CONDITIONS THAT MAY CAUSE HEMOLYSIS IN NEONATES

The reduced life span of normal newborn RBCs (70–90 days as opposed to 120 days in the adult)[77,78] contributes to enhanced bilirubin production in neonates. Heritable hemolytic disorders accelerate RBC turnover and are major risk factors for severe hyperbilirubinemia.[3] The heritable causes of hemolysis in the newborns are many, but can be broadly grouped into: (i) defects of RBC metabolism, of which G6PD and pyruvate kinase (PK) deficiency are notable causes; (ii) defects of RBC membrane structure, of which congenital spherocytosis is an important and underrecognized contributor; (iii) defects

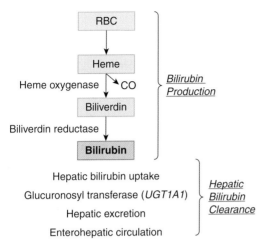

FIGURE 1-3. Schematic of bilirubin production and hepatic bilirubin clearance in neonates. Heme, produced largely by the breakdown of red blood cells (RBCs), is catabolized by heme oxygenase (HO) to produce an equimolar amount of carbon monoxide (CO) and biliverdin; the latter is reduced to unconjugated bilirubin by biliverdin reductase. Unconjugated bilirubin is taken up by the hepatocyte via facilitated diffusion, bound to glutathione S-transferase (ligandin), and conjugated with glucuronic acid by UGT1A1. Conjugated bilirubin is excreted into bile via multidrug resistance protein 2, a portion of which may be deconjugated by intestinal β-glucuronidases and reabsorbed into the portal circulation enhancing the hepatic bilirubin load (enterohepatic circulation).

of hemoglobin production of which α-thalassemia syndromes are the most likely to be clinically apparent in newborns; and (iv) immune-mediated hemolytic disease inherited as a Mendelian trait.

Heritable Causes of Hemolysis— Defects of RBC Metabolism

G6PD Mutations

G6PD (OMIM *305900) deficiency is a common X-linked enzymopathy affecting hemizygous males, homozygous females, and a subset of heterozygous females (via nonrandom X chromosome inactivation).[13] G6PD is critical to the redox metabolism of RBCs and G6PD deficiency may be associated with acute hemolysis in newborns following exposure to oxidative stress. It is an important cause of severe neonatal hyperbilirubinemia and kernicterus.[13,57,79–83] The prevalence of G6PD deficiency has spread widely from its population origins in tropical malaria-laden latitudes to a global distribution over centuries of immigration and intermarriage.[13,79,80,82,83] The highest G6PD deficiency prevalence rates in the United States are in African American males (12.2%), African American females (4.1%), and Asian males (4.3%) (Table 1-3).[84] However, even among an ethnicity subset characterized as "unknown/other" in a current large United States–based cohort, G6PD deficiency prevalence was of 3.0% in males and 1.8% in females (Table 1-3).[84] Recent global migration patterns in North American and Europe where immigrant populations have grown by 80% and 41%, respectively, during the past 20 years alone (Table 1-4)[85,86] suggest that current G6PD deficiency prevalence rates in these regions will be sustained or possibly increase in decades to come.

G6PD is remarkable for its genetic diversity[13,82] and those mutations most frequently seen in the United States

	G6PD Deficient[a]		
Ethnicity	Female	Male	Total
American Indian/Alaskan	112 (0.9)	492 (0.8)	604 (0.8)
Asian	465 (0.9)	1658 (4.30)	2123 (3.6)
African American	2763 (4.1)	8513 (12.2)	11,276 (10.2)
Hispanic	842 (1.2)	4462 (2.0)	5304 (1.9)
Caucasian	4018 (0.0)	38,108 (0.3)	42,126 (1.3)
Unknown/other	228 (1.8)	1641 (3.0)	1869 (2.9)

■ TABLE 1-3. Presence of G6PD Deficiency in US Military Personnel by Sex and Self-Reported Ethnicity

[a]Number tested (percent deficient).

From Chinevere TD, Murray CK, Grant E, Johnson GA, Duelm F, Hospenthal DR. Prevalence of glucose-6-phosphate dehydrogenase deficiency in U.S. Army personnel. *Mil Med.* 2006;171:906, with permission.

■ **TABLE 1-4.** Estimated Number of International Migrants

Year	World	North America	Europe
1990	155,518,065	27,773,888	49,400,661
1995	165,968,778	33,595,046	54,717,864
2000	178,498,563	40,395,432	57,639,114
2005	195,245,404	45,597,061	64,398,585
2010	213,943,812	50,042,408	69,819,282

Data from United Nations, Department of Economic and Social Affairs, Population Division (2009). *Trends in International Migrant Stock: The 2008 Revision.* (United Nations database, POP/DB/MIG/Stock/Rev.2008).

include the: (i) *African A–* variants, a group of double-site mutations all of which share the A376G variant (also known as G6PD A+ when expressed alone, a nondeficient variant) coupled most commonly with the G202A mutation (G202A;A376G), but on occasion with the T968C variant (T968C;A376G, also known as G6PD Betica), or the G680T mutation (G680T;A376G); (ii) the *Mediterranean* (C563T) mutation; (iii) the *Canton* (G1376T) mutation; and (iv) the *Kaiping* (G1388A) variant.[13,53] These four mutations account for ~90% of G6PD deficiency in the United States.[87]

G6PD deficiency is reported in 20.8% of kernicterus cases in the United States, the majority of which are African American neonates.[3,5] G6PD-deficient infants of Asian, Hispanic, and Caucasian heritage were also reported in the US Pilot Kernicterus Registry.[3,5] Several recent papers have highlighted the importance of G6PD deficiency in the genesis of neonatal hyperbilirubinemia in African American newborns[57,80,88–90] as contrasted with earlier reports.[91–93] That *G6PD African A–* mutations of intermediate enzyme activity (i.e., class III with 10–60% normal activity), often thought to pose minimal hemolytic risk, can lead to hazardous hyperbilirubinemia is supported by the high incidence of associated hemolysis and kernicterus in Nigerian neonates in whom this variant is widely encountered.[80,94]

Two modes of hyperbilirubinemia presentation have classically been described in G6PD-deficient neonates.[79,80] The first is characterized by an acute hemolytic event, precipitated by an environmental trigger (e.g., naphthalene in moth balls or infection) with a resultant rapid exponential rise in TSB to potentially hazardous levels.[13,57,79,80] This mode may be difficult to predict and therefore anticipate and it is often a challenge to ascertain the trigger.[57,79,80,95,96] As underscored by Kaplan and Hammerman,[80] such

G6PD deficiency-associated hyperbilirubinemia can result in kernicterus that may not always be preventable. Seventeen of the 26 G6PD-deficient newborns in the US Pilot Kernicterus Registry were anemic (Hct ≤ 40%) and/or had a history of hemolytic trigger exposure (i.e., mothball, sepsis, or urosepsis) consistent with the assertion that this mode may place neonates at particular risk.[5] Peak TSB ranged from 28.0 to 50.1 mg/dL (479–857 µmol/L) in this cohort.[5]

The second mode of hyperbilirubinemia presentation in G6PD-deficient neonates couples low-grade hemolysis with genetic polymorphisms of the *UGT1A1* gene that reduce *UGT1A1* expression and thereby limit hepatic bilirubin conjugation. The $(TA)_7$ [*UGT1A1*28*] and $(TA)_8$ [*UGT1A1*37*] dinucleotide variant alleles within the $A(TA)_nTAA$ repeat of the *UGT1A1* TATAA box promoter, which usually consists of $(TA)_6$ repeats, account for these polymorphisms in Caucasians and African Americans, and, when expressed in the homozygous form and/or coexpressed with each other, a Gilbert syndrome genotype.[58,97] In newborns Gilbert syndrome is associated with accelerated jaundice development[98] and prolonged indirect hyperbilirubinemia in breastfed infants.[41,45,99] A dose-dependent genetic interaction between the *UGT1A1*28* promoter variant and G6PD deficiency enhances neonatal hyperbilirubinemia risk,[12,90] a phenomenon originally described by Kaplan et al. with the *G6PD Mediterranean* mutation (Figure 1-4)[12] and more recently noted in a cohort of African American neonates with a TSB >95th percentile on the Bhutani nomogram[100] who carried the *G6PD African A–* mutation.[16] In addition, the *UGT1A1* PBREM promoter polymorphism T-3279G (*UGT1A1*60*), a variant itself associated with reduced *UGT1A1* expression,[101] may contribute an icterogenic effect. Coexpression of the *UGT1A1*60* and *UGT1A1*28*

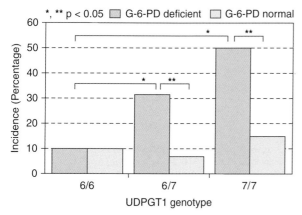

FIGURE 1-4. Hyperbilirubinemia (TSB >15 mg/dL [257 μmol/L]) incidence in G6PD-deficient (G6PD *Mediterranean* mutation) neonates and normal controls as a function of UGT1A1*28 promoter genotype. (Reprinted from Kaplan M, Renbaum P, Levy-Lahad E, Hammerman C, Lahad A, Beutler E. Gilbert syndrome and glucose-6-phosphate dehydrogenase deficiency: a dose-dependent genetic interaction crucial to neonatal hyperbilirubinemia. *Proc Natl Acad Sci U S A.* 1997;94:12128–12132, with permission. Copyright (1997) National Academy of Sciences, USA.)

promoter variant alleles is frequent and every hyperbilirubinemic (>95th percentile on the Bhutani nomogram) African American neonate in the aforementioned cohort who was homozygous for (TA)$_7$ was homozygous for T-3279G as well;[16] that is, in the context of a Gilbert genotype, (TA)$_7$ and T-3279G were in linkage disequilibrium. The higher allele frequencies of *UGT1A1*28* (0.426) and *UGT1A1*37* (0.069) variants in African Americans may predispose African American neonates to significant hyperbilirubinemia when coexpressed with *G6PD African A−* mutations.[57,95] If *G6PD African A−* and *UGT1A1* promoter polymorphisms are inherited independently, one would estimate that ~3% of African American males and ~1% of African American females will be G6PD deficient *and* carry a Gilbert genotype.[57] In a similar fashion, homozygous carriage of the *UGT1A1*6* Gilbert genotype prevalent in East Asian populations coexpressed with G6PD mutations is reported to enhance neonatal hyperbilirubinemia risk (Figure 1-5).[42]

On occasion, G6PD-deficient neonates with Gilbert syndrome may experience an acute hemolytic event with potentially devastating consequences as would be predicted in the coupling of a marked unconjugated bilirubin production secondary to severe hemolysis with a reduced

bilirubin conjugating capacity secondary to low *UGT1A1* enzyme activity.[57,95] Two recent case reports of kernicterus in G6PD-deficient newborns who carried Gilbert alleles underscore this risk.[57,95]

Gene polymorphisms of *SLCO1B1*, a putative bilirubin transporter[102,103] localized to the sinusoidal membrane of hepatocytes, that is, the blood–hepatocyte interface, have also been reported in association with *G6PD African A−*[104] and may predispose to neonatal hyperbilirubinemia by limiting hepatic bilirubin uptake and thereby hepatic bilirubin clearance.[102] Indeed, of neonates who carry G6PD *African A−*, those with a TSB >95th percentile on the Bhutani nomogram more often were homozygous for the nonsynonymous *SLCO1B1* A388G polymorphism (*SLCO1B1*1b*) than those who carried *G6PD African A−* with a TSB <40th percentile.[16] That coexpression of *UGT1A1* and/or *SLCO1B1* variants plays a clinically relevant role in modulating hyperbilirubinemia risk in African American infants is supported by the observation that the presence of *G6PD African A−* mutation *alone* (sans acute hemolytic event) is not associated with an increased risk of marked hyperbilirubinemia in a large cohort of African American neonates.[22] The genetic interaction(s) among *UGT1A1*, *SLCO1B1*, and *G6PD* variant alleles illustrate the importance of coupling gene polymorphisms that impair hepatic bilirubin clearance with genetically determined hemolytic conditions in determining the genetic architecture of neonatal hyperbilirubinemia generally and in African Americans in particular.[16,17,57,83,90,95]

Female Neonates Heterozygous for G6PD Mutations

Female neonates heterozygous for the *G6PD* mutations represent a *unique* at-risk group that merit special comment. X-linkage of the *G6PD* gene coupled with random X-inactivation results in a subpopulation of G6PD-deficient RBCs in *every* female heterozygote; that is, each heterozygous female is a mosaic of *two RBC populations* including one that is G6PD deficient.[105] In a given heterozygous female, nonrandom X-inactivation (i.e., a significant deviation from the theoretical 1:1 ratio between the paternal and maternal X-linked alleles) will skew the proportions of deficient and sufficient populations and depending on the relative proportion of each, a heterozygous female may appear enzymatically normal or deficient. It is important to note that standard biochemical G6PD enzyme tests assay *both* RBC populations in a single sample. The assayed G6PD enzyme activity therefore represents an average of the deficient and sufficient

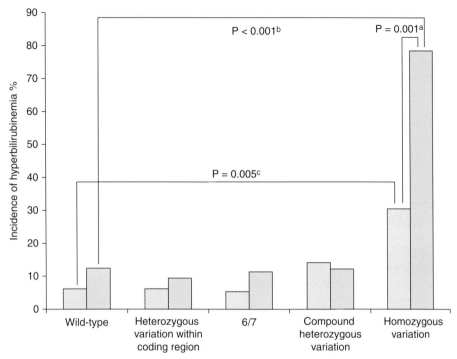

FIGURE 1-5. Hyperbilirubinemia (TSB >15 mg/dL [257 μmol/L]) incidence in G6PD-deficient (green bars) and G6PD-normal (tan bars) Taiwanese male neonates as a function of UGT1A1 genotype. Homozygous variation for *UGT1A1* polymorphisms (predominantly *UGT1A1*6*) was associated with a higher relative risk for hyperbilirubinemia in both G6PD-deficient and -normal neonates as compared with wild-type controls. Among those homozygous for *UGT1A1* variants, the prevalence of significant hyperbilirubinemia and level of peak TSB were greater in G6PD-deficient neonates than for their G6PD-normal counterparts. (Reprinted from Huang CS, Change PF, Huang MJ, Chen ES, Chen WC. Glucose-6-phosphate dehydrogenase deficiency, the UDP-glucuronosyl transferase 1A1 gene, and neonatal hyperbilirubinemia. *Gastroenterology.* 2002;123:127–133, with permission from Elsevier, copyright 2002.)

RBC populations and may give a falsely normal reading. Even the use of intermediate enzyme activity thresholds is associated with the misclassification of female heterozygotes as sufficient in over 50% of cases.[106] More importantly, a heterozygous female may be reported as enzymatically normal, yet harbor a sizable population of G6PD-deficient, potentially hemolyzable RBCs that represent a substantial reservoir of bilirubin. A recent case report of an African American female neonate heterozygous for *G6PD A*− who evidenced a steep TSB trajectory from 28.9 mg/dL (494 μmol/L) at 98 hours of life to 46.2 mg/dL (790 μmol/L) 6 hours later, and resultant kernicterus, underscores this potential.[57] As such, the reported G6PD deficiency prevalence of 4.1% in African American females[84] may underestimate the proportion of African American females at hyperbilirubinemia risk. There is no

reliable biochemical assay to detect G6PD heterozygotes; only DNA analysis meets this requirement.

Pyruvate Kinase Deficiency

PK deficiency (OMIM #266200) is an uncommon (~1:20,000),[107] but important RBC glycolytic enzymopathy most often characterized by autosomal recessive transmission, jaundice, anemia, and reticulocytosis.[108–110] In RBCs, which are devoid of mitochondria, PK plays a central role in the regulation of glycolysis and ATP production.[108] RBC-specific PK is derived from the *PKLR* gene[108] and at least 158 different *PKLR* mutations have been reported.[110] The three most common mutations demonstrate region-specific population distributions: 1529A in the United States and Northern and Central Europe, 1456T in Southern Europe (Spain, Portugal, Italy), and

1468T in Asia.[110] Communities with considerable consanguinity can evidence higher PK deficiency prevalence rates and include Old Order Amish in Pennsylvania[111] and Ohio[112] and a recently reported polygamist community in Utah.[113] Neonatal jaundice may be severe; in two separate series one third[114] to almost one half[110] of affected infants required exchange transfusion to control their hyperbilirubinemia, and kernicterus in the context of PK deficiency has been described.[115] These authors are aware of at least one recent case of kernicterus in a PK-deficient Old Order Amish neonate with a peak TSB of 46 mg/dL (787 μmol/L). The diagnosis of PK deficiency is often difficult as the enzymatic abnormality is frequently not simply a quantitative defect, but in many cases involves abnormal enzyme kinetics or an unstable enzyme that decreases in activity as the RBC ages.[108] The diagnosis of PK deficiency should be considered whenever persistent jaundice and a picture of nonspherocytic, Coombs-negative hemolytic anemia are observed.

Heritable Causes of Hemolysis— RBC Membrane Defects

Of the many RBC membrane defects that lead to hemolysis, only hereditary spherocytosis, elliptocytosis, stomatocytosis, and infantile pyknocytosis have manifested themselves in the newborn period.[116–118] A high level of diagnostic suspicion is required for their detection as newborns normally exhibit a marked variation in RBC membrane size and shape.[116,119,120] Spherocytes, however, are not often seen on RBC smears of hematologically normal newborns and this morphologic abnormality, when prominent, may yield a diagnosis of hereditary spherocytosis in the immediate neonatal period. Given that approximately 75% of families affected with hereditary spherocytosis manifest an autosomal dominant transmission, a positive family history can often be elicited and provide further support for this diagnosis. Hereditary spherocytosis may result from mutations of several genes that encode RBC membrane proteins including the *SPTA1* (α-spectrin) gene (OMIM +182860), the *SPTB* (β-spectrin) gene (OMIM +182870), the *ANK1* (ankyrin-1) gene (OMIM +182900), *SLC4A1* (band 3) gene (OMIM +109270), and EPB42 (protein 4.2) gene (OMIM *177070).[121,122] It has been reported across all racial and ethnic groups, but is most frequently seen in Northern European populations (~1 per 5000).[122] Almost one half of patients diagnosed with hereditary

spherocytosis have a history of neonatal jaundice,[123] which can be severe[122,124,125] and lead to kernicterus.[126,127] Coexpression of hereditary spherocytosis with a Gilbert *UGT1A1* variant genotype enhances hyperbilirubinemia risk.[126,128] Recent data suggest that hereditary spherocytosis is underdiagnosed in neonates and underrecognized as a cause of severe hyperbilirbinemia.[124] A mean corpuscular hemoglobin concentration (MCHC) of ≥36.0 g/dL alone should alert caregivers to this diagnostic possibility.[124] Ascertainment can be further enhanced by dividing MCHC by the mean corpuscular volume (MCV); the latter index tends to be low in hereditary spherocytosis (personal communication, R.D. Christensen). An MCHC:MCV ratio ≥0.36 is almost diagnostic of the condition. The actual diagnosis of hereditary spherocytosis can be confirmed using the incubated osmotic fragility test, which is a reliable diagnostic tool in newborns after the first weeks of life when coupled with fetal RBC controls. One must rule out symptomatic ABO hemolytic disease by performing a direct Coombs test as infants so affected may also manifest prominent microspherocytosis.[122] Moreover, hereditary spherocytosis and symptomatic ABO hemolytic disease can occur in the same infant and result in severe anemia and hyperbilirubinemia.[129]

Hereditary elliptocytosis and stomatocytosis are rare, but reported causes of hemolysis in the newborn period.[116] Infantile pyknocytosis, a transient RBC membrane abnormality manifesting itself during the first few months of life, is more common. The pyknocyte, an irregularly contracted RBC with multiple spines, can normally be observed in newborns, particularly premature infants where up to ~5% of RBCs may manifest this morphologic variant.[118] In newborns affected with infantile pyknocytosis, up to 50% of RBCs exhibit the morphologic abnormality and this degree of pyknocytosis is associated with jaundice, anemia, and a reticulocytosis. Infantile pyknocytosis can cause significant hyperbilirubinemia as demonstrated in one recent cohort (mean TSB: 19.2 ± 6.1 mg/dL [328 ± 104 μmol/L]; range 7.0–25.3 mg/dL [120–433 μmol/L])[130] and may be severe enough to require control by exchange transfusion.[118] RBCs transfused into affected infants become pyknocytic and have a shortened life span suggesting that an extracorpuscular factor mediates the morphologic alteration.[118,131,132] Recent descriptions of a familial predisposition[130] including three siblings with infantile pyknocytosis born to consanguineous parents[133] suggest a possible autosomal recessive genetic inheritance. The disorder tends to resolve after several months of life. Pyknocytosis may also occur in other conditions including G6PD deficiency and hereditary elliptocytosis.

Heritable Causes of Hemolysis— Hemoglobinopathies

Defects in hemoglobin structure or synthesis infrequently manifest themselves in the neonatal period. Of these, the α-thalassemia syndromes are the most likely to be clinically apparent in newborns. Thalassemias are inherited disorders of hemoglobin synthesis. Each human diploid cell contains four copies of the α-globin gene and, thus, four α-thalassemia syndromes have been described reflecting the presence of defects in one, two, three, or four α-globin genes. Silent carriers have one abnormal α-globin chain and are asymptomatic. α-Thalassemia trait is associated with two α-thalassemia mutations, can be detected by a low MCV of <95 μ^3 (normal infants 100–120 μ^3),[134] and in neonates is not associated with hemolysis. Hemoglobin H disease, prevalent in Asian and Mediterranean populations, results from the presence of three α-thalassemia mutations and can cause hemolysis and anemia in neonates.[135] An increasing number of infants with Hemoglobin H disease have been reported in the United States since the early 1990s reflecting recent immigration patterns.[136,137] Homozygous α-thalassemia (total absence of α-chain synthesis) often results in profound hemolysis, anemia, hydrops fetalis, and almost always stillbirth or death in the immediate neonatal period, although survival throughout childhood has been reported.[136]

The pure β-thalassemias do not manifest themselves in the newborn period and the γ-thalassemias are: (i) incompatible with life (homozygous form); (ii) associated with transient mild to moderate neonatal anemia if one or two genes are involved that resolves when β-chain synthesis begins; or (iii) in combination with impaired β-chain synthesis, associated with severe hemolytic anemia and marked hyperbilirubinemia.[138]

Immune-Mediated Hemolytic Disease of the Newborn

Immune-mediated hemolytic disease can develop in the neonate of a heterospecific RBC antigen mother/infant pair when maternally derived antibody binds to the neonatal RBC antigen. The ABO (OMIM #110300) and RHD/CE (OMIM #111680 and 111700) blood group systems are the most commonly encountered in this regard, albeit minor RBC groups can also be associated with immune-mediated hemolytic disease of the newborn. ABO antigen status is under the control of at least three alleles on chromosome 9q34; A and B are codominant; O is recessive. The antibody type is also under genetic control. For all intents and purposes, symptomatic ABO hemolytic disease is limited to infants of blood group A or B born to mothers of blood group O, who show marked jaundice, a positive direct Coombs test, and often microspherocytosis on an RBC smear.[139] It is of interest that the frequency distribution of blood types A, B, and O differs across populations. Some previous studies suggest that ABO hemolytic disease is more frequent in African American newborns,[140–143] including evidence that a positive direct Coombs test is more common in African American heterospecific mother/infant pairs.[141]

The RH antigen types are determined by three closely linked loci on chromosome 1p34–36 each with two alleles: Cc, Dd, and Ee. The lower case letters do not indicate recessitivity; each allele determines the presence of an antigen (C, c, D, E, e), sans d which does not exist.[32,144] Most symptomatic RH hemolytic disease (~90%) is related to RHD incompatibility although maternally derived alloantibodies to C, c, E, and e can lead to hemolytic disease of the newborn.[144] The incidence of common RH haplotypes differs significantly across populations,[144] the resultant ratio of RHD-positive to RHD-negative phenotypes being ~0.84:0.16 in Caucasians, ~0.92:0.08 in African American, and ~0.99:<0.01 in Asians.[144] Although RH isoimmunization can still lead to severe neonatal hyperbilirubinemia, the prevalence of RH hemolytic disease has decreased markedly as a result of effective immunoprophylaxis with anti-RH (anti-D) gamma-globulin.[144]

Heme Oxygenase-1 (HO-1) Promoter Variants

HO is the initial and rate-limiting enzymatic step in the conversion of heme to bilirubin. Two isoenzymes HO-1 (OMIM *141250) and HO-2 (OMIM *1412451) are expressed in a tissue-specific fashion with HO-1 the inducible and HO-2 the constitutive forms, respectively. There is evidence that HO-1 expression is developmentally regulated and greater in the immediate neonatal period relative to the adult.[145] Variant length $(GT)_n$ dinucleotide repeat microsatellite polymorphisms in the HO-1 promoter sequence numbering from ~12 to 40 tandem repeats modulate HO-1 transcription.[146] Short alleles (<27 GT repeats) are reported in association with higher TSB levels in adults.[147–149] This association is consistent with functional studies demonstrating greater basal HO-1 expression and HO-1 inducibility by oxidative stimuli in short $(GT)_n$ repeat alleles as compared with their longer counterparts.[150] To date, only two studies has explored the relationship between HO-1 $(GT)_n$ repeats and TSB levels in neonates and no effect of $(GT)_n$ number was observed on peak hyperbilirubinemia risk,[151,152] albeit in one of these reports, short (<24 GT) alleles were associated with prolonged breast milk jaundice.[152] A recent case report of a boy with hazardous hyperbilirubinemia, autoimmune hemolytic disease, and homozygosity for short $(GT)_n$ repeats[153] suggests the potential modulatory role of HO-1 promoter polymorphisms on TSB in neonates merits further study, particularly when short HO-1 (GT) repeat alleles are coexpressed with a genetic predisposition to hemolysis and increased heme production (e.g., G6PD deficiency, ABO hemolytic disease, hereditary spherocytosis).[153]

Biliverdin Reductase Polymorphisms

Biliverdin reductase A (*BLVRA*; OMIM *109750) efficiently reduces biliverdin to bilirubin. In theory, *BLVRA* polymorphisms might affect hyperbilirubinemia risk in newborns. However, only one common nonsynonymous *BLVRA* gene variant (rs699512:A>G) has been reported in the dbSNP database (allele frequency 0.23 Caucasians, 0.08 African Americans, 0.27 Chinese, and 0.40 Japanese) and this variant is not associated with adult TSB levels across three Asian populations.[147] This *BLVRA* variant allele has not been studied in neonates. A recent case report of two unrelated Inuit women with a homozygous nonsense *BLVRA* mutation indicates that complete absence of BLVRA activity is a nonlethal condition, characterized phenotypically by green jaundice during episodes of cholestasis.[154]

SLCO1B1 Polymorphisms

Recent evidence suggests that unconjugated bilirubin may be a substrate for the *SLCO1B1* (alternative gene symbols include *OATP1B1*, *OATP-2*, *OATP-C*, *LST-1*),[102] a sinusoidal transporter that facilitates the hepatic uptake of numerous endogenous substrates and xenobiotics in an ATP-independent fashion. This issue remains unsettled[155,156] and unconjugated bilirubin hepatocyte entry is at least in part passive in nature.[157] Nevertheless, the developmental expression of *SLCO1B1*[158] and evolving data on nonsynonymous gene variants suggest SLCO1B1 may impact unconjugated bilirubin hepatic uptake kinetics and metabolism in neonates.[15,102,158,159] *SLCO1B1* polymorphisms are numerous (Figure 1-6) and several have

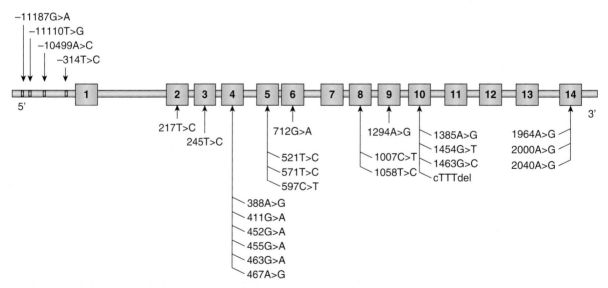

FIGURE 1-6. Schematic of *SLCO1B1* gene and identified polymorphisms in promoter (above) and coding (below) sequences. The 388A>G nonsynonymous polymorphism (*SLCO1B1*1b*) has been reported in association with significant neonatal hyperbilirubinemia in some populations.[15] (Reprinted from Jada SR, Xiaochen S, Yan LY, et al. Pharmacogenetics of *SLCO1B1*: haplotypes, htSNPs and hepatic expression in three distinct Asian populations. *Eur J Clin Pharmacol.* 2007;63:555–563, Figure 1, with kind permission from Springer Science and Business Media, copyright 2007.)

been studied in human neonates.[15,16] Their coexpression with other icterogenic genes is also common.[16,17,104] As detailed above, the *SLCO1B1*1b* variant allele is associated with increased risk for severe hyperbilirubinemia in Taiwanese newborns[15] and coupling of *UGT1A1* with *SLCO1B1* variant alleles further enhances that risk.[15] Although homozygosity for *SLCO1B1*1b* was not observed at greater frequency in neonates with TSB >95th percentile in a United States–based cohort,[16] *SLCO1B1*1b* coexpression with *G6PD A–* was.[16] Some adult genome-wide association studies suggest that *SLCO1B1* polymorphisms are directly associated with higher TSB levels, albeit they account for only ~1% of the TSB variance, as contrasted with *UGT1A1* polymorphisms that account for ~18% of TSB variance.[160]

Glutathione S-transferase (Ligandin) Polymorphisms

Human cytosolic GSTs are a superfamily of multifunctional proteins that in addition to their catalytic function also demonstrate high-capacity ligand binding for a variety of nonsubstrate compounds. Although several different GST gene classes evidence a ligandin function, the class alpha (A) GSTs *hGSTA1-1* and *hGSTA2-2* appear to be the major ligand-binding and transporter proteins for unconjugated bilirubin in the hepatocyte.[161] Hepatic uptake of unconjugated bilirubin is enhanced by increasing concentrations of ligandin.[162] As such, the low hepatic ligandin concentration observed at birth[163] may contribute to the early hyperbilirubinemia risk in neonates. Moreover, a variant *hGSTA1-1* allele (G-52A) within a polymorphic SP-1 binding site of the proximal promoter is associated with 4-fold lower mean hepatic expression than the referent allele[161,164] and presumably decreased hepatic unconjugated bilirubin binding, although the latter has not been confirmed in functional assay. To date, only Muslu et al. have studied *hGST* polymorphisms in neonatal hyperbilirubinemia, specifically two non-α-GST isoenzymes *hGSTT1* and *hGSTM1*, and found no relationship between these allelic variants and neonatal hyperbilirubinemia risk.[165] However, proteins of the theta (T) and mu (M) classes bind bilirubin with a lower affinity than alpha-class GSTs so the aforementioned findings do not preclude an impact of *hGSTA1-1* (or *hGSTA2-2*) variant alleles on neonatal hyperbilirubinemia risk. It is clinically notable that induction of both *hGSTA1* and *hGSTA2* occurs in response to phenobarbital treatment.[166]

UGT1A1 Polymorphisms

Once bilirubin enters the hepatocyte, it is conjugated with glucuronic acid to form the polar, water-soluble, and readily excretable bilirubin monoglucuronides and diglucuronides. The formation of these derivatives is catalyzed by hepatic *UGT1A1*, an endoplasmic reticulum membrane protein isoenzyme that arises from the *UGT1* gene complex on chromosome 2(2q37). In addition to the A1 exon, the *UGT1* gene locus contains: (i) nine variable exons that encode functional proteins (exons 3–10, 13); (ii) three pseudogenes (exons 2, 11, 12); and (iii) the exon 2–5 sequence common to all *UGT1* transcripts (Figure 1-7).[167,168]

UGT1A1 isoenzyme expression is modulated in a developmental manner such that its activity is 0.1% of adult levels at 17–30 weeks gestation, increasing to 1% of adult values between 30 and 40 weeks gestation, and reaching adult levels by 14 weeks of postnatal life.[169,170] This graded upregulation of hepatic *UGT1A1* activity over the first few days of life is induced by unconjugated bilirubin itself and noted following birth regardless of the newborn's gestational age. Multifunctional nuclear receptors mediate *UGT1A1* induction (e.g., constitutive androstane receptor [CAR] and aryl hydrocarbon receptor [AhR]) via the PBREM in the *UGT1A1* gene promoter element (Figure 1-7).[171]

In addition to the developmentally modulated postnatal transition in hepatic bilirubin *UGT1A1* activity, there are congenital inborn errors of *UGT1A1* expression, commonly referred to as the indirect hyperbilirubinemia syndromes.[172] To date, 113 *UGT1A1* gene variants have been identified.[173] These include Crigler–Najjar type I (CN-I; OMIM *218800) and II (CN-II; Arias; OMIM *616785) syndromes, and Gilbert syndrome (OMIM *143500) (Table 1-5). Infants with CN-I have complete absence of bilirubin *UGT1A1* activity and are at significant risk for hyperbilirubinemic encephalopathy.[174] Although inherited in an autosomal recessive pattern, CN-I has marked genetic heterogeneity.[11,167] More than 30 different genetic mutations have been identified in CN-I and coding sequence defects common to both the *UGT1A1* exon and those comprising the constant domain (exons 2–5) underlie most cases.[11,167] Such gene defects are typically nonsense or "stop" mutations that result in premature termination codons and an inactive UGT1A1 enzyme. CN-II is typified by more moderate levels of indirect hyperbilirubinemia as well as low, but detectable, hepatic bilirubin *UGT1A1*

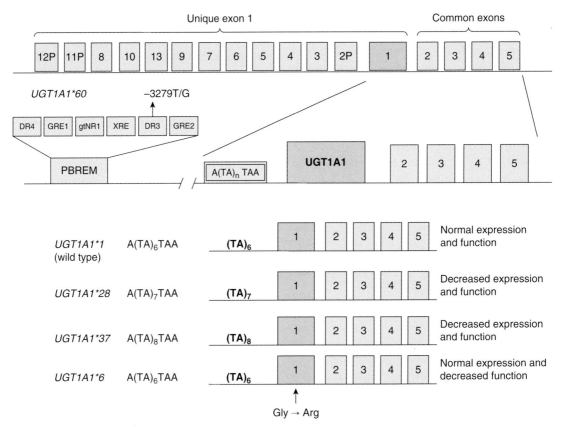

FIGURE 1-7. Schematic of the *UGT1A1* gene. The uppermost panel represents the entire *UGT1A* gene complex encompassing: (i) the A1 exon, (ii) nine additional exons that encode functional proteins (exons 3–10, 13), (iii) three pseudogenes (exons 2P, 11P, 12P), and (iv) the common domain exon 2–5 sequence shared across all *UGT1A1* transcripts. The *UGT1A1* locus and common exons 2–5 are shown in middle panel including the upstream (i) phenobarbital-responsive enhancer module (PBREM) encompassing six nuclear receptor motifs (and hypomorphic variant *UGT1A1*60*) and (ii) TATA box promoter sequences. Lower panels show wild-type *UGT1A1*1* and *UGT1A1*28*, *UGT1A1*37*, and *UGT1A1*6* variant alleles and relevant change in expression–function. (Adapted from Clarke DJ, Moghrabi N, Monaghan G, et al. Genetic defects of the UDP-glucuronosyltransferase-1 (UGT1) gene that cause familial nonhemolytic unconjugated hyperbilirubinemias. *Clin Chim Acta*. 1997;166:63–74, with permission from Elsevier Science; Perera MA, Innocenti F, Ratain MJ. Pharmacogenetic testing for uridine diphosphate glucuronosyltransferase 1A1 polymorphisms. Are we there yet? *Pharmacotherapy*. 2008;28:755–768, with permission from *Pharmacotherapy*; Li Y, Buckely D, Wang S, Klaassen CD, Zhong X. Genetic polymorphisms in the TATA box and upstream phenobarbital-responsive enhancer module of the *UGT1A1* promoter have combined effects on UDP-glucuronosyltransferase 1A1 transcription mediated by constitutive androstane receptor, pregnane X receptor, or glucocorticoid receptor in human liver. *Drug Metab Dispos*. 2009;37:1978–1986, with permission.)

activity and appears in the majority of cases to be mediated by missense mutations in the *UGT1A1* gene.[11,167] Phenobarbital can be trialed to induce residual *UGT1A1* activity via PBREM. These rare, but important, clinical syndromes must be included in the differential diagnosis of prolonged marked indirect hyperbilirubinemia.

Gilbert syndrome, originally described at the turn of the century,[175] is far more common.[58,97] Hepatic *UGT1A1* activity is reduced by ~70%, and >95% of TSB is unconjugated.[40,58,97] In adults, the indirect hyperbilirubinemia associated with Gilbert syndrome is often seen during fasting associated with an intercurrent illness.

■ **TABLE 1-5.** Congenital Nonhemolytic Unconjugated Hyperbilirubinemia Syndromes

	Clinical Severity		
Characteristic	Marked Crigler–Najjar Type I	Moderate Crigler–Najjar Type II	Mild Gilbert Syndrome
Steady-state serum total bilirubin	>20 mg/dL	<20 mg/dL	<5 mg/dL
Range of bilirubin values	14–50 mg/dL	5.3–37.6 mg/dL	0.8–10 mg/dL
Total bilirubin in bile	<10 mg/dL (increased with phototherapy)	50–100 mg/dL	Normal
Conjugated bilirubin in bile	Absent	Present (only monoglucuronide)	Present (50% monoglucuronide)
Bilirubin clearance	Extremely decreased	Markedly decreased	20–30% of normal
Hepatic bilirubin uptake	Normal	Normal	Reduced
Bilirubin UGT1A1 activity	None detected	None detected	Decreased
Genetics	Autosomal recessive	Heterogeneity of defect distinctly possible	Genetic polymorphisms (see Table 1-6): 1. Thymine-adenine $(TA)_7$ and $(TA)_8$ repeats in the *UGT1A1* promoter region 2. G211A (Gly71Arg) *UGT1A1* coding sequence variant identified in Asian populations 3. Linkage disequilibrium between $(TA)_7/(TA)_7$ and T-3279G PBREM *UGT1A1* promoter polymorphisms 4. Other variants, generally not polymorphic

UGT1A1, uridine diphosphate glucuronosyltransferase 1A1 isoenzyme.

Adapted from Valaes T. Bilirubin metabolism: review and discussion of inborn errors. *Clin Perinatol.* 1976;3:177. Copyright Elsevier 1976.

Interestingly, in about half of patients there is also an unexplained, shortened RBC life span and increased bilirubin production.[176]

In addition to the four coding sequence variants (*UGT1A1*6, UGT1A1*7, UGT1A1*27,* and *UGT1A1*73*) in East Asian populations detailed above, several other hypomorphic *UGT1A1* promoter and coding sequence polymorphisms have been described in association with Gilbert syndrome (Table 1-6).[182] Of these the $(TA)_7$ [*UGT1A1*28*] dinucleotide variant allele within the $A(TA)_n$TAA repeat element of the *UGT1A1* TATAA box promoter is the most common in Caucasians and African Americans[58,97] differing from the wild-type $A(TA)_6$TAA promoter element (Figure 1-7; Tables 1-6 and 1-7). The $(TA)_8$ [*UGT1A1*37*] dinucleotide variant allele is also observed, most often in African Americans[58] (Table 1-7). The extra $(TA)_n$ repeats in the *UGT1A1*28* and *UGT1A1*37* alleles impair proper message transcription and account for a reduced *UGT1A1* activity;[58,97] indeed as the number of repeats increases, *UGT1A1* activity declines.[58] In contrast, the $A(TA)_5$TAA allele (*UGT1A1*36*) is associated with increased UGT1A1 activity[58] and a reduced risk of significant neonatal hyperbilirubinemia;[16] similarly the −3156G>A promoter variant (*UGTA1A*93*) is hypothesized to enhance UGT1A1 activity and reduce TSB levels.[189] *UGT1A1*

■ **TABLE 1-6.** *UGT1A1* Gene Variants Reported in Gilbert Syndrome

Allele	Nucleotide	Amino Acids	Location	Reference
UGT1A1*1	A(TA)$_6$TAA	Wild type	Promoter	
UGT1A1*6	211(G>A)	G71R	Exon 1	177
UGT1A1*7	1456(T>G)	Y486D	Exon 5	177
UGT1A1*27	686(C>A)	P229Q	Exon 1	39
UGT1A1*28	A(TA)$_6$TAA to A(TA)$_7$TAA	n/a	Promoter	97
UGT1A1*29	1099(C>G)	R367G	Exon 4	177
UGT1A1*37	A(TA)$_6$TAA to A(TA)$_8$TAA	n/a	Promoter	58
UGT1A1*60	−3279(T>G)	n/a	Promoter	101
UGT1A1*62	247(T>C)	F83L	Exon 1	178
UGT1A1*64	488–491 dupACCT	Frameshift	Exon 1	179
UGT1A1*65	−1126(C>T)	n/a	Promoter	179
UGT1A1*66	997−82(T>C)	n/a	Intron 2	179
UGT1A1*67	−85 to −83 ins CAT	n/a	Promoter	180
UGT1A1*68	−63(G>C)	n/a	Promoter	180
UGT1A1*69	476(T>C)	I159T	Exon 1	180
UGT1A1*70	962(C>G)	A321G	Exon 2	180
UGT1A1*72	1075(G>A)	D359N	Exon 3	180
UGT1A1*73	1091(C>T)	P364L	Exon 4	180
UGT1A1*81	−64(G>C)	n/a	Promoter	181

Alleles highlighted in gray are polymorphic.

Adapted, updated, and modified from Strassburgh CP, Kalthoff S, Ehmer U. Variability and function of family 1 uridine-5′-diphosphate glucuronosyltransferases (UGT1A). *Crit Rev Clin Lab Sci.* 2008;45:485–530. Reproduced with permission of Taylor & Francis Inc.

Gilbert nonsynonymous coding sequence variants (e.g., *UGT1A1*6, UGT1A1*62*) by contrast result in reduced bilirubin conjugation via suboptimal substrate orientation to coenzyme reactive sites.[190]

Investigators have long speculated that Gilbert syndrome would contribute to indirect hyperbilirubinemia in the newborn period.[171,191,192] Identification of genotypes underlying Gilbert syndrome provided an

■ **TABLE 1-7.** Frequency of Polymorphic *UGT1A1* Allele Variants Associated with Gilbert Syndrome Across Various Populations

Allele	European	African	Hispanic	Chinese	Indian	Japanese	Korean
UGT1A1*6	Absent	Absent	Absent	0.23[183]	0[184]–0.03[44]	0.13[183]	0.23[183,187]
UGT1A1*28	0.26–0.36[58,185]	0.42–0.56[58,185,186]	0.39[185]	0.11[44]	0.29[184]–0.37[44]	0.09[185]	0.07[187]
UGT1A1*37	Absent	0.04–0.07[58,185,186]	Absent	Absent	0.06[184]	Absent	Absent
UGT1A1*60	0.39–0.57	0.15	n/a	0.32[188]	n/a	0.42[101]	0.24[187]

n/a, not available.

Reprinted from Watchko JF, Lin Z. Exploring the genetic architecture of neonatal hyperbilirubinemia. *Semin Fetal Neonatal Med.* 2010;15: 169–175, with permission from Elsevier, copyright 2010.

important tool to study the role of this condition in the pathogenesis of neonatal jaundice. Bancroft et al: were the first to explore this relationship and observed that newborn infants with the A(TA)$_7$TAA *UGT1A1* promoter polymorphism had accelerated jaundice and decreased fecal excretion of bilirubin monoglucuronides and diglucuronides.[98] Although some subsequent studies demonstrated that *UGT1A1*28* and/or *UGT1A1*37* alleles are associated with modest[193] to more significant postnatal TSB elevation,[184,194] others have failed to demonstrate a clinically significant effect of *UGT1A1*28 alone* on neonatal hyperbilirubinemia risk[16,183,195] including a TSB >95th percentile on the Bhutani nomogram[16] or need for phototherapy.[184] The latter may reflect in part the incomplete penetrance of the *UGT1A1*28* genotype.[97] Indeed in adults only about 50% of subjects homozygous for the *UGT1A1*28* allele display a Gilbert phenotype; as stated by Bosma et al., the *UGT1A1*28* variant allele is necessary, but not sufficient for complete phenotypic expression.[97] However, the coupling of *UGT1A1*28* and/or *UGT1A1*37* with other icterogenic conditions, for example, G6PD deficiency and hereditary spherocytosis, appears to markedly increase a newborn's hyperbilirubinemia risk.[12,16,128] Several reports also convincingly demonstrate that *UGT1A1*28* is prevalent in breastfed infants who develop prolonged indirect hyperbilirubinemia.[45,99,193] In East Asian populations the *UGT1A1*6* coding sequence variant described above appears to underlie a Gilbert phenotype and contribute to their widely recognized increased neonatal hyperbilirubinemia risk[15,36,37,41,44,51,183,195,196] (Table 1-7).

The PBREM is located ~3 kb upstream to the TATA box on the *UGT1A1* promoter (Figure 1-7) and is a composite of six nuclear receptor motifs: DR4 (CAR), gtNR1 (CAR, pregnane X receptor [PXR]), DR3 (CAR, PXR), two glucocorticoid-receptor response elements (GRE1 and GRE2), and the receptor-type transcription factor AhR (xenobiotic response element [XRE]).[171] These nuclear receptor regulatory motifs modulate the expression of an overlapping set of target genes involved in the detoxification and transport of drugs and endogenous substances including bilirubin and impact neonatal hyperbilirubinemia risk.[76] A single nucleotide polymorphism *T-3279G* (*UGT1A1*60*) in the DR3 site of PBREM (Figure 1-7) significantly reduces *UGT1A1* transcription and is associated with an increased risk of hyperbilirubinemia.[101,171] It is of clinical interest that coexpression of *UGT1A*60* with *UGT1A1*28* is frequent and subjects with a Gilbert genotype are often homozygous for both *UGT1A1*28* and *UGT1A1*60*.[16,104,197] Some investigators suggest such linkage is essential to the pathogenesis of Gilbert syndrome,[185] whereas others do not.[198,199] Recent reports also suggest that compound heterozygosity for *UGT1A1*60* and *UGT1A1*6* is associated with a Gilbert phenotype in Japanese patients.[101] Another promoter polymorphism *UGT1A1*81* (–64[G>C])[181] may also be associated with decreased *UGT1A1* expression and in recent study, although expressed only in the heterozygous state, was found more frequently in neonates with a TSB >95th percentile versus those with a TSB <40th percentile on the Bhutani nomogram.[16]

Of physiologic note, the monoconjugated bilirubin fraction predominates over the diconjugated bilirubin fraction in Gilbert syndrome[200] and thereby enhances the enterohepatic circulation of bilirubin given that hydrolysis of monoglucoronides back to unconjugated bilirubin occurs at rates four to six times that of the diglucuronide.[201] These studies taken together demonstrate that Gilbert syndrome is a contributing factor to neonatal jaundice particularly when coexpressed with other icterogenic conditions. The role Gilbert syndrome may play in the genesis of extreme hyperbilirubinemia remains unclear, although a possible contribution is suggested by the low direct bilirubin fraction and evidence of poor feeding and prominent weight loss (i.e., a state resembling fasting) reported in several kernicterus cases.[3,202]

Compound and Synergistic Heterozygosity

Coexpression of variant alleles for genes involved in bilirubin metabolism is common.[11,12,15,16,104] In one recent study of *G6PD*, *UGT1A1*, and *SLCO1B1* allele frequencies in 450 anonymous DNA samples of US residents with genetic ancestry from all the major regions of the world, more than three quarter of subjects demonstrated two or more variants.[104] This broad array of polymorphisms and high degree of variant coexpression underscore the potential for compound and/or synergistic heterozygosity to enhance hyperbilirubinemia risk, contributing to the etiologic heterogeneity and complex nature of neonatal hyperbilirubinemia.[16,17,104]

Compound heterozygosity, that is, the expression of two different disease-causing alleles at a particular locus, has been reported in association with neonatal hyperbilirubinemia risk and even kernicterus.[203] In particular, compound heterozygosity of a Gilbert-type promoter and coding region mutation of *UGT1A1* has been reported in the genesis of CN-I and CN-II syndromes.[11,203–206] In addition, heterozygosities *across* different genes can also combine to produce subtle to more severe phenotypes, a process termed "synergistic heterozygosity."[207] Two recent reports of kernicterus in females heterozygous for both *G6PD* mutations and *UGT1A1*28*[57,95] underscore the clinical potential of synergistic heterozygosity to impact the genesis of hazardous hyperbilirubinemia.[17]

Gene–Diet and Gene–Environment Interactions

No discussion of the genetics of neonatal hyperbilirubinemia would be complete without alluding to potential gene–diet and gene–environment interactions, the most notable being exclusive breast milk feedings and environmental factors capable of triggering hemolysis in G6PD-deficient RBCs, respectively. We will consider exclusive breast milk feedings first. It is likely no coincidence that almost every reported case of kernicterus over the past three decades has been in breastfed infants.[3] As such, exclusive breast milk feeding, particularly if nursing is not going well and weight loss is excessive, is listed as a major hyperbilirubinemia risk factor in the 2004 AAP practice guideline.[34] What does the association between exclusive breast milk feeding and kernicterus imply with respect to the etiopathogenesis of marked neonatal jaundice? Numerous studies have reported an association between breastfeeding and an increased incidence and severity of hyperbilirubinemia, both during the first few days of life and in prolonged neonatal jaundice.[55,208–211] A pooled analysis of 12 studies comprising over 8000 neonates showed a 3-fold greater incidence in TSB of ≥12.0 mg/dL (205 µmol/L), and a 6-fold greater incidence in levels of ≥15 mg/dL (257 µmol/L) in breastfed infants as compared with their formula-fed counterparts.[210] Others, however, report that if adequate breastfeeding is established and sufficient lactation support is in place, breastfed infants should be at no greater risk for hyperbilirubinemia than their formula-fed counterparts.[26,212–214] The later studies suggest that many breastfed infants who develop marked neonatal jaundice do so in the context of a delay in lactation or varying degrees of lactation failure. Indeed, an appreciable percentage of the breastfed infants who develop kernicterus have been noted to have inadequate intake, and variable, but substantial, degrees of dehydration and weight loss.[202,215]

Inadequate breast milk intake, in addition to contributing to dehydration, can further enhance hyperbilirubinemia by increasing the enterohepatic circulation of bilirubin, and resultant hepatic bilirubin load. The enterohepatic circulation of bilirubin is already exaggerated in the neonatal period, in part because the newborn gastrointestinal tract is not yet colonized with bacteria that convert conjugated bilirubin to urobilinogen and because intestinal β-glucuronidase activity is high.[216,217] Earlier studies in newborn humans and primates suggest that the enterohepatic circulation of bilirubin may account for up to 50% of the hepatic bilirubin load in neonates.[218,219] Fasting hyperbilirubinemia is largely due to intestinal reabsorption of unconjugated bilirubin,[220,221] a potential mechanism by which inadequate lactation and/or poor enteral intake may contribute to marked hyperbilirubinemia in some newborns. In the context of limited hepatic conjugation capacity in the immediate postnatal period, any further increase in hepatic bilirubin load secondary to enhanced enterohepatic bilirubin recirculation will likely result in worsening hyperbilirubinemia. Recent study confirms that early breastfeeding-associated jaundice is associated with a state of relative caloric deprivation[222] and resultant enhanced enterohepatic recirculation of bilirubin.[20,222] Breastfeeding-associated jaundice, however, is not associated with increased bilirubin production.[223,224]

Lactation failure, however, is not uniformly present in affected infants, suggesting that other mechanism(s) may be operative in breastfeeding-associated jaundice, a finding that merits further clinical study. Breast milk feeding may act as an environmental modifier for selected genotypes and thereby potentially predispose to the development of marked neonatal jaundice.[8,225] A recent report lends credence to this possibility demonstrating that the risk of developing a TSB ≥20 mg/dL (342 µmol/L) associated with breast milk feeding was enhanced 22-fold when combined with expression of either a coding sequence gene polymorphism of the *UGT1A1* (*UGT1A1*6*) or *SLCO1B1* (*SLCO1B1*1b*).[15] This hyperbilirubinemia risk increased to 88-fold when breast milk feedings were combined with both *UGT1A1* and *SLCO1B1* variants.[15] Others have previously reported an association between prolonged (>14 days) breast milk jaundice and expression of the *UGT1A1* gene promoter variant *UGT1A1*28*[41] and coding sequence variant *UGT1A1*6*.[43] The mechanism driving this gene–environment augmentation of hyperbilirubinemia risk is not clear, but likely relates to enhanced enterohepatic recirculation as detailed above. While recognizing the relationship between breast milk feeding and jaundice, the benefits of breast milk feeds far outweigh the related risk of hyperbilirubinemia. Cases of severe neonatal hyperbilirubinemia with suboptimal breast milk feedings underscore the need for effective lactation support and timely follow-up exams.

The classic example of gene–environment interaction in the genesis of neonatal hyperbilirubinemia is oxidant-induced hemolysis of G6PD-deficient RBCs. Although acute hemolysis is not an absolute prerequisite for hazardous hyperbilirubinemia development in G6PD-deficient neonates, an oxidative stress exposure history is evident in many such cases including several with kernicterus.[3,5,79,80,83,95,226,227] Agents reported to produce hemolysis in G6PD-deficient RBCs include: (i) antimalarials, (ii) sulfonamides, (iii) fava beans (in utero exposure via maternal ingestion[228] or postnatal exposure via breast milk feedings[229]), (iv) naphthalene (used in mothballs), (v) napthaquinones (used in mothballs), (vi) paradichlorobenzenes (moth repellent, car freshener, bathroom deodorizer), (vii) henna (traditional cosmetic), and (viii) methylene blue among others.[79,83,109,229] These compounds differ in their chemical composition, but each is capable of inducing a chain of events including NADPH and glutathione oxidation, resulting in hemolysis of the G6PD-deficient RBC.[229] Another important hemolytic trigger in G6PD-deficient newborns is infection.[79,83,229] Regardless of the trigger, it is evident that environmental conditions can play a pivotal role in modulating neonatal hyperbilirubinemia risk in the context of G6PD deficiency. Other potential gene–environment interactions including epigenetic programming have not been studied in neonatal hyperbilirubinemia but merit investigation.[230,231]

■ SUMMARY

Adult studies suggest that up to ~50% of TSB variance can be explained by genetic variables.[232–234] Although incomplete penetrance of allelic variants and developmental modulation of *UGT1A1* and *SLCO1B1* may partially mask genetic contributors in newborns, a growing literature shows the important modulatory role genetic variation across bilirubin metabolism genes can have on neonatal hyperbilirubinemia risk. Future study will further clarify the interactions among multiple bilirubin metabolism gene loci, other genes, and nongenetic factors to neonatal hyperbilirubinemia.

REFERENCES

1. Keren R, Tremont K, Luan X, Cnaan A. Visual assessment of jaundice in term and late preterm infants. *Arch Dis Child Fetal Neonatal Ed.* 2009;94:F317–F322.
2. Maisels MJ, Kring E. Length of stay, jaundice and hospital readmission. *Pediatrics.* 1998;101:995–998.
3. Bhutani VK, Johnson LH, Maisels MJ, et al. Kernicterus: epidemiological strategies for its prevention through systems-based approaches. *J Perinatol.* 2004;24:650–662.
4. Newman TB, Escobar GJ, Gonzales VM, et al. Frequency of neonatal bilirubin testing and hyperbilirubinemia in a large health maintenance organization. *Pediatrics.* 1999;104:1198–1203.
5. Johnson L, Bhutani VK, Karp K, Sivieri EM, Shapiro SM. Clinical report from the Pilot USA Kernicterus Registry (1992 to 2004). *J Perinatol.* 2009;29:S25–S45.
6. Perlstein MA. The late clinical syndrome of posticteric encephalopathy. *Pediatr Clin North Am.* 1960;7:665–687.
7. Watchko JF, Daood MJ, Biniwale M. Understanding neonatal hyperbilirubinemia in the era of genomics. *Semin Neonatol.* 2002;7:143–152.
8. Watchko JF. Vigintiphobia revisited. *Pediatrics.* 2005;115:1747–1753.
9. Kaplan M, Hammerman C. Bilirubin and the genome: the hereditary basis of unconjugated neonatal hyperbilirubinemia. *Curr Pharmacogenomics.* 2005;3:21–42.
10. Bosma PJ. Inherited disorders of bilirubin metabolism. *J Hepatol.* 2003;38:107–117.
11. Kadakol A, Ghosh SS, Sappal BS, et al. Genetic lesions of bilirubin uridine-diphosphoglucuronate glucuronosyltransferase (*UGT1A1*) causing Crigler–Najjar and Gilbert syndromes: correlation of genotype to phenotype. *Hum Mutat.* 2000;16:297–306.
12. Kaplan M, Renbaum P, Levy-Lahad E, et al. Gilbert syndrome and glucose-6-phosphate dehydrogenase deficiency: a dose-dependent genetic interaction crucial to neonatal hyperbilirubinemia. *Proc Natl Acad Sci USA.* 1997;94:12128–12132.
13. Beutler E. G6PD deficiency. *Blood.* 1994;84:3613–3636.
14. Huang CS, Huang MJ, Lin MS, et al. Genetic factors related to unconjugated hyperbilirubinemia amongst adults. *Pharmacogenet Genomics.* 2005;15:43–50.
15. Huang MJ, Kua KE, Teng HC, et al. Risk factors for severe hyperbilirubinemia in neonates. *Pediatr Res.* 2004;56:682–689.
16. Watchko JF, Lin Z, Clark RH, et al. Complex multifactorial nature of significant hyperbilirubinemia in neonates. *Pediatrics.* 2009;124:e868–e877.
17. Watchko JF, Lin Z. Exploring the genetic architecture of neonatal hyperbilirubinemia. *Semin Fetal Neonatal Med.* 2010;15:169–175.

18. Bomprezzi R, Kovanen PE, Martin R. New approaches to investigating heterogeneity in complex traits. *J Med Genet.* 2003;40:553–559.

19. Kidd KK, Kidd JR. Human genetic variation of medical significance. In: Stearns SC, Koella JC, eds. *Evolution in Health and Disease.* New York, NY: Oxford University Press; 2008:51–62.

20. Maisels MJ. Epidemiology of neonatal jaundice. In: Maisels MJ, Watchko JF, eds. *Neonatal Jaundice.* Amsterdam, The Netherlands: Harwood Academic Publishers; 2000:37–49.

21. Dolan SM, Moore C. Linking family history in obstetric and pediatric care: assessing risk for genetic disease and birth defects. *Pediatrics.* 2007;120:S66–S70.

22. Keren R, Luan X, Friedman S, et al. A comparison of alternative risk-assessment strategies for predicting significant neonatal hyperbilirubinemia in term and near term infants. *Pediatrics.* 2008;121:e170–e179.

23. Gale R, Seidman DS, Dollberg S, Stevenson DK. Epidemiology of neonatal jaundice in the Jerusalem population. *J Pediatr Gastroenterol Nutr.* 1990;10:82–86.

24. Newman TB, Xiong B, Gonzales VM, Escobar GJ. Prediction and prevention of extreme neonatal hyperbilirubinemia in a mature health maintenance organization. *Arch Pediatr Adolesc Med.* 2000;154:1140–1147.

25. Khoury MJ, Calle EE, Joesoef RM. Recurrence risk of neonatal hyperbilirubinemia in siblings. *Am J Dis Child.* 1988;142:1065–1069.

26. Nielsen H, Hasse P, Blaabjerg J, Stryhn H, Hilden J. Risk factors and sib correlation in physiological neonatal jaundice. *Acta Paediatr Scand.* 1987;76:504–511.

27. Boomsma D, Busjahn A, Peltonen L. Classical twin studies and beyond. *Nat Rev Genet.* 2002;3:872–882.

28. Ebbesen F, Mortensen BB. Difference in plasma bilirubin concentration between monozygotic and dizygotic newborn twins. *Acta Paediatr.* 2003;92:569–573.

29. Tan KL. Neonatal jaundice in twins. *Aust Paediatr J.* 1980;16:70–72.

30. Newman TB, Easterling MJ, Goldman ES, Stevenson DK. Laboratory evaluation of jaundice in newborns. *Am J Dis Child.* 1990;144:364–368 [erratum in: *Am J Dis Child.* 1992;146:1420–1421].

31. Setia S, Villaveces A, Dhillon P, Mueller BA. Neonatal jaundice in Asian, white and mixed-race infants. *Arch Pediatr Adolesc Med.* 2002;156:276–279.

32. Molnar S. *Human Variation. Races, Types and Ethnic Groups.* 6th ed. Upper Saddle River, NJ: Pearson Prentice Hall; 2006.

33. Risch N, Burchard E, Ziv E, Tang H. Categorization of humans in biomedical research: genes, race and disease. *Genome Biol.* 2002;3: comment 2007.

34. American Academy of Pediatrics, Subcommittee on Hyperbilirubinemia. Management of hyperbilirubinemia in the newborn infant 35 or more weeks of gestation. *Pediatrics.* 2004;114:297–316.

35. Ho NK. Neonatal jaundice in Asia. *Baillieres Clin Hematol.* 1992;5:131–142.

36. Huang CS, Luo GA, Huang MJ, Yu SC, Yang SS. Variations of the bilirubin uridine-glucuronosyl transferase 1A1 gene in healthy Taiwanese. *Pharmacogenetics.* 2000;10:539–544.

37. Huang CS, Chang PF, Huang MJ, et al. Relationship between bilirubin UDP-glucuronosyl transferase 1A1 gene and neonatal hyperbilirubinemia. *Pediatr Res.* 2002;52:601–605.

38. Yamamoto K, Sato H, Fujiyama Y, et al. Contribution of two missense mutations (G71R and Y486D) of the bilirubin UDP glycosyltransferase (*UGT1A1*) gene to phenotypes of Gilbert's syndrome and Crigler–Najjar syndrome type II. *Biochim Biophys Acta.* 1998;1406:267–273.

39. Koiwai O, Nishizawa M, Hasada K, et al. Gilbert's syndrome is caused by a heterozygous missense mutation in the gene for bilirubin UDP-glucuronosyltransferase. *Hum Mol Genet.* 1995;4:1183–1186.

40. Gourley GR. Disorders of bilirubin metabolism. In: Suchy FJ, ed. *Liver Disease in Children.* St. Louis: Mosby-Yearbook; 1994:401–413.

41. Maruo Y, Nishizawa K, Sato H, Doida Y, Shimada M. Association of neonatal hyperbilirubinemia with bilirubin UDP-glucuronosyltransferase polymorphism. *Pediatrics.* 1999;103:1224–1227.

42. Huang CS, Chang PF, Huang MJ, Chen ES, Chen WC. Glucose-6-phosphate dehydrogenase deficiency, the UDP-glucuronosyl transferase 1A1 gene, and neonatal hyperbilirubinemia. *Gastroenterology.* 2002;123:127–133.

43. Kang H, Lim JH, Kim JS, et al. The association of neonatal hyperbilirubinemia with UGT1A1 and CYP1A2 gene polymorphism in Korean neonate. *Korean J Pediatr.* 2005;48:380–386.

44. Zhou YY, Lee LY, Ng SY, et al. UGT1A1 haplotype mutation among Asians in Singapore. *Neonatology.* 2009;96:150–155.

45. Maruo Y, Nishizawa K, Sato H, et al. Prolonged unconjugated hyperbilirubinemia associated with breast milk and mutations of the bilirubin uridine diphosphate-glucuronosyltransferase gene. *Pediatrics.* 2000;106:e59.

46. Sun G, Wu M, Cao J, Du L. Cord blood bilirubin level in relation to bilirubin UDP-glucuronosyltransferase gene missense allele in Chinese neonates. *Acta Paediatr.* 2007;96:1622–1625.

47. Gao ZY, Zhong DN, Liu Y, Liu YN, Wei LM. Roles of *UGT1A1* gene mutation in the development of neonatal

hyperbilirubinemia in Guangxi. *Zhonghua Er Ke Za Zhi.* 2010;48:646–649.

48. Ramirez J, Ratain MJ, Innocenti F. Uridine 5′-diphospho-glucuronosyltransferase genetic polymorphisms and response to cancer chemotherapy. *Future Oncol.* 2010;6: 563–585.

49. Pasanen M, Neuvonen PJ, Niemi M. Global analysis of genetic variation in SLCO1B1. *Pharmacogenomics.* 2008;9:19–33.

50. Prachukthum S, Nunnarumit P, Pienvichit P, et al. Genetic polymorphisms in Thai neonates with hyper-bilirubinemia. *Acta Paediatr.* 2009;98:1106–1110.

51. Wong FL, Boo MY, Ainoon O, Wang MK. Variants of organic anion transporter polypeptide 2 gene are not risk factors associated with severe neonatal hyperbiliru-binemia. *Malays J Pathol.* 2009;31:99–104.

52. Chou SC, Palmer RH, Ezhuthachan S, et al. Management of hyperbilirubinemia in newborns: measuring per-formance by using a benchmarking model. *Pediatrics.* 2003;112:1264–1273.

53. Newman TB, Kuzniewicz, Liljestrand P, et al. Num-bers needed to treat with phototherapy according to American Academy of Pediatrics guidelines. *Pediatrics.* 2009;123:1352–1359.

54. Hardy JB, Drage JS, Jackson EE. *The First Year of Life. The Collaborative Perinatal Project of the National Institute of Neurological and Communicative Disorders and Stroke.* Baltimore: Johns Hopkins University Press; 1979:104.

55. Brown AK, Kim MH, Wu PYK, Bryla DA. Efficacy of phototherapy in prevention and management of neona-tal hyperbilirubinemia. *Pediatrics.* 1985;75:393–441.

56. Linn S, Schoenbaum SC, Monson RR, et al. Epidemiol-ogy of neonatal hyperbilirubinemia. *Pediatrics.* 1985;75: 770–774.

57. Watchko JF. Hyperbilirubinemia in African American neonates: clinical issues and current challenges. *Semin Fetal Neonatal Med.* 2010;15:176–182.

58. Beutler E, Gelbert T, Demina A. Racial variability in the UDP-glucuronosyltransferase 1 (*UGT1A1*) pro-moter: a balanced polymorphism for regulation of bili-rubin metabolism. *Proc Natl Acad Sci U S A.* 1998;95: 8170–8174.

59. Li R, Darling N, Maurice E, Barker L, Grummer-Strawn LM. Breastfeeding rates in the United States by charac-teristics of the child, mother, or family: the 2002 National Immunization Survey. *Pediatrics.* 2005;115:e31–e37.

60. McDowell MM, Wang CY, Kennedy-Stephenson J. Breastfeeding in the United States: findings from the national health and nutrition examination surveys, 1999–2006. *NCHS Data Brief.* 2008;5:1–8.

61. Manning D, Todd P, Maxwell M, Platt MJ. Prospective surveillance study of severe hyperbilirubinaemia in the newborn in the UK and Ireland. *Arch Dis Child Fetal Neonatal Ed.* 2007;92:342–346.

62. Nock ML, Johnson EM, Krugman RR, et al. Imple-mentation and analysis of a pilot in-hospital newborn screening program for glucose-6-phosphate dehy-drogenase deficiency in the United States. *J Perinatol.* 2011;31:112–117.

63. Maisels MJ, Gifford K, Antle CE, et al. Jaundice in the healthy newborn infant: a new approach to an old prob-lem. *Pediatrics.* 1988;81:505–511.

64. Fattah MA, Ghany EA, Adel A, Mosallam D. Glucose-6-phosphate dehydrogenase and red cell pyruvate kinase deficiency in neonatal jaundice cases in Egypt. *Pediatr Hematol Oncol.* 2010;27:262–271.

65. Adekunle-Ojo AO, Smitherman HF, Parker R, Ma L, Caviness AC. Managing well-appearing neonates with hyperbilirubinemia in the emergency department obser-vation unit. *Pediatr Emerg Care.* 2010;26:343–348.

66. Haymaker W, Margoles C, Pentschew A, et al. Pathol-ogy of kernicterus and posticteric encephalopathy. In: *Kernicterus and its Importance in Cerebral Palsy.* A con-ference presented by the American Academy for Cere-bral Palsy. Springfield, IL: Charles C Thomas; 1961: 21–228.

67. Sieg A, Arab L, Schlierf G, et al. Prevalence of Gilbert's syndrome in Germany. *Dtsch Med Wochenschr.* 1987; 112:1206–1208.

68. Diamond LK, Vaughn VC, Allen FH Jr. Erythroblastosis fetalis. III. Prognosis in relation to clinical and serologic manifestations at birth. *Pediatrics.* 1950;6:630–637.

69. Armitage P, Mollison PL. Further analysis of controlled trials of treatment of haemolytic disease of the newborn. *J Obstet Gynecol Br Emp.* 1953;60:605–620.

70. Walker W, Mollison PL. Haemolytic disease of the new-born: deaths in England and Wales during 1953 and 1955. *Lancet.* 1957;1:1309–1314.

71. Crosse VM. The incidence of kernicterus (not due to haemolytic disease) among premature babies. In: Sass-Kortsak A, ed. *Kernicterus.* Toronto: University of Toronto Press; 1961:4–9.

72. Johnson L, Garcia ML, Figueroa E, et al. Kernicterus in rats lacking glucuronyl transferase. *Am J Dis Child.* 1961;101:322–349.

73. Cannon C, Daood MJ, Watchko JF. Sex specific regional brain bilirubin content in hyperbilirubinemic Gunn rat pups. *Biol Neonate.* 2006;90:40–45.

74. Becu-Villabos D, Gonzalez Iglesias A, Diaz-Torga G, et al. Brain sexual differentiation and gonadotropins secretion in the rat. *Cell Mol Neurobiol.* 1997;17:699–715.

75. Du L, Bayir H, Lai Y, et al. Innate gender-based proclivity in response to cytotoxicity and programmed cell death pathway. *J Biol Chem.* 2004;279:38563–38570.

76. Huang W, Zhang J, Chua SS, et al. Induction of bilirubin clearance by the constitutive androstane receptor (CAR). *Proc Natl Acad Sci U S A*. 2003;100:4156–4161.

77. Pearson HA. Life-span of the fetal red blood cell. *J Pediatr*. 1967;70:166–171.

78. Vest MF, Grieder HR. Erythrocyte survival in the newborn infant, as measured by chromium 51 and its relation to the postnatal serum bilirubin level. *J Pediatr*. 1961;59:194–199.

79. Valaes T. Severe neonatal jaundice associated with glucose-6-phosphate dehydrogenase deficiency: pathogenesis and global epidemiology. *Acta Paediatr Suppl*. 1994;394:58–76.

80. Kaplan M, Hammerman C. Glucose-6-phosphate dehydrogenase deficiency: a hidden risk for kernicterus. *Semin Perinatol*. 2004;28:356–364.

81. Ogunlesi TA, Ogunfowora OB. Predictors of acute bilirubin encephalopathy among Nigerian term babies with moderate-to-severe hyperbilirubinemia. *J Trop Pediatr*. 2011;57:80–86 [Epub ahead of print June 15, 2010].

82. Beutler E. Glucose-6-phosphate dehydrogenase deficiency: a historical perspective. *Blood*. 2008;111:16–24.

83. Kaplan M, Hammerman C. Glucose-6-phosphate dehydrogenase deficiency and severe neonatal hyperbilirubinemia: a complexity of interactions between genes and environment. *Semin Fetal Neonatal Med*. 2010;15:148–156.

84. Chinevere TD, Murray CK, Grant E, et al. Prevalence of glucose-6-phosphate dehydrogenase deficiency in U.S. Army personnel. *Mil Med*. 2006;171:905–907.

85. United Nations, Department of Economic and Social Affairs, Population Division. *Trends in International Migrant Stock: The 2008 Revision*. United Nations database, POP/DB/MIG/Stock/Rev.2008; 2009.

86. DeParle J. A world on the move. *New York Times*. June 27, 2010.

87. Lin Z, Fontaine JM, Freer DE, et al. Alternative DNA-based newborn screening for glucose-6-phosphate dehydrogenase deficiency. *Mol Genet Metab*. 2005;86:212–219.

88. Kaplan M, Herschel M, Hammerman C, Hoyer JD, Stevenson DK. Hyperbilirubinemia among African American, glucose-6-phosphate dehydrogenase-deficient neonates. *Pediatrics*. 2004;114:e213–e219.

89. Kaplan M, Herschel M, Hammerman C, et al. Neonatal hyperbilirubinemia in African American males: the importance of glucose-6-phosphate dehydrogenase deficiency. *J Pediatr*. 2006;149:83–88.

90. Herschel M, Ryan M, Gelbart T, Kaplan M. Hemolysis and hyperbilirubinemia in an African American neonate heterozygous for glucose-6-phosphate dehydrogenase deficiency. *J Perinatol*. 2002;22:577–579.

91. O'Flynn ME, Hsia DY. Serum bilirubin levels and glucose-6-phosphate dehydrogenase deficiency in newborn American Negroes. *J Pediatr*. 1963;63:160–161.

92. Wolff JA, Grossman BH, Paya K. Neonatal serum bilirubin and glucose-6-phosphate dehydrogenase. *Am J Dis Child*. 1967;113:251–254.

93. Zinkham WH. Peripheral blood and bilirubin values in normal full term primaquine-sensitive Negro infants. Effect of vitamin K. *Pediatrics*. 1963;31:983–995.

94. Slusher TM, Vreman HJ, McLaren DW, et al. Glucose-6-phosphate dehydrogenase deficiency and carboxyhemoglobin concentrations associated with bilirubin-related morbidity and death in Nigerian infants. *J Pediatr*. 1995;126:102–108.

95. Zangen S, Kidron D, Gelbart T, et al. Fatal kernicterus in a girl deficient in glucose-6-phophate dehydrogenase: a paradigm of synergistic heterozygosity. *J Pediatr*. 2009;154:616–619.

96. Washington EC, Ector W, Abbound M, Ohning B, Holden K. Hemolytic jaundice due to G6PD deficiency causing kernicterus in a female newborn. *South Med J*. 1995;88:776–779.

97. Bosma PJ, Roy Chowdhury J, Bakker C, et al. The genetic basis of the reduced expression of bilirubin UDP-glucuronosyltransferase 1 in Gilbert's syndrome. *N Engl J Med*. 1995;333:1171–1175.

98. Bancroft JD, Kreamer B, Gourley GR. Gilbert syndrome accelerates development of neonatal jaundice. *J Pediatr*. 1998;132:656–660.

99. Monaghan G, McLellan A, McGeehan A, et al. Gilbert's syndrome is a contributory factor in prolonged unconjugated hyperbilirubinemia of the newborn. *J Pediatr*. 1999;134:441–446.

100. Bhutani V, Johnson L, Sivieri EM, et al. Predictive ability of a predischarge hour-specific serum bilirubin for subsequent significant hyperbilirubinemia in healthy term and near-term newborns. *Pediatrics*. 1999;103:6–14.

101. Sugatani J, Yamakawa K, Yoshinari K, et al. Identification of a defect in the UGT1A1 gene promoter and its association with hyperbilirubinemia. *Biochem Biophys Res Commun*. 2002;292:492–497.

102. Cui Y, Konig J, Leier I, et al. Hepatic uptake of bilirubin and its conjugates by the human organic anion transporter SLC21A6. *J Biol Chem*. 2001;276:9626–9630.

103. Briz O, Serrano MA, MacIas RI, et al. Role of organic anion-transporting polypeptides, OATP-A, OATP-C and OATP-8, in the human placenta–maternal liver tandem excretory pathway for foetal bilirubin. *Biochem J*. 2000;371:897–905.

104. Lin Z, Fontaine J, Watchko, JF. Coexpression of gene polymorphisms involved in bilirubin production and metabolism. *Pediatrics*. 2008;122:e156–e162.

105. Beutler E, Baluda MC. The separation of glucose-6-phosphate dehydrogenase deficient erythrocytes from the blood of heterozygotes for glucose-6-phosphate dehydrogenase deficiency. *Lancet.* 1964;1:189–192.

106. May J, Meyer CG, Grossterlinden L, et al. Red cell glucose-6-phosphate dehydrogenase status and pyruvate kinase activity in a Nigerian population. *Trop Med Int Health.* 2000;5:119–123.

107. Beutler E, Gelbart T. Estimating the prevalence of pyruvate kinase deficiency from the gene frequency in the general white population. *Blood.* 2000;95:3585–3588.

108. Mentzer WC Jr. Pyruvate kinase deficiency and disorders of glycolysis. In: Nathan DG, Orkin SH, Ginsburgh D, Look AT, eds. *Hematology of Infancy and Childhood.* 6th ed. Philadelphia: WB Saunders; 2003: 685–720.

109. Oski, FA. Disorders of red cell metabolism. In: Oski FA, Naiman JL, eds. *Hematologic Problems in the Newborn.* Philadelphia: WB Saunders; 1982:97–136.

110. Zanella A, Fermo E, Bianchi P, Valentini G. Red cell pyruvate kinase deficiency: molecular and clinical aspects. *Br J Haematol.* 2005;130:11–25.

111. Bowman HS, McKusick VA, Dronamraju KR. Pyruvate kinase deficient hemolytic anemia in an Amish isolate. *Am J Hum Genet.* 1965;17:1–8.

112. Muir WA, Beutler E, Watson C. Erythrocyte pyruvate kinase deficiency in the Ohio Amish: origin and characterization of the mutant enzyme. *Am J Hum Genet.* 1984;36:634–639.

113. Christensen RD, Eggert LD, Baer VL, Smith KN. Pyruvate kinase deficiency as a cause of extreme hyperbilirubinemia in neonates from a polygamist community. *J Perinatol.* 2010;30:233–236.

114. Matthay KK, Mentzer WC. Erythrocyte enzymopathies in the newborn. *Clin Hematol.* 1981;10:31–55.

115. Oski FA, Nathan DG, Sidel VW, et al. Extreme hemolysis and red-cell distortion in erythrocyte pyruvate kinase deficiency. I. Morphology, erythrokinetics and family enzyme studies. *New Engl J Med.* 1964;270: 1023–1030.

116. Oski FA. The erythrocyte and its disorders. In: Nathan DG, Oski FA, eds. *Hematology of Infancy and Childhood.* Philadelphia: WB Saunders; 1993:18–43.

117. Caprari P, Maiorana A, Marzetti G, et al. Severe neonatal hemolytic jaundice associated with pyknocytosis and alterations of red cell skeletal proteins. *Prenat Neonatal Med.* 1997;2:140–145.

118. Tuffy P, Brown AK, Zuelzer WW. Infantile pyknocytosis: common erythrocyte abnormality of the first trimester. *Am J Dis Child.* 1959;98:227–241.

119. Stockman JA. Physical properties of the neonatal red blood cell. In: Stockman JA, Pochedly C, eds.

120. Zipursky A, Brown E, Palko J. The erythrocyte differential count in the newborn infant. *Am J Pediatr Hematol Oncol.* 1983;5:45–51.

121. Delaunay J. The molecular basis of hereditary red cell membrane disorders. *Blood Rev.* 2007;21:1–20.

122. Gallagher PG, Lux SE. Disorders of the erythrocyte membrane. In: Nathan, DG, Orkin SH, Ginsburgh D, Look AT, eds. *Hematology of Infancy and Childhood.* 6th ed. Philadelphia: WB Saunders; 2003:560–684.

123. Stamey CC, Diamond LK. Congenital hemolytic anemia in the newborn. *Am J Dis Child.* 1957;94:616–622.

124. Christensen RD, Henry E. Hereditary spherocytosis in neonates with hyperbilirubinemia. *Pediatrics.* 2010;125:120–125.

125. Sgro M, Campbell D, Shah V. Incidence and causes of severe neonatal hyperbilirubinemia in Canada. *CMAJ.* 2006;175:587–590.

126. Berardi A, Lugli L, Ferrari F, et al. Kernicterus associated with hereditary spherocytosis and UGT1A1 promoter polymorphism. *Biol Neonate.* 2006;90: 243–246.

127. Burman D. Congenital spherocytosis in infancy. *Arch Dis Child.* 1958;33:335–338.

128. Iolascon A, Faienza MF, Moretti A, Perrotta S, Miraglia del Giudice E. UGT1 promoter polymorphism accounts for increased neonatal appearance of hereditary spherocytosis. *Blood.* 1998;91:1093.

129. Trucco JI, Brown AK. Neonatal manifestations of hereditary spherocytosis. *Am J Dis Child.* 1967;113:263–270.

130. Eyssette-Guerreau S, Bader-Meunier B, Garcon L, Guitton C, Cynober T. Infantile pyknocytosis: a cause of haemolytic anemia of the newborn. *Br J Haematol.* 2006;133:439–442.

131. Keimowitz R, Desforges JF. Infantile pyknocytosis. *N Engl J Med.* 1965;273:1152–1155.

132. Ackerman BD. Infantile pyknocytosis in Mexican-American infants. *Am J Dis Child.* 1969;117:417–423.

133. Dahoui HA, Abboud MR, Saab R, et al. Familial infantile pyknocytosis in association with pulmonary hypertension. *Pediatr Blood Cancer.* 2008;51:290–292.

134. Schmaier A, Maurer HM, Johnston CL, et al. Alpha thalassemia screening in neonates by mean corpuscular volume and mean corpuscular hemoglobin concentration. *J Pediatr.* 1973;83:794–797.

135. Pearson HA. Disorders of hemoglobin synthesis and metabolism. In: Oski FA, Naiman JL, eds. *Hematologic Problems in the Newborn.* Philadelphia: WB Saunders; 1982:245–282.

136. Vichinsky EP, MacKlin EA, Waye JS, Lorey F, Olivieri NF. Changes in the epidemiology of thalassemia in

Developmental and Neonatal Hematology. New York, NY: Raven Press; 1988:297–323.

North America: a new minority disease. *Pediatrics.* 2005;116:e818–e825.

137. Benz EJ. Newborn screening for α-thalassemia—keeping up with globalization. *N Engl J Med.* 2011;364:770–771.

138. Oort M, Heerspink W, Roos D, et al. Haemolytic disease of the newborn and chronic anaemia induced by gamma-beta thalassemia in a Dutch family. *Br J Haematol.* 1981;48:251–262.

139. Watchko JF. Indirect hyperbilirubinemia in the neonate. In: Maisels MJ, Watchko JF, eds. *Neonatal Jaundice.* Amsterdam: Harwood Academic Publisher; 2000:51–66.

140. Bucher KA, Patterson AM, Elston RC, Jones CA, Kirkman HN. Racial difference in incidence of ABO hemolytic disease. *Am J Public Health.* 1976;66:854–858.

141. Toy PTCY, Reid ME, Papenfus L, Yeap HH, Black D. Prevalence of ABO maternal–infant incompatibility in Asians, blacks, Hispanics, and Caucasians. *Vox Sang.* 1988;54:181–183.

142. Naiman JL. Erythroblastosis fetalis. In: Oski FA, Naiman JL, eds. *Hematologic Problems in the Newborn.* Philadelphia: WB Saunders; 1982:326–332.

143. Kirkman HN. Further evidence for a racial difference in frequency of ABO hemolytic disease. *J Pediatr.* 1977;90:717–721.

144. Liley HG. Immune hemolytic disease. In: Nathan DG, Orkin SH, Ginsburgh D, Look AT, eds. *Hematology of Infancy and Childhood.* 6th ed. Philadelphia: WB Saunders; 2003:56–85.

145. Zhao H, Wong R, Nguyen X, et al. Expression and regulation of heme oxygenase isozymes in the developing mouse cortex. *Pediatr Res.* 2006;60:518–523.

146. Exner M, Minar E, Wagner O, Schillinger M. The role of heme oxygenase-1 promoter polymorphisms in human disease. *Free Radic Biol Med.* 2004;37:1097–1104.

147. Lin R, Wang X, Wang Y, et al. Association of polymorphisms in four bilirubin metabolism genes with serum bilirubin in three Asian populations. *Hum Mutat.* 2009;30:609–615.

148. Endler G, Exner M, Schillinger M, et al. A microsatellite polymorphism in the heme oxygenase-1 gene promoter is associated with increased bilirubin and HDL levels but not with coronary artery disease. *Thromb Haemost.* 2004;91:155–161.

149. D'Silva S, Borse V, Colah RB, Ghosh K, Mukherjee MB. Association of (GT)*n* repeats promoter polymorphism of heme oxygenase-1 gene and serum bilirubin levels in healthy Indian adults. *Genet Test Mol Biomarkers.* 2011;15:215–218 [Epub ahead of print].

150. Yamda N, Yamaya M, Okinaga S, et al. Microsatellite polymorphism in the heme oxygenase-1 gene promoter is associated with susceptibility to emphysema. *Am J Hum Genet.* 2000;66:187–195.

151. Kanai M, Akaba K, Sasaki A, et al. Neonatal hyperbilirubinemia in Japanese neonates: analysis of the heme oxygenase-1 gene and fetal hemoglobin composition in cord blood. *Pediatr Res.* 2003;54:165–171.

152. Bozkaya OG, Kumral A, Yesilirmak DC, et al. Prolonged unconjugated hyperbilirubinemia associated with the haem oxygenase-1 gene promoter polymorphism. *Acta Paediatr.* 2010;99:679–683.

153. Immenschuh S, Shan Y, Kroll H, et al. Marked hyperbilirubinemia associated with the heme oxygenase-1 gene promoter microsatellite polymorphism in a boy with autoimmune hemolytic anemia. *Pediatrics.* 2007;119:e764–e767.

154. Nytofte NS, Serrano MA, Monte MJ, et al. A homozygous nonsense mutation (c.214C → A) in the biliverdin reductase alpha gene (BLVRA) results in accumulation of biliverdin during episodes of cholestasis. *J Med Genet.* 2011;48:219–225 [Epub ahead of print].

155. Wang P, Kim RB, Chowdhury JR, Wolkoff AW. The human organic anion transport protein SLC21A6 is not sufficient for bilirubin transport. *J Biol Chem.* 2003;278:20695–20699.

156. McDonagh A. Controversies in bilirubin biochemistry and their clinical relevance. *Semin Fetal Neonatal Med.* 2010;15:141–147.

157. Zucker SD, Goessling W, Hoppin AG. Unconjugated bilirubin exhibits spontaneous diffusion through model lipid bilayers and native hepatocyte membranes. *J Biol Chem.* 1999;274:10852–10862.

158. Daood MJ, Watchko JF. Ontogeny of human and murine solute carrier organic anion transporter 1B1 (SLCO1B1) expression in liver. *EPAS.* 2006;59:5575.484.

159. van der Deure WM, Friesema EC, de Jong FJ, et al. Organic anion transporter 1B1: an important factor in hepatic thyroid and estrogen transport and metabolism. *Endocrinology.* 2008;149:4695–4701.

160. Johnson AD, Kavousi M, Smith AV, et al. Genome-wide association meta-analysis for total serum bilirubin levels. *Hum Mol Genet.* 2009;18:2700–2710.

161. Coles BF, Kadlubar FF. Human alpha class glutathione S-transferases: genetic polymorphism, expression and susceptibility to disease. *Methods Enzymol.* 2005;401:9–42.

162. Wolkoff AW, Goresky CA, Sellin J, Gatmaitan Z, Aria I. Role of ligandin in transfer of bilirubin from plasma to liver. *Am J Physiol.* 1979;236:142–149.

163. Levi AJ, Gatmaitan Z, Aria IM. Deficiency of hepatic organic anion-binding protein, impaired organic anion uptake by liver and "physiologic" jaundice in newborn monkeys. *N Engl J Med.* 1970;283:1136–1139.

164. Morel F, Rauch C, Coles B, Le Ferrec E, Guillouzo A. The human glutathione transferase alpha locus:

genomic organization of the gene cluster and functional characterization of the genetic polymorphism in the *hGSTA1* promoter. *Pharmacogenetics.* 2002;12: 277–286.

165. Muslu N, Dogruer ZN, Eskandari G, et al. Are glutathione *S*-transferase gene polymorphisms linked to neonatal jaundice. *Eur J Pediatr.* 2008;167:57–61.

166. Morel F, Fardel O, Meyer DJ, et al. Preferential increase of glutathione *S*-transferase class α transcripts in cultured human hepatocytes by phenobarbital, 3-methylcholanthrene, and dithioethiones. *Cancer Res.* 1993;53:231–234.

167. Clarke DJ, Moghrabi N, Monaghan G, et al. Genetic defects of the UDP-glucoronosyltransferase-1 (UGT1) gene that cause familial non-haemolytic unconjugated hyperbilirubinemias. *Clin Chim Acta.* 1997;266:63–74.

168. Perera MA, Innocenti F, Ratain MJ. Pharmacogenetic testing for uridine diphosphate glucuronosyltransferase 1A1 polymorphisms. Are we there yet? *Pharmacotherapy.* 2008;28:755–768.

169. Kawade N, Onishi S. The prenatal and postnatal development of UDP glucuronyltransferase activity towards bilirubin and the effect of premature birth on this activity in human liver. *Biochem J.* 1981;196:257–260.

170. Coughtrie MW, Burchell B, Leakey JE, Hume R. The inadequacy of perinatal glucuronidation: immunoblot analysis of the developmental expression of individual UDP-glucuronosyltransferase isoenzymes in rat and human liver microsomes. *Mol Pharmacol.* 1988;34:729–735.

171. Sugatani J, Mizushima K, Osabe M, et al. Transcriptional regulation of human *UGT1A1* gene expression through distal and proximal promoter motifs: implication of defects in the *UGT1A1* promoter. *Naunyn Schmiedebergs Arch Pharmacol.* 2008;377:597–605.

172. Valaes T. Bilirubin metabolism: review and discussion of inborn errors. *Clin Perinatol.* 1976;3:177–209.

173. Bock KW, Burchell B, Guillemette C, et al. *UGT Alleles Nomenclature Home Page.* Available at: http://www.ugtalleles.ulaval.ca. Accessed April 11, 2010.

174. Crigler JF Jr, Najjar VA. Congenital familial nonhemolytic jaundice with kernicterus. *Pediatrics.* 1952;10:169–180.

175. Gilbert A, Lereboullet P. La cholemia simple familiale. *Semaine Med.* 1901;21:241–243.

176. Powell LW, Hemingway E, Billing BH, et al. Idiopathic unconjugated hyperbilirubinemia (Gilbert's syndrome): a study of 42 families. *N Engl J Med.* 1967;277: 1108–1112.

177. Aono S, Yamada Y, Keino H, et al. Identification of defect in the genes for bilirubin UDP-glucuronosyl-transferase in a patient with Crigler–Najjar syndrome type II. *Biochem Biophys Res Commun.* 1993;197:1239–1244.

178. Sutomo R, Laosombat V, Sadewa AH, et al. Novel missense mutation of the UGT1A1 gene in Thai siblings with Gilbert's syndrome. *Pediatr Int.* 2002;44: 427–432.

179. Costa E, Vieira E, Martins M, et al. Analysis of the UDP-glucuronosyltransferase gene in Portuguese patients with a clinical diagnosis of Gilbert and Crigler–Najjar syndromes. *Blood Cells Mol Dis.* 2006;36:91–97.

180. Farheen S, Sengupta S, Santra A, et al. Gilbert's syndrome: high frequency of the (TA)7 TAA allele in India and its interaction with a novel CAT insertion in promoter of the gene for bilirubin UDP-glucuronosyltransferase 1 gene. *World J Gastroenterol.* 2006;12:2269–2275.

181. Sai K, Saeki M, Saito Y, et al. UGT1A1 haplotypes associated with reduced glucuronidation and increased serum bilirubin in irinotecan-administered Japanese patients with cancer. *Clin Pharmacol Ther.* 2004;75:501–515.

182. Strassburgh CP, Kalthoff S, Ehmer U. Variability and function of family 1 uridine-5′-diphosphate glucuronosyltransferases (UGT1A). *Crit Rev Clin Lab Sci.* 2008;45:485–530.

183. Akaba K, Kimura T, Sasaki A, et al. Neonatal hyperbilirubinemia and mutation of the bilirubin uridine diphosphate-glucuronosyltransferase gene: a common missense mutation among Japanese, Koreans and Chinese. *Biochem Mol Biol Int.* 1998;46:21–26.

184. Agrawal SK, Kumar P, Rathi R, et al. UGT1A1 gene polymorphisms in North Indian neonates presenting with unconjugated hyperbilirubinemia. *Pediatr Res.* 2009;65:675–680.

185. Hall D, Ybazeta G, Destro-Bisol G, Petzl-Erler ML, Di Rienzo A. Variability at the uridine diphosphate glucuronosyltransferase 1A1 promoter in human populations and primates. *Pharmacogenetics.* 1999;9: 591–599.

186. Haverfield EV, McKenzie CA, Forrester T, et al. UGT1A1 variation and gallstone formation in sickle cell disease. *Blood.* 2005;105:968–972.

187. Han JY, Lim HS, Shin ES, et al. Comprehensive analysis of UGT1A1 polymorphisms predictive for pharmacokinetics and treatment outcome in patients with non-small-cell lung cancer treated with irinotecan and cisplatin. *J Clin Oncol.* 2006;24:2237–2244.

188. Saito Y, Maekawa K, Ozawa S, Sawada J. Genetic polymorphisms and haplotypes of major drug metabolizing enzymes in East Asians and their comparison with other ethnic populations. *Curr Pharmacogenomics.* 2007; 5:49–78.

189. Innocenti F, Undevia SD, Iyer L, et al. Genetic variants in the *UDP-glucuronosyltransferase 1A1* gene predict the risk of sever neutropenia of irinotecan. *J Clin Oncol.* 2004;22:1382–1388.

190. Takaoka Y, Ohta M, Takeuchi A, et al. Ligand orientation governs conjugation capacity of UDP-glucuronosyltransferase 1A1. *J Biochem.* 2010;148:25–28.

191. Odell GB. *Neonatal Hyperbilirubinemia.* New York, NY: Grune and Stratton; 1980.

192. Oski FA. Unconjugated hyperbilirubinemia. In: Avery ME, Taeusch HW, eds. *Diseases of the Newborn.* Philadelphia: WB Saunders; 1984:630–632.

193. Roy-Chowdury N, Deocharan B, Bejjanki HR, et al. Presence of the genetic marker for Gilbert syndrome is associated with increased level and duration of neonatal jaundice. *Acta Paediatr.* 2002;91:100–102.

194. Ergin H, Bican M, Atalay OE. A causal relationship between UDP-glucuronosyltransferase 1A1 promoter polymorphism and idiopathic hyperbilirubinemia in Turkish newborns. *Turk J Pediatr.* 2010;52:28–34.

195. Boo NY, Wong FL, Wang MK, Othman A. Homozygous variant of *UGT1A1* gene mutation and severe neonatal hyperbilirubinemia. *Pediatr Int.* 2009;51:488–493.

196. Huang A, Tai BC, Wong LY, Lee J, Yong EL. Differential risk for early breastfeeding jaundice in a multi-ethnic Asian cohort. *Ann Acad Med Singapore.* 2009;38:217–224.

197. Maruo Y, Addario CD, Mori A, et al. Two linked polymorphic mutations (A(TA)7TAA and T-3279G) of *UGT1A1* as principal cause of Gilbert syndrome. *Hum Genet.* 2004;115:525–526.

198. Jirsa M, Petrasek J, Vitek L. Linkage between A(TA)7TAA and −3279T>G mutations in UGT1A1 is not essential for pathogenesis of Gilbert syndrome. *Liver Int.* 2006;26:1302–1303.

199. Costa E, Vieira E, dos Santos R. The polymorphism c.−3279T>G in the phenobarbital responsive enhancer module of the bilirubin UDP-glucuronosyltransferase gene is associated with Gilbert syndrome. *Clin Chem.* 2005;51:2204–2206.

200. Muraca M, Fevery J, Blanckaert N. Relationships between serum bilirubins and production and conjugation of bilirubin. Studies in Gilbert's syndrome, Crigler–Najjar disease, hemolytic disorders and rat models. *Gastroenterology.* 1987;92:309–317.

201. Spivak W, DiVenuto D, Yuey W. Non-enzymatic hydrolysis of bilirubin mono- and diglucuronide to unconjugated bilirubin in model and native bilirubin systems. *Biochem J.* 1987;242:323–329.

202. Maisels MJ, Newman TB. Kernicterus in otherwise healthy, breast-fed term newborns. *Pediatrics.* 1995;96:730–733.

203. Kadakol A, Sappal BS, Ghosh SS, et al. Interaction of coding region mutations and the Gilbert-type promoter abnormality of the UGT1A1 gene causes moderate degrees of unconjugated hyperbilirubinemia and may lead to neonatal kernicterus. *J Med Genet.* 2001;38:244–249.

204. Chalasani N, Roy-Chowdhury N, Roy-Chowdhury J, Boyer TD. Kernicterus in an adult who is heterozygous for Crigler–Najjar syndrome and homozygous for Gilbert-type genetic defect. *Gastroenterology.* 1997;112:2099–2103.

205. Ciotti M, Chen F. Rubatelli FF, Owens IS. Coding and a TATA box mutation at the bilirubin UDP-glucuronosyl transferase gene cause Crigler–Najjar syndrome type I disease. *Biochim Biophys Acta.* 1998;1407:40–50.

206. Yamamoto K, Soeda Y, Kamisako T, et al. Analysis of bilirubin uridine 5′-diphosphate (UDP)-glucuronosyltransferase gene mutations in seven patients with Crigler–Najjar syndrome type II. *J Hum Genet.* 1998;43:111–114.

207. Vockley J, Rinaldo P, Bennett MJ, Matern D, Vladutiu GD. Synergistic heterozygosity: disease resulting from multiple partial defects in one or more metabolic pathways. *Mol Genet Metab.* 2000;71:10–18.

208. Kivlahan C, James EJP. The natural history of neonatal jaundice. *Pediatrics.* 1984;74:364–370.

209. Maisels MJ, Gifford K, Antle CE, et al. Normal serum bilirubin levels in the newborn and the effect of breast feeding. *Pediatrics.* 1986;78:837–843.

210. Schneider AP. Breast milk jaundice in the newborn. A real entity. *JAMA.* 1986;255:3270–3274.

211. Hansen TWR. Bilirubin production, breast-feeding and neonatal jaundice. *Acta Paediatr.* 2001;90:716–723.

212. Rubaltelli FF. Unconjugated and conjugated bilirubin pigments during perinatal development. IV: the influence of breast-feeding on neonatal hyperbilirubinemia. *Biol Neonate.* 1993;64:104–109.

213. De Carvalho M, Klaus MH, Merkatz RB. Frequency of breastfeeding and serum bilirubin concentration. *Am J Dis Child.* 1982;136:737–738.

214. Yamauchi Y, Yamanouchi I. Breast-feeding frequency during the first 24 hours after birth in full term neonates. *Pediatrics.* 1990;86:171–175.

215. Johnson LH, Bhutani VK, Brown AK. System-based approach to management of neonatal jaundice and prevention of kernicterus. *J Pediatr.* 2002;140:396–403.

216. Takimoto M, Matsuda I. β-Glucuronidase activity in the stool of newborn infant. *Biol Neonate.* 1971;18:66–70.

217. Gourley GR. Perinatal bilirubin metabolism. In: Gluckman PD, Heymann MA, eds. *Perinatal and Pediatric Pathophysiology. A Clinical Perspective.* Boston: Hodder and Stoughton; 1993:437–439.

218. Poland RD, Odell GB. Physiologic jaundice: the enterohepatic circulation of bilirubin. *N Engl J Med.* 1971;284:1–6.

219. Gartner LM, Lee K-S, Vaisman S, et al. Development of bilirubin transport and metabolism in the newborn rhesus monkey. *J Pediatr.* 1977;90:513–531.

220. Gartner U, Goeser T, Wolkoff AW. Effect of fasting on the uptake of bilirubin and sulfobromopthalein by the isolated perfused rat liver. *Gastroenterology.* 1997;113:1707–1713.

221. Fevery J. Fasting hyperbilirubinemia. Unraveling the mechanism involved. *Gastroenterology.* 1997;113:1798–1800.

222. Bertini G, Carlo C, Tronchin M, Rubaltelli FF. Is breastfeeding really favoring early neonatal jaundice. *Pediatrics.* 2001;107:e41. Available at: http://www.pediatrics.org/cgi/content/full/107/3/e41.

223. Stevenson DK, Bartoletti AL, Ostrander CR, et al. Pulmonary excretion of carbon monoxide in the human infant as an index of bilirubin production. IV: effects of breast-feeding and caloric intake in the first postnatal week. *Pediatrics.* 1980;65:1170–1172.

224. Hintz SR, Gaylord, TD, Oh W, et al. Serum bilirubin levels at 72 hours by selected characteristics in breastfed and formula-fed term infants delivered by cesarean section. *Acta Paediatr.* 2001;90:776–781.

225. Watchko JF. Genetics and the risk of neonatal hyperbilirubinemia. *Pediatr Res.* 2004;56:677–678.

226. Kaplan M, Hammerman C, Vreman HJ, Wong RJ, Stevenson DK. Severe hemolysis with normal blood count in a glucose-6-phosphage dehydrogenase deficient neonate. *J Perinatol.* 2008;28:306–309.

227. Valaes T. Neonatal jaundice in glucose-6-phosphate dehydrogenase deficiency. In: Maisels MJ, Watchko JF, eds. *Neonatal Jaundice.* Amsterdam: Harwood Academic Publisher; 2000:67–72.

228. Corchia C, Balata A, Meloni GF, Meloni T. Favism in a female newborn infant whose mother ingested fava beans before delivery. *J Pediatr.* 1995;127:807–808.

229. Luzatto L. G6PD deficiency and hemolytic anemia. In: Nathan GD, Oski FA, eds. *Hematology of Infancy and Childhood.* Philadelphia: WB Saunders; 1993: 674–695.

230. Guillemette C, Levesque E, Harvey M, Bellemare J, Menard V. UGT genomic diversity: beyond gene duplication. *Drug Metab Rev.* 2010;42:24–44.

231. Gagnon JF, Bernard O, Villeneuve L, Tetu B, Guillemette C. Irinotecan inactivation is modulated by epigenetic silencing of UGT1A1 in colon cancer. *Clin Cancer Res.* 2006;12:1850–1858.

232. Lin JP, Cupples LA, Wilson PW, Heard-Costa N, O'Donnell CJ. Evidence for a gene influencing serum bilirubin on chromosome 2q telomere: a genomewide scan in the Framingham study. *Am J Hum Genet.* 2003;72:1029–1034.

233. Hunt SC, Wu LL, Hopkins PN, Williams RR. Evidence for a major gene elevating serum bilirubin concentration in Utah pedigree. *Arterioscler Thromb Vasc Biol.* 1996;16:912–917.

234. Ki CS, Lee KA, Lee SY, et al. Haplotype structure of the UDP-glucuronosyltransferase A1A (UGT1A1) gene and its relationship to serum total bilirubin concentration in a male Korean population. *Clin Chem.* 2003;49:2078–2081.

Bilirubin Production and Its Measurement

David K. Stevenson, Hendrik J. Vreman, and Ronald J. Wong

Neonatal jaundice is one of the first and perhaps the most common problem encountered by the practicing pediatrician. It is a natural phenomenon occurring in the majority of full-term infants and virtually in all preterm infants.[1,2] Neonatal jaundice reflects the presence of pigment in the skin and sclera, although little is known about the exact location of the pigment and to what it might be bound in those locations.[3] Nonetheless, it is related to hyperbilirubinemia in the transition after birth, which occurs in all babies, except those lacking albumin, which is an extremely rare condition. This transitional phenomenon is usually benign and may have a physiological role in development, but under some conditions bilirubin outside the circulation can be dangerous, such as its accumulation in the brain, contributing to neurologic dysfunction and, sometimes, permanent injury.[1,4]

The syndrome of neonatal jaundice results from an imbalance between bilirubin production and bilirubin elimination,[1,2,5] which is temporarily exacerbated during the transition after birth. This imbalance can be understood by analogy to a sink where the turned on spigot represents the process of bilirubin production and the drain represents the process of bilirubin elimination (Figure 2-1). If the rate at which bilirubin is produced in the body exceeds the rate at which bilirubin is eliminated, then the level in the body increases. In the analogy, the size of the sink represents the capacity of the circulation to contain bilirubin, and this is dependent mainly on the albumin concentration and the affinity of albumin to bind bilirubin. In the newborn, the capacity of the sink is decreased, and thus the likelihood that bilirubin will escape the circulation and move into tissues such as the brain is increased. The situation is worse in this regard in the preterm infant where the capacity is even lower because of a decreased albumin concentration and lower affinity for binding bilirubin, especially in the first days after birth and further compromised by any illness reflected in physiological instability.[6] A more general discussion of the physiology of neonatal unconjugated hyperbilirubinemia and the epidemiology of neonatal jaundice is contained in other chapters. However, the biochemistry of bilirubin production is fundamental to the problem of neonatal jaundice, which cannot occur without the existence of the pigment.[7]

■ THE SOURCE OF BILIRUBIN

There is a single biochemical source of bilirubin in the body, which is the enzymatic two-step process of heme catabolism.[8] The reaction is ubiquitous, occurring in all nucleated cells, and thus in all tissues including the nucleated cells in blood. The substrate for the reaction, heme, is a part of many important proteins, but is present in large amounts in the hemoglobin of red blood cells (RBCs). The first step in the process is catalyzed by heme oxygenase (HO) (Figure 2-2).[8] This is the rate-limiting step in the process and is a membrane-bound event with requirements for NADPH donated from the cytochrome P450 system and molecular oxygen and involving a series of oxidations and reductions ultimately resulting in the

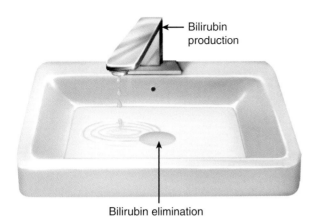

FIGURE 2-1. Diagram of bilirubin production and elimination. (Modified from Stevenson DK, Dennery PA, Hintz SR. Understanding newborn jaundice. *J Perinatol.* 2001;21:S22. Modified by permission from Macmillan Publishers Ltd., copyright 2001.)

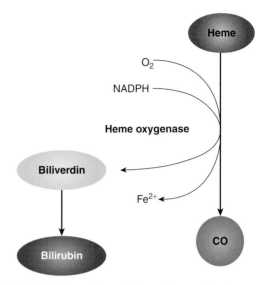

FIGURE 2-2. Heme degradation pathway. The turnover of hemoglobin and other hemoproteins yields heme, which is metabolized to equimolar quantities of carbon monoxide (CO), iron (Fe^{2+}), and biliverdin. Biliverdin is subsequently reduced to form bilirubin. (Modified from Stevenson DK. American Pediatric Society Presidential Address 2006: science on the edge with life in the balance. *Pediatr Res.* 2006;60:630–635. Reprinted with permission.)

breaking of the IXα methene bridge of the porphyrin macrocycle, yielding equimolar amounts of carbon monoxide (CO), biliverdin, and ferrous iron (Fe^{2+}). Biliverdin is further reduced enzymatically by biliverdin reductase to bilirubin, which thus is also produced in equimolar amounts with the intermediate products in the same process. The one gaseous product of the first step, CO, diffuses from the cell and is bound to hemoglobin forming carboxyhemoglobin (COHb), which is carried in the circulation to the lungs. CO is excreted in breath in exchange for oxygen, reflecting the total-body production from all sources. Because of the equimolar production of bilirubin and CO in the catabolism of heme, total CO production can be used as an index of total bilirubin production.[9,10]

The rate of bilirubin formation is highly regulated, in particular by HO. HO is present in tissues in two main isoforms, HO-1 and HO-2.[11] The former is inducible and the latter is constitutive. The ratio of these isoforms of HO to each other varies in tissues, with one or the other usually predominating. The expression of HO is also regulated developmentally.[12] There are many inducers of HO-1, which has a promoter reflecting its many different roles in biology, probably accumulated over millions of years. Thus, it is important to understand HO as not simply a cause of jaundice, neurologic disturbances, and kernicterus, CO not simply as a toxin capable of causing mitochondrial dysfunction, and Fe^{2+} not simply as a participant in the Fenton reaction and generator of reactive oxygen species (ROS) production.[13] In fact, the same

enzymatic system has many potential important biologic effects, some of them clearly beneficial. For example, the biliverdin–bilirubin shuttle[14,15] may have important antioxidant,[16] anti-inflammatory,[14] and antiapoptotic[14] effects. CO has a role in many physiological processes.[17] It can act directly to cause vessel relaxation and also indirectly through increases in soluble guanylyl cyclase (sGC) and cyclic GMP to cause vessel relaxation[17,18] and antiplatelet,[19] antiapoptotic,[20] and antiproliferative[21,22] effects (the latter in vascular smooth muscle cells) (Figure 2-3). It also may have a role in neurotransmission,[21,22] and by acting through p38 MAPK, CO may have an inhibitory effect on proinflammatory cytokines.[23] Working through increases vascular endothelial growth factor (VEGF),[24] CO may have a role in angiogenesis as well. Even Fe^{2+} under some conditions may participate in antioxidant, anti-inflammatory, and antiapoptotic processes.[25] Thus, the process by which bilirubin is produced needs to be understood in the context of other complex interactions between this enzymatic system and others. Such interactions include the biochemical pathways containing hemoproteins, with one of the most notable examples being the nitric oxide synthase (NOS) system.[17,26] The resulting interactions are

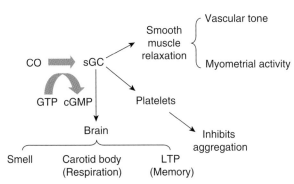

FIGURE 2-3. Physiological roles of carbon monoxide (CO). In this simplified overview, CO binds to sGC, stimulating the production of cGMP, which then further activates a number of signaling pathways, which in turn mediates a variety of processes: smooth muscle relaxation, which leads to changes in vascular and visceral tones; inhibition of platelet aggregation; and neuronal transmission, affecting processes such as smell, respiration, and long-term potentiation (LTP).

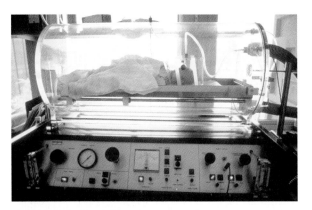

FIGURE 2-4. Flow-through system. Flow-through used to estimate total body endogenous CO production (VeCO) can be used as an index of total bilirubin production at Stanford University (circa 1979).

not always predictable or intuitive and are dependent on the timing and context, including developmental time frame. Relevant to the ensuing discussion about the use of CO measurements to estimate total bilirubin formation, it is always important to understand that there are a variety of nonenzymatic sources of CO in the body.[27] Under some pathologic conditions these sources can be quite large. Two very important sources, which we have described, are photo-oxidation[27–29] and lipid peroxidation.[13] Nonetheless, under most conditions encountered in the newborn, except in the case of high supplemental oxygen exposure, severe infection, or intense light exposure in the smallest infants, estimates of total CO production can be used as an index of total bilirubin production.[10] In this regard, heme degradation accounts for over 80% of all the endogenous sources of CO with 70% of heme degradation represented by senescing RBCs, 10% by ineffective erythropoiesis, and the remaining 20% by the degradation of other hemoproteins.[13,27] Under usual conditions, less than 20% of endogenous CO comes from nonheme source, such as lipid peroxidation and photo-oxidation.[13,27]

■ ESTIMATING BILIRUBIN PRODUCTION

Thus, estimates of total body endogenous CO production (VeCO) can be used as estimates of total bilirubin production. Measurements were made in human infants as

early as 1949 by Sjöstrand[30] and in 1968 by Fällström.[31] These investigators used a flow-through system similar to the one used later by investigators at Stanford in the 1970s (Figure 2-4).[32] Most of this earlier work was limited by detector technology, and it was understood that these CO measurements could only serve as an index of total body bilirubin formation because of the inability to account for alternative sources of CO in the clinical setting. In a laboratory, however, the stoichiometric relationship between CO production from heme catabolism and bilirubin production could be validated. This was demonstrated in a rat model using a gas collection apparatus connected to a reduction gas detector, which replaced the earlier infrared CO detectors and had much greater sensitivity.[33–35] The new detector depended on a mercuric oxide reaction bed, which would react with a reducing gas, such as CO, to produce carbon dioxide (CO_2) and mercury vapor (Hg), the latter measurable using an optical detection system.[36] Other reducing gases, such as H_2, could also be detected after separation by a gas chromatograph. The detection limit for CO was less than 1 part per billion using such a CO analyzer, making it possible to study CO production by small animals, such as rats and mice, as well as by tissue slices and even collections of cells. The new reduction gas detector could also be adapted for a gas chromatographic HO assay,[37] replacing the Tenhunen assay,[8] and making it possible to assess directly the activity level of the first and rate-limiting enzyme in the two-step catabolic process of heme in a variety of tissues. In the validation experiment, 100% of heme was recovered as CO in the breath of the

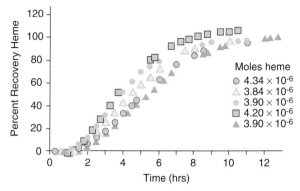

FIGURE 2-5. Percent recovery of injected heme over time. The cumulative percent of the total injected heme recovered as expired carbon monoxide (CO) in a given experiment was calculated for each determination in that experiment and plotted as a function of time. (Reproduced from Stevenson DK, Ostrander CR, Johnson JD. Effect of erythrocyte destruction on the pulmonary excretion rate of carbon monoxide in adult male Wistar rats. *J Lab Clin Med.* 1979;94:649–654, with permission from *Journal of Laboratory and Clinical Medicine*, copyright Elsevier 1979.)

animals after injection of a known amount of heme as damaged RBCs over a time frame of 8–12 hours reflecting RBC sequestration, destruction, and heme degradation (Figure 2-5).[38]

A large number of infants were studied in the 1970s[32,39] and 1980s[40–42] at Stanford using this older, yet elegant, flow-through system to measure VeCO. This work affirmed earlier reports demonstrating that the term infant produced

bilirubin at a rate two to three times higher than the human adult on a bodyweight basis. The technology was also able to distinguish infants with known risk factors for jaundice, such as hematoma and polycythemia (Figure 2-6).[43] Nonventilated preterm infants were also observed to have a slightly higher VeCO, probably related to an even shorter RBC lifespan compared with the term infant. Small, ventilated preterm infants had even higher CO excretion rates,[44] but it is now known that such infants might also have had a pathologic source of CO related to oxygen exposure and mechanical ventilation, that is, lipid peroxidation in their lungs.[45] Although the latter possibility is only speculation at this point in time, circumstantial evidence is supportive of this interpretation. Also, the Stanford group was the first to report that increased bilirubin production was an important contributing cause to the jaundice observed in infants of diabetic mothers.[32] In some cases this was related to polycythemia, but in others, because of the absence of erythrocytosis, it was most likely related to ineffective erythropoiesis probably occurring in the liver. Companion studies demonstrated that infants of diabetic mothers also had impaired elimination of the pigment after controlling for bilirubin production.[42] Finally, infants with hemolytic conditions were easily identified, with Rh disease demonstrating the highest VeCO measurements (Figure 2-6).[43]

VeCO measurements conducted using the large chamber or using a smaller hood with a neck seal were cumbersome and limited in application in the clinical setting (Figure 2-4).[40] New techniques were developed to measure

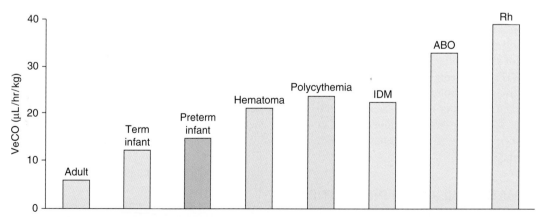

FIGURE 2-6. End-tidal carbon monoxide levels in infants with known risk factors for jaundice. End-tidal carbon monoxide (CO) levels, corrected for ambient CO (ETCOc) in infants with known risk factors for jaundice. IDM, infant of diabetic mother.

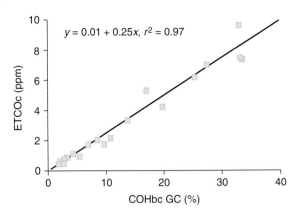

$y = 0.01 + 0.25x, r^2 = 0.97$

FIGURE 2-7. Correlation of end-tidal carbon monoxide and carboxyhemoglobin levels, both corrected for ambient CO (ETCOc and COHbc, respectively) in infants.

end-tidal CO concentration corrected for ambient carbon monoxide (ETCOc).[9,46–48] Equations predicted a direct relationship between the VeCO and ETCOc as well as carboxyhemoglobin corrected for ambient carbon monoxide (COHbc).[40,41] The relationship between COHbc and ETCOc was validated (Figure 2-7), and currently either technique, with appropriate correction for ambient CO, can be used to estimate endogenous CO production and thus total body bilirubin formation.[44,49] In fact, a COHbc measurement had been considered the standard approach because it involved a simple blood sample technique and avoided cumbersome technology.[27,36,50] Earlier elegant studies conducted by Maisels et al. using a rebreathing system also used a COHb measurement over time to estimate bilirubin production rates.[51] Nonetheless, ETCO measurements represent the easiest and least invasive of the techniques for estimating endogenous CO production and can be used to study large numbers of infants, providing for the first time data on the distribution of ETCOc in a large population of infants, most of them normal but some with conditions known to be associated with neonatal jaundice. In fact, the hour-specific bilirubin nomogram[52] (Figure 2-8), which is used for decision-

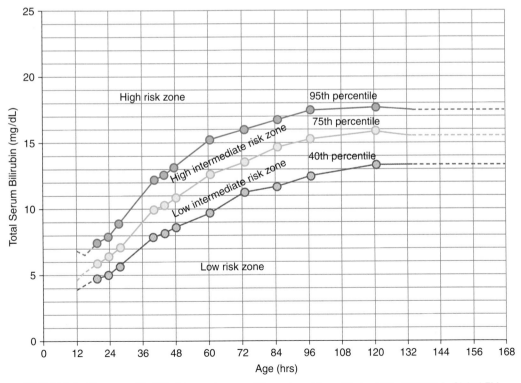

FIGURE 2-8. Hour-specific bilirubin nomogram. (Reproduced from Bhutani VK, Johnson L, Sivieri EM. Predictive ability of a predischarge hour-specific serum bilirubin for subsequent significant hyperbilirubinemia in healthy term and near-term newborns. *Pediatrics.* 1999;103:6–14, with permission from *Pediatrics*, copyright 1999 by the American Association of Pediatrics.)

making about treatment for late preterm and term infants, is further informed by information about total bilirubin formation, with infants in the highest risk quartile having a much greater likelihood of having increased bilirubin production as an important contributing cause of their neonatal jaundice. Thus, not only does bilirubin help to define risk for the normal population, but it is also now known that hemolysis represents an important risk factor for neurologic dysfunction and permanent injury caused by bilirubin.[53] In this regard, the diagnosis of hemolysis is paramount in the management strategy for neonatal jaundice, with intervention being recommended at lower bilirubin levels for a given postnatal age in hours. Because estimates of endogenous CO production can be used to index total bilirubin production, estimates of endogenous CO production can be used to identify infants at high risk for neurologic dysfunction or injury in the presence of jaundice. As a case in point, only about half of infants with a positive Coombs' test are hemolyzing at the time of the test.[54] CO detection technology can identify the half who are hemolyzing and moreover might be useful in gauging the magnitude of the risk not only for jaundice but also for neurologic dysfunction or permanent injury in this group.

Because of the tremendous variation in the ability to conjugate, the use of estimates of endogenous CO production to predict onset of jaundice is limited and not particularly useful, except perhaps in some subgroups known to have increased production as an important contributing cause. However, because most of the pathologic jaundice observed in the newborn period is associated with increased bilirubin production, the combination of estimates of endogenous CO production and bilirubin levels at various postnatal ages might provide a better understanding of the imbalance of bilirubin production and bilirubin elimination that may contribute to dangerous jaundice in a particular infant.[9]

■ POTENTIAL TOXICITY OF PHOTOTHERAPY

Phototherapy has been the mainstay of treatment for hyperbilirubinemia for approximately half a century.[55] Recent improvements in technology have narrowed the wavelength spectrum and introduced alternative light sources, such as light-emitting diodes (LEDs).[56,57] Amazingly, phototherapy was only studied in one randomized controlled trial in the late 1970s. In this trial,

it was proven that phototherapy could reduce the need for exchange transfusion, which was a major advance.[58] There were very few infants less than 1000 g enrolled in that study. A worrisome observation was that these smaller preterm infants appeared to have a higher death rate, although this finding did not reach statistical significance and the study was not powered for this purpose. Recently, however, a study was conducted to assess aggressive versus conservative phototherapy in infants with extremely low birth weight (ELBW ≤1000 g).[59] The primary outcome of this study was that aggressive phototherapy treatment did not significantly reduce the rate of death or neurodevelopmental impairment (NDI). Ironically, planned secondary outcomes, however, suggested that the rate of NDI alone was significantly reduced with aggressive phototherapy. However, this reduction appeared to be offset by an increase in mortality among infants weighing 501–750 g at birth. In a follow-up study, risk-adjusted outcomes at 18–22 months corrected age were assessed in these small infants who received any phototherapy compared with those who did not.[60] It appeared that phototherapy was not independently associated with death or NDI for the overall ELBW group. Whether phototherapy increases mortality could not be excluded due to bias from deaths before reaching conservative treatment threshold. Nonetheless, the finding that there was a higher rate of Mental Development Index (MDI) <50 in the 501–750 g infants not receiving phototherapy is concerning. Because these very small, translucent preterm infants were not surviving in large numbers 30 years ago, there was little opportunity to assess the safety of even commonly used therapies such as phototherapy. Phototherapy was simply assumed to be safe and its application was extended universally to this part of the preterm population with essentially no one escaping exposure. The question has now been raised whether visible light might have adverse effects in ELBW premature infants who have reduced antioxidant defenses and might be more vulnerable to photo-oxidation, not only in the skin but also in deeper tissues such as the brain, as it is obvious that light can penetrate beyond the skin surface to deeper tissues, even being used for detection of chemical reactions and imaging inside the brain or other body tissues.[29] Thus, the rationale for inhibiting bilirubin production as an alternative to enhancing bilirubin elimination with the use of phototherapy is further substantiated by these findings.[61]

■ CONTROLLING BILIRUBIN PRODUCTION

This makes the first enzymatic step in the two-step catabolic process of heme catabolism a target for controlling the process of bilirubin production.[62–64] A variety of heme analogs, metalloporphyrins, have been evaluated for this purpose.[65–67] Metalloporphyrins vary, depending on the metal in the center of the porphyrin macrocycle and the various ring substituents. The heme analogs differ from iron protoporphyrin (hemin) by such alterations in the central metal and ring substituents. The most promising compounds to date include tin mesoporphyrin (SnMP),[61] which is currently being studied in human trials,[68,69] zinc deuteroporphyrin IX bis glycol (ZnBG),[70,71] and chromium mesoporphyrin.[72,73] Zinc protoporphyrin (ZnPP), a naturally occurring heme analog, is less potent, but also effective in controlling hemolytic jaundice as modeled in the Rhesus newborn primate.[74,75] Criteria for potential antihyperbilirubinemia drugs include a biocompatible central metal, potent HO inhibition, negligible degradation, negligible inhibition of other enzymes, negligible photoreactivity at an effective dose, optimal duration of action (short), and negligible HO-1 upregulation.[61,76] In vivo bioluminescence imaging (BLI) technology has been used to evaluate the metalloporphyrins with respect to the last criterion.[61,77–79] ZnBG seems to be the most promising in this regard while it is also an extremely potent and orally absorbable heme analog.[67,76] Its one drawback is that it is photoreactive under some conditions,[65,80] although, because of its potency and the lack of activation within the narrow blue wavelength part of the spectrum,[81] it remains an attractive drug candidate, perhaps even more so than SnMP.

Because of the fundamental importance of increased bilirubin production in all kinds of neonatal jaundice, inhibition of bilirubin production remains a promising preventive and therapeutic approach to the problem. Even in the cases where impaired elimination is an important contributing cause, as encountered with several genetic polymorphisms, prevention or modulation of neonatal jaundice might be possible with this singular approach, if the drug had no, or few, toxic effects. This might provide the rationale for treating a whole population in a preventive manner, if a significant proportion of the population had such polymorphisms or other risk factors contributing to the risk for increased bilirubin production, such as glucose-6-phosphate dehydrogenase (G6PD) deficiency,[82] and also lacked access to more standard therapies, such as phototherapy and exchange transfusion, which might present unreasonable risks (e.g., because of unreliable electricity or contaminated blood supplies). Nonetheless, in developed countries, a more targeted approach to the use of HO inhibitors would be warranted.[61,64] Such an approach would necessarily use estimates of CO production as an index of bilirubin production to identify individual infants with increased bilirubin production as a major contributing cause to their propensity for neonatal jaundice. The targeting could be made even more specific by combining such screening after birth with antenatal information about genetic polymorphisms that might contribute to inherited increased production of bilirubin or impaired conjugation (see Chapter 1).[82–84] Such a gene interaction has been suggested by Kaplan et al. related to G6PD deficiency and Gilbert disease.[85–92]

■ ANTENATAL SCREENING FOR THE RISK OF HYPERBILIRUBINEMIA

The possibility of antenatal screening for various polymorphisms putting infants at risk for increased bilirubin production or impaired elimination might provide practitioners with anticipatory guidance toward postnatal screening for increased bilirubin production and impaired elimination, using minimally invasive devices, probably optical in nature. Jaundice risk profiles developed antenatally could identify infants with low or high bilirubin production potential and fast or slow elimination capacity, the highest risk group being identified as high producers and slow eliminators (Figure 2-9). The hour-specific production and elimination profile would provide early identification of individual infants, who are at either low or high risk and could be managed differently. Individuals

Bilirubin Production	Bilirubin Elimination: Fast	Bilirubin Elimination: Slow
Low	Low	Medium
High	Medium	High

FIGURE 2-9. Jaundice risk profiles. These profiles obtained antenatally could identify infants with low or high bilirubin production potential and fast or slow elimination capacity, the highest risk group being identified as high producers and slow eliminators.

in the high-risk category could be targeted for inhibition of bilirubin production and prevention of the postnatal syndromes putting infants at risk for neurologic disturbances and kernicterus and driving their postnatal bilirubin trajectory into the normal percentile ranges.

Thus, there would be the potential for a new therapeutic paradigm. The ability to identify and isolate a single fetal cell from the maternal circulation early in gestation is technically feasible. Using a single cell, a genetic profile of jaundice risk could be ascertained. The anticipated pathophysiology could be confirmed rapidly after birth in the postnatal period with noninvasive optical monitoring. Individuals producing the pigment at a high rate or showing impaired elimination by rapidly rising bilirubin levels or, most dangerous, a combination of both problems would be a target for HO inhibition, avoiding the need for phototherapy (Figure 2-7). This would be particularly desirable for the smallest infants, who might, in fact, be at high risk for bilirubin-induced neurologic dysfunction, kernicterus, or death, or, ironically, also neurologic injury or death caused by phototoxicity.[59] In this way, toxic effects of the HO system could be avoided and beneficial effects might be maintained in the transitional period after birth. This personalized approach to management of neonatal jaundice would be the ultimate solution, which is now technically possible, although not currently available with all of its components implementable in routine practice. Nonetheless, it seems highly likely that the day is coming when the possibility of targeted prevention of neonatal hyperbilirubinemia will be a reality.

REFERENCES

1. Stevenson DK, Wong RJ, Hintz SR, Vreman HJ. The jaundiced newborn: understanding and managing transitional hyperbilirubinemia. *Minerva Pediatr.* 2002;54:373–382.

2. Cohen RS, Wong RJ, Stevenson DK. Understanding neonatal jaundice: a perspective on causation. *Pediatr Neonatol.* 2010;51:143–148.

3. Narendran V, Pickens WL, Visscher M, Alta SK, Hoath SB. Binding of unconjugated bilirubin to human epidermis and vernix caseosa: the physiological basis of jaundice. *E-PAS2010:*2851.338.

4. American Academy of Pediatrics. Management of hyperbilirubinemia in the newborn infant 35 or more weeks of gestation. *Pediatrics.* 2004;114:297–316.

5. Kaplan M, Muraca M, Hammerman C, et al. Imbalance between production and conjugation of bilirubin: a fundamental concept in the mechanism of neonatal jaundice. *Pediatrics.* 2002;110:e47.

6. Oh W, Tyson JE, Fanaroff AA, et al. Association between peak serum bilirubin and neurodevelopmental outcomes in extremely low birth weight infants. *Pediatrics.* 2003;112:773–779.

7. Wong RJ, Stevenson DK, Ahlfors CE, Vreman HJ. Neonatal jaundice: bilirubin physiology and clinical chemistry. *NeoReviews.* 2007;8:e58–e67.

8. Tenhunen R, Marver HS, Schmid R. The enzymatic conversion of heme to bilirubin by microsomal heme oxygenase. *Proc Natl Acad Sci USA.* 1968;61:748–755.

9. Stevenson DK, Fanaroff AA, Maisels MJ, et al. Prediction of hyperbilirubinemia in near-term and term infants. *Pediatrics.* 2001;108:31–39.

10. Stevenson DK, Vreman HJ, Oh W, et al. Bilirubin production in healthy term infants as measured by carbon monoxide in breath. *Clin Chem.* 1994;40:1934–1939.

11. Maines MD. The heme oxygenase system: a regulator of second messenger gases. *Annu Rev Pharmacol Toxicol.* 1997;37:517–554.

12. Zhao H, Wong RJ, Nguyen X, et al. Expression and regulation of heme oxygenase isozymes in the developing mouse cortex. *Pediatr Res.* 2006;60:518–523.

13. Vreman HJ, Wong RJ, Sanesi CA, Dennery PA, Stevenson DK. Simultaneous production of carbon monoxide and thiobarbituric acid reactive substances in rat tissue preparations by an iron-ascorbate system. *Can J Physiol Pharmacol.* 1998;76:1057–1065.

14. Baranano DE, Rao M, Ferris CD, Snyder SH. Biliverdin reductase: a major physiologic cytoprotectant. *Proc Natl Acad Sci USA.* 2002;99:16093–16098.

15. Foresti R, Green CJ, Motterlini R. Generation of bile pigments by haem oxygenase: a refined cellular strategy in response to stressful insults. *Biochem Soc Symp.* 2004;(71):177–192.

16. Stocker R, Yamamoto Y, McDonagh AF, Glazer AN, Ames BN. Bilirubin is an antioxidant of possible physiological importance. *Science.* 1987;235:1043–1046.

17. Marks GS, Brien JF, Nakatsu K, McLaughlin BE. Does carbon monoxide have a physiological function? *Trends Pharmacol Sci.* 1991;12:185–188.

18. Furchgott RF, Jothianandan D. Endothelium-dependent and -independent vasodilation involving cyclic GMP: relaxation induced by nitric oxide, carbon monoxide and light. *Blood Vessels.* 1991;28:52–61.

19. Brune B, Ullrich V. Inhibition of platelet aggregation by carbon monoxide is mediated by activation of guanylate cyclase. *Mol Pharmacol.* 1987;32:497–504.

20. Brouard S, Otterbein LE, Anrather J, et al. Carbon monoxide generated by heme oxygenase 1 suppresses endothelial cell apoptosis. *J Exp Med.* 2000;192:1015–1026.

21. Prabhakar NR, Dinerman JL, Agani FH, Snyder SH. Carbon monoxide: a role in carotid body chemoreception. *Proc Natl Acad Sci USA.* 1995;92:1994–1997.

22. Leinders-Zufall T, Shepherd GM, Zufall F. Regulation of cyclic nucleotide-gated channels and membrane excitability in olfactory receptor cells by carbon monoxide. *J Neurophysiol.* 1995;74:1498–1508.

23. Ryter SW, Otterbein LE, Morse D, Choi AM. Heme oxygenase/carbon monoxide signaling pathways: regulation and functional significance. *Mol Cell Biochem.* 2002;234–235:249–263.

24. Cudmore M, Ahmad S, Al-Ani B, et al. Negative regulation of soluble Flt-1 and soluble endoglin release by heme oxygenase-1. *Circulation.* 2007;115:1789–1797.

25. Loboda A, Jazwa A, Grochot-Przeczek A, et al. Heme oxygenase-1 and the vascular bed: from molecular mechanisms to therapeutic opportunities. *Antioxid Redox Signal.* 2008;10:1767–1812.

26. Odrcich MJ, Graham CH, Kimura KA, et al. Heme oxygenase and nitric oxide synthase in the placenta of the guinea pig during gestation. *Placenta.* 1998;19:509–516.

27. Vreman HJ, Wong RJ, Stevenson DK. Sources, sinks, and measurements of carbon monoxide. In: *Carbon Monoxide and Cardiovascular Functions.* Boca Raton, FL: CRC Press; 2001.

28. Vreman HJ, Gillman MJ, Downum KR, Stevenson DK. *In vitro* generation of carbon monoxide from organic molecules and synthetic metalloporphyrins mediated by light. *Dev Pharmacol Ther.* 1990;15:112–124.

29. Vreman HJ, Knauer Y, Wong RJ, Chan ML, Stevenson DK. Dermal carbon monoxide excretion in neonatal rats during light exposure. *Pediatr Res.* 2009;66:66–69.

30. Sjöstrand T. Endogenous formation of carbon monoxide in man. *Nature.* 1949;164:580–581.

31. Fällström SP. Endogenous formation of carbon monoxide in newborn infants. IV. On the relation between the blood carboxyhaemoglobin concentration and the pulmonary elimination of carbon monoxide. *Acta Paediatr Scand.* 1968;57:321–329.

32. Stevenson DK, Bartoletti AL, Ostrander CR, Johnson JD. Pulmonary excretion of carbon monoxide in the human infant as an index of bilirubin production. II. Infants of diabetic mothers. *J Pediatr.* 1979;94:956–958.

33. Ostrander CR, Stevenson DK, Neu J, Kerner JA, Moses SW. A sensitive analytical apparatus for measuring hydrogen production rates. I. Application to studies in small animals. Evidence of the effects of an alpha-glucosidehydrolase inhibitor in the rat. *Anal Biochem.* 1982;119:378–386.

34. Stevenson DK, Salomon WL, Moore LY, et al. Pulmonary excretion rate of carbon monoxide as an index of total bilirubin formation in adult male Wistar rats with common bile duct ligation. *J Pediatr Gastroenterol Nutr.* 1984;3:790–794.

35. Salomon WL, Vreman HJ, Kwong LK, Stevenson DK. Red cell destruction and bilirubin production in adult rats with short-term biliary obstruction. *J Pediatr Gastroenterol Nutr.* 1986;5:806–810.

36. Vreman HJ, Wong RJ, Stevenson DK. Carbon monoxide in breath, blood, and other tissues. In: Penney DG, ed. *Carbon Monoxide Toxicity.* Boca Raton, FL: CRC Press; 2000:19–60.

37. Vreman HJ, Stevenson DK. Heme oxygenase activity as measured by carbon monoxide production. *Anal Biochem.* 1988;168:31–38.

38. Stevenson DK, Ostrander CE, Johnson JD. Effect of erythrocyte destruction on the pulmonary excretion rate of carbon monoxide in adult male Wistar rats. *J Lab Clin Med.* 1979;94:649–654.

39. Stevenson DK, Bartoletti AL, Ostrander CR, Johnson JD. Pulmonary excretion of carbon monoxide in the human newborn infant as an index of bilirubin production: III. Measurement of pulmonary excretion of carbon monoxide after the first postnatal week in premature infants. *Pediatrics.* 1979;64:598–600.

40. Smith DW, Hopper AO, Shahin SM, et al. Neonatal bilirubin production estimated from "end-tidal" carbon monoxide concentration. *J Pediatr Gastroenterol Nutr.* 1984;3:77–80.

41. Ostrander CR, Cohen RS, Hopper AO, Cowan BE, Stevens GB, Stevenson DK. Paired determinations of blood carboxyhemoglobin concentration and carbon monoxide excretion rate in term and preterm infants. *J Lab Clin Med.* 1982;100:745–755.

42. Stevenson DK, Ostrander CR, Hopper AO, Cohen RS, Johnson JD. Pulmonary excretion of carbon monoxide as an index of bilirubin production. IIa. Evidence for possible delayed clearance of bilirubin in infants of diabetic mothers. *J Pediatr.* 1981;98:822–824.

43. Stevenson DK, Wong RJ, DeSandre GH, Vreman HJ. A primer on neonatal jaundice. *Adv Pediatr.* 2004;51:263–288.

44. Fischer AF, Ochikubo CG, Vreman HJ, Stevenson DK. Carbon monoxide production in ventilated premature infants weighing less than 1500 g. *Arch Dis Child.* 1987;62:1070–1072.

45. Krediet TG, Cirkel GA, Vreman HJ, et al. End-tidal carbon monoxide measurements in infant respiratory distress syndrome. *Acta Paediatr.* 2006;95:1075–1082.

46. Vreman HJ, Stevenson DK, Oh W, et al. Semiportable electrochemical instrument for determining carbon monoxide in breath. *Clin Chem.* 1994;40:1927–1933.

47. Vreman HJ, Wong RJ, Harmatz P, Fanaroff AA, Berman B, Stevenson DK. Validation of the Natus CO-Stat™ End

Tidal Breath Analyzer in children and adults. *J Clin Monit Comput.* 1999;15:421–427.

48. Vreman HJ, Baxter LM, Stone RT, Stevenson DK. Evaluation of a fully automated end-tidal carbon monoxide instrument for breath analysis. *Clin Chem.* 1996;42: 50–56.

49. Kaplan M, Hammerman C, Vreman HJ, Wong RJ, Stevenson DK. Severe hemolysis with normal blood count in a glucose-6-phosphate dehydrogenase deficient neonate. *J Perinatol.* 2008;28:306–309.

50. Vreman HJ, Kwong LK, Stevenson DK. Carbon monoxide in blood: an improved microliter blood-sample collection system, with rapid analysis by gas chromatography. *Clin Chem.* 1984;30:1382–1386.

51. Maisels MJ, Pathak A, Nelson NM, Nathan DG, Smith CA. Endogenous production of carbon monoxide in normal and erythroblastotic newborn infants. *J Clin Invest.* 1971;50:1–8.

52. Bhutani VK, Johnson L, Sivieri EM. Predictive ability of a predischarge hour-specific serum bilirubin for subsequent significant hyperbilirubinemia in healthy term and near-term newborns. *Pediatrics.* 1999;103:6–14.

53. Kuzniewicz M, Newman TB. Interaction of hemolysis and hyperbilirubinemia on neurodevelopmental outcomes in the collaborative perinatal project. *Pediatrics.* 2009;123:1045–1050.

54. Kaplan M, Na'amad M, Kenan A, et al. Failure to predict hemolysis and hyperbilirubinemia by IgG subclass in blood group A or B infants born to group O mothers. *Pediatrics.* 2009;123:e132–e137.

55. Cremer RJ, Perryman PW, Richards DH. Influence of light on the hyperbilirubinaemia of infants. *Lancet.* 1958;1:1094–1097.

56. Vreman HJ, Wong RJ, Stevenson DK. Phototherapy: current methods and future directions. *Semin Perinatol.* 2004;28:326–333.

57. Vreman HJ, Wong RJ, Stevenson DK, et al. Light-emitting diodes: a novel light source for phototherapy. *Pediatr Res.* 1998;44:804–809.

58. Brown AK, Kim MH, Wu PY, Bryla DA. Efficacy of phototherapy in prevention and management of neonatal hyperbilirubinemia. *Pediatrics.* 1985;75:393–400.

59. Morris BH, Oh W, Tyson JE, et al. Aggressive vs. conservative phototherapy for infants with extremely low birth weight. *N Engl J Med.* 2008;359:1885–1896.

60. Hintz SR, Stevenson DK, Yao Q, et al. Is the lack of phototherapy exposure associated with better or worse outcomes in 501–1000 gram birth weight infants? *Acta Pediatr.* 2011;100:960–965.

61. Wong RJ, Bhutani VK, Vreman HJ, Stevenson DK. Tin mesoporphyrin for the prevention of severe neonatal hyperbilirubinemia. *NeoReviews.* 2007;8:e77–e84.

62. Drummond GS, Kappas A. Prevention of neonatal hyperbilirubinemia by tin protoporphyrin IX, a potent competitive inhibitor of heme oxidation. *Proc Natl Acad Sci U S A.* 1981;78:6466–6470.

63. Maines MD. Zinc-protoporphyrin is a selective inhibitor of heme oxygenase activity in the neonatal rat. *Biochim Biophys Acta.* 1981;673:339–350.

64. Stevenson DK, Rodgers PA, Vreman HJ. The use of metalloporphyrins for the chemoprevention of neonatal jaundice. *Am J Dis Child.* 1989;143:353–356.

65. Vreman HJ, Ekstrand BC, Stevenson DK. Selection of metalloporphyrin heme oxygenase inhibitors based on potency and photoreactivity. *Pediatr Res.* 1993;33:195–200.

66. Vreman HJ, Wong RJ, Stevenson DK. Alternative metalloporphyrins for the treatment of neonatal jaundice. *J Perinatol.* 2001;21(suppl 1):S108–S113.

67. Wong RJ, Vreman HJ, Schulz S, Kalish FS, Pierce NW, Stevenson DK. *In vitro* inhibition of heme oxygenase isoenzymes by metalloporphyrins. *J Perinatol.* 2011. In press.

68. Martinez JC, Garcia HO, Otheguy LE, Drummond GS, Kappas A. Control of severe hyperbilirubinemia in full-term newborns with the inhibitor of bilirubin production Sn-mesoporphyrin. *Pediatrics.* 1999;103:1–5.

69. Valaes T, Petmezaki S, Henschke C, Drummond GS, Kappas A. Control of jaundice in preterm newborns by an inhibitor of bilirubin production: studies with tin-mesoporphyrin. *Pediatrics.* 1994;93:1–11.

70. Campbell CM, Morisawa T, Zhao H, Wong RJ, Stevenson DK. Dose-dependent effects of zinc bis glycol porphyrin on the expression of heme oxygenase in newborn mice. *J Invest Med.* 2009;57:177 (#287).

71. He CX, Campbell CM, Zhao H, et al. Effects of zinc deutroporphyrin bis glycol on newborn mice after heme loading. *Pediatr Res.* 2011;70:467–472.

72. Morisawa T, Wong RJ, Xiao H, Bhutani VK, Vreman HJ, Stevenson DK. Inhibition of heme oxygenase activity by chromium mesoporphyrin in the heme-loaded newborn mouse. *E-PAS2008*:6130.9.

73. Xiao H, Morisawa T, Wong RJ, Stevenson DK. Short- and long-term effects of heme oxygenase activity by chromium mesoporphyrin in newborn mice. *E-PAS2008*:6130.8.

74. Vreman HJ, Rodgers PA, Stevenson DK. Zinc protoporphyrin administration for suppression of increased bilirubin production by iatrogenic hemolysis in rhesus neonates. *J Pediatr.* 1990;117:292–297.

75. Rodgers PA, Vreman HJ, Stevenson DK. Heme catabolism in rhesus neonates inhibited by zinc protoporphyrin. *Dev Pharmacol Ther.* 1990;14:216–222.

76. Stevenson DK, Wong RJ. Metalloporphyrins in the management of neonatal hyperbilirubinemia. *Semin Fetal Neonatal Med.* 2010;15:164–168.

77. Morioka I, Wong RJ, Abate A, Vreman HJ, Contag CH, Stevenson DK. Systemic effects of orally-administered zinc and tin (IV) metalloporphyrins on heme oxygenase expression in mice. *Pediatr Res.* 2006;59:667–672.

78. Hajdena-Dawson M, Zhang W, Contag PR, et al. Effects of metalloporphyrins on heme oxygenase-1 transcription: correlative cell culture assays guide *in vivo* imaging. *Mol Imaging.* 2003;2:138–149.

79. Zhang W, Contag PR, Hardy J, et al. Selection of potential therapeutics based on *in vivo* spatiotemporal transcription patterns of heme oxygenase-1. *J Mol Med.* 2002;80:655–664.

80. Vreman HJ, Lee OK, Stevenson DK. *In vitro* and *in vivo* characteristics of a heme oxygenase inhibitor: ZnBG. *Am J Med Sci.* 1991;302:335–341.

81. Schulz-Geske S, Kalish FS, Zhao H, et al. The effect of fluorescent light exposure on metalloporphyrin-treated newborn mice. *J Invest Med.* 2011;59:126 (#37).

82. Kaplan M, Hammerman C, Maisels MJ. Bilirubin genetics for the nongeneticist: hereditary defects of neonatal bilirubin conjugation. *Pediatrics.* 2003;111:886–893.

83. Akaba K, Kimura T, Sasaki A, et al. Neonatal hyperbilirubinemia and mutation of the bilirubin uridine diphosphate-glucuronosyltransferase gene: a common missense mutation among Japanese, Koreans and Chinese. *Biochem Mol Biol Int.* 1998;46:21–26.

84. Yamamoto K, Sato H, Fujiyama Y, Doida Y, Bamba T. Contribution of two missense mutations (G71R and Y486D) of the bilirubin UDP glycosyltransferase (UGT1A1) gene to phenotypes of Gilbert's syndrome and Crigler–Najjar syndrome type II. *Biochim Biophys Acta.* 1998;1406: 267–273.

85. Kaplan M, Beutler E, Vreman HJ, et al. Neonatal hyperbilirubinemia in glucose-6-phosphate dehydrogenase-deficient heterozygotes. *Pediatrics.* 1999;104:68–74.

86. Kaplan M, Hammerman C. Glucose-6-phosphate dehydrogenase deficiency: a hidden risk for kernicterus. *Semin Perinatol.* 2004;28:356–364.

87. Kaplan M, Hammerman C, Feldman R, Brisk R. Predischarge bilirubin screening in glucose-6-phosphate dehydrogenase-deficient neonates. *Pediatrics.* 2000;105:533–537.

88. Kaplan M, Hammerman C, Renbaum P, Klein G, Levy-Lahad E. Gilbert's syndrome and hyperbilirubinaemia in ABO-incompatible neonates. *Lancet.* 2000;356: 652–653.

89. Kaplan M, Hammerman C, Vreman HJ, Stevenson DK, Beutler E. Acute hemolysis and severe neonatal hyperbilirubinemia in glucose-6-phosphate dehydrogenase-deficient heterozygotes. *J Pediatr.* 2001;139:137–140.

90. Kaplan M, Herschel M, Hammerman C, Karrison T, Hoyer JD, Stevenson DK. Studies in hemolysis in glucose-6-phosphate dehydrogenase-deficient African American neonates. *Clin Chim Acta.* 2006;365:177–182.

91. Kaplan M, Renbaum P, Levy-Lahad E, Hammerman C, Lahad A, Beutler E. Gilbert syndrome and glucose-6-phosphate dehydrogenase deficiency: a dose-dependent genetic interaction crucial to neonatal hyperbilirubinemia. *Proc Natl Acad Sci U S A.* 1997;94: 12128–12132.

92. Kaplan M, Rubaltelli FF, Hammerman C, et al. Conjugated bilirubin in neonates with glucose-6-phosphate dehydrogenase deficiency. *J Pediatr.* 1996;128:695–697.

Bilirubin and Its Various Fractions

Jane E. Brumbaugh and Glenn R. Gourley

■ INTRODUCTION

In the human fetus, as in the adult, biliverdin-IXα and any small amounts of non-IXα isomers that are formed are reduced to the corresponding bilirubins. Of these, bilirubin-IXα is uniquely hydrophobic and lipophilic, and ready to cross the placenta for elimination by the mother. In utero, residual non-IXα isomers too polar to cross the placenta, particularly the IXβ isomer, accumulate and are detectable in bile and meconium by 15 weeks gestation.[1] This observation has led some to conclude erroneously that heme catabolism in the fetus yields predominantly the IXβ isomer. The major form of bilirubin generated in infants and adults alike is bilirubin-IXα, and can be measured in various forms (Table 3-1).

The poor solubility of bilirubin can be explained by considering its chemical three-dimensional structure.[2] Although often represented as a linear structure for convenience (Figure 3-1, structure 5), bilirubin has a folded flexible structure in which the weakly acidic propionic acid side chains can stretch and form internal hydrogen bonds with spatially proximate nitrogen and oxygen groups. This results in a compact structure in which the surface is lipophilic and the polar parts of the molecule are protected from interactions with solvent water. The stereochemical configuration of the two double bonds between the rings in bilirubin is the same as in heme from which the bilirubin was derived and is designated unambiguously in current organic chemistry nomenclature as *Z* (from *zusammen*, German: together) (in contradistinction to *E* [*entgegen*: opposite], the other possible configuration). Because of its low solubility in water at physiologic pH, bilirubin requires a carrier molecule for transport from the reticuloendothelial system to the liver for excretion.[3] In blood and extravascular fluid, bilirubin is bound noncovalently to albumin that possesses a single high-affinity binding site ($K_a = 7 \times 10^7/M$) for bilirubin as well as secondary binding sites of lower affinity.[4] Due to the strong binding affinity and relatively high concentration of albumin at physiologic levels, most bilirubin is bound to albumin and the relative concentration of free, unbound bilirubin is negligible.

■ MEASUREMENT OF BILIRUBIN FRACTIONS

Total Serum Bilirubin Measurement

From a historical perspective, recognition of the complexity of bilirubin has evolved over the past century (Figure 3-2). Measurement of the total serum bilirubin (TSB) concentration allows quantification of jaundice. TSB measurements are commonplace in the newborn nursery, and in one study were made at least once in 61% of full-term newborns[5] although the frequency may be decreasing with advances in transcutaneous bilirubinometry (TcB). Most clinical laboratories use a modified diazo reaction to measure TSB. In this assay, bilirubin in the sample is exposed to the diazo reagent.[6] The conjugated bilirubin in the sample reacts quickly, or directly, with the diazo reagent, hence the term direct bilirubin. Meanwhile, the TSB level can only be measured after

■ TABLE 3-1. Bilirubin Nomenclature and Chemical Behavior

Terms	Description
Unconjugated bilirubin or indirect bilirubin	Produced from heme degradation by HO; indirect bilirubin requires an "accelerator" to react with diazo reagents
Conjugated bilirubin	Bilirubin conjugated with one or two glucuronic acid molecules
Direct bilirubin	Forms diazo derivatives immediately after addition of diazo reagents; includes conjugated and albumin-bound delta-bilirubin
Albumin-bound bilirubin or bound bilirubin	Usually refers to bilirubin bound to albumin, but bilirubin monoglucuronide or bilirubin diglucuronides also bind to albumin
Unbound bilirubin or free bilirubin or nonalbumin-bound bilirubin	Usually refers to bilirubin not bound to albumin but would also include bilirubin monoglucuronide or bilirubin diglucuronides not bound to albumin
Delta-bilirubin	Bilirubin covalently bound to albumin (reacts with direct bilirubin fraction of the diazo test)
Configurational bilirubin photoisomers	Photolabile isomers of bilirubin occurring on exposure to light of wavelength 400–525 nm
Lumirubin; structural bilirubin photoisomers	Photolabile isomers of bilirubin occurring on exposure to light of wavelength 400–525 nm

HO, heme oxygenase.

Reproduced and modified with permission from Wong RJ, Stevenson DK, Ahlfors CE, Vreman HJ. Neonatal jaundice: bilirubin physiology and clinical chemistry. *NeoReviews.* 2007;8:e58–e67. Copyright 2007 by the American Association of Pediatrics.

the addition of an accelerant in the diazo method. The unconjugated, or indirect, fraction is then calculated by determining the difference between the total and direct reacting fractions. Using the diazo method, the normal value for unconjugated bilirubin in adults is less than 1 mg/dL and that for conjugated bilirubin is less than 0.3 mg/dL.[7] Any elevation of conjugated bilirubin should be considered potentially pathologic, although the majority of such elevations in the neonate resolve spontaneously and are unexplained.[8]

In conjugated hyperbilirubinemia, the accumulated glucuronides undergo hydrolysis and rearrangement to a large number of isomers and also undergo spontaneous (i.e., nonenzymatic) transesterification with amino groups on albumin. This leads to covalent amide linkages between one of the propionic acid side chains of bilirubin glucuronide and albumin.[9] The resulting bilirubin–protein complex is known as "delta-bilirubin."[10] It is impossible to present a single structure for delta-bilirubin since it is not a homogeneous substance but rather a mixture of compounds and because the location(s) of the covalent binding of bilirubin glucuronide to albumin is not certain. Delta-bilirubin is not formed in the absence of an elevated conjugated bilirubin fraction.

Similar nonenzymatic reactions have been demonstrated between albumin and various drugs.[9,11–13]

The presence of delta-bilirubin explains the clinical conundrum of a persistently elevated TSB level in the infant who has experienced a clinical recovery from cholestatic jaundice. The direct-reacting fraction of bilirubin includes both conjugated bilirubin and delta-bilirubin. The terms direct and indirect are often used interchangeably with conjugated and unconjugated bilirubin, respectively, in the clinical setting. However, this is inaccurate from a biochemical standpoint. Direct bilirubin measurements include both conjugated and albumin-bound delta-bilirubin.[14] Because of the strong covalent bond, the half-life of delta-bilirubin approximates that of albumin (~3 weeks).[15] Recognition and understanding of the difference between direct and conjugated bilirubin measurements is critical to prevent the unnecessary evaluation of an infant recovering from a hepatic insult, who continues to have a high delta-bilirubin and, therefore, an elevated direct bilirubin measurement. Conjugated bilirubin measurement is an earlier indicator of recovery from biliary cholestasis compared with direct bilirubin measurement because of the long half-life of delta-bilirubin.[16] Due to the more timely response, conjugated bilirubin measurement

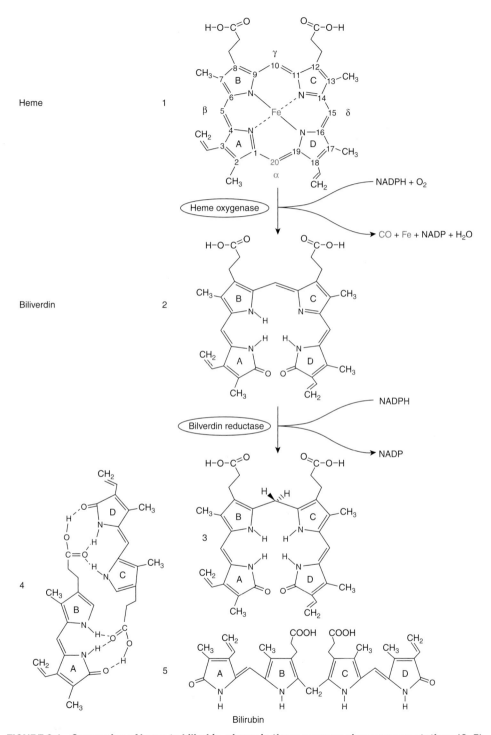

FIGURE 3-1. Conversion of heme to bilirubin, shown in three common planar representations (3–5). (Reproduced from Gourley GR. Neonatal jaundice and disorders of bilirubin metabolism. In: Suchy FJ, Sokol RJ, Balistreri WF, eds. *Liver Disease in Children*. 3rd ed. New York, NY: Cambridge University Press; 2007. Reprinted with the permission of Cambridge University Press.)

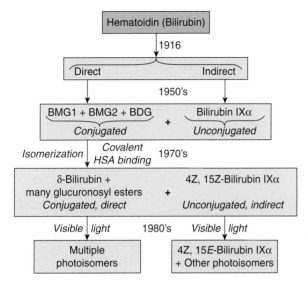

FIGURE 3-2. Historical recognition of the complexity of bilirubin species that can occur in infants with conjugated or unconjugated hyperbilirubinemia. (Reproduced from McDonagh AF. Controversies in bilirubin biochemistry and their clinical relevance. *Semin Fetal Neonatal Med.* 2010;15:141–147. Copyright 2010, with permission from Elsevier.)

is preferred over direct bilirubin measurement for the neonate.[17]

There is a long history of undesirable variability in the measurement of TSB fractions.[18,19] One problem is the ditaurobilirubin surrogate standard provided by the College of American Pathologists (CAP),[18] which influences measurement of TSB fractions variably because of protein matrix differences related to the specific bilirubin measurement used. This has prompted the suggestion that standards consisting of human serum enriched solely with unconjugated bilirubin rather than bovine serum containing a mixture of unconjugated bilirubin and ditaurobilirubin should be used.[20]

The automated laboratory methods now used to measure TSB have been reviewed elsewhere.[14,21–23] The Jendrassik–Grof procedure has been suggested as the method of choice for TSB measurement, although this method has limitations.[24] When the TSB level is high, factitious elevation of the direct fraction has been reported.[25] Three newer methods have been developed that can more accurately determine the various bilirubin fractions (unconjugated, monoconjugated, diconjugated, and delta-bilirubin; Table 3-1): high-performance liquid chromatography (HPLC),[26] multilayered slides,[27,28] and use of bilirubin oxidase.[29] HPLC analysis is the superior method and is considered by some to be the "gold standard,"[30,31] but is too expensive and time consuming for the clinical laboratory.[14] Furthermore, there are no published data of interlaboratory comparisons of HPLC analysis as there are with the other laboratory methods. HPLC analysis of serum from healthy neonates showed that unconjugated and conjugated bilirubin levels rose in parallel in the first 4 days of life with the conjugated fraction making up only 1.2–1.6% of total pigment.[32] Although the absolute concentration of conjugates was two to six times higher in neonates compared with adults, only 20% were diconjugates (54% in adults). These sensitive HPLC data are consistent with the increased bilirubin production and relatively deficient glucuronidation seen in the neonate. Analysis with automated multilayered slide technology (Vitros, Ortho Clinical Diagnostics, Raritan, NJ) used in many clinical laboratories allows measurement of conjugated and unconjugated bilirubin fractions without inclusion of delta-bilirubin. Analysis of the bilirubin oxidase method concluded that measurement of neonatal TSB was not advanced by this method.[33]

Newer methods of TSB measurement (Twin Beam, Ginevri, Rome, Italy; ABL 735, Radiometer, Copenhagen, Denmark; Roche OMNI S, Roche Diagnostics, Graz, Austria) using nonenzymatic photometric analysis offer the convenience of bilirubin quantitation outside of the clinical laboratory setting (i.e., blood gas analyzer in the nursery) with a smaller blood sample than traditional serum analysis. However, these measurements must be interpreted with caution as the instruments tend to underestimate the TSB concentration at levels >15 mg/dL.[34]

There are conflicting data regarding the accuracy of capillary versus venous TSB levels.[35,36] However, the literature regarding kernicterus, phototherapy, and exchange transfusion is based on bilirubin measurement from capillary samples, and treatment should not be delayed for a confirmatory measurement from a venous specimen.[37] While it is acknowledged that TSB may not be the most important factor related to neurotoxicity, there is not an alternative laboratory test that is broadly accepted and widely available that better identifies infants at risk for bilirubin-induced neurologic dysfunction (BIND).

Clinical laboratories that perform newborn bilirubin testing are required to perform proficiency testing. The proficiency testing program offered through the CAP is the most commonly used program by laboratories in

■ **TABLE 3-2.** Bilirubin Concentrations from the 2010 Proficiency Testing Survey by the College of American Pathologists (CAP)

Sample Identity[a]	Total Labs	Mean TSB Concentration, mg/dL (µmol/L)	Standard Deviation, mg/dL (µmol/L)	% CV
NB-11	2274	23.42 (400.5)	1.05 (18.0)	4.5
NB-12	2291	10.19 (174.3)	0.98 (16.8)	9.7
NB-13	1876	19.49 (333.3)	1.01 (17.2)	5.2
NB-14	1863	10.19 (174.3)	1.01 (17.3)	9.9
NB-15	1862	14.96 (255.8)	0.99 (17.0)	6.6
CHM-06	6219	4.32 (73.9)	0.33 (5.6)	7.6
CHM-07	6213	3.17 (54.2)	0.28 (4.8)	8.9
CHM-08	6242	1.70 (29.1)	0.23 (4.0)	13.7
CHM-09	6257	0.71 (12.1)	0.21 (3.6)	29.9
CHM-10	6237	1.68 (28.8)	0.23 (4.0)	13.9

[a]Samples NB-11 to NB-15 are from the 2010 neonatal bilirubin, cycle C (NB-C) proficiency testing survey. Samples CHM-06 to CHM-10 are from the 2010 chemistry, cycle B (C-B) proficiency testing survey.

Data from College of American Pathologists. *Participant Summary Report, CAP 2010 C-B Survey;* 2010; College of American Pathologists. *Participant Summary Report, CAP 2010 NB-C Survey;* 2010.

the United States. The 2010 neonatal bilirubin, cycle C (NB-C) and 2010 chemistry, cycle B (C-B) participant summary reports from CAP assessed the different methods for measurement of neonatal bilirubin and TSB concentrations currently in use (see Table 3-2).[38,39] For the survey of neonatal TSB measurements, approximately 2000 laboratories participated in the 2010 NB-C survey. Each laboratory received five unknown samples for measurement of neonatal TSB, ranging in concentration from 10.2 to 23.4 mg/dL. There were 9 different methods used to measure bilirubin on 17 different instrument platforms. The most common method used was a diazo-caffeine/benzoate coupling with a blank (26%) or without a blank (23%). A spectrophotometric method was used by 24%, and an additional 17% of laboratories used a diazonium salt/diazonium ion method. The samples used in the CAP NB-C survey contained high concentrations of TSB because accurate measurements of increased bilirubin concentrations are critical in the neonatal period.

The CAP chemistry survey was taken by clinical laboratories that perform measurement of TSB (not limited to the neonatal population). Approximately 6200 laboratories completed the chemistry survey for proficiency testing. Like the neonatal survey described previously, each laboratory received five unknown samples for measurement of TSB. The laboratories that participated in the CAP C-B survey used 15 different methods on 22 different platforms. Bilirubin concentrations in the five different samples ranged from 0.7 to 4.3 mg/dL. Table 3-2 summarizes the bilirubin concentrations measured by all instruments and methods in samples from the 2010 NB-C and 2010 C-B proficiency testing surveys.

Transcutaneous Bilirubinometry

Jaundice presents in the face and progresses in a cephalocaudal pattern.[40] Kramer determined the range of serum unconjugated bilirubin levels as jaundice progressed: head and neck (4–8 mg/dL), upper trunk (5–12 mg/dL), lower trunk and thighs (8–16 mg/dL), arms and lower legs (11–18 mg/dL), and finally the palms and soles (>15 mg/dL).[41] However, visual assessment is not reliable among providers and patient populations. Darker skin tones can make jaundice difficult to assess visually.[42] Heel stick is the most common means to collect a specimen for TSB measurement. In addition to being traumatic to the newborn and parents, heel stick is a suboptimal technique due to the potential for hemolysis and resultant interference in bilirubin measurement depending on the laboratory method used.[43] An inexpensive, noninvasive method

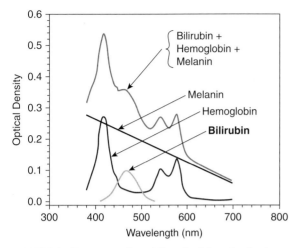

FIGURE 3-3. Demonstration of the principles of reflectance spectrophotometry used in the BiliChek bilirubinometer to measure bilirubin by correcting for differences in melanin, hemoglobin, and other interfering factors. (Reproduced from Jacques SL. *SPIE Proceedings of laser-tissue interactions*; February 1997; San Jose, CA; Vol. 2975, pp. 115–124.)

useful in assessing jaundice utilizes a Plexiglas color chart pressed against the baby's nose (Ingram icterometer, Thos. A. Ingram and Co Ltd, Birmingham, England).[44–46] However, today other noninvasive methods, specifically TcB, to assess jaundice have become routine practice in the newborn nursery as a screening method more sensitive than visual assessment for jaundice.[47]

There are two commercially available transcutaneous instruments approved by the Food and Drug Administration (FDA) to measure TcB in neonates: the Philips Children's Medical Ventures BiliChek (Respironics, Inc, Murrysville, PA)[30,31] and the Konica Minolta Air-Shields Transcutaneous Jaundice Meter 103 (JM-103, Draeger Medical Systems, Inc, Telford, PA).[48] The BiliChek utilizes principles of reflectance spectrophotometry, has been validated against both HPLC and clinical laboratory measures,[30,31] and has been advocated by the American Academy of Pediatrics (AAP).[42] BiliChek uses light from multiple wavelengths, captures the light reflected, and corrects for differences in melanin, hemoglobin, and other interfering factors (Figure 3-3). The device touches the skin in a painless manner and provides an almost immediate point-of-care measurement of TcB. The JM-103 measures the difference in the optical densities of reflected light at 450 and 550 nm. Two optical paths are incorporated into a probe that minimizes interference by melanin, and the

reflected light is collected by photodiodes. One limitation of the two devices currently available on the market is their inability to interface with the neonate's electronic medical record leaving documentation of the TcB reading subject to human error inherent with manual entry.[43,49]

TcB measurements have been incorporated into clinical practice as an alternative to heel stick for screening jaundice in the newborn nursery. This has the potential to reduce the incidence of heel stick by 40–60%[50–52] and to reduce potential serious, albeit rare, complications of blood collection, including infection and osteomyelitis.[53] Serum bilirubin testing may be done more frequently since the introduction of TcB testing potentially as a result of more neonates being monitored for hyperbilirubinemia after identification of clinically significant jaundice by TcB.[54] However, use of TcB measurements decreases TSB measurements and saves money.[55] The combination of peak predischarge TcB with two clinical risk factors for pathologic hyperbilirubinemia, exclusive breastfeeding and gestational age, improves prediction of subsequent hyperbilirubinemia meriting treatment.[55] Significant TcB levels (>14 mg/dL) should prompt measurement of a TSB level for confirmation.[42,56–58]

The body site used for TcB impacts the accuracy of the results with measurements taken on the sternum and forehead correlating best with TSB.[31,50,59] Because the sternum is less often exposed to ambient light, it may prove to be the preferred site of measurement for TcB.[59] With evidence of the reliability and safety of TcB screening measurements in term neonates, research has shifted toward the evaluation of TcB as a method of screening preterm neonates with promising prospects in neonates weighing ≥1000 g or born at ≥28 weeks gestation.[60–65]

The nomograms published by the AAP based on TSB measurements may not be appropriate for use with TcB measurements. As a result, hour-specific nomograms for TcB measurements to identify neonates in need of additional monitoring for hyperbilirubinemia have been developed using North American, Thai, and European neonates.[66–68] The reliability of these new TcB nomograms is under evaluation, and a standard TcB nomogram is expected to become the clinical practice standard pending validation[69] and has already been incorporated into practice in at least one institution in the United States.[55]

Screening neonates with TcB incurs additional costs in the form of the meters, disposable materials, and staff training. The costs associated with neonatal TcB screening may be offset by the savings of reduced TSB measurements[55] and neonatal hospital readmissions for hyperbilirubinemia.[54] In addition, the operational costs of TcB are potentially offset by the improvement in patient comfort.[43] A transcutaneous meter that does not contact the neonate's skin has been developed (BiliMed, Medick SA, Paris, France) and does not require disposable tips resulting in lower cost. However, the BiliMed device has reduced accuracy compared with the BiliChek meter and as such does not have a role in clinical practice at present.[62,70]

Currently, TcB measurements are used to screen for hyperbilirubinemia but are not followed sequentially during phototherapy. Phototherapy bleaches the skin and, thus, TcB is an unreliable method for assessing jaundice in exposed skin during phototherapy. The negative impact of phototherapy on the correlation between TcB and TSB has been documented in the literature.[71,72] The manufacturer of BiliChek makes a photo-opaque patch to be applied to the skin during phototherapy (BiliEclipse, Respironics, Inc). When assessing jaundice in this patched skin, Zecca et al.[73] found no significant difference between TSB and TcB during phototherapy for up to 96 hours. This suggests that TcB on patched skin may be a safe method to monitor hyperbilirubinemia and to determine when phototherapy may be discontinued. This would expand the role of TcB from exclusively screening to both screening and monitoring hyperbilirubinemia. While the National Academy of Clinical Biochemistry (NACB) recommends the adoption of the BiliChek or JM-103 devices for TcB measurement in the management of neonatal jaundice, it does not have clear recommendations regarding the use of TcB during phototherapy.[43]

Free Bilirubin and Kernicterus

Nonalbumin-bound unconjugated bilirubin-IXα, also referred to as "free bilirubin" or unbound bilirubin, has the potential for devastating neurotoxicity if sufficient amounts enter the brain and remain there long enough to cause damage. The relationship between TSB and neurotoxicity, referred to as BIND presenting as acute bilirubin encephalopathy (ABE) or kernicterus depending on the clinical scenario, is complicated and far from a perfect correlation. Newborn jaundice has traditionally been monitored by TSB levels, which consist of three fractions: unconjugated, conjugated, and delta-bilirubin. Delta-bilirubin is covalently bound to albumin and present in negligible amounts in the newborn period.

Concentrations of conjugated bilirubin are also low and of no toxicological significance. The largest fraction, unconjugated bilirubin, is almost entirely bound reversibly to albumin. Since the blood–brain barrier is impermeable to albumin, bilirubin has to dissociate from albumin to enter the brain and cause toxicity. There is evidence that the minute concentration of bilirubin in blood that is not bound to albumin, which is the free bilirubin fraction, correlates with BIND better than the TSB level. This is clinically relevant as there are individuals with kernicterus whose TSB levels never exceeded 25 mg/dL.[74,75] The unpredictable relationship between total bilirubin and kernicterus in Gunn rats was described by Johnson et al. in 1959.[76] Sulfisoxazole administered to congenitally jaundiced Gunn rats induced kernicterus secondary to disruption of bilirubin–albumin binding.[76] Previously, preterm infants administered sulfisoxazole as infection prophylaxis developed kernicterus and died with low TSB levels before it was recognized that sulfisoxazole competes with unconjugated bilirubin for protein-binding sites.[77]

A potentially helpful laboratory measurement to obtain when a neonate is approaching the threshold for exchange transfusion to prevent BIND is the serum albumin level.[42] Albumin essentially acts as a bilirubin-binding sponge. Bilirubin bound to albumin in the vasculature cannot easily enter tissues. Because of its high-affinity binding to bilirubin, the AAP guideline supports the use of the TSB to albumin ratio for risk assessment and management planning in hyperbilirubinemia.[42] Bilirubin–albumin binding and neonatal jaundice have been reviewed by Ahlfors and Wennberg.[74] A low albumin level may alert the clinician to consider intervention for hyperbilirubinemia at a lower TSB level.[74] Albumin has a high-affinity binding site for bilirubin in addition to other sites with much lower affinity constants.[4,78] Changes in the albumin concentration and its affinity for bilirubin are two reasons why total bilirubin does not predict bilirubin-related neurotoxicity as well as free bilirubin.[79] Drugs and organic anions also bind to albumin and can displace bilirubin, thereby increasing the free bilirubin fraction that can diffuse into cells causing toxicity.[80,81] The most notable example of this is the kernicterus that occurred in the setting of low TSB levels when sulfisoxazole was given to premature infants described previously.[77]

The peroxidase method allows measurement of free bilirubin by oxidation.[82,83] Horseradish peroxidase catalyzes oxidation of nonprotein-bound unconjugated bilirubin by peroxide, while albumin-bound unconjugated bilirubin is protected from oxidation. Jacobsen and Wennberg introduced the peroxidase test assay in 1974,[83] and there has been renewed interest in the method recently. The motivation for introducing free bilirubin measurement into the clinical toolbox is to better identify infants in need of treatment of jaundice and to minimize unnecessary intervention, which can disrupt breastfeeding and maternal–infant bonding in the early neonatal period. With the adoption of a low threshold for intervention in order to prevent neurotoxicity, there is a risk of subjecting a small number of newborns to the potential morbidity and mortality of exchange transfusion.[74] But Wennberg et al.[84] speculate that enhanced sensitivity and specificity of free bilirubin measurement may improve risk assessment for BIND, and, therefore, reduce unnecessary aggressive intervention (i.e., exchange transfusion) and its associated cost and morbidity.

While there is an FDA-evaluated device that measures free bilirubin using the peroxidase test (UB-A1 Analyzer, Arrows Co Ltd, Osaka, Japan), it has primarily been used in the research setting and is not currently marketed in the United States.[74,79] There is no established gold standard control for free bilirubin measurement. The peroxidase test remains problematic requiring manual manipulation and sample dilution, which alters the state of bilirubin–albumin binding. Ahlfors et al.[85] have described the use of zone fluidics to measure free bilirubin to overcome some of the challenges with free bilirubin measurement. Even with an automated device, moderate to severe hemolysis compromises accurate measurement of free bilirubin. Hemolysis adds peroxidase activity and falsely lowers the concentration of free bilirubin measured. In addition to the limitation posed by hemolysis, the presence of conjugated bilirubin >1 mg/dL falsely elevates the free bilirubin concentration because conjugated bilirubin is more readily oxidized than unconjugated bilirubin.[79] At present, reference thresholds for phototherapy and exchange transfusion that use free bilirubin rather than the TSB level are not available, which continues to relegate the measurement of free bilirubin to the research setting.

TSB remains at the core of the current clinical algorithms designed to treat newborn jaundice and prevent BIND in part because measurement of free bilirubin was not available until 20 years after free bilirubin was first considered to be a cause of BIND. In the interim, RhoGAM prophylaxis and phototherapy had reduced the occurrence of exchange transfusion dramatically such that it was not feasible or ethical to conduct prospective studies on the relationship between free bilirubin and BIND.[79,86] Renewed interest in free bilirubin measurement in management of newborn jaundice developed in the 1980s with the introduction of auditory brainstem response (ABR) for assessment of newborn hearing, which provided a noninvasive outcome measure to assess BIND.[87] Again the congenitally jaundiced Gunn rat served as an animal model for assessment of BIND in the form of central auditory pathway dysfunction.[88] Unbound bilirubin was shown to induce reversible ABR signal changes.[89,90] Bilirubin-induced ABR changes correlate better with free bilirubin than TSB levels.[79,91–93] In addition to ABR, magnetic resonance imaging (MRI) now provides another tool to document BIND or neurotoxicity.[94] Shapiro and Nakamura[95] reviewed the relationship between bilirubin and the auditory system as a window into the central nervous system and bilirubin-induced pathology.

Ahlfors and Wennberg[74] have made the analogy of free bilirubin to pH on a blood gas determination. In the same manner that pH helps interpret the respiratory status of a patient at a given pCO_2, the free bilirubin level helps interpret the risk of bilirubin toxicity for a patient at a given TSB concentration. The introduction of free bilirubin measurement to the clinical setting has the potential to demonstrate bilirubin toxicity across a wider range of TSB level than often recognized as Johnson et al.[96] noted in the congenitally jaundiced Gunn rats exposed to sulfisoxazole in 1959. Free bilirubin used in conjunction with ABR has been proposed to improve identification of newborns at risk of BIND. The goal in measuring TSB levels is not to prevent hyperbilirubinemia but rather to prevent BIND.

Photoisomers and Free Bilirubin

While free bilirubin measurements have been advocated as possibly superior to TSB measurement for monitoring the risk of kernicterus, the potential interference by photoisomers (Table 3-1) may limit accurate free bilirubin measurement. Photoisomers are isomeric forms of bilirubin that are produced on exposure of infants to phototherapy or ambient light and with incidental exposure of blood specimens during the collection or measurement process. These configurational isomers are formed on absorption of light by bilirubin (Figure 3-4). A premise of the peroxidase assay used to measure free bilirubin is that unconjugated 4Z,15Z-bilirubin-IXα is the only form of bilirubin

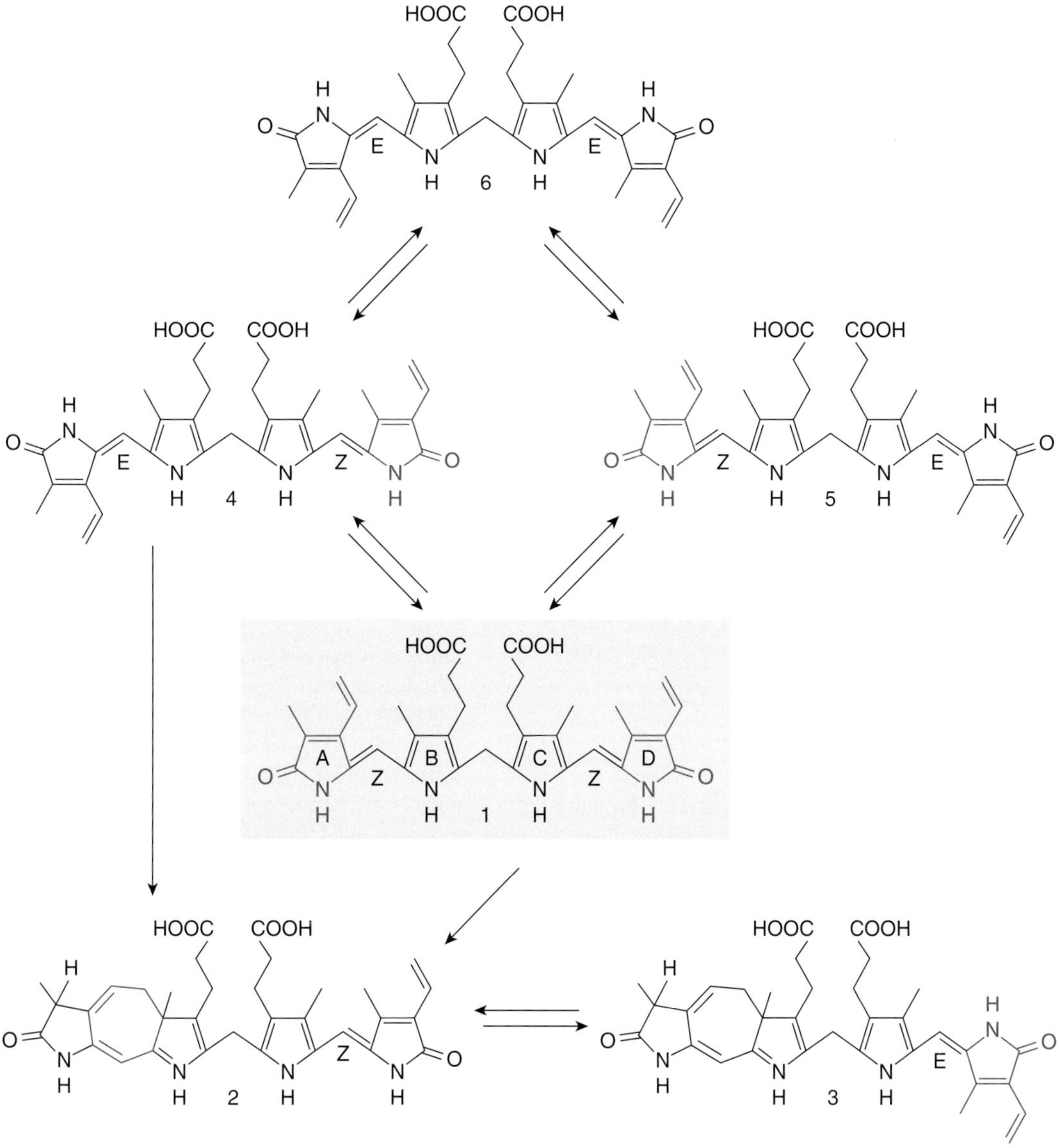

FIGURE 3-4. The products of phototherapy. Light induces an isomerization of 4Z,15Z-bilirubin (1) to produce the configurational isomers 4E,15Z-bilirubin (4), 4Z,15E-bilirubin (5), 4E,15E-bilirubin (6), and the structural isomers, Z-lumirubin (2) and E-Lumirubin (3) as shown. Isomerization exposes one or both of the propionic acid side chains, increasing the polarities of the isomers with respect to biosynthetic bilirubin (1) and allowing excretion in bile without hepatic glucuronidation. Formation of 4E,15Z-bilirubin, 4Z,15E-bilirubin, and 4E,15E-bilirubin is reversible and these isomers spontaneously revert to the parent 4Z,15Z-bilirubin (1) isomer after excretion in bile. The predominant isomer present in the circulation of infants exposed to light or phototherapy is 4Z,15E-bilirubin (5). Although the structural isomers (2 and 3) are formed more slowly than the configurational isomers, they may contribute more to the overall effect of the treatment because of their relatively faster excretion. (Reproduced from McDonagh AF. Phototherapy: from ancient Egypt to the new millenium. *J Perinatol.* 2001;21:S7–S12. Reprinted by permission from Macmillan Publishers Ltd., copyright 2001.)

found in neonatal serum. This is the predominant bilirubin form in jaundiced neonates. However, photoisomers constitute a significant fraction of bilirubin in neonates undergoing phototherapy. Up to 30% of bilirubin may be the 4Z,15E-isomer, which is more polar and less hydrophobic than the predominant 4Z,15Z-bilirubin isomer.[97] These chemical features make the 4Z,15E-isomer less able to cross the blood–brain barrier and presumably less neurotoxic as a result. This has significant clinical implications since photoisomers are thought to be less neurotoxic than unconjugated 4Z,15Z-bilirubin-IXα. The presence of photoisomers may limit accurate measurement of free bilirubin by the peroxidase method, a concern identified by McDonagh et al.[98] in 1980. Investigation into the impact of photoisomers on measurement of bilirubin fractions, including free bilirubin, has demonstrated inconclusive results.[97,99–104] A very small fraction of bilirubin exists in the free form unbound to albumin. However, there is a constant ongoing equilibrium between different forms of bilirubin, so that to only consider the free bilirubin fraction at a single time point would be a gross underestimation of the potential toxicity.[103]

■ SUMMARY

This chapter reviewed the biochemistry and measurement of the various bilirubin fractions with a historical perspective. Prevention of BIND continues to be the underlying goal when measuring neonatal bilirubin levels. In the clinical setting, TcB is increasing in frequency and being used in conjunction with TSB measurement. Free bilirubin may be a better predictor for BIND than TcB or TSB. However, the use of phototherapy rapidly produces configurational photoisomers that interfere with reliable measurement of free bilirubin. At present, the measurement of free bilirubin remains a research tool only in the United States.

■ ACKNOWLEDGMENTS

The authors would like to thank Antony F. McDonagh, Steven Kazmierczak, and Scott Kerr for their assistance in preparing this chapter.

REFERENCES

1. Blumenthal SG, Stucker T, Rasmussen RD, et al. Changes in bilirubins in human prenatal development. *Biochem J.* 1980;186:693–700.

2. Bonnett R, Davies JE, Hursthouse MB. Structure of bilirubin. *Nature.* 1976;262:327–328.

3. Bennhold H. Uber die vehikelfunktion der serumeiweisskorper. *Engeb Inn Med Kinderheilkd.* 1932;42:273–375.

4. Jacobsen J. Binding of bilirubin to human serum albumin—determination of the dissociation constants. *FEBS Lett.* 1969;5:112–114.

5. Newman TB, Easterling MJ, Goldman ES, Stevenson DK. Laboratory evaluation of jaundice in newborns. Frequency, cost, and yield. *Am J Dis Child.* 1990;144:364–368.

6. Zieve L, Hill E, Hanson M, Falcone AB, Watson CJ. Normal and abnormal variations and clinical significance of the one-minute and total serum bilirubin determinations. *J Lab Clin Med.* 1951;38:446–469.

7. Bloomer JR, Berk PD, Howe RB, Berlin NI. Interpretation of plasma bilirubin levels based on studies with radioactive bilirubin. *JAMA.* 1971;218:216–220.

8. Davis AR, Rosenthal P, Escobar GJ, Newman TB. Interpreting conjugated bilirubin levels in newborns. *J Pediatr.* 2011;158:562–565.e1.

9. Weiss JS, Gautam A, Lauff JJ, et al. The clinical importance of a protein-bound fraction of serum bilirubin in patients with hyperbilirubinemia. *N Engl J Med.* 1983;309:147–150.

10. Brett EM, Hicks JM, Powers DM, Rand RN. Delta bilirubin in serum of pediatric patients: correlations with age and disease. *Clin Chem.* 1984;30:1561–1564.

11. Stogniew M, Fenselau C. Electrophilic reactions of acyl-linked glucuronides. Formation of clofibrate mercapturate in humans. *Drug Metab Dispos.* 1982;10:609–613.

12. van Breeman RB. *Electrophilic Reactions of 1-O-Acyl Glucuronides.* Baltimore: Johns Hopkins University; 1985.

13. van Breemen RB, Fenselau C. Acylation of albumin by 1-O-acyl glucuronides. *Drug Metab Dispos.* 1985;13:318–320.

14. Rutledge JC, Ou CN. Bilirubin and the laboratory. Advances in the 1980s, considerations for the 1990s. *Pediatr Clin North Am.* 1989;36:189–198.

15. Berson SA, Yalow RS, Schreiber SS, Post J. Tracer experiments with I131 labeled human serum albumin: distribution and degradation studies. *J Clin Invest.* 1953;32:746–768.

16. Arvan D, Shirey TL. Conjugated bilirubin: a better indicator of impaired hepatobiliary excretion than direct bilirubin. *Ann Clin Lab Sci.* 1985;15:252–259.

17. Ou CN, Buffone GJ, Herr Calomeni PJ, Finegold MJ, Shirey TL. Conjugated bilirubin versus direct bilirubin in neonates. *Am J Clin Pathol.* 1986;85:613–616.

18. Lo SF, Doumas BT, Ashwood ER. Performance of bilirubin determinations in US laboratories—revisited. *Clin Chem.* 2004;50:190–194.

19. Schreiner RL, Glick MR. Interlaboratory bilirubin variability. *Pediatrics*. 1982;69:277–281.

20. Lo SF, Doumas BT, Ashwood ER. Bilirubin proficiency testing using specimens containing unconjugated bilirubin and human serum: results of a College of American Pathologists study. *Arch Pathol Lab Med*. 2004;128:1219–1223.

21. Rosenthal P, Keefe MT, Henton D, et al. Total and direct-reacting bilirubin values by automated methods compared with liquid chromatography and with manual methods for determining delta bilirubin. *Clin Chem*. 1990;36:788–791.

22. Vreman HJ, Verter J, Oh W, et al. Interlaboratory variability of bilirubin measurements. *Clin Chem*. 1996;42:869–873.

23. Westwood A. The analysis of bilirubin in serum. *Ann Clin Biochem*. 1991;28(pt 2):119–130.

24. Schlebusch H, Axer K, Schneider C, Liappis N, Rohle G. Comparison of five routine methods with the candidate reference method for the determination of bilirubin in neonatal serum. *J Clin Chem Clin Biochem*. 1990;28:203–210.

25. Mair B, Klempner LB. Abnormally high values for direct bilirubin in the serum of newborns as measured with the DuPont aca. *Am J Clin Pathol*. 1987;87:642–644.

26. Blanckaert N, Kabra PM, Farina FA, Stafford BE, Marton LJ, Schmid R. Measurement of bilirubin and its monoconjugates and diconjugates in human serum by alkaline methanolysis and high-performance liquid chromatography. *J Lab Clin Med*. 1980;96:198–212.

27. Wu TW, Dappen GM, Powers DM, Lo DH, Rand RN, Spayd RW. The Kodak Ektachem clinical chemistry slide for measurement of bilirubin in newborns: principles and performance. *Clin Chem*. 1982;28:2366–2372.

28. Wu TW, Dappen GM, Spayd RW, Sundberg MW, Powers DM. The Ektachem clinical chemistry slide for simultaneous determination of unconjugated and sugar-conjugated bilirubin. *Clin Chem*. 1984;30:1304–1309.

29. Mullon CJ, Langer R. Determination of conjugated and total bilirubin in serum of neonates, with use of bilirubin oxidase. *Clin Chem*. 1987;33:1822–1825.

30. Bhutani VK, Gourley GR, Adler S, Kreamer B, Dalin C, Johnson LH. Noninvasive measurement of total serum bilirubin in a multiracial predischarge newborn population to assess the risk of severe hyperbilirubinemia. *Pediatrics*. 2000;106:E17.

31. Rubaltelli FF, Gourley GR, Loskamp N, et al. Transcutaneous bilirubin measurement: a multicenter evaluation of a new device. *Pediatrics*. 2001;107:1264–1271.

32. Muraca M, Rubaltelli FF, Blanckaert N, Fevery J. Unconjugated and conjugated bilirubin pigments during perinatal development. II. Studies on serum of healthy newborns and of neonates with erythroblastosis fetalis. *Biol Neonate*. 1990;57:1–9.

33. Schlebusch H, Schneider C. Enzymatic determination of bilirubin in serum of newborns—any advantage over previous methods? *Ann Clin Biochem*. 1991;28 (pt 3):290–296.

34. Grohmann K, Roser M, Rolinski B, et al. Bilirubin measurement for neonates: comparison of 9 frequently used methods. *Pediatrics*. 2006;117:1174–1183.

35. Eidelman AI, Schimmel MS, Algur N, Eylath U. Capillary and venous bilirubin values: they are different—and how! *Am J Dis Child*. 1989;143:642.

36. Leslie GI, Philips JB 3rd, Cassady G. Capillary and venous bilirubin values. Are they really different? *Am J Dis Child*. 1987;141:1199–1200.

37. Maisels MJ. Capillary vs venous bilirubin values. *Am J Dis Child*. 1990;144:521–522.

38. College of American Pathologists. *Participant Summary Report: CAP 2010 NB-C Survey*; 2010.

39. College of American Pathologists. *Participant Summary Report: CAP 2010 C-B Survey*; 2010.

40. Knudsen A. The cephalocaudal progression of jaundice in newborns in relation to the transfer of bilirubin from plasma to skin. *Early Hum Dev*. 1990;22:23–28.

41. Kramer LI. Advancement of dermal icterus in the jaundiced newborn. *Am J Dis Child*. 1969;118:454–458.

42. American Academy of Pediatrics. Management of hyperbilirubinemia in the newborn infant 35 or more weeks of gestation. *Pediatrics*. 2004;114:297–316.

43. Carceller-Blanchard A, Cousineau J, Delvin EE. Point of care testing: transcutaneous bilirubinometry in neonates. *Clin Biochem*. 2009;42:143–149.

44. Bilgen H, Ince Z, Ozek E, Bekiroglu N, Ors R. Transcutaneous measurement of hyperbilirubinaemia: comparison of the Minolta jaundice meter and the Ingram icterometer. *Ann Trop Paediatr*. 1998;18:325–328.

45. Schumacher RE, Thornbery JM, Gutcher GR. Transcutaneous bilirubinometry: a comparison of old and new methods. *Pediatrics*. 1985;76:10–14.

46. Gossett IH, Oxon BM. A Perspex icterometer for neonates. *Lancet*. 1960;i:87–88.

47. Tayaba R, Gribetz D, Gribetz I, Holzman IR. Noninvasive estimation of serum bilirubin. *Pediatrics*. 1998;102: E28.

48. Maisels MJ, Ostrea EM Jr, Touch S, et al. Evaluation of a new transcutaneous bilirubinometer. *Pediatrics*. 2004;113:1628–1635.

49. el-Beshbishi SN, Shattuck KE, Mohammad AA, Petersen JR. Hyperbilirubinemia and transcutaneous bilirubinometry. *Clin Chem*. 2009;55:1280–1287.

50. Ebbesen F, Rasmussen LM, Wimberley PD. A new transcutaneous bilirubinometer, BiliCheck, used in the

neonatal intensive care unit and the maternity ward. *Acta Paediatr.* 2002;91:203–211.

51. Holland L, Blick K. Implementing and validating transcutaneous bilirubinometry for neonates. *Am J Clin Pathol.* 2009;132:555–561.

52. Samanta S, Tan M, Kissack C, Nayak S, Chittick R, Yoxall CW. The value of Bilicheck as a screening tool for neonatal jaundice in term and near-term babies. *Acta Paediatr.* 2004;93:1486–1490.

53. Lilien LD, Harris VJ, Ramamurthy RS, Pildes RS. Neonatal osteomyelitis of the calcaneus: complication of heel puncture. *J Pediatr.* 1976;88:478–480.

54. Petersen JR, Okorodudu AO, Mohammad AA, Fernando A, Shattuck KE. Association of transcutaneous bilirubin testing in hospital with decreased readmission rate for hyperbilirubinemia. *Clin Chem.* 2005;51:540–544.

55. Maisels MJ, Deridder JM, Kring EA, Balasubramaniam M. Routine transcutaneous bilirubin measurements combined with clinical risk factors improve the prediction of subsequent hyperbilirubinemia. *J Perinatol.* 2009;29:612–617.

56. Leite MG, Granato Vde A, Facchini FP, Marba ST. Comparison of transcutaneous and plasma bilirubin measurement. *J Pediatr (Rio J).* 2007;83:283–286.

57. Maisels MJ, Engle WD, Wainer S, Jackson GL, McManus S, Artinian F. Transcutaneous bilirubin levels in an outpatient and office population. *J Perinatol.* 2011;31:621–624.

58. Engle WD, Jackson GL, Stehel EK, Sendelbach DM, Manning MD. Evaluation of a transcutaneous jaundice meter following hospital discharge in term and near-term neonates. *J Perinatol.* 2005;25:486–490.

59. Randeberg LL, Roll EB, Nilsen LT, Christensen T, Svaasand LO. In vivo spectroscopy of jaundiced newborn skin reveals more than a bilirubin index. *Acta Paediatr.* 2005;94:65–71.

60. Ahmed M, Mostafa S, Fisher G, Reynolds TM. Comparison between transcutaneous bilirubinometry and total serum bilirubin measurements in preterm infants <35 weeks gestation. *Ann Clin Biochem.* 2010;47:72–77.

61. De Luca D, Zecca E, de Turris P, Barbato G, Marras M, Romagnoli C. Using BiliCheck for preterm neonates in a sub-intensive unit: diagnostic usefulness and suitability. *Early Hum Dev.* 2007;83:313–317.

62. Karen T, Bucher HU, Fauchere JC. Comparison of a new transcutaneous bilirubinometer (Bilimed) with serum bilirubin measurements in preterm and full-term infants. *BMC Pediatr.* 2009;9:70.

63. Namba F, Kitajima H. Utility of a new transcutaneous jaundice device with two optical paths in premature infants. *Pediatr Int.* 2007;49:497–501.

64. Schmidt ET, Wheeler CA, Jackson GL, Engle WD. Evaluation of transcutaneous bilirubinometry in preterm neonates. *J Perinatol.* 2009;29:564–569.

65. Stillova L, Matasova K, Mikitova T, Stilla J, Kolarovszka H, Zibolen M. Evaluation of transcutaneous bilirubinometry in preterm infants of gestational age 32–34 weeks. *Biomed Pap Med Fac Univ Palacky Olomouc Czech Repub.* 2007;151:267–271.

66. De Luca D, Romagnoli C, Tiberi E, Zuppa AA, Zecca E. Skin bilirubin nomogram for the first 96 h of life in a European normal healthy newborn population, obtained with multiwavelength transcutaneous bilirubinometry. *Acta Paediatr.* 2008;97:146–150.

67. Maisels MJ, Kring E. Transcutaneous bilirubin levels in the first 96 hours in a normal newborn population of > or = 35 weeks' gestation. *Pediatrics.* 2006;117:1169–1173.

68. Sanpavat S, Nuchprayoon I, Smathakanee C, Hansuebsai R. Nomogram for prediction of the risk of neonatal hyperbilirubinemia, using transcutaneous bilirubin. *J Med Assoc Thai.* 2005;88:1187–1193.

69. Rodriguez-Capote K, Kim K, Paes B, Turner D, Grey V. Clinical implication of the difference between transcutaneous bilirubinometry and total serum bilirubin for the classification of newborns at risk of hyperbilirubinemia. *Clin Biochem.* 2009;42:176–179.

70. De Luca D, Zecca E, Corsello M, Tiberi E, Semeraro C, Romagnoli C. Attempt to improve transcutaneous bilirubinometry: a double-blind study of Medick BiliMed versus Respironics BiliCheck. *Arch Dis Child Fetal Neonatal Ed.* 2008;93:F135–F139.

71. Jangaard K, Curtis H, Goldbloom R. Estimation of bilirubin using BiliChektrade mark, a transcutaneous bilirubin measurement device: effects of gestational age and use of phototherapy. *Paediatr Child Health.* 2006;11:79–83.

72. Tan KL, Dong F. Transcutaneous bilirubinometry during and after phototherapy. *Acta Paediatr.* 2003;92:327–331.

73. Zecca E, Barone G, De Luca D, Marra R, Tiberi E, Romagnoli C. Skin bilirubin measurement during phototherapy in preterm and term newborn infants. *Early Hum Dev.* 2009;85:537–540.

74. Ahlfors CE, Wennberg RP. Bilirubin–albumin binding and neonatal jaundice. *Semin Perinatol.* 2004;28:334–339.

75. Wennberg RP, Ahlfors CE, Aravkin AY. Intervention guidelines for neonatal hyperbilirubinemia: an evidence based quagmire. *Curr Pharm Des.* 2009;15:2939–2945.

76. Johnson L, Sarmiento F, Blanc WA, Day R. Kernicterus in rats with an inherited deficiency of glucuronyl transferase. *AMA J Dis Child.* 1959;97:591–608.

77. Harris RC, Lucey JF, Maclean JR. Kernicterus in premature infants associated with low concentrations of bilirubin in the plasma. *Pediatrics.* 1958;21:875–884.

78. Ahlfors CE, Parker AE. Evaluation of a model for brain bilirubin uptake in jaundiced newborns. *Pediatr Res.* 2005;58:1175–1179.

79. Ahlfors CE, Wennberg RP, Ostrow JD, Tiribelli C. Unbound (free) bilirubin: improving the paradigm for evaluating neonatal jaundice. *Clin Chem.* 2009;55:1288–1299.

80. Odell GB. The dissociation of bilirubin from albumin and its clinical implications. *J Pediatr.* 1959;55:268–279.

81. Wadsworth SJ, Suh B. In vitro displacement of bilirubin by antibiotics and 2-hydroxybenzoylglycine in newborns. *Antimicrob Agents Chemother.* 1988;32:1571–1575.

82. Ahlfors CE. Measurement of plasma unbound unconjugated bilirubin. *Anal Biochem.* 2000;279:130–135.

83. Jacobsen J, Wennberg RP. Determination of unbound bilirubin in the serum of newborns. *Clin Chem.* 1974;20:783.

84. Wennberg RP, Ahlfors CE, Bhutani VK, Johnson LH, Shapiro SM. Toward understanding kernicterus: a challenge to improve the management of jaundiced newborns. *Pediatrics.* 2006;117:474–485.

85. Ahlfors CE, Marshall GD, Wolcott DK, Olson DC, Van Overmeire B. Measurement of unbound bilirubin by the peroxidase test using Zone Fluidics. *Clin Chim Acta.* 2006;365:78–85.

86. Wennberg R. Unbound bilirubin: a better predictor of kernicterus? *Clin Chem.* 2008;54:207–208.

87. Nakamura H, Takada S, Shimabuku R, Matsuo M, Matsuo T, Negishi H. Auditory nerve and brainstem responses in newborn infants with hyperbilirubinemia. *Pediatrics.* 1985;75:703–708.

88. Shapiro SM, Hecox KE. Development of brainstem auditory evoked potentials in heterozygous and homozygous jaundiced Gunn rats. *Brain Res.* 1988;469:147–157.

89. Kaga K, Kitazumi E, Kodama K. Auditory brain stem responses of kernicterus infants. *Int J Pediatr Otorhinolaryngol.* 1979;1:255–264.

90. Wennberg RP, Ahlfors CE, Bickers R, McMurtry CA, Shetter JL. Abnormal auditory brainstem response in a newborn infant with hyperbilirubinemia: improvement with exchange transfusion. *J Pediatr.* 1982;100:624–626.

91. Ahlfors CE, Parker AE. Unbound bilirubin concentration is associated with abnormal automated auditory brainstem response for jaundiced newborns. *Pediatrics.* 2008;121:976–978.

92. Amin SB, Ahlfors C, Orlando MS, Dalzell LE, Merle KS, Guillet R. Bilirubin and serial auditory brainstem responses in premature infants. *Pediatrics.* 2001;107:664–670.

93. Funato M, Tamai H, Shimada S, Nakamura H. Vigintiphobia, unbound bilirubin, and auditory brainstem responses. *Pediatrics.* 1994;93:50–53.

94. Govaert P, Lequin M, Swarte R, et al. Changes in globus pallidus with (pre)term kernicterus. *Pediatrics.* 2003;112:1256–1263.

95. Shapiro SM, Nakamura H. Bilirubin and the auditory system. *J Perinatol.* 2001;21(suppl 1):S52–S55 [discussion S9–S62].

96. Ahlfors CE, Amin SB, Parker AE. Unbound bilirubin predicts abnormal automated auditory brainstem response in a diverse newborn population. *J Perinatol.* 2009;29:305–309.

97. Myara A, Sender A, Valette V, et al. Early changes in cutaneous bilirubin and serum bilirubin isomers during intensive phototherapy of jaundiced neonates with blue and green light. *Biol Neonate.* 1997;71:75–82.

98. McDonagh AF, Palma LA, Lightner DA. Blue light and bilirubin excretion. *Science.* 1980;208:145–151.

99. Ahlfors CE, Shwer ML, Wennberg RP. Absence of bilirubin binding competitors during phototherapy for neonatal jaundice. *Early Hum Dev.* 1982;6:125–130.

100. Ebbesen F, Madsen P, Stovring S, Hundborg H, Agati G. Therapeutic effect of turquoise versus blue light with equal irradiance in preterm infants with jaundice. *Acta Paediatr.* 2007;96:837–841.

101. Itoh S, Kawada K, Kusaka T, et al. Influence of glucuronosyl bilirubin and (*EZ*)-cyclobilirubin on determination of serum unbound bilirubin by UB-analyser. *Ann Clin Biochem.* 2002;39:583–588.

102. Itoh S, Yamakawa T, Onishi S, Isobe K, Manabe M, Sasaki K. The effect of bilirubin photoisomers on unbound-bilirubin concentrations estimated by the peroxidase method. *Biochem J.* 1986;239:417–421.

103. McDonagh AF, Vreman HJ, Wong RJ, Stevenson DK. Photoisomers: obfuscating factors in clinical peroxidase measurements of unbound bilirubin? *Pediatrics.* 2009;123:67–76.

104. Roca L, Calligaris S, Wennberg RP, et al. Factors affecting the binding of bilirubin to serum albumins: validation and application of the peroxidase method. *Pediatr Res.* 2006;60:724–728.

Bilirubin Metabolism and Transport

Cristina Bellarosa, Lucie Muchova, Libor Vitek, and Claudio Tiribelli

■ TRANSPORT OF BILIRUBIN: AN OVERVIEW

Unconjugated bilirubin (UCB), the principal mammalian bile pigment, is the end intravascular product of heme catabolism. Like many weakly polar, poorly soluble compounds, UCB is transported in blood tightly bound to albumin, with less than 0.01% of total bilirubin circulating in an unbound form (free bilirubin [Bf]). This fraction governs UCB tissue flux, and is responsible for its pathophysiological effects on cells and tissues.

The transport mechanisms of different organic anions across the hepatocyte membrane have been the subject of extensive investigation over the last three decades. The primary reason for this interest is the crucial role played by the liver in the biotransformation of several endogenous and exogenous substances and their secretion via the biliary system. UCB is no exception since this endogenous organic anion is taken up rapidly and selectively by the liver and secreted into the bile after metabolic biotransformation (conjugation).

The uptake of UCB across the basolateral membrane of the hepatocyte may be a carrier-mediated process based on experiments performed with different experimental models ranging from isolated basolateral plasma membrane–enriched vesicles to isolated and perfused liver. It is generally accepted that UCB enters the liver cells via a saturable, possibly carrier-mediated mechanism at low concentration (<40–50 nM) while its transport across the basolateral plasma membrane is passive and concentration dependent when the Bf

concentration increases above certain levels (≈70 nM). Spontaneous diffusion accounts for the observation that UCB may enter any cell when its plasma concentration reaches a certain threshold. Evidence has accrued that the spontaneous transmembrane UCB diffusion is rapid and efficient, and that the overall transfer is mainly determined by the dissociation rate of UCB from albumin.

Diffusion across the cell plasma membrane is particularly important to account the entry of UCB in cells other than the hepatocyte that has a unique mechanism for conjugating the pigment. As high concentrations of UCB in the cell are toxic, it is important to understand the mechanisms by which UCB diffused into the cell can be eliminated therefrom.

■ PUTATIVE TRANSPORTERS FOR THE CELLULAR UPTAKE OF UCB

In the 1990s, an extensive debate took place on the nature and the existence of UCB transporter(s) involved in the transmembrane passage of the pigment, particularly in the hepatocyte. At least four different putative transporters were suggested (bilirubin/BSP-binding protein [BBBP], organic anion–binding protein [OABP], bilitranslocase, and organic anion–transporting polypeptide [OATP])[1] but the use of surrogate dyes instead of bilirubin limited the conclusive nature of these studies. More recently data have been provided indicating that one member of the OATP family, human SLC01B1 (OATP1B1), also known as SLC21A6, OATP2, OATPC, and LST-1, may mediate hepatic bilirubin transport.[2] This conclusion was not confirmed in a subsequent study, however, leaving the issue of OATP1B1-mediated bilirubin membrane transport still unsettled. Data obtained in isolated liver cells, however, do indicate that UCB enters the cells in a saturable, carrier-mediated mechanism at low concentration. However, the molecular species involved in this function requires further investigation.[3] The role of another putative transport protein in UCB uptake by the liver, SLC01B3 (OATP8), is not clear. The available studies indicate that when expressed in HEK293 cells, this carrier is able to transport at least monoglucuronosyl bilirubin.[2,4] The carrier-mediated transport of UCB was also assessed in placenta with regard to the potential involvement of three members of the SLC21A family of carriers described at the level of the liver cell (SLC01A2, also known as OATP-A; SLC01B1 [OATP1B1], also known as OATP-C; and SLC01B3, also known as OATP8). Results suggested that SLC01B3 (OATP8) may play a role in the carrier-mediated uptake of the fetal UCB by the placental trophoblast, whereas both SLC01B3 (OATP8) and SLC01B1 (OATP1B1), also known as OATP-C, may substantially contribute to UCB uptake by adult hepatocytes.[5] Collectively these data suggest the possible involvement of one or more members of the large OATP family (see Figure 4-1) although the nature of the transporter(s) is still unsettled.

By contrast, Zucker et al. have presented evidence that uptake of bilirubin is a carrier-independent (diffusion) process.[6] Regarding placental transport McDonagh showed that, if the mother has elevated levels of UCB in her blood (as for Crigler–Najjar patients or Gunn rat model), bilirubin transport is consistent with passive bidirectional diffusion and does not reflect active transport against a concentration gradient.[7]

■ ROLE OF THE ABC TRANSPORTERS IN UCB TRANSPORT

The ATP-binding cassette (ABC) superfamily is the largest transporter family reported,[8] and one or more of its members have been found in almost all organisms. The ABC proteins bind intracellularly ATP, and use the energy to drive the transport of various molecules across the plasma membrane as well as intracellular membranes of the endoplasmic reticulum (ER), peroxisomes, and mitochondria against a concentration gradient. These proteins translocate a wide variety of substrates including sugars, amino acids, metal ions, peptides, and proteins, and a large number of hydrophobic compounds.[8] Based on organization of domains and amino acid homology, *ABC* genes can be divided into seven families: *ABCA*, *ABCB*, *ABCC*, *ABCD*, *ABCE*, *ABCF*, and *ABCG*.[9] These genes are essential for many processes in the cell. Mutations in some of the ABC genes cause or contribute to many genetic disorders, including cystic fibrosis, anemia, neurological disease, cholesterol and bile acid transport defects, and retinal degeneration.

Multidrug resistance proteins (MRPs), together with the cystic fibrosis conductance transmembrane regulator (CFTR/ABCC7) and the sulfonylurea receptors

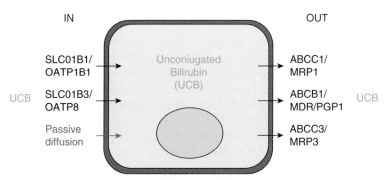

FIGURE 4-1. Putative transporters implicated in unconjugated bilirubin entrance and extrusion of the cell. Two members of the large OATP family are possibly involved in active bilirubin transport inside the cell: SLC01B1 (OATP1B1), also known as SLC21A6, OATP2, OATPC, and LST-1; and SLC01B3, also known as OATP8. There is also evidence that uptake of bilirubin is a carrier-independent (diffusion) process. Putative ABC transporters involved in UCB extrusion are ABCC1, also known as MRP1; ABCC3, also known as MRP3; and ABCB1, also known as MDR or PGP1.

(SUR1/ABCC8 and SUR2/ABCC9), comprise the 13 members of the human ATP-binding cassette C (ABCC) family. Establishing the substrate specificities of the MRPs has been, and remains, an area of considerable research activity. Many studies have focused on xenobiotic substrates because of the potential role of the MRPs in clinical drug resistance and in protection against a wide range of environmental potentially toxic compounds. Other studies investigated the involvement of MRPs in the transport of endogenous substrates, including UCB, in order to gain insight into possible physiological functions of the proteins.[10] It was shown that UCB undergoes ATP-dependent export from trophoblastic BeWo cells and that the transport activity is somehow proportional to the level of expression and activity of ABCC1 (MRP1).[11] Studies using membrane vesicles obtained from MRP1-transfected MDCKII kidney cells confirmed that UCB is a substrate for ABCC1.[12] The transport was ATP and GSH dependent, with an apparent K_m of 10 nM, by the lowest K_m for any known substrate of this transporter.[12] By contrast, MDCKII cells overexpressing multidrug resistance-related protein 2 (MRP2) did not transport UCB, indicating that MRP2 is not involved in the excretion of UCB.[12] These data demonstrate that MRP1 transports UCB suggesting a physiological role of MRP1 in the cellular export of UCB.[12]

Belonging to the same family, ABCC3 (also known as multidrug resistance protein 3 [MRP3]) shares the highest degree of amino acid homology with MRP1 (58%).[13] The presence of MRP3 protein has been confirmed in the liver, kidneys, the intestines, adrenals, pancreas, gallbladder, and spleen.[14] In polarized epithelial cells, MRP3 localizes to the basolateral membrane.[14] Higuchi et al.[15] investigated the expression of MRP3 in the hyperbilirubinemic Gunn rat. The hepatic expression of MRP3 mRNA (RT-PCR) and protein (Western blot and immunohistochemical staining) was significantly higher in Gunn rats than in normal rats, in agreement with findings of Ogawa et al.[16] Evidence regarding MRP3 transport of conjugated bilirubin will be discussed in the next paragraph.

Another ABC protein claimed to be involved in transport of endogenous compounds is ABCB1 (MDR/PGP1/P-glycoprotein 1) that belongs to the ABCB subfamily. The ABCB subfamily is unique in that it contains both four full transporters and seven half transporters. PGP1 was the first human ABC transporter cloned and characterized through its ability to confer a multidrug resistance phenotype to cancer cells.[9] Watchko et al. suggested that UCB is a substrate for PGP1 based on the observation following an intravenous bilirubin load; mdr1a[–/–], Pgp-deficient mice showed a significantly greater bilirubin content in the brain than wild-type littermates.[17] Further support for the concept that PGP1 may be involved in UCB transport is derived from Caco-2 cells overexpressing the protein at the apical membrane. These cells showed basal-to-apical vectorial transport of UCB that was significantly attenuated by the P-glycoprotein 1 inhibitor, verapamil.[18]

Although PGP1 probably has a lower affinity for the UCB than does MRP1, these data may be interpreted as evidence that UCB may be a substrate for both PGP1 and MRP1, and both may be involved in the extrusion from the cell of UCB thus contributing to prevent bilirubin cellular toxicity.

■ BILIRUBIN CONJUGATION AND EXCRETION FROM THE LIVER CELL

The naturally occurring UCB in adults is IXα isomer with internal hydrogen bonding engaging all polar groups and giving UCB its hydrophobic properties. These hydrogen bonds can be disrupted by configurational isomerization of bilirubin, which occurs on exposure to light. Unlike UCB, the photoisomers and photodegradation products behave as more polar molecules and are readily secreted into bile without conjugation.

In the liver cell, UCB is transported within the cell bound to a group of cytosolic proteins (Figure 4-2), preferentially to glutathione S-transferase B (ligandin or protein Y) and fatty acid–binding protein 1 (FABP1 or protein Z), which serve as an intracellular storage (sink) for UCB. In addition, almost half of the intracellular UCB may be membrane bound.[19] In the ER, UCB is conjugated for efficient elimination as a water-soluble molecule into the bile.

UCB is principally conjugated with glucuronic acid catalyzed by microsomal enzyme bilirubin uridine diphosphate-5'-glucuronosyltransferase type 1 (UGT1A1). Of the large UGT superfamily, UGT1A1 is the only physiologically relevant isoenzyme that catalyzes the transfer of the glucuronosyl moiety from uridinediphosphoglucuronate (UDPGA) to one or both propionic acid side chains of bilirubin, forming monoglucuronosyl and bisglucuronosyl bilirubins. UDPGA is severely limited in neonatal period or by the action of several drugs,[20] and only 1% of adult level of UGT1A1 enzyme activity

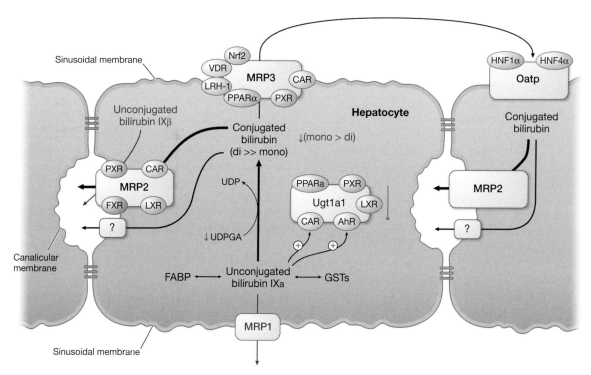

FIGURE 4-2. Intracellular metabolism and excretion of unconjugated bilirubin from liver cells. Hydrophobic UCB-IXα binds to cytosolic proteins glutathion-S-transferases (GSTs) and fatty acid–binding protein 1 (FABP1) within the hepatocyte. A specific isoform of microsomal enzyme uridine diphosphate-5′-glucuronosyltransferase (Ugt1a1) catalyzes the transfer of the glucuronosyl moiety from uridinediphosphoglucuronate (UDPGA) to form monoglucuronosyl and bisglucuronosyl bilirubins (mono, di). *Ugt1a1* expression might be activated via nuclear hormone receptors including constitutive androstane receptor (CAR), aryl hydrocarbon receptor (AhR), pregnane X receptor (PXR), liver X receptor (LXR), or peroxisome proliferator-activated receptor α (PPARα). UCB might induce its own conjugation via CAR and AhR activation. Conjugated bilirubin is secreted across canalicular membrane to bile by an active ATP-utilizing transporter multidrug resistance–related protein 2 (MRP2, ABCC2). An alternative transport to bile might occur by another yet unidentified transporter. Putative candidate is breast cancer resistance protein (BCRP, ABCG2). A part of conjugated bilirubin might be transported back to sinusoidal blood via multidrug resistance protein 3 transporter (MRP3, ABCC3) and subsequently taken up again by organic anion–transporting polypeptides (Oatp) of downstream hepatocytes to prevent oversaturation of canalicular excretion mechanisms in periportal hepatocytes. The distinctiveness of bilirubin transport and metabolism in neonatal hepatocytes are depicted in orange. In neonates, Ugt1a1 activity and UDPGA concentrations are severely limited and monoglucuronosyl bilirubin is a predominant bilirubin conjugate in neonatal bile (mono > di). In high concentrations, UCB might be transported from hepatocyte by a multidrug resistance–related protein 1 (MRP1, ABCC2). Furthermore, UCB-IXβ exclusively present in fetal and neonatal period is eliminated to bile without conjugation. Depicted pathways are based on data from both animal and human studies. For sake of simplicity, all gene/transporter symbols are used in small letters.

is present at birth. UGT1A1 activity matures early in the postnatal period reaching adult values at 6–14 weeks of life. The majority of bilirubin conjugates are secreted into bile as bisglucuronosyl bilirubin (80%) in adults while monoglucuronosyl bilirubin predominates in newborns;

UCB accounts for only 1–2% of total biliary bilirubin formed by limited hydrolysis of the conjugated bilirubin in the gallbladder.[21]

Given the uniqueness of UGT1A1 in bilirubin glucuronosylation, quantitative or functional deficiency of this enzyme results in an accumulation of UCB in plasma. To date, three types of familial unconjugated hyperbilirubinemic syndromes have been characterized. Structural mutations in any of five exons of *UGT1A1* result in Crigler–Najjar syndrome type 1 (complete absence of UGT1A1 activity with hyperbilirubinemia 20–50 mg/dL [342–855 μmol/L]) or type 2 (more or less severe disruption of UGT1A1 activity with serum bilirubin 7–20 mg/dL [103–342 μmol/L]). Gilbert syndrome is the mildest form of inherited hyperbilirubinemia with serum bilirubin levels fluctuating from normal to 5 mg/dL and UGT1A1 activity reduced to about 30%. This disorder results (mostly in Caucasian and African population) from a variant TA element within the *UGT1A1* promoter leading to a reduced *UGT1A1* transcription.[22] However, the structural mutations within the coding regions of *UGT1A1* (i.e., G71R or Y486D) consistent with the clinical diagnosis of Gilbert syndrome have been described primarily in Asians. In neonates, the presence of the variant *UGT1A1* promoter has been shown to increase the incidence of neonatal hyperbilirubinemia when in combination with additional icterogenic factors, such as glucose-6-phosphate dehydrogenase deficiency, *OATP1B1* variants, hereditary spherocytosis, or ABO incompatibility.[23]

Recently, it has been shown that UCB can induce its own conjugation through induction of nuclear hormone receptors (constitutive androstane receptor [CAR] or aryl hydrocarbon receptor [AhR]) of the phenobarbital-responsive enhancer module (PBREM) UGT1A1 promoter element activating the *UGT1A1* expression.[24] Several other ligand-dependent transcriptional regulators have also been reported to contribute to bilirubin detoxification via UGT1A1 activation including pregnane X receptor (PXR), glucocorticoid receptor, hepatocyte nuclear receptor 1α, or PPARα (Figure 4-2).

In patients with decreased UGT1A1 activity as well as in hyperbilirubinemic Gunn rats (mutant strain of Wistar rats with the inherited deficiency of UGT1A1), the biliary secretion of bilirubin is considerably decreased, but still remains significant. There is in vitro evidence of ATP-dependent transport of UCB by canalicular membranes of hepatocyte,[25] although the particular transporter and its role in vivo remains to be elucidated. Moreover, alternative pathways of UCB catabolism within hepatocyte have been proposed; they include bilirubin oxidation mediated by induced cytochromes P_{450} (mainly CYP1A1, CYP1A2), but the proof of its biological relevance in UCB disposal is still lacking.

Bilirubin conjugates are secreted against concentration gradient through the canalicular membrane of hepatocyte into the bile by an active transporter, ABCC2 (MRP2), belonging to the ABCC subfamily of transporters[26] (Figure 4-2). The substrate specificity of MRP2 is broad and includes glutathione, sulfate, and glucuronide conjugates of many drugs and organic anions and some neutral and positively charged xenobiotics. Accordingly, mutations in a coding sequence of *MRP2* and absence of a corresponding protein in the canalicular membrane cause conjugated hyperbilirubinemia and have been reported in Dubin–Johnson syndrome.[27] This autosomal recessive disorder described by Dubin and Johnson in 1954[28] is characterized by mild conjugated/mixed hyperbilirubinemia and deposition of a dark pigment in hepatocytes without further hepatic or hematological abnormalities and is considered a benign disorder without need for treatment. Unlike Dubin–Johnson, Rotor syndrome, also characterized by mild conjugated/mixed hyperbilirubinemia, demonstrates normal MRP2 expression and function. The mode of inheritance of Rotor syndrome is also autosomal recessive but the association to a specific gene remains to be elucidated.

The absence of MRP2 is usually compensated by the upregulation of sinusoidal transporters mediating efflux of organic anions from hepatocyte to blood. The main transporter responsible for reflux of bilirubin glucuronides back to systemic circulation has been identified as MRP3, an ATP-binding cassette transporter (ABCC3)[29] (Figure 4-2).

The presence of bilirubin glucuronides in the bile of MRP2-deficient animals suggests that other transporters of bilirubin glucuronides might exist in the canalicular membrane. Putative candidate is a canalicular transporter breast cancer resistance protein (BCRP, also named ABCG2), a member of ABC transporter superfamily with a broad substrate specificity substantially overlapping with MRP2.[30]

Recently, a novel view on the physiological elimination of conjugated bilirubin from the liver has been proposed.[31] It is assumed that a part of conjugated bilirubin is not transported directly from hepatocyte to bile, but rather moves back to sinusoidal blood via MRP3 transporter and subsequently re-taken up by OATP transporters (see above) of downstream hepatocytes. This "hepatocyte hopping" should prevent oversaturation of canalicular excretion mechanisms in periportal hepatocytes. Further studies, however, are needed to prove this mechanism.

■ UCB TRANSFER ACROSS BLOOD–BRAIN BARRIERS AND NEUROTOXICITY

The sophisticated system of bilirubin elimination described above maintains plasma bilirubin within a relatively narrow concentration range (up to 17 µmol/L) in adults and even mild unconjugated hyperbilirubinemia, as in Gilbert syndrome, does not represent any risk. By contrast, markedly elevated serum UCB levels, especially in neonates or patients with severe congenital impairment of UCB conjugation (as in the Crigler–Najjar type I syndrome), may cause deposition of bilirubin in different tissues but most importantly in the nervous system causing severe neurological damage.

Blood–Brain Barriers

The central nervous system (CNS) is well protected from penetration of drugs and other compounds by two barriers: the endothelial cells of brain capillaries and microvessels forming the blood–brain barrier (BBB) and the epithelium of the choroid plexuses forming the blood–cerebrospinal fluid barrier (BCSFB) (Figure 4-3).[32] The cerebral endothelium offers a very large surface area for exchange of endogenous compounds as well as xenobiotics between blood and brain. However, this process is strictly regulated, since the endothelial cells are sealed by an elaborate network of interconnecting complex tight junctions, which restrict the paracellular passage of blood-borne compounds into the adjacent neurons and astrocytes. Together with the absence of fenestrae and a very low pinocytotic activity, which inhibits transcellular passage of molecules, a very low permeability of BBB is present. Likewise, the paracellular entry of blood-borne compounds into the CSF through the choroid plexus is also restricted by the presence of apical tight junctions interconnecting choroidal epithelial cells.[33] Although there is lingering debate,[34] several lines of evidence suggest that blood–brain and blood–CSF interfaces are more permeable in newborns.[35] These include, in

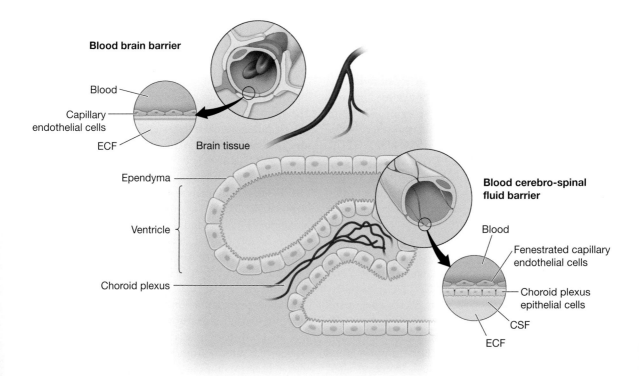

FIGURE 4-3. Schematic representation of blood–brain barrier and blood–cerebrospinal fluid barrier. The central nervous system (CNS) is protected from penetration of drugs and other compounds by two barriers: the endothelial cells of brain capillaries and microvessels forming the blood–brain barrier (BBB) and the epithelium of the choroid plexuses forming the blood–cerebrospinal fluid barrier (BCSFB).

particular, protein concentrations in CSF that are substantially elevated in newborns compared with adults and even higher in prematures.[36]

Factors Affecting Blood–Brain Transfer of UCB

The blood–CNS interfaces protect the brain from UCB transport by several mechanisms.[36] The tight junctions efficiently restrict the entry of blood-borne polar compounds, or compounds bound to plasma proteins. The penetration of more lipid-soluble molecules capable of diffusing across the cell membranes like UCB is limited by binding to albumin and/or other transporting molecules in the intravascular compartment, as well as UCB-binding molecules in the BBB epithelial cell cytoplasm and/or CSF. In human adults, 90% of UCB in the circulation is bound to albumin, and the remaining 10% mainly to the apolipoprotein D in high-density lipoprotein.[37,38] In the neonates, α1-fetoprotein is an additional high-affinity transporter for UCB. Human serum albumin (HSA), the major UCB transporter in the blood, has one primary high-affinity site for UCB, and one or more sites with lower affinity. These secondary sites contribute significantly to overall UCB binding at higher UCB/HSA molar ratios. UCB can also be competitively displaced from the binding sites on albumin by numerous drugs resulting in an increase of the plasma concentration of Bf. The binding capacity of human plasma for UCB is primarily dependent on the affinity constant, which at the mean serum HSA concentration in full-term newborns (450 μmol/L) is approximately 3.1×10^6 L/mol. The binding of UCB in neonatal plasma, however, may be even lower, as the affinity of additional UCB binders in neonatal plasma is weaker. If the Bf exceeds its aqueous solubility (70 nmol/L), UCB becomes cytotoxic in vitro.[39] Since several variables influence the binding of UCB to HSA and any other binders, the measurement of Bf may be more clinically relevant than that of total bilirubin.[40,41]

As described above, however, UCB can passively diffuse across the plasma membrane of any cell. Thus, membranes of the BBB cells do not appear to be a significant barrier to the entry of UCB into brain.[37,38] It is estimated that a single-pass blood–brain bilirubin extraction ranges from 8% to 28% depending on biological conditions, especially the Bf concentration. The passive diffusion of UCB across the BBB may be countered in part by the metabolism of UCB and active secretion of UCB into the plasma by the brain capillary endothelium.[37,38]

Metabolic Disturbances and Brain Bilirubin Flux

The risk of bilirubin transfer into CNS increases with disordered acid–base equilibrium, plasma osmolality, or systemic inflammation.

a. *Blood pH*: UCB, present in human plasma as a dianion, preferentially binds to HSA. The proportion of dianion decreases as pH falls; hence, binding of UCB decreases with decreasing pH, thus contributing to the increased risk of bilirubin neurotoxicity. Respiratory acidosis appears to be more dangerous compared with metabolic causes of acid–base disequilibrium.[42] This might be due to the additional contributing pathogenic factors, such as hypercapnia-induced increased cerebral blood flow in severely asphyctic neonates, or hypoxemia-induced increased protein transport across the BBB. It is also likely that brain pH is as important as blood pH in facilitating bilirubin uptake, and brain pH is better protected against metabolic acidosis than it is against respiratory acidosis.[36]

b. *Increased plasma osmolality*: Hyperosmolality causes capillary leakage of BBB and hence increases the transport of UCB/HSA into brain, as repeatedly reported in experimental animals exposed to urea or other osmotically active agents. Although it is unlikely that massive BBB disruption occurs in human newborns, the presence of a generalized increase in brain capillary leak, for example, following asphyxia, could enhance UCB transfer across BBB.[36]

c. *Systemic inflammation*: Many inflammatory agents and other endogenous compounds increase both endothelial permeability and vessel diameter, contributing to a significant leakage across the BBB. These agents include bacterial lipopolysaccharide, free oxygen radicals, inflammatory cytokines (IL-1β, IL-6), bradykinin, histamine, and serotonin, indicating that neonates with bacterial infections, sepsis, meningitis, or encephalitis are at higher risk of increased bilirubin neurotoxicity.[43]

d. *Immaturity of BBB*: Based on animal data there is a maturational effect on bilirubin uptake by brain, since susceptibility of the brainstem auditory evoked response to bilirubin is dependent on gestational age, and the BBB permeability to bilirubin decreases with the postnatal age.[44] Similarly, maturational decrease in albumin transport across the BBB has been observed.[45] All these observations are consistent with the clinical experience, suggesting that the risk for bilirubin neurotoxicity is higher in premature neonates compared with term infants.[42]

Other Factors Affecting Bilirubin Influx Into Brain

UCB flux into brain is also regulated by additional important factors[36] including: (a) the transit time through the capillary bed (prolonged in patients with increased venous pressure)[42]; (b) the dissociation rate of UCB/HSA (altered in neonates with high total plasma bilirubin or those treated with competitive inhibitors of UCB/HSA binding)[42]; (c) cerebral blood flow (increased in hypercapnia)[46]; (d) the ABC efflux transport proteins present in both the BBB and BCSF barriers capable of exporting UCB back to plasma[47]; (e) availability of ligandin and other UCB-binding proteins in the cytosol of CNS cells[36]; (f) ability of CNS cells to metabolize UCB to nontoxic products, by conjugation and/or oxidation[48]; and potentially (g) UCB production within the brain by catabolism of heme-containing proteins. Unfortunately, the relative role of each is hard to assess particularly in the clinical setting.

■ CONCLUDING REMARKS AND PERSPECTIVES

The understanding of the molecular events governing the passage of bilirubin across the cell membrane, the intracellular processing, and extrusion may help provide a more rational approach in the diagnosis, treatment, and prevention of bilirubin-induced neurotoxicity in the newborn. In spite of the several studies performed and the clinical relevance of the bilirubin-induced neurological damage, several points remain to be elucidated. We still do not have definitive clues on how bilirubin enters cells and how the cell can reduce the concentration of the pigment to a nontoxic level. We also do not have easy and widely applicable methods to measure the Bf concentration, in cells and in the CNS in vivo. Future study is necessary to clarify these and related issues regarding the pathogenesis of bilirubin encephalopathy and kernicterus.

■ ACKNOWLEDGMENTS

Supported by grant no. SVV 262513 and LH11030 given by the Czech Ministry of Education, NT 11327-4/2010 given by the Czech Ministry of Health, grant NTB on L.R. 26/05 given by Regione Autonoma Friuli Venezia Giulia, Italy, and grant no. GGP10051 given by Telethon.

REFERENCES

1. Adachi Y, Kamisako T, Okuyama Y, Miya H. Hepatic metabolism and transport of bilirubin and other organic anions. *Nippon Rinsho*. 1996;54:2276–2290.

2. Cui Y, Konig J, Leier I, Buchholz U, Keppler D. Hepatic uptake of bilirubin and its conjugates by the human organic anion transporter SLC21A6. *J Biol Chem*. 2001;276:9626–9630.

3. Wang P, Kim RB, Chowdhury JR, Wolkoff AW. The human organic anion transport protein SLC21A6 is not sufficient for bilirubin transport. *J Biol Chem*. 2003;278:20695–20699.

4. Konig J, Cui Y, Nies AT, Keppler D. A novel human organic anion transporting polypeptide localized to the basolateral hepatocyte membrane. *Am J Physiol Gastrointest Liver Physiol*. 2000;278:G156–G164.

5. Briz O, Serrano MA, MacIas RI, Gonzalez-Gallego J, Marin JJ. Role of organic anion-transporting polypeptides, OATP-A, OATP-C and OATP-8, in the human placenta–maternal liver tandem excretory pathway for foetal bilirubin. *Biochem J*. 2003;371:897–905.

6. Zucker SD, Goessling W, Hoppin AG. Unconjugated bilirubin exhibits spontaneous diffusion through model lipid bilayers and native hepatocyte membranes. *J Biol Chem*. 1999;274:10852–10862.

7. McDonagh AF. Controversies in bilirubin biochemistry and their clinical relevance. *Semin Fetal Neonatal Med*. 2010;15:141–147.

8. Dean M, Hamon Y, Chimini G. The human ATP-binding cassette (ABC) transporter superfamily. *J Lipid Res*. 2001;42:1007–1017.

9. Dean M, Rzhetsky A, Allikmets R. The human ATP-binding cassette (ABC) transporter superfamily. *Genome Res*. 2001;11:1156–1166.

10. Cole SP, Deeley RG. Multidrug resistance-associated protein: sequence correction. *Science*. 1993;260:879.

11. Pascolo L, Fernetti C, Garcia-Mediavilla MV, Ostrow JD, Tiribelli C. Mechanisms for the transport of unconjugated bilirubin in human trophoblastic BeWo cells. *FEBS Lett*. 2001;495:94–99.

12. Rigato I, Pascolo L, Fernetti C, Ostrow JD, Tiribelli C. The human multidrug-resistance-associated protein MRP1 mediates ATP-dependent transport of unconjugated bilirubin. *Biochem J*. 2004;383:335–341.

13. Kool M, van der Linden M, de Haas M, et al. MRP3, an organic anion transporter able to transport anti-cancer drugs. *Proc Natl Acad Sci U S A*. 1999;96:6914–6919.

14. Scheffer GL, Kool M, de Haas M, et al. Tissue distribution and induction of human multidrug resistant protein 3. *Lab Invest.* 2002;82:193–201.

15. Higuchi K, Kobayashi Y, Kuroda M, et al. Modulation of organic anion transporting polypeptide 1 and multidrug resistance protein 3 expression in the liver and kidney of Gunn rats. *Hepatol Res.* 2004;29:60–66.

16. Ogawa K, Suzuki H, Hirohashi T, et al. Characterization of inducible nature of MRP3 in rat liver. *Am J Physiol Gastrointest Liver Physiol.* 2000;278:G438–G446.

17. Watchko JF, Daood MJ, Hansen TW. Brain bilirubin content is increased in P-glycoprotein-deficient transgenic null mutant mice. *Pediatr Res.* 1998;44:763–766.

18. Watchko JF, Daood MJ, Mahmood B, Vats K, Hart C, Ahdab-Barmada M. P-glycoprotein and bilirubin disposition. *J Perinatol.* 2001;21(suppl 1):S43–S47.

19. Gollan JL, Zucker SD. A new voyage of discovery: transport through the hepatocyte. *Trans Am Clin Climatol Assoc.* 1996;107:48–55.

20. Crawford JM, Hauser SC, Gollan JL. Formation, hepatic metabolism, and transport of bile pigments: a status report. *Semin Liver Dis.* 1988;8:105–118.

21. Vitek L, Ostrow JD. Bilirubin chemistry and metabolism; harmful and protective aspects. *Curr Pharm Des.* 2009;15:2869–2883.

22. Bosma PJ, Chowdhury JR, Bakker C, et al. The genetic basis of the reduced expression of bilirubin UDP-glucuronosyltransferase 1 in Gilbert's syndrome. *N Engl J Med.* 1995;333:1171–1175.

23. Schmid R. Gilbert's syndrome—a legitimate genetic anomaly? *N Engl J Med.* 1995;333:1217–1218.

24. Huang W, Zhang J, Chua SS, et al. Induction of bilirubin clearance by the constitutive androstane receptor (CAR). *Proc Natl Acad Sci U S A.* 2003;100:4156–4161.

25. Pascolo L, Bayon EJ, Cupelli F, Ostrow JD, Tiribelli C. ATP-dependent transport of unconjugated bilirubin by rat liver canalicular plasma membrane vesicles. *Biochem J.* 1998;331(pt 1):99–103.

26. Kamisako T, Leier I, Cui Y, et al. Transport of monoglucuronosyl and bisglucuronosyl bilirubin by recombinant human and rat multidrug resistance protein 2. *Hepatology.* 1999;30:485–490.

27. Kartenbeck J, Leuschner U, Mayer R, Keppler D. Absence of the canalicular isoform of the MRP gene-encoded conjugate export pump from the hepatocytes in Dubin–Johnson syndrome. *Hepatology.* 1996;23:1061–1066.

28. Dubin IN, Johnson FB. Chronic idiopathic jaundice with unidentified pigment in liver cells; a new clinicopathologic entity with a report of 12 cases. *Medicine (Baltimore).* 1954;33:155–197.

29. Lee YM, Cui Y, Konig J, et al. Identification and functional characterization of the natural variant MRP3-Arg1297His of human multidrug resistance protein 3 (MRP3/ABCC3). *Pharmacogenetics.* 2004;14:213–223.

30. Vlaming ML, Pala Z, van Esch A, et al. Functionally overlapping roles of Abcg2 (Bcrp1) and Abcc2 (Mrp2) in the elimination of methotrexate and its main toxic metabolite 7-hydroxymethotrexate in vivo. *Clin Cancer Res.* 2009;15:3084–3093.

31. van de Steeg E, Wagenaar E, van der Kruijssen CM, et al. Organic anion transporting polypeptide 1a/1b-knockout mice provide insights into hepatic handling of bilirubin, bile acids, and drugs. *J Clin Invest.* 2010;120:2942–2952.

32. Ghersi-Egea JF, Gazzin S, Strazielle N. Blood–brain interfaces and bilirubin-induced neurological diseases. *Curr Pharm Des.* 2009;15:2893–2907.

33. Engelhardt B, Sorokin L. The blood–brain and the blood–cerebrospinal fluid barriers: function and dysfunction. *Semin Immunopathol.* 2009;31:497–511.

34. Johansson PA, Dziegielewska KM, Liddelow SA, Saunders NR. The blood–CSF barrier explained: when development is not immaturity. *Bioessays.* 2008;30:237–248.

35. Wenzel D, Felgenhauer K. The development of the blood–CSF barrier after birth. *Neuropadiatrie.* 1976;7:175–181.

36. Ostrow JD, Pascolo L, Shapiro SM, Tiribelli C. New concepts in bilirubin encephalopathy. *Eur J Clin Invest.* 2003;33:988–997.

37. Suzuki N, Yamaguchi T, Nakajima H. Role of high-density lipoprotein in transport of circulating bilirubin in rats. *J Biol Chem.* 1988;263:5037–5043.

38. Goessling W, Zucker SD. Role of apolipoprotein D in the transport of bilirubin in plasma. *Am J Physiol Gastrointest Liver Physiol.* 2000;279:G356–G365.

39. Dore S, Snyder SH. Neuroprotective action of bilirubin against oxidative stress in primary hippocampal cultures. *Ann N Y Acad Sci.* 1999;890:167–172.

40. Calligaris SD, Bellarosa C, Giraudi P, Wennberg RP, Ostrow JD, Tiribelli C. Cytotoxicity is predicted by unbound and not total bilirubin concentration. *Pediatr Res.* 2007;62:576–580.

41. Ahlfors CE, Wennberg RP, Ostrow JD, Tiribelli C. Unbound (free) bilirubin: improving the paradigm for evaluating neonatal jaundice. *Clin Chem.* 2009;55:1288–1299.

42. Wennberg RP. The blood–brain barrier and bilirubin encephalopathy. *Cell Mol Neurobiol.* 2000;20:97–109.

43. Abbott NJ, Patabendige AA, Dolman DE, Yusof SR, Begley DJ. Structure and function of the blood–brain barrier. *Neurobiol Dis.* 2010;37:13–25.

44. Lee C, Stonestreet BS, Oh W, Outerbridge EW, Cashore WJ. Postnatal maturation of the blood–brain barrier for unbound bilirubin in newborn piglets. *Brain Res.* 1995;689:233–238.

45. Lee C, Oh W, Stonestreet BS, Cashore WJ. Permeability of the blood brain barrier for 125I-albumin-bound bilirubin in newborn piglets. *Pediatr Res.* 1989;25:452–456.

46. Burgess GH, Oh W, Bratlid D, Brubakk AM, Cashore WJ, Stonestreet BS. The effects of brain blood flow on brain bilirubin deposition in newborn piglets. *Pediatr Res.* 1985;19:691–696.

47. Gazzin S, Berengeno AL, Strazielle N, et al. Modulation of Mrp1 (ABCc1) and Pgp (ABCb1) by bilirubin at the blood–CSF and blood–brain barriers in the Gunn rat. *PLoS One.* 2011;6:e16165.

48. Hansen TW. Bilirubin oxidation in brain. *Mol Genet Metab.* 2000;71:411–417.

Physiology of Neonatal Unconjugated Hyperbilirubinemia

Thor Willy Ruud Hansen and Dag Bratlid

■ BILIRUBIN PRODUCTION IN THE FETUS AND NEWBORN

Development of Bilirubin Production by Heme Catabolism

Bilirubin is formed in the organism by oxidation–reduction reactions. It is the end product of heme catabolism (Figure 5-1). The heme comes mainly from aging red blood cells (RBCs), but muscle myoglobin and some liver enzymes such as cytochromes and catalases are a partial source.[1] Production of erythrocytes is first observed in the fetal yolk sac at 2–3 weeks of gestation. RBC production in the liver is seen at about 6 weeks of gestation and in the marrow at 20 weeks.[2] The mean life span of RBCs in the term newborn infant is around 45–90 days, and about 35–50 days in premature infants.[3] Fetal and adult hemoglobin are structurally different. Together with a higher hemoglobin concentration, this explains the increased oxygen-carrying capacity in the fetus. Postnatally, these mechanisms are no longer needed. Production of adult hemoglobin starts in the last trimester of pregnancy, and in the absence of certain hemoglobinopathies the production of fetal hemoglobin is turned off at birth.[3]

Bilirubin-IXβ appears in the human fetus at 14 weeks of gestation.[4] Two weeks later unconjugated bilirubin-IXα appears in bile. By 20 weeks of gestation IXα constitutes 6% of bilirubin in bile, IXβ 87%, IXγ 0.5%, and IXδ 6%.[5]

By 38 weeks gestation, bilirubin-IXα has replaced IXβ as the main isomer.[4]

In fetal hemolytic disease, such as Rhesus immunization, the concentration of total serum bilirubin (TSB) can increase from 1.5 mg/dL at 20 weeks of gestation to 4.1 mg/dL at 32 weeks. Weiner described an inverse relationship between TSB and hemoglobin concentrations.[6] Thus, when fetuses became severely anemic (hematocrit <30), 82% had TSB concentrations exceeding the 97.5th percentile on the Bhutani nomogram.[7] Increased TSB could be detected weeks before the development of anemia. A TSB >3 mg/dL was associated with a high likelihood of severe fetal anemia. Goodrum et al. studied the effect of repeated intrauterine transfusions and found a mean TSB value of 5.6 mg/dL (1.3–10.8 mg/dL) at the time of the third transfusion, almost all unconjugated.[8] Thus, although bilirubin can pass the placenta (see below), fetal hemolytic disease is accompanied by fetal hyperbilirubinemia. It therefore appears that the placenta has a limited capacity for transfer of bilirubin, which is exceeded in fetal hemolytic disease.

The first step in the breakdown of heme is catalyzed by heme oxygenase (HO), and is the rate-limiting step in heme degradation (Figure 5-1).[9,10] This enzyme is found in the reticuloendothelial system, and also in tissue macrophages and in gut mucosa.[11] Formation of

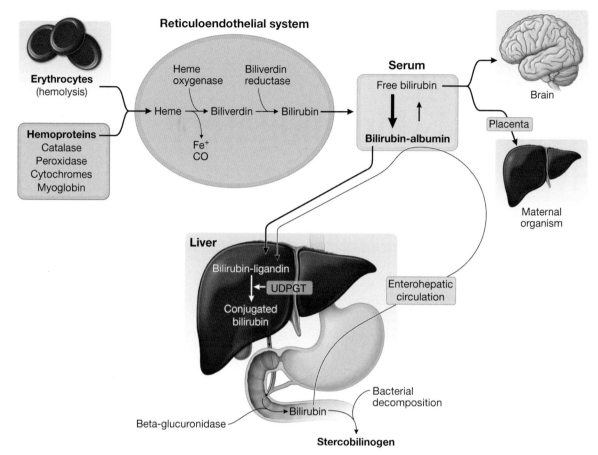

FIGURE 5-1. Diagram of bilirubin metabolism. Fe^{2+}, iron; CO, carbon monoxide; UDPGT (UGT), uridine diphosphoglucuronyltransferase.

biliverdin is an intermediate step in bilirubin production. Because carbon monoxide (CO) is a by-product of this process, measurement of CO in exhaled breath, corrected for ambient CO (ETCOc), can be used to estimate bilirubin production (see Chapter 2). The production rate in the neonate was estimated to be about 8.5 mg/kg per day, about double the rate of 4 mg/kg per day in adults.[12]

Reduction of biliverdin-IXα to bilirubin-IXα takes place in the cytosol and is catalyzed by biliverdin reductase.[13] Biliverdin has a blue-green color and is water soluble, while bilirubin has a strong yellow-to-orange color. Bilirubin-IXα occurs in several isomeric forms, but in the absence of skin exposure to strong light is found mostly as the (4Z,15Z) isomer in the serum of humans. This bilirubin isomer appears to be lipophilic,

which may be explained by intramolecular hydrogen bonds between the side groups (Z, zusammen—German for "together").[13,14] It is this solubility characteristic that allows bilirubin to cross tissue membranes and explains its ability to enter the brain. A sketch of bilirubin metabolism is shown in Figure 5-1.

Heme Oxygenase Activity in the Fetus, Placenta, and Newborn

Heme catabolism releases the iron bound to heme for renewed use by the body, and CO for release through the respiration. HO is needed to convert heme to biliverdin. Therefore, it must be active when bilirubin first appears in the fetus at 14 weeks gestation.[4] HO has a broad range of substrate affinities, but the oxidative degradation of heme is alpha-specific.

Three functional isoforms of HO (HO-1, HO-2, and HO-3) have been described in humans. Of these, HO-2 and HO-3 are constitutive and HO-1 is inducible. HO-1 and HO-2 have roles in heme catabolism, but the role of HO-3 has not been well elucidated.[15,16] HO may be inhibited by a number of metalloporphyrins, a phenomenon which has a therapeutic potential.[17]

In the fetus, microsomal HO activity in the liver may be as much as eight times higher than in the adult.[18] This suggests that the increased catabolism of heme in neonates may be associated with an increased transcription of the inducible HO isoform, HO-1. However, in a study of healthy mature and premature infants HO-1 was induced until day 2 or 3 after birth, possibly suggesting oxidative stress, but by the end of the first week the HO-1 mRNA level had dropped below the level at birth.[19] HO-1 levels and inducibility were not dependent on gestational age, at least down to the 26 weeks gestation which was investigated. Deficiency of HO-1 has been described in one single patient who suffered from growth failure, anemia, tissue iron deposition, lymphadenopathy, leukocytosis, and increased sensitivity to oxidant injury.[20]

HO is expressed in human placenta, where it contributes to normal placental function. The amounts of mRNA in placenta that encode both the HO-1 and HO-2 isoforms have been measured, showing an elevated expression of HO-2 relative to HO-1.[21] Furthermore, the expression of both HO-1 and HO-2 in the placenta increased with gestational age.[21]

■ TRANSPORT AND EXCRETION OF BILIRUBIN IN THE FETUS AND NEWBORN

Hepatic Uptake and Transport of Bilirubin in the Fetus and Newborn

Unconjugated bilirubin (UCB) is transported in plasma bound to albumin with a binding affinity of 10^7–10^8/M at the primary binding site.[22] There is also a secondary binding site with lower affinity.[22,23] Because of the high affinity of albumin for bilirubin, equilibrium concentrations of free (unbound) bilirubin in plasma are only in the low nanomolar range, even in significant hyperbilirubinemia.[24,25] However, when the molar concentration of bilirubin exceeds that of albumin, free bilirubin concentrations may increase significantly.[22,24,26] Binding of bilirubin to albumin increases with postnatal age but is reduced in sick infants

and in the presence of exogenous or endogenous binding competitors.[27–30] In addition to albumin, bilirubin can also bind to other proteins (e.g., α-fetoprotein and ligandin), as well as to lipoproteins and to erythrocytes.[31–34]

When the bilirubin–albumin complex comes in contact with hepatocytes, bilirubin is transported into the cell. Three different transport proteins may be involved.[35,36] These appear to be dominant at different substrate concentrations, as well as having different driving forces. It has been suggested that the apparent receptor effect may be due to clusters of membrane proteins with high affinities for specific classes of ligands.[35] These protein clusters may be located in the sinusoidal liver cell plasma membrane.

In liver cells about 60% of bilirubin is found in the cytosol and about 25% in microsomes.[37] Ligandin, a glutathione S-transferase (GST), binds bilirubin in the hepatocytes. In fetal rat liver, the activity of GST is <5% of adult values on day 16 of pregnancy and ~10% on day 20.[38] Basic monomers of GST are present in human fetal liver cytosol at 21 weeks gestation, while near-neutral isoenzymes do not appear until 30 weeks.[39]

Lysine may be involved in bilirubin binding to both albumin and ligandin, as well as to other proteins.[40,41] It has been suggested that binding to lysine may play a role in the mediation or modulation of bilirubin toxicity.[42]

Bilirubin and the Placenta

Bilirubin metabolism is different in the fetus compared with the neonate. UCB in a mammalian fetus can be disposed of either by crossing the placenta into the maternal circulation or by excretion into fetal bile. Excretion into bile causes bilirubin to accumulate in meconium, but only in an amount that corresponds to 5–10 times daily production.[43] Therefore, elimination across the placenta is the major route for excretion of fetal UCB.[44] Placental membranes are more or less impermeable to such polar compounds as biliverdin and bilirubin conjugates,[44] but nonpolar compounds such as UCB can diffuse across.[44,45] Evidence obtained using plasma membrane vesicles from human placental trophoblast[46] and an in vivo experimental model of in situ perfused rat placenta at term[47] point to an important role for carrier-mediated transport of UCB across the placenta. OATP8 may play an important role in this context.[48]

Inside trophoblast cells, bilirubin may be bound in part to lipids and proteins (e.g., GST).[49] Bilirubin export across the apical pole of the trophoblast may occur via an ATP-dependent mechanism.[46] Several isoforms of multidrug resistance proteins (MRPs) are expressed in human[50] and rat[51,52] placentas. Whether these are involved in bilirubin export is as yet not known. MRP2, possibly also MRP1, is able to transport bilirubin glucuronides.[53] However, UDP-glucuronosyl transferase (UGT) activity in fetal liver is low, and biotransformation of UCB appears not to occur during transplacental transfer.[54] Thus, MRP2 and MRP1 may not play an important role in bilirubin transfer across the placenta.

Comparing TSB levels in samples from umbilical artery and vein as well as from maternal serum, Rosenthal found that the bilirubin concentration in the artery was nearly double that of the vein.[55] Thus, bilirubin appears to be cleared quite efficiently from fetal blood during passage through the placenta. In Rosenthal's study the transplacental gradient of bilirubin from fetus to mother was ~10:1, while Monte et al. found a gradient of ~5:1.[56]

Bilirubin has been found in amniotic fluid from the 12th week of gestation. However, it gradually disappears as the volume of amniotic fluid increases, and normally near-term amniotic fluid does not contain measurable bilirubin.[57] Bilirubin was first found in amniotic fluid from rhesus immunized women.[58] The levels of amniotic fluid bilirubin correlated with the degree of fetal affection.[59] Amniotic fluid is primarily a fetal product; thus, bilirubin in this fluid most likely comes from the fetus itself. Although several modes of transfer are possible, recent data support the intramembranous pathway as the only one that is compatible with the observed amniotic fluid/fetal blood ratios, and it is therefore likely to be the most important.[60]

Medical literature contains a few reports of infants who have been exposed to significant maternal hyperbilirubinemia in utero. An infant born to a mother with the Crigler–Najjar syndrome had a cord TSB of 24 mg/dL of which 12.7 mg/dL was unconjugated. Although neurological symptoms were absent in the newborn period, follow-up at 18 months revealed quadriplegia.[61]

Two infants born to women with the Crigler–Najjar syndrome received exchange transfusions soon after birth and had normal neurodevelopmental outcomes at 18 months and 4 years of age, respectively.[62] Of note, a brain magnetic resonance imaging (MRI) of one of these infants performed on the fifth day of life showed a high T1 signal in the globus pallidus bilaterally, consistent with acute bilirubin encephalopathy (ABE), apparently without clinical neurological symptoms. His TSB at birth was 18.9 mg/dL. Brain MRI of the other infant was normal, although a cord TSB at birth had been 24.6 mg/dL. Evidence for reversibility of ABE has recently been published,[63] and the above infant with MRI changes, but normal outcome, appears to add to such cases.

Conjugation and Excretion of Bilirubin

There appears to be marked interspecies differences in fetal handling of bilirubin. Therefore, extrapolating from animal data to humans requires caution.[64] For example, fetal dog and sheep livers excrete about 50% of injected radiolabeled bilirubin as conjugates, while the fetal monkey liver excretes only about 5% of the dose, and very little as conjugates.[65,66] In rats monoconjugates appear in the intestines on fetal day 18, while diconjugates show up 2 days later.[67] On day 18, 80% of intestinal bilirubin is unconjugated, while from day 20, the conjugated pigment predominates. Thus, in this species there appears to be a rapid development of the conjugation mechanisms in the last few days of fetal life.

An organism can excrete heme directly in bile,[68] a phenomenon which is currently being exploited in the prevention and treatment of neonatal jaundice through the use of metalloporphyrins, inhibitors of HO[17] (see Chapter 2). However, direct excretion of heme in the bile would result in the loss of iron, whereas conversion of heme to biliverdin conserves this valuable resource for the body. Biliverdin can also be excreted in bile,[69] and although it makes sense for the fetus to reduce biliverdin to bilirubin that can cross the placenta, it is something of a biological puzzle why we continue after birth to produce and excrete potentially toxic bilirubin rather than stop the process at nontoxic biliverdin. Birds appear to lack biliverdin reductase in their reticuloendothelial system and thus excrete biliverdin rather than bilirubin.[13] The discovery that bilirubin is a free radical quencher could possibly be a piece in this puzzle.[70,71]

The last step of the bilirubin conjugation process takes place at the cell membrane.[72] Excretion of conjugated bilirubin into bile occurs against a concentration gradient, thus requiring energy. In rabbits excretion of conjugated bilirubin into bile is enhanced by the intravenous (IV) infusion of glucose.[73] The Dubin–Johnson syndrome is caused by a defect in the gene encoding the hepatocyte bilirubin conjugate export pump (MRP2).[74,75] Clearance of bilirubin from the hepatocyte is a saturable process, and after the first week of life appears to be the rate-limiting step in the excretion of bilirubin.[76,77] The transport maximum can be increased by drugs that stimulate bile flow (e.g., barbiturates).[78]

Glucuronosyl Transferase in the Fetus and Newborn

When bilirubin is conjugated with glucuronic acid, the reaction is catalyzed by uridine diphosphoglucuronosyl transferase (UDPGT or UGT, EC 2.4.1.17). Conjugation makes bilirubin water soluble and permits transfer of bilirubin into bile. UGT activity is low at birth but increases to adult values by 1–2 months. As for ligandin, certain drugs (phenobarbital, dexamethasone, clofibrate) increase UGT activity (see below).

The activity of UGT in fetuses has been measured to be 0.1% at 16–32 weeks gestation, increasing to ~1% of adult values at term.[79] Conjugated bile pigments were found in the liver of fetuses with Rhesus incompatibility.[80] Bilirubin-IXα glycosyl conjugates appear in human fetal bile at 20 weeks gestation, while monoglucuronide is first seen 2–3 weeks later.[81] Monoconjugates of bilirubin-IXα are the predominant bilirubins in human fetal bile from around 30 weeks gestation, but only at term do bilirubin-IXα monoconjugates with glucuronic acid, that is, monoglucuronides, constitute the major pigment.[81] In comparison, adult bile contains about 80% bilirubin-IXα diglucuronide and 18% monoglucuronide.[82] Premature birth accelerates the development of UGT activity in human liver.[79] In the first days of life, conjugated bilirubin constitutes <2% of total bile pigment in serum.[83] Diconjugates make up about 20% of the total conjugated fraction in babies, less than half of the estimated >50% in adults.[83]

In the endoplasmic reticulum of the microsomes, UGT catalyzes the binding first of one molecule of glucuronic acid to bilirubin, forming bilirubin monoglucuronide.[78] Human bilirubin UDP-glucuronosyl transferase is a tetramer with molecular weight 209 kD.[84] The monomer can convert UCB to the monoglucuronide, but only the tetramer can convert the monoglucuronide to the diglucuronide.[84] The importance of this process is that the essentially water-insoluble UCB is converted to a water-soluble form, which can be excreted in the bile. Conjugation of bilirubin in the liver is controlled by a gene complex on chromosome 2, at 2q37.[85] Mutations and amino acid substitutions are responsible for genetic errors in bilirubin conjugation such as the Crigler–Najjar

syndrome types I and II, and Gilbert syndrome (see elsewhere in this chapter as well as Chapter 1).

Inducibility of UGT Activity

Giving phenobarbital to pregnant women increases conjugation in the neonate.[86] Therefore, phenobarbital has been used both before and after birth to prevent and/or treat neonatal jaundice.[87] UGT activity is also increased by administration of a thyroid analog,[88] dexamethasone,[89] and clofibrate.[90]

Development of Intrahepatic Transport Proteins

The principal intracellular bilirubin binding protein in the liver is ligandin, a GST.[91] Uptake of bilirubin into hepatocytes seems to increase with increasing concentrations of ligandin.[37] Ligandin has two binding sites for bilirubin, one with high ($K_a = 5 \times 10^7/M$) and one with lower ($K_a = 3 \times 10^5/M$) affinity.[97] The high-affinity site is not the same as the catalytic site, but binding to the low-affinity site is associated with competitive inhibition of the enzymatic activity of ligandin.[92]

The neonate is relatively deficient in ligandin, thus decreasing the ability to retain bilirubin inside the hepatocyte. This may cause bilirubin to reflux into the circulation. The concentration of ligandin in hepatocytes can be increased by pharmacological agents such as phenobarbital.[37] Recent evidence points to the possibility that polymorphisms of the GST gene GSTM1 may affect ligandin functions in hepatocytes, and individuals with the GSTM1-null genotype may have higher TSB levels in the neonatal period.[93]

Enterohepatic Circulation of Bilirubin

In the intestines bilirubin is reduced to colorless tetrapyrroles by microbes in the colon. The infant is born with a sterile gut, and the intestinal microbial flora normally contributes to further breakdown of bilirubin, which is established during the first days and weeks of life. Some deconjugation may occur in the proximal small intestine through β-glucuronidases located in the brush border.[93] UCB can be reabsorbed into the circulation, increasing the total plasma bilirubin pool. This cycle of uptake, conjugation, excretion, deconjugation, and reabsorption is called "enterohepatic circulation" (Figure 5-1). Enterohepatic circulation may be significant in the newborn infant, in part due to limited nutrient intake in the first days of life, which delays intestinal transit. There is also a lack of a binding vehicle in the intestinal lumen to transport bilirubin conjugates through the gut.

In addition, it is thought that in some mother/infant dyads factors in breast milk, which have not been unequivocally identified, may contribute to increased enterohepatic circulation in so-called breast milk–associated jaundice. The risk of breast milk jaundice appears to be increased in infants who have genetic polymorphisms in the coding sequences of the UGT1A1 or OATP2 genes.[94] The mechanisms that cause this phenomenon are still uncertain. However, it appears that supplementation with breast milk substitutes may reduce the degree of breast milk jaundice.[95]

Meconium contains a significant amount of bilirubin, estimated to be about 5–10 times the daily production.[78] Half of this is UCB and thus capable of being reabsorbed. Bilirubin-IXβ is the predominant bile pigment in the first excreted batch of meconium. It decreases subsequently, and is a biochemical marker of meconium, as is zinc coproporphyrin.[96]

Early Feeding, Intestinal Malformations
Enterohepatic circulation is increased by any condition that causes delayed or interrupted passage of intestinal contents. This is evident in intestinal atresias,[97] in infants kept off oral feeds for reasons of severe illness, and in infants receiving inadequate nutrition due to difficulties in establishing lactation ("lack-of-breast milk jaundice"). Conversely, enterohepatic circulation is reduced by establishment of enteral nutrition, by increasing the frequency of feeding,[98] by oral feeding of agar, which binds bilirubin in the gut,[99] and by oral administration of bilirubin oxidase.[100] It should be noted that the latter two treatments must be considered "off-label" and have not been subjected to any approval process of which we are aware.

Delayed passage of meconium has been believed to be associated with hyperbilirubinemia. In a study, 84 healthy term neonates were randomly assigned to a suppository group and a nonsuppository group.[101] The suppositories resulted in earlier evacuation of meconium. However, no significant effect was noted on TSB levels in the first 3 days of life. In another study, early evacuation of meconium through glycerin enemas given within 30 minutes after birth, and 12 hours after birth, had no effect on peak TSB levels or on TSB concentrations in the first 7 days of life.[102] Thus, routine use of suppositories or enemas to decrease TSB levels is unlikely to be effective and cannot be recommended for term healthy neonates.

■ PRESENTATION OF JAUNDICE IN THE NEWBORN

Development of Jaundice in the Newborn
Neonatal *hyperbilirubinemia* affects nearly all newborns, in the sense that TSB levels above the range considered as normal during the remainder of an individual's life cycle are typically present in neonates. Thus, almost all newborn infants will develop a TSB >1.8 mg/dL during the first week of life.[103] Neonatal *jaundice* occurs when TSB increases to a level where the accumulation of bilirubin in skin becomes visible to the unaided eye in daylight conditions (or similar quality artificial light). Such visual detection is possible when TSB exceeds 5–6 mg/dL, but actual detection will vary between observers and depend on lighting conditions. The type of feeding also influences the expected course of jaundice in the neonate. Some infants affected by breast milk jaundice may remain visibly jaundiced for weeks after birth ("breast milk jaundice").

Jaundice typically first becomes visible on the forehead (Figure 5-2A). With time, jaundice moves further down the body.[104] This may be clinically useful because visible jaundice in the hands or feet may suggest a significantly elevated TSB level that one should consider checking by appropriate tests (Figure 5-2B). In most infants, yellow color is the only finding on physical examination, although infants who have pronounced jaundice may be drowsy.

Physiological versus Nonphysiological Jaundice
Textbooks may refer to neonatal jaundice as either *physiological* or *nonphysiological* (or *pathologic*). *Physiological jaundice* is due to the normal occurrences of increased breakdown of RBCs in the presence of a low capacity for uptake, conjugation, and excretion of bilirubin in the liver. Reabsorption of bilirubin from the bowel because of relatively low nutrient intake and reduced intestinal transit in the first days of life must be said to be part of this normal phenomenon. *Nonphysiological* or *pathologic* jaundice refers to situations where hyperbilirubinemia is accentuated by diseases or conditions such as genetic variations, leading, for example, to increased hemolysis or reduced excretion of bilirubin (or both combined). It is important to note that there is often not a clear-cut distinction between physiological and pathologic jaundice in newborns. Each of the normal mechanisms that produce hyperbilirubinemia may

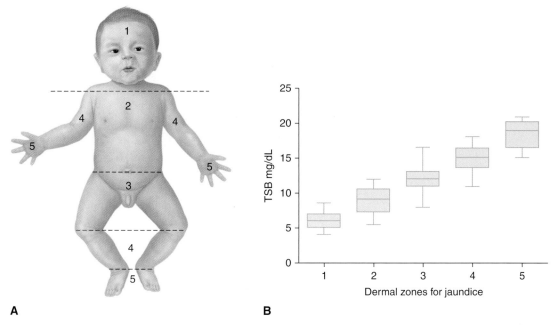

FIGURE 5-2. Zones of dermal jaundice. A. Location of dermal jaundice zones 1–5. **B.** Box and whisker plots of relation between TSB values and dermal jaundice zones 1–5. (Based on recalculated data abstracted from Kramer.[104])

be affected. A priori an infant with a very high serum bilirubin level is more likely to have a pathologic cause contributing to his or her jaundice than an infant with a low serum bilirubin level, but a simple measurement of serum bilirubin is not enough to ascertain this. From a didactic perspective we have found it helpful to compare this situation with measuring the height of a mountain that is topped by an ice cap. The measurement obtained at the summit will not tell you how many meters (or feet) is contributed by the rock (i.e., "physiology") and how many by ice (i.e., "pathology").

■ CLINICAL AND LABORATORY EVALUATION OF JAUNDICE IN THE NEWBORN

Physiological Jaundice

As mentioned, jaundice is a very common phenomenon in neonates, and a frequent reason for clinical concern and investigation. In a study of 490 term and near-term infants from a racially diverse background, 80% of infants were found to have TSB concentrations greater

than 5 mg/dL.[105] This is approximately the value at which the human eye can detect jaundice due to unconjugated hyperbilirubinemia by looking at the skin. In contrast, as shown in Figure 5-3, conjugated hyperbilirubinemia,

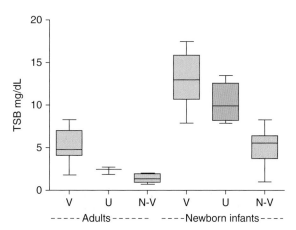

FIGURE 5-3. Visual identification of jaundice. Box and whisker plots of relationship between visible (V), uncertain (U), and not visible (N-V) dermal jaundice and TSB values in adults and infants. (Recalculated from data from With.[106])

such as in cholestatic jaundice in the adult, is readily detected at levels as low as 1.8 mg/dL.[106]

Most surveys of the range of normal TSB levels in North American newborns identify peak TSB in normal newborns to be 14–15 mg/dL at the third to fifth days of life. It has been estimated that bilirubin production in the neonate is about 8.5 mg/kg per day,[12] equaling 30 mg per day (50 μmol per day) in a 3.5-kg term infant. Thus, if no bilirubin conjugation and excretion took place, 90 mg (150 μmol) of bilirubin would have accumulated in the body at day 3 of life. If we assume that albumin-bound UCB distributes only in the plasma volume, peak TSB levels in these infants would readily reach 64 mg/dL on average instead of the usual normal peak value of 15 mg/dL. This suggests that the liver of the newborn infant, in spite of decreased ability to take up, conjugate, and excrete bilirubin, is still able to dispose most of the bilirubin produced in the early neonatal period.

Initial Assessment of the Jaundiced Newborn

When presentation of jaundice occurs during the first 24 hours of life or later than days 3–4 of life, it is likely that factors in addition to those involved in the normal physiological adaptation of the newborn may contribute. This is discussed further in section "Jaundice as a Sign of Disease."

The diagnosis of jaundice in a newborn typically begins with the mother or caregivers recognizing the yellow color of the infant's skin. Targeted screening has, however, become more common, and has been recommended in guidelines.[107–109] Jaundice in the neonate is first visible in the face and forehead, but can be difficult to assess in polycythemic infants or in infants with a reddish or dark hue. Pressure on the skin helps to reveal the underlying color. However, visual inspection might not be reliable for assessing the degree of jaundice as pointed out in several studies.[110–112]

In most infants, yellow color is the only finding on physical examination, although infants who have pronounced jaundice may also appear drowsy and feed poorly. When called upon to assess a newborn infant for jaundice, the physician should consider whether: (i) the infant looks generally healthy; (ii) it is necessary to measure a TSB level; (iii) treatment is indicated, and (iv) elements in the history or physical examination suggest that nonphysiological factors may contribute to jaundice (see section "Jaundice as a Sign of Disease").

Measurement of Bilirubin

If an infant appears more than mildly jaundiced by visual inspection, an objective measurement of a TSB level should be measured. In most infants who develop a moderate jaundice on second or third day of life, and without any history and/or physical findings suggestive of a pathologic process, a TSB measurement is the only necessary test. Bilirubin can be measured noninvasively in the skin by transcutaneous bilirubinometry (TcB). This technique is commonly used as a screening instrument to decide whether there is a need to measure TSB.[113]

Measurement of TSB is necessary for determining whether therapy should be instituted since therapeutic guidelines mostly refer to TSB values. Measurement of TcB using handheld devices performs better than visual assessment. In the presence of apparently mild jaundice, this may be sufficient to assure that TSB levels are safely below intervention levels. In a recent study of a 1-year cohort of infants in a normal newborn nursery, blood tests for TSB determinations were performed in 598 (16.4%) of 3648 infants,[114] and phototherapy was instituted in 45% of infants tested.

It is well known that measurement of TSB in a routine clinical setting represents a challenge. The test results can be significantly affected by the technique for blood sampling, transport time, and conditions, as well as the analytical method.[115] Recent studies indicate, however, that variation in analytical quality of TSB measurements within and between hospitals is acceptable, and does not represent a critical factor in the diagnosis and treatment of jaundiced newborn infants.[116]

Although it has been shown that TcB correlates relatively well with TSB, the difference between these two measurements can be significant in individual infants[109] (Figure 5-4). It has therefore been recommended that infants with a TcB within 2.9 mg/dL of treatment indication or with a TcB >14.6 mg/dL should have TSB measured before treatment is evaluated.[117] Since it has been shown that TcB measurements can be inaccurate in infants with darkly pigmented skin, it is also recommended that TSB should be measured routinely in such infants around 24 hours of age. It should also be emphasized that TcB is not useful during and in the first hours after phototherapy has been discontinued due to fading of the skin.

Measurement of conjugated bilirubin in serum is not necessary in most infants. However, in the presence of an enlarged liver or spleen, petechiae, thrombocytopenia, or other findings suggesting liver or biliary

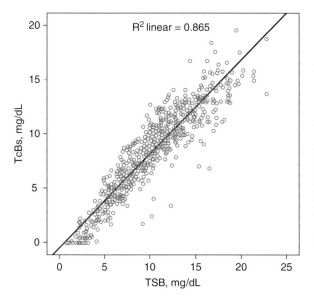

FIGURE 5-4. Correlation between total serum bilirubin (TSB) and transcutaneous bilirubin (TcB) measurements. TSB and TcB (mg/dL) was measured simultaneously (within 1 hour) in infants in normal newborn nursery. TcB was measured at the sternum.

disease, metabolic disease, or congenital infection, bilirubin fractions should be measured. Measurement of the conjugated bilirubin fraction is also indicated in infants who remain jaundiced beyond the first 2 weeks of life and infants whose TSB levels repeatedly rebound following treatment.

From a methodological point of view, conjugated bilirubin is not a precise term. This is partly due to the fact that both monoglucuronides and diglucuronides as well as other conjugates are produced.[118] There are also several different methods available for bilirubin determinations, which include or exclude different bilirubin conjugates.[118,119] However, in clinical use determination of so-called direct-reacting bilirubin is often used as a substitute for conjugated bilirubin. When obtaining separate values for UCB and conjugated bilirubin is desirable, the value for direct-reacting bilirubin (conjugated bilirubin) is subtracted from the total bilirubin to give the value for UCB. However, this is also not very precise, since the delta fraction of UCB will be included in the measurement of direct-reacting bilirubin.[120] Thus, even in a strictly unconjugated hyperbilirubinemia, a significant fraction of the TSB will be determined as conjugated bilirubin. Studies in newborn infants with

erythroblastosis indicate that a direct-reacting fraction of 5–10% of the TSB should be considered normal, and not indicative of any increase in conjugated bilirubin in the sample.[118] Situations in which additional laboratory studies may be indicated are further discussed in section "Jaundice as a Sign of Disease."

Bilirubin toxicity is related to the nonalbumin-bound or "free" bilirubin. Since several physiological substances and conditions as well as drugs might displace bilirubin from albumin,[33,34,121] the concentration of unbound bilirubin often does not correspond to TSB.[28,122,123] The concentration of unbound bilirubin is, however, rarely measured in the clinical setting. This is mainly due to methodology not suited for routine analysis. An important step in improving treatment indications and the prevention of bilirubin toxicity in the newborn would be to develop a methodology suitable for routine clinical use.

Assessment of the Jaundiced Infant at Discharge

When an infant is about to be discharged, the American Academy of Pediatrics (AAP) recommends a risk assessment as far as development of jaundice.[107] This may consist of a measurement of TcB or TSB, with plotting of the TcB/TSB value on a nomogram for hour-specific values. The nomogram recommended by the AAP is shown in Figure 2-8. An infant whose hour-specific bilirubin value is in the low-risk zone of the nomogram is at low risk of developing severe jaundice after discharge. Recently published Norwegian guidelines recommend that all infants discharged before 24–48 hours of age should be screened with measurement of TcB or TSB.[117] Infants with a TSB less than 1.8 mg/dL below treatment indication should be seen again. In Norway this is usually done in connection with return to the hospital for the routine metabolic screen at 60–72 hours of age.[124] Parents of infants with identified risk factors for hyperbilirubinemia (large cephalhematoma, previous sibling treated for jaundice, late preterm infants, Asian ethnicity) should be given written information about jaundice in the newborn as well as oral and written information to return to the maternity ward if the infant becomes more jaundiced and/or feeds poorly. When parents call on the phone with such problems, the situation should not be discussed over the phone, but be told that the infant needs to be seen at the hospital immediately.

Assessment of Infants Readmitted for Prolonged Jaundice

The most common cause of prolonged jaundice in newborn infants is probably so-called breast milk–associated jaundice.[125] In the absence of specific diagnostic tests, the diagnosis of breast milk–associated jaundice can only be presumptive, and more serious conditions need to be ruled out, as discussed in section "Jaundice as a Sign of Disease." Follow-up must be close with careful instruction of the parents. Interruption of breastfeeding for 24–48 hours and/or feeding with breast milk substitutes may help to reduce the TSB level. Supplementing breast milk feeds with 5 mL of a breast milk substitute also reduces the level and duration of jaundice in breast milk–fed infants.[95] Because this latter intervention causes less interference with the establishment of the breastfeeding dyad, this approach tends to be our first step.

When jaundice continues beyond the first 2 weeks of life, obtaining the lactation/nutrition history is a first priority since hypogalactia and dehydration of the infant may play a role. The infant's weight curve should be evaluated. Delay to regain birth weight may be associated with prolongation of jaundice through increased enterohepatic circulation of bilirubin. The mother's impressions as far as adequacy of her breastfeeding may be erroneous, particularly in primiparous women.

The family history should also be explored. The risk of breast milk jaundice appears to be increased in infants who have genetic polymorphisms in the coding sequences of the UGT1A1 or OATP2 genes; prolonged and/or pronounced jaundice in older siblings may also be significant, and may suggest Gilbert syndrome.[126] The result of the newborn metabolic screening for congenital hypothyroidism and galactosemia, if that condition is included in the screening program, should be checked. A gray/whitish stool may suggest intrahepatic or extrahepatic biliary atresia. The threshold should be low for ordering supplementary studies as outlined in section "Jaundice as a Sign of Disease."

■ PHARMACOLOGICAL DANGERS IN TREATMENT OF JAUNDICED INFANTS

The Role of Drugs that Act as Binding Competitors

An epidemic of kernicterus, which occurred in the 1950s when sulfonamides were used for infection prophylaxis in newborn nurseries, led to the recognition that kernicterus in these infants was caused by the drug displacing bilirubin from its binding to albumin.[127] Since then, several other drugs have also been shown to compete with bilirubin for the binding site on albumin.[128,129] Some stabilizers used with IV drugs may also cause bilirubin displacement.[130,131] Therefore, all drugs to be used in sick infants should be tested for their ability to displace bilirubin from its binding to albumin; any drug that has this characteristic must be avoided, at least as long as TSB levels remain significantly elevated.

Recent data on ibuprofen, a drug used to close the ductus arteriosus in preterm infants and approved as an orphan drug on the European market for this purpose, provide worrisome evidence that bilirubin displacement is not taken seriously enough at present. Thus, ibuprofen may be a competitive displacer of bilirubin in vitro and should therefore be used with caution in premature infants with significant hyperbilirubinemia.[132–134] Soligard et al. found that ibuprofen showed a competitive displacement of bilirubin from albumin and increased the dissociation constant of the bilirubin–albumin complex from 3.9×10^{-8} to 9.9×10^{-8} M.[134]

Theoretically, free fatty acids have the ability to displace bilirubin from albumin.[135] For this reason, there has been some concern regarding the use of lipid solutions in total parental nutrition. When lipid doses are less than 1 g/kg, the effect is not significant,[136] and it may even enhance the effect of phototherapy.[137]

The Role of Drugs with Other Mechanisms of Action

More recent data have further suggested that some drugs used in jaundiced infants, and which do not affect bilirubin binding, may nevertheless increase the risk of bilirubin neurotoxicity. Posphoglycoprotein P (PGP) may play a role in restricting the entry of bilirubin into the brain.[138,139] PGP, when expressed in cancer cells, limits the entry of several cytostatic drugs into these cells, and seems to confer increased resistance to such drugs.[140–142] The fact that PGP function may be inhibited or downregulated by a number of commonly used drugs has therefore excited interest among oncologists. Similarly, drugs that are used in the neonate, which are tested for bilirubin displacement, may also need to be tested for their effect on PGP. One important example is the drug ceftriaxone, which is *both* a PGP inhibitor and a bilirubin displacer;

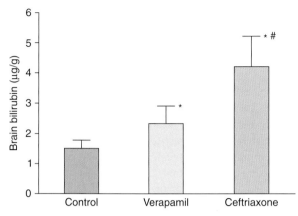

FIGURE 5-5. Brain bilirubin and posphoglycoprotein P. Brain bilirubin values from rats given an IV bolus of bilirubin after administration of verapamil (a PGP inhibitor) or ceftriaxone (both a PGP inhibitor and a bilirubin displacer). (*) $P < .05$ compared with controls; (#) $P < .05$ compared with verapamil. (Based on data recalculated from Hankø.[138])

it is therefore particularly potent for increasing bilirubin entry into the brain (Figure 5-5).[138] This issue clearly requires further research.

MRP1 mediates the ATP-dependent cellular export of bilirubin, appears to play a role as far as protecting cells from bilirubin toxicity,[143] and can be inhibited by a number of drugs.[144] Inhibitors of PGP also appear able to inhibit MRP1.[144]

The Role of Herbal/Traditional Medicine

Herbal medicines are commonly used in some countries and population groups. Yin et al. studied the impact of *yin zhi huang*, a decoction of four plants, which is widely used in Asia to treat neonatal jaundice, on induction of hepatic drug and bilirubin-metabolizing enzymes in rats.[145] The effect of the individual constituents of the decoction was compared with that of phenobarbital, a well-known inducer. *Artemisia*, *Rheum*, and phenobarbital increased UGT activity. Phenobarbital was the most effective inducer of GST activity. Both phenobarbital and gardenia induced delta 5-3-ketosteroid isomerase activity, a marker for the Ya subunit of GST, responsible for intracellular bilirubin transport in liver. Thus, the possibility that there may be some benefits in treating neonatal jaundice with these plant extracts cannot be ruled out, although safety studies would clearly be required.

On the other hand, Yeung et al.[146] studied Chinese goldthread (*Coptis chinensis*), also commonly given to newborn infants in China. This herb, which is taken as a tea, was shown to have a significant effect in displacing bilirubin from its albumin binding. The authors strongly caution against the use of this herb in southern Chinese neonates, where neonatal jaundice is very common. Other Chinese herbal drugs (purified constituents LZX-A, QTJ, YHS, and SQZG) were, however, without displacing properties.[147]

Can Hyperbilirubinemia Impact Drug Therapy?

While it is well established that drug therapy in jaundiced infants requires caution because of the risk of both increased brain bilirubin entry secondary to binding competition and inhibition of membrane pumps, the question of whether jaundice can affect drug therapy has not been well studied. Although it has been shown that significant jaundice (TSB >11.7 mg/dL) can delay gastric emptying,[148] whether this has any impact on the absorption or metabolism of drugs administered enterally can at present only be speculated. Similarly, the possible effect on drug absorption of the secretory diarrhea observed in jaundiced infants receiving phototherapy[149] appears not to have been studied. The normal increase in blood flow to the bowel seen postprandially in infants is blunted during phototherapy for neonatal jaundice.[150] This might also theoretically influence the absorption of drugs given by mouth, but no studies addressing this question appear to be on record. Finally, when drugs and bilirubin compete for binding to serum albumin, depending on the specificity and competitive nature of binding, conceivably free drug concentrations might be increased.

■ BILIRUBIN–BRAIN INTERACTION

After more than 50 years of research into the mechanisms of bilirubin-induced neurological dysfunction (BIND), the specific nature of this phenomenon remains elusive.[151] Experimentally, bilirubin has diverse toxic, intracellular effects, which in vitro have appeared to be mainly inhibitory. It has been suggested that the diversity of effects might be understood in terms of inhibition of a common regulatory mechanism such as protein phosphorylation.[151] However, McDonagh has recently proposed that bilirubin may be a so-called promiscuous inhibitor, cautioning that effects observed in vitro may be nonspecific and not related to in vivo mechanism(s) of toxicity.[152] "Promiscuous inhibitors" have high hydrophobicity, high molecular flexibility, and the ability to form microaggregates, properties also shared by bilirubin. For a more detailed discussion of these vexing problems, please see Chapter 7.

For bilirubin to affect the brain, it must gain entry. Different conditions and mechanisms for bilirubin entry into the brain are shown in Figure 5-6. The chemistry and solubility characteristics of bilirubin may to some extent explain how this happens. The main bilirubin isomer, bilirubin-IXα (Z,Z), may occur as a charged dianion or as bilirubin acid. The dianion has some water solubility

at neutral pH, whereas the acid, due to intramolecular hydrogen bonds, is nearly insoluble in water.[14,23] It has been believed that the hydrophobic isomer is responsible for the toxic effects, while the water-soluble isomers are thought to be nontoxic.[153,154] However, there are weaknesses in the experimental approaches to these questions, and the issue cannot be said to be fully resolved.

Bilirubin-IXα (Z,Z) is an amphipathic molecule, but is lipophilic with respect to membranes (i.e., it crosses phospholipid membranes).[155,156] It is assumed that this characteristic enables bilirubin to cross an intact blood–brain barrier and enter the brain. The serum to brain bilirubin gradient with an intact blood–brain barrier is

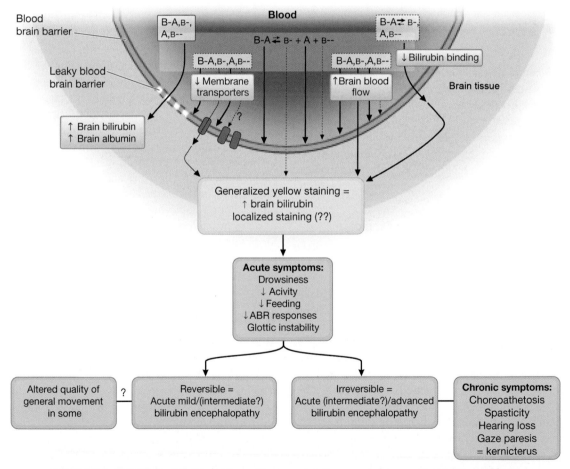

FIGURE 5-6. Bilirubin–brain interaction. Diagram showing mechanisms of bilirubin entry into brain, acute symptoms, and chronic sequelae. B, bilirubin; A, albumin; B-A, albumin-bound bilirubin; B-, bilirubin acid; B--, bilirubin dianion.

considerable; the brain bilirubin concentration in study animals is only 1–2% of their TSB concentration,[157,158] much less than would be expected for, for example, a lipophilic drug. However, it seems that specific barrier mechanisms may be responsible for maintaining a lower than expected concentration of bilirubin in the brain. PGP is an ATP-dependent plasma membrane efflux pump, expressed inter alia in the blood–brain barrier, and is thought to have a role in protecting the organism against potentially toxic compounds.[141] Watchko et al. have shown that mutant mice who were deficient in PGP had significantly increased brain bilirubin concentrations following an IV bolus of bilirubin when compared with control mice with normal PGP expression.[139]

Bilirubin bound to albumin probably does not cross the blood–brain barrier as long as this is intact.[159-161] According to the "free bilirubin theory" it is the unbound bilirubin molecule that enters the brain to produce neuronal injury.[162] Increased concentrations of unbound bilirubin in the blood will shift more bilirubin into the tissues, including the brain. Factors that cause increased concentrations of unbound bilirubin may include altered albumin characteristics[163] and the presence of exogenous or endogenous binding competitors.[29]

Blood–Brain Barrier

The blood–brain barrier in neonates may be more permeable to bilirubin than that of more mature subjects, whereas albumin permeability is equally restricted in young and old subjects.[164,165] The concept of an "immature" blood–brain barrier seems supported by data on PGP function.[140] The blood–brain barrier is functionally closed to albumin, and consequently also to albumin-bound bilirubin. However, any condition that involves increased permeability of the blood–brain barrier may cause increased[159,160,166] and/or prolonged exposure of the brain to bilirubin.[159] Such conditions include hyperosmolarity, hypercarbia, hypoxia, asphyxia, and acidosis. Hypoxia may also increase the risk of kernicterus via blood–brain barrier permeability.[167] Whether this should influence the management of jaundice in infants with cyanotic congenital heart disease is not clear. Hyperoxia was proposed as a risk factor for kernicterus but has not been verified experimentally.[168]

When conditions that affect blood–brain barrier integrity are present in a jaundiced neonate, it is prudent to institute treatment at lower TSB levels. Thus, in our

Norwegian national guidelines for management of neonatal jaundice intervention levels are reduced by 3 mg/dL in sick infants.[117]

In vitro studies have suggested that bilirubin affects membrane function and permeability.[169,170] Bilirubin toxicity to glial cells might also translate into effects on barrier function.[171,172] Some studies have addressed bilirubin effects on the blood–brain barrier directly; preexposure to bilirubin increased the permeability of the blood–brain barrier to a dye[173] and to bilirubin itself.[165]

Brain Blood Flow

The impact of brain blood flow on bilirubin entry into the brain is illustrated by the studies of hypercarbia, which increases brain blood flow.[174,175] In experimental animals increased brain blood flow increases bilirubin entry into brain. A speculation is that with increased brain blood flow, each circulating bilirubin molecule passes the blood–brain barrier more often and has more opportunities to equilibrate with bilirubin in the brain.

Bilirubin Metabolism in the Brain

Bilirubin that enters the brain is also cleared from the brain. Levine et al. estimated the half-life of bilirubin in brain to be 1.7 hours.[176] Other studies have shown a more rapid clearance, with a half-life of 16–18 minutes in rat brain.[158,159] A meta-analysis of data from several rat studies showed that clearance from brain was more rapid than from blood, suggesting that mechanisms in addition to transport across the blood–brain barrier might influence bilirubin kinetics in brain.[177]

Brodersen and Bartels studied an enzyme capable of oxidizing bilirubin, and which could be found inter alia on the inner mitochondrial membrane of brain cells.[178] Further studies of this enzyme have shown that it shares some of the characteristics of the cytochrome oxidases, but it has not been fully identified.[179] The activity was found to be lower in immature versus mature brain, and lower in neurons versus glia, as well as subject to genetic variability. More studies will be necessary to elucidate the role, if any, of this enzyme on modulation of brain bilirubin toxicity.

The Role of Infection/Septicemia

Intervention limits for jaundice are commonly lowered in infants who are infected or otherwise appear ill.[180] Infection is believed to increase the risk for BIND.[181] Both clinical and laboratory data point to increased risk for BIND in infants who appear ill or have significant physiological abnormality.[123,181,182] The mechanisms behind this elevated risk are not clear. Thus, in animal experiments neither infection nor endotoxemia significantly affected the entry of bilirubin into the brain.[183] Nevertheless, it appears prudent to be vigilant when managing jaundice in infants with suspected or confirmed infection.

What is a Neurotoxic Bilirubin Level?

The "basic mechanism" of kernicterus and BIND remains an enigma. Even the apparently simple question about the level of TSB at which one should intervene with therapy is answered by "expert opinion" more than scientific data.[107] In fact, there is not a single, simple TSB level that is safe for every newborn. There are probably interindividual differences in vulnerability to BIND of which we are currently ignorant. Some term or near-term infants appear to tolerate TSB levels of up to 29.2–35.1 mg/dL without harm,[68,184,185] while others may suffer permanent damage at much lower levels.[184,186–188] Thus, every jaundiced newborn must be evaluated individually, paying attention to circumstances that point to increased risk or decreased tolerance.

Any experimental animal with significant unconjugated hyperbilirubinemia has bilirubin in its brain.[138,160,166,183] Changes in neurophysiological function (e.g., decreased amplitudes in the auditory brainstem response [ABR]) did not translate into permanent damage of neurons.[189] Similarly, changes in the ABRs of jaundiced infants were reversed after lowering the TSB.[190] Therefore, measuring ABRs or other neurophysiological functions in jaundiced infants does not help us decide on clinical management of these infants.

In practical terms, an infant who has both a low risk of developing significant jaundice and low vulnerability to BIND is probably at very low risk of kernicterus. Conversely, an infant at high risk of severe jaundice and with high vulnerability to BIND should be managed with the assumption that he or she is at high risk of kernicterus. Risk factors for development of severe jaundice and for neurotoxicity are listed in Table 5-1.

Reversibility of Bilirubin Effects on Brain

Mild ABE should be reversible with treatment. However, the intermediate to advanced acute stages have hitherto been considered largely irreversible.[191] This impression is tempered by recent data, which suggest that reversibility may be possible in some such infants who have been treated aggressively and urgently.[63] The specific circumstances or individual characteristics that allow such reversal remain to be characterized. Whether neuronal death by bilirubin toxicity is the end point of a continuum in which the earlier stages are characterized by clinical somnolence and electrophysiological changes, or whether cell death is an all-or-none phenomenon, which has no relation to these processes, remains an open question. The clinical challenge in risk evaluation of the individual infant is probably the presence of a concentration range of TSB where all outcomes are possible (Figure 5-7).

■ BILIRUBIN AS AN ANTIOXIDANT

Biochemical Evidence of Antioxidative Effects of Bilirubin

Development of ABE in the newborn and later BIND in survivors has designated bilirubin as a toxic waste product.[192] However, the fact that hyperbilirubinemia is physiological and seen in all newborn infants suggests that bilirubin might also have a positive function in the organism.

On this background, researchers have long been looking for a physiologically useful role for bilirubin. HO has been shown to be induced by a number of conditions known to represent oxidative stress.[193,194] Also, more than 50 years ago, German researchers showed that bilirubin protected against oxidation of fatty acids and vitamin A.[195] Later research has confirmed that bilirubin is an effective scavenger of free oxygen radicals, and equally effective as α-tocopherol and vitamin E, which are regarded as the best antioxidants in the body.[70] Bilirubin concentrations in serum (μmol/L) are high enough to account for a substantial part of the antioxidant effect of serum, particularly in the newborn period.[196] Intracellular and tissue concentrations of bilirubin are, however, very low (nmol/L) and related to the concentration of unbound bilirubin. It has nevertheless been shown that nanomolar concentrations of bilirubin are sufficient to protect hippocampal and cortical neuronal cells from toxic effects of a 10,000-fold molar increase of H_2O_2.[197] It has therefore been suggested that the antioxidant activity of bilirubin is related to a biliverdin reductase antioxidant cycle.[71] In this cycle, lipophilic oxygen radicals react directly with bilirubin and oxidize bilirubin to biliverdin. NADPH/biliverdin reductase then catalyzes the reduction of biliverdin

■ TABLE 5-1. Risk Factors for Severe Jaundice and Bilirubin Neurotoxicity in Term and Preterm Infants

Risk for Neonatal Jaundice	Risk for Bilirubin Neurotoxicity

Significantly increased risk for jaundice
 • Family history
   • Phototherapy given to older sibling
   • Known Gilbert syndrome in family
   • Known hemolytic disease in family
   • East Asian ethnicity
 • Preterm (including late preterm) infant
 • Jaundice noted on the first day of life
 • Blood group incompatibility
 • Extravasation of blood (cephalhematoma, fractures, bruising)
 • Exclusive breastfeeding with or without excessive weight loss
 • TSB or TcB level at discharge is in the high-risk zone (Figure 2-8)
	Significantly increased risk for neurotoxicity
	 • Prematurity
	 • Hemolysis
	 • Sick infant
	   • Acidosis (respiratory or metabolic)
	   • Infection
	   • Asphyxia
	   • Reduced bilirubin–albumin binding
	 • Immature albumin (as in prematurity)
	 • Binding competitors
	   • Bilirubin displacement by certain drugs
	   • Bilirubin displacement by endogenous substances (i.v. lipids >1–2 g/kg)
	 • More permeable blood–brain barrier
	   • Hypercapnia (increased brain blood flow)
	   • Hyperosmolality (hypernatremia, hyperglycemia)
	 • Interference with membrane transporters
	   • Inhibition of P-glycoprotein (certain drugs)

Moderately increased risk for jaundice
 • Family and pregnancy history
   • Older sibling jaundiced but no phototherapy
   • Macrosomic infant of a diabetic mother
   • Maternal age ≥25 years
   • Gestational age 37–38 weeks
   • Male gender
 • Jaundice observed before discharge or predischarge TSB or TcB level in the high intermediate-risk zone (Figure 2-8)	

Decreased risk for significant jaundice[a] • Gestational age >41 weeks • African ethnicity • Exclusive bottle feeding • Discharge from hospital after 72 h • TSB or TcB level at discharge in the low-risk zone (Figure 2-8)	

[a]When factors indicating lower risk coexist with factors indicating increased risk, individual assessment in needed and caution is advised.

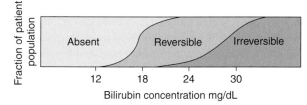

FIGURE 5-7. Reversibility of bilirubin toxicity. Schematic presentation of the association between bilirubin concentrations and outcome, as no toxicity, reversible toxicity, and irreversible toxicity. Note the presence of a concentration range where all outcomes are possible.

back to bilirubin, and the speed of the reactions in this cycle permits bilirubin to detoxify a 10,000-fold excess of oxidants. The experimental basis for this hypothesis has, however, recently been questioned.[198]

Antioxidative Effects of Bilirubin in Adult Diseases

Several studies in adults have confirmed that high normal TSB levels might be protective in different conditions. In a study with more than 10,000 cancer patients, higher TSB levels were associated with lower risk of death.[199] Reduced risk of ischemic heart disease has also been shown in individuals with increased TSB concentrations.[200,201] It has also been shown that patients with Gilbert syndrome who have moderately elevated TSB levels have significantly reduced risk for coronary artery disease compared with normal controls, and this was not related to the genetic mutations but to TSB levels.[202] Recent studies on a similar population have, however, not been able to confirm a reduced incidence of myocardial infarction in individuals with Gilbert syndrome.[203]

Bilirubin as an Antioxidant in the Newborn

There is also evidence that mildly to moderately elevated TSB levels in the newborn are associated with better outcome in diseases involving oxidative stress. In a study of infants with five illnesses thought to enhance free radical production, mean TSB rise was significantly lower in the combined illness group than in the control group.[204] The authors concluded that the findings confirmed the hypothesis that bilirubin is consumed in vivo as an antioxidant.

Most studies relating protective effects of bilirubin to specific diseases have focused on retinopathy of prematurity (ROP). Several studies have not been able to find a protective effect of bilirubin on the development of ROP,[205–208] while others have confirmed such an association.[209,210] In a recent study on the association between breast milk, hyperbilirubinemia, and ROP, a significantly reduced incidence of ROP was found in hyperbilirubinemic infants, OR = 0.82 per 1 mg/dL change in TSB concentration, 95% confidence interval = 0.66, 1.01.[211] No association between breast milk feeding and ROP was found.

The somewhat conflicting findings regarding the protective effects of bilirubin in the clinical setting are difficult to evaluate. In the normal newborn, the greatest oxidative stress is probably seen in the first neonatal hours, when TSB levels are low. Significant hyperbilirubinemia is usually seen only from the second to the seventh day of life when oxidative stress should be less. Further studies on the antioxidant effects of bilirubin in the newborn are therefore needed. The results might have significant impact on treatment strategies for hyperbilirubinemia, particularly in the extremely premature infant.

■ JAUNDICE IN THE VERY PREMATURE INFANT

Several developmental and clinical characteristics of jaundice in the premature infant differ from term or near-term newborns. First, bilirubin production is increased due to increased hemolysis and increased HO activity. Second, biliary excretion of bilirubin is reduced in premature infants compared with term infants as a result of reduced ligandin and reduced UGT activity in hepatocytes (see sections "Bilirubin Production in the Fetus and Newborn" and "Transport and Excretion of Bilirubin in the Fetus and Newborn"). As a consequence of increased production and decreased biliary excretion of bilirubin, jaundice in premature infants reaches significantly higher levels and lasts longer than in term infants. Since enteral feeding often is delayed in very premature infants, increased enterohepatic circulation of bilirubin might also add to this. Many premature infants are still clearly jaundiced at 2 weeks of age, and might even be jaundiced at 6 weeks of age, a time where jaundice would normally be considered a sign of disease (see section "Jaundice as a Sign of Disease").

Bilirubin toxicity is related to the concentration of unbound bilirubin. Since serum albumin concentrations increase throughout gestation, the concentration of unbound bilirubin is inversely related to gestational age.[27] Also, sick infants have significantly higher levels of unbound bilirubin.[122,123] Experimental data also suggest that the blood–brain barrier is more permeable to bilirubin in more immature subjects.[140,164] The ability of brain cells to metabolize bilirubin also increases with maturation.

As immature organisms seem to have increased risk for bilirubin toxicity, most treatment guidelines advocate start of phototherapy at lower TSB concentrations.[117,180] As a result of this, premature infants rarely reach TSB levels previously seen and normally accepted in term or near-term infants. Thus, in a national cohort study of extremely premature infants (gestational age 22^0–27^6 weeks and/or birth weight 500–999 g), 85% of infants received phototherapy and no significant difference in peak TSB concentrations was found in relation to birth weight or gestational age.[212] Mean peak TSB levels were 10.3 ± 2.5 mg/dL and TSB levels ≥14.6 mg/dL were seen in only 4.3% of infants. Mean duration of TSB ≥11.7 mg/dL was only 1.9 ± 1.7 days and showed no relation to gestational age.

Interestingly, ABO blood group immunization in this cohort was diagnosed in only one infant (0.3%).[212] This might indicate that ABO immunization is significantly underdiagnosed in extremely premature infants. Another possibility is that erythrocyte A and B antigens are significantly less expressed in very immature infants. The study also revealed that peak TSB concentrations were significantly reduced by maternal prenatal steroid treatment ($P < .05$), while initial postnatal acidosis increased peak TSB concentrations.

Kernicterus has been reported at very low TSB levels in premature infants,[213] and premature infants are generally considered to be at increased risk for BIND, particularly with respect to adverse neurodevelopmental outcome. However, as reviewed by Watchko and Maisels not all studies have been able to confirm hyperbilirubinemia as a significant risk factor for adverse outcome in premature infants.[214] More recent studies seem to challenge this view.[215,216] In these studies, both increased peak TSB concentrations and peak unbound bilirubin concentrations were directly correlated with adverse neurodevelopmental outcome and death. Furthermore, adverse outcome in relation to TSB concentrations was more frequent in unstable than in stable infants. While moderate hyperbilirubinemia in the premature infant might to some extent be protective due to its antioxidant effect, there is little doubt that high TSB levels are toxic in the premature infant.

Although the guidelines for treatment of term infants, which are largely empirically based, result in considerable overtreatment of healthy newborns, they seem to do well in preventing BIND and kernicterus.[117] Treatment guidelines for premature infants are even less evidence based than for term infants,[117] and differ considerably nationally as well as internationally.[117,180,217] A balance between overtreatment and preventive treatment is probably even more important than in the term infant. Development of more evidence-based treatment guidelines for these vulnerable infants should therefore have high priority.

■ JAUNDICE AS A SIGN OF DISEASE

Moderately increased early jaundice or moderately prolonged later jaundice is often related to infant feeding.[125] It is also well known that infants of diabetic mothers might have significantly early and increased jaundice. Extravasation of blood such as in cephalhematomas and bruising is accompanied by increased RBC lysis and higher bilirubin production, which also often results in exaggeration of the physiological jaundice. However, when significant jaundice occurs very early, particularly during the first 24 hours of life, or reaches significantly higher levels than usually seen, it is likely that factors in addition to those involved in the normal physiology or mentioned above may contribute.

Jaundice in the Early Neonatal Period

Immune Hemolytic Disease

The most common cause of marked early jaundice is blood group incompatibilities between the mother and infant leading to hemolytic disease of the newborn (HDN).[218] After the introduction in the 1970s of routine prophylactic postnatal treatment of RhD-negative women with anti-D immunoglobulin, this condition as a cause of neonatal disease has been reduced dramatically.[218] As a result, ABO incompatibility is now the most common cause of HDN in industrialized countries. Affected neonates will usually be direct antiglobulin test (DAT) positive, but, in contrast with the clinical picture with anti-Rh antibodies, ABO HDN rarely causes significant anemia because neonatal RBCs have relatively few group A or B antigenic sites, allowing the antibody-coated cells to remain in the circulation for a longer period than in RhD disease. HDN due to ABO immunization is therefore usually diagnosed by a rapidly increasing jaundice shortly after birth in an otherwise healthy infant and is, in most cases, successfully treated with phototherapy alone. However, close monitoring of the affected neonate is essential, and exchange transfusion is occasionally required. Studies have shown that ABO HDN due to anti-B IgG seems to be more aggressive than anti-A IgG.[219] Racial differences with a more severe disease in mothers and neonates of black African origin have also been reported.[218]

In all infants with marked early jaundice ABO immunization should be considered. Determination of ABO blood group as well as a DAT (Coombs') test should therefore be performed on all infants with early onset of jaundice. If an infant has blood group A or B or a positive DAT, the blood group of the mother should be determined if not already known. If the mother has blood group O and a positive DAT, the jaundice can be diagnosed as an ABO isoimmunization. However, in several cases, the DAT might be negative even in the presence of high levels of anti-A or -B hemolysins.[219] If the clinical picture is compatible with an isoimmunization, determination of the level of anti-A or -B hemolysins should be performed in order to make a definite diagnosis. If there is no evidence of ABO incompatibility, HDN due to minor blood groups (Rh c, Rh E, Kell, Kidd, Lewis, and Duffy or others) should be considered.[220]

Nonimmune Hemolytic Disorders

Nonimmune hemolytic disorders may also cause increased neonatal jaundice.[218] This could be due to genetic mutations of RBC enzymes such as glucose-6-phosphate dehydrogenase (G6PD) deficiency, which is common in infants of African or Mediterranean ethnicity,[221] or pyruvate kinase (PK) deficiency, which is the second most common RBC enzymopathy in neonates. Disorders of the RBC membrane such as congenital hereditary spherocytosis must also be considered in infants with unexplained significant neonatal jaundice. This is the most common inherited hemolytic disease among people of Northern European descent, and the condition is probably significantly underdiagnosed as a cause of jaundice in the newborn.[222] Other less common RBC membrane disorders such as hereditary poikilocytosis and elliptocytosis are mainly associated with severe anemia in the newborn and less with hyperbilirubinemia.[218] Hemoglobinopathies do not usually present in the neonatal period, except for α-thalassemia as a cause of severe anemia.[218]

Early Jaundice as a Sign of Infection

It is commonly believed that newborns with generalized infections and septicemia often present with jaundice. This can probably be related to increased activity of HO-1, which is inducible by inflammatory or oxidative stress.[223,224] This latter effect seems to be a cytoprotective response by converting the pro-oxidant molecule heme to biliverdin and bilirubin, both of which have antioxidant properties.[70,71,225] It has also recently been shown that biliverdin more specifically has direct antiviral effects by increasing the interferon response to viral infections.[226]

The extra bilirubin production resulting from the induction of HO-1 as a stress response to an infection will further increase the already high bilirubin load caused by the normal downregulation of the fetal erythrocyte pool, which exceeds the excretory capacity of the liver. As a consequence of this, newborns with marked and seemingly unexpected jaundice should routinely be evaluated for any underlying infectious disease.

Prolonged Neonatal Jaundice

Prolonged hyperbilirubinemia may be the first indicator of several rare diseases. In many of these the etiology is complex and includes not only related bilirubin metabolism but also inborn errors of metabolism and endocrinological conditions.

Jaundice Related to Genetic Variations in Bilirubin Conjugation

More than 50 mutations and polymorphisms in the gene for UGT1A1 have been identified in association with severe, prolonged, or recurrent unconjugated hyperbilirubinemia.[126,227,228] In general, these mutations have an autosomal recessive pattern of inheritance, but combinations of different heterozygous mutations may produce clinical disease in some infants. Several mutations of UGT1A1 have distinctive clinical phenotypes, whereas others show variable patterns of unconjugated hyperbilirubinemia. The age of onset and severity of clinical jaundice may be influenced by the rate of bilirubin production and excretion, nutritional status, and intercurrent illness, as well as specific mutations in the conjugating enzyme. All mutations and polymorphisms of clinical importance can cause severe or prolonged neonatal jaundice, particularly in combination with increased hemolysis.[229] For a detailed discussion, see Chapter 1.

Crigler–Najjar Syndrome Type I

Crigler–Najjar syndrome type I is a rare autosomal recessive disorder where no activity of the UGT enzyme can be found. Several nonsense mutations that stop synthesis or delete key amino acid sequences of the UGT enzyme have been described in these infants.[227,228] Severe, prolonged unconjugated hyperbilirubinemia begins in infancy and persists throughout life, usually at levels of 20–45 mg/dL or higher, and with eventual signs of central nervous system injury in nearly all cases. Gene replacement and liver transplantation are the only effective long-term therapies, although brain damage has been avoided by daily and extensive phototherapy in some.

Crigler–Najjar Syndrome Type II

In patients with Crigler–Najjar syndrome type II, a partial conjugating defect is caused by numerous single-site missense or insertion mutations that may retard the synthesis of the UGT enzyme or may impair the glucuronide binding of its COOH-terminal.[228] Although small amounts of bilirubin conjugates may be found in hepatocytes and bile, unconjugated hyperbilirubinemia may be severe in the newborn period and may persist or recur in adulthood. Peak or intermittent TSB levels are usually 6–20 mg/dL, but they are occasionally higher in newborns. UGT enzyme synthesis or activity may be induced or enhanced by phenobarbital, with an increase in bilirubin conjugates and a decrease in TSB and UCB.

Gilbert Syndrome

Gilbert syndrome is a milder form of unconjugated hyperbilirubinemia. The most common genotype associated with Gilbert syndrome is an insertion of two extra bases (TA) in the 5′ promoter region of the gene for UGT, resulting in a sequence of $A(TA)_7TAA$ instead of the normal $A(TA)_6TAA$.[126,228] This polymorphism has a high carrier rate in some families and ethnic groups, and polymorphisms incorporating other numbers of five to eight TA repeat sequences in the TATAA portion of the promoter have been described.[229,230]

Newborns with Gilbert syndrome mutations may have severe hyperbilirubinemia and develop kernicterus, especially if they have a concurrent hemolytic disorder such as ABO incompatibility or G6PD deficiency.[231] Enzyme synthesis and activity can be induced by administration of phenobarbital.

Other Causes of Prolonged Jaundice

Prolonged and/or severe hyperbilirubinemia can also be the first symptom in infants with hypothyroidism.[232,233] Prolonged jaundice has further been observed in infants with hypertrophic pyloric stenosis. This may be due to a Gilbert-type genetic variant. Genetic polymorphism for ligandin (OATP2) also increases the risk of developing significant neonatal jaundice. When this is combined with a variant UGT1A1 gene, the risk is augmented 22-fold.[94,126]

Cholestatic Jaundice in the Newborn

Neonatal cholestasis is not uncommon in neonates and should always be considered in infants with prolonged jaundice.[234] Measurement of bilirubin fractions (conjugated vs. unconjugated) is therefore required in infants who remain jaundiced beyond the first 2 weeks of life and in infants whose TSB levels repeatedly rebound following treatment. This is particularly important since phototherapy of an infant with jaundice caused by conjugated bilirubin may be harmful by resulting in the bronze baby syndrome.[235] There are several different methods available

for determination of conjugated bilirubin. In clinical use determination of direct-reacting bilirubin is often used as a substitute for conjugated bilirubin. However, since this method includes the delta fraction of UCB, 5–10% of the TSB will be determined as conjugated bilirubin even in a strictly unconjugated hyperbilirubinemia.[118,120]

Measurement of conjugated hyperbilirubinemia should also be done in the presence of an enlarged liver or spleen, petechiae, thrombocytopenia, or other findings suggesting congenital infection (cytomegalovirus infection, toxoplasmosis, bacterial septicemia), acquired or congenital liver or biliary disease (hepatitis, choledochus cyst, biliary atresia), as well as metabolic diseases (galactosemia, tyrosinemia). Such infants should also be observed for clinical signs of cholestasis such as pale stools and dark urine. Since only traces of UCB (<0.03 mg/dL) can be found in normal urine even at high TSB concentrations,[145] determination of bilirubin in the urine by reagent strip test for conjugated bilirubin (Urobilistix®) is a rapid and simple qualitative substitute for determination of conjugated bilirubin in the blood.

In a recent study, 27 out of 1289 infants admitted to a neonatal intensive care unit were diagnosed with cholestasis and conjugated hyperbilirubinemia.[236] In most of these infants, cholestasis had a multifactorial cause, in many of these particularly related to complications of prolonged parenteral nutrition in preterm infants.

In conclusion, when an infant presents with severe and/or prolonged jaundice in the neonatal period, several different and potentially severe conditions must be considered. Differences in clinical and laboratory examinations as well as maternal and neonatal history will often be a diagnostic clue to the cause of the jaundice and need for immediate treatment, before a more specific diagnosis can be made. Such differences between the different causes of jaundice are listed in Table 5-2.

■ ASSOCIATION OF NEONATAL HYPERBILIRUBINEMIA TO LATER DISEASE

Recently, it has been shown that bilirubin modulates the monolayer paracellular permeability in Caco-2 intestinal cells in vitro.[237] This effect was reversible, redox dependent, and mediated by a redistribution of tight junction occlusion. Previously, Jährig et al. found decreased gut transmural potential differences in jaundiced newborn

■ TABLE 5-2. Differences in Physical Findings, Maternal and Family History, and Laboratory Results in Newborn Infants with Pathologic Jaundice, in Relation to Possible Etiology and Postnatal Age

	Jaundice <24 h of Age[a]			Jaundice 1–10 Days of Age[b]			Prolonged Jaundice[c]	
	Immune Hemolytic Disease[d]	Nonimmune Hemolytic Disease[e]	Polycythemia	UDPGT-1 Mutations[f]	Neonatal Infections	Inborn Errors of Metabolism[g]	Endocrine-Related Disorders[h]	Cholestatic Jaundice[i]
Physical findings								
Hepatosplenomegaly	Occasional	Unusual	Unusual	Not related	Occasional	Unusual	Unusual	Common
Large for gestation	Not related	Not related	Common	Not related	Not related	Not related	Not related	Not related
Loss of stool color	Not related	Not related	Not related	Never	Occasional	Occasional	Not related	Common
Bilirubinuria	Unusual	Never	Never	Never	Occasional	Occasional	Never	Common
Maternal history								
Blood group O, Rh-negative	Common	Not related	Not related	Not related	Not related	Not related	Not related	Not related
Antibody screen +	Common	Unusual	Unusual	Unusual	Unusual	Unusual	Unusual	Unusual
Fever, infection	Not related	Not related	Not related	Not related	Occasional	Not related	Not related	Unusual
Diabetes	Not related	Not related	Common	Not related	Not related	Not related	Occasional	Unusual
Family history								
Jaundice in siblings and relatives	Common	Common	Unusual	Occasional	Unusual	Occasional	Occasional	Occasional
Splenectomy	Not related	Occasional	Not related	Not related	Not related	Not related	Not related	Not related
Liver disease	Not related	Occasional	Not related	Not related	Not related	Not related	Not related	Occasional
Laboratory results								
DAT positive	Common	Unusual	Unusual	Not related	Not related	Not related	Not related	Not related
Conjugated bilirubin	Occasional	Unusual	Unusual	Not related	Occasional	Occasional	Not related	Always
Anemia	Common	Occasional	Never	Not related	Occasional	Not related	Not related	Occasional
Increased CRP	Unusual	Unusual	Unusual	Not related	Always	Not related	Not related	Occasional
Hypoglycemia	Not related	Not related	Occasional	Not related	Common	Occasional	Occasional	Occasional

TSB, total serum bilirubin concentration.

[a] TSB usually 5.9–11.8 mg/dL.
[b] TSB usually 11.8–23.6 mg/dL.
[c] TSB usually 11.8–17.6 mg/dL.
[d] Includes Rh and ABO incompatibility as well as others.
[e] Includes congenital spherocytosis, pyruvate kinase deficiency, G6PD, and others.
[f] Includes Crigler–Najjar syndrome types I and II and Gilbert syndrome.
[g] Includes maternal diabetes, galactosemia, tyrosinemia, and others.
[h] Includes congenital hypothyroidism, Down syndrome, breast milk jaundice, and others.
[i] Includes biliary atresia, gastrointestinal obstruction, hepatitis, Dubin–Johnson syndrome, Rotor syndrome, and others.

infants with increased biliary excretion of bilirubin during phototherapy.[238] Since this potential is an indirect marker of the tightness of the intestinal barrier, they suggested that bilirubin could affect the permeability of the intestinal wall. Later studies have confirmed that jaundiced newborn infants had significantly higher intestinal permeability compared with that of nonjaundiced newborns when measured with the dual probe (lactulose/mannitol) sugar absorption test.[239] A significant correlation was also found between TSB levels and intestinal permeability. The authors speculate that this increased gut permeability in jaundiced newborn infants might increase the passage of different antigens and food allergens with later clinical implications. On this background, it is interesting that several studies indicate a link between intestinal barrier function and human disease.[240–245] In addition to possible long-term neurotoxic effects of bilirubin,[197] neonatal hyperbilirubinemia might therefore also be a risk factor for later development of common infantile diseases where the etiology is associated with increased intestinal permeability.

Neonatal Hyperbilirubinemia and Later Cow's Milk Intolerance

In a study by Raimondi et al., 353 jaundiced infants were compared with 339 infants without significant neonatal jaundice.[246] In a subset of 20 case–control pairs, intestinal permeability was studied at days 6–9 of life by determination of fecal a1AT, a serum antiprotease not catalyzed by digestive enzymes. Hyperbilirubinemic infants with peak TSB levels of 14.3 ± 1.9 mg/dL had significantly higher levels of a1AT in stools compared with control infants with peak TSB levels of 4.6 ± 2.0 mg/dL. Furthermore, a1AT concentrations in stool showed a significant correlation to TSB levels. At 12 months of age, the infants were examined for symptoms and signs of cow's milk protein intolerance (CMPI). Infants with hyperbilirubinemia in the neonatal period had significantly higher incidence of CMPI, 14/353 versus 4/339, $P = .045$. The authors conclude that jaundiced newborns have an increased risk for later CMPI caused by increased intestinal permeability in the neonatal period.

Neonatal Hyperbilirubinemia and Later Diabetes Type 1

An association between neonatal jaundice and later development of diabetes type 1 has also been reported, in both national and multinational studies.[247] In a European collaborative study on 892 cases of diabetes type 1 and 2291 controls, neonatal jaundice came out as a significant risk factor for diabetes type 1 (OR = 1.44; 95% CI = 1.19–1.75, $P < .001$) and was seen in all age-at-diagnosis groups, with a tendency toward higher ORs in the age group 5–9 years.[252] By subgroup analyses, the strongest correlation was found in infants with ABO incompatibility (OR = 3.78; 95% CI = 2.17–6.58, $P < .001$), and also for jaundice not related to maternal–fetal blood group incompatibility (OR = 1.39; 95% CI = 1.09–1.77, $P < .008$). The authors were not able to rule out an effect of phototherapy treatment for neonatal jaundice. However, in a recent case–control study of 361 infants with diabetes type 1 and 1083 controls, no significant association could be found between development of diabetes type 1 and neonatal jaundice, phototherapy, and other neonatal risk factors.[248]

Neonatal Hyperbilirubinemia and Later Development of Asthma

Studies have also found an association between neonatal hyperbilirubinemia and later development of asthma.[249] In a study from Sweden, 61,256 singleton 12- to 15-year-old children who had been prescribed asthma medication, maternal and perinatal events were compared with a control group of 1,338,319 children who had not been prescribed such medication. A statistically significant correlation to development of asthma was found for several perinatal risk factors, such as prematurity, low birth weight, mechanical ventilation, and infections, as well as jaundice and phototherapy. After extensive exclusion of children with other risk factors, the association between asthma and phototherapy and/or jaundice was still significant with an OR of 1.41 and 95% CI of 1.32–1.50.

Neonatal Hyperbilirubinemia and Later Neuropsychiatric and Cognitive Disabilities

Bilirubin toxicity to the brain might in addition to kernicterus also result in milder and less defined BIND.[192] Several studies have thus examined the association between neonatal hyperbilirubinemia and later IQ and neuropsychiatric or cognitive disorders.[250–255] The findings have not been uniform, and a possible reason for this could be the inclusion in many studies of both preterm infants and infants with Rhesus isoimmunization. The largest of the studies, which only included term infants, comprised 21,324 newborns and found no association between hyperbilirubinemia and IQ recorded at the age of 2–13 years. Recently Ebbesen et al. studied a cohort of 463 singleton men at a mean age of 18.8 years who had been diagnosed with neonatal jaundice (TSB levels from 6.1 to 28.2 mg/dL).[256] Cases of jaundice related to known diseases such as blood group isoimmunization, spherocytosis, and hypothyroidism were excluded. They found no difference in the incidence of neuropsychiatric disorders, low IQ, or cognitive performance compared with 13,370 controls. Moderate to severe uncomplicated jaundice in term infants therefore seems not to be related to such problems in later life.

Several investigators have also studied more specifically a possible relationship between neonatal hyperbilirubinemia and later development of autism spectrum disorders (ASD). The demonstrated effect of bilirubin on intestinal permeability is in this connection interesting, since a possible link between autism and intestinal dysfunction, particularly increased intestinal permeability, has been demonstrated.[244,245] Croen et al. compared 338 children with ASD with 1817 controls.[257] No correlation between hyperbilirubinemia and ASD could be found, not even in infants with very high TSB levels (≥24.9 mg/dL). This conclusion has recently been challenged by others. In a study of 473 children with autism and 473 matched controls born in Denmark in 1990–1999, an almost 4-fold risk for infantile autism was found in infants with gestational age ≥37 weeks who had been hyperbilirubinemic after birth (OR = 3.7; 95% CI = 1.5–10.5). No association was found to low Apgar scores, acidosis, or hypoglycemia.[258] In a recent study of all living children in Denmark born between 1994 and 2004 (n = 733,826), similar results were found for both autism and other psychological development disorders diagnosed in patients treated in somatic Danish hospitals. No association was, however, found when only patients diagnosed with ASD at the mental hospitals were added.[259] This study has also been criticized by others,[260] and a recent meta-analysis of all studies published on this issue found no association between neonatal hyperbilirubinemia and later autism.[261]

In conclusion, UCB has significant effects on cellular functions both in the brain and in other organs such as the gut. However, on the basis of present research findings it still seems difficult to conclude on any causative relationships between physiological neonatal hyperbilirubinemia and later development of conditions such as diabetes, asthma, and autism. These questions need further research. Any such causative relationship will significantly challenge the current clinical approach to the jaundiced newborn infant.

REFERENCES

1. Robinson SH. The origins of bilirubin. *N Engl J Med.* 1968;279:143–149.
2. Sieff CA, Nathan DG. The anatomy and physiology of hematopoiesis. In: Nathan DG, Oski FA, eds. *Hematology of Infancy and Childhood.* Philadelphia: WB Saunders Company; 1993:156–215.
3. Oski FA. The erythrocyte and its disorders. In: Nathan DG, Oski FA, eds. *Hematology of Infancy and Childhood.* Philadelphia: WB Saunders Company; 1993:18–43.
4. Blumenthal SG, Taggart DB, Rasmussen RD, Ikeda RM, Ruebner BH. Conjugated and unconjugated bilirubins in humans and rhesus monkeys: structural identity of bilirubins from biles and meconiums of newborn humans and rhesus monkeys. *Biochem J.* 1979;179:537–547.
5. Yamaguchi T, Nakajima H. Changes in the composition of bilirubin-IXα isomers during human prenatal development. *Eur J Biochem.* 1995;233:467–472.
6. Weiner CP. Human fetal bilirubin levels and fetal hemolytic disease. *Am J Obstet Gynecol.* 1992;166:1449–1454.
7. Bhutani VK, Johnson L, Sivieri EM. Predictive ability of a predischarge hour-specific serum bilirubin for subsequent significant hyperbilirubinemia in healthy term and near-term newborns. *Pediatrics.* 1999;103;6–14.
8. Goodrum LA, Saade GR, Belfort MA, Carpenter RJ, Moise KJ. The effect of intrauterine transfusion on fetal bilirubin in red cell alloimmunization. *Obstet Gynecol.* 1997;89:57–60.
9. Tenhunen R, Marver HS, Schmid R. Microsomal heme oxygenase. Characterization of the enzyme. *J Biol Chem.* 1969;244:6388–6394.
10. Maines MD. Heme oxygenase: function, multiplicity, regulatory mechanisms, and clinical applications. *FASEB J.* 1988;2:2557–2568.
11. Raffin SB, Woo CH, Roost KT, Price DC, Schmid R. Intestinal absorption of hemoglobin iron–heme cleavage by mucosal heme oxygenase. *J Clin Invest.* 1974;54:1344–1352.
12. Bartoletti AL, Stevenson DK, Ostrander CR, Johnson JD. Pulmonary excretion of carbon monoxide in the human infant as an index of bilirubin production. I. Effects of gestational and postnatal age and some common neonatal abnormalities. *J Pediatr.* 1979;94:952–955.
13. Colleran E, O'Carra P. Enzymology and comparative physiology of biliverdin reduction. In: Berk PD, Berlin

NR, eds. *International Symposium on Chemistry and Physiology of Bile Pigments*. Washington, DC: US Government Printing Office; 1977:69.

14. Fog J, Jellum E. Structure of bilirubin. *Nature*. 1963;198:88–89.

15. McCoubrey WK Jr, Huang TJ, Maines MD. Isolation and characterization of a cDNA from the rat brain that encodes hemoprotein heme oxygenase-3. *Eur J Biochem*. 1997; 247:725–732.

16. Donnelly LE, Barnes PJ. Expression of heme oxygenase in human airway epithelial cells. *Am J Respir Cell Mol Biol*. 2001;24:295–303.

17. Drummond GS, Kappas A. Prevention of neonatal hyperbilirubinemia by tin protoporphyrin IX, a potent competitive inhibitor of heme oxidation. *Proc Natl Acad Sci U S A*. 1981;78:6466–6470.

18. Abraham NG, Lin JH, Mitrione SM, et al. Expression of heme oxygenase gene in rat and human liver. *Biochem Biophys Res Commun*. 1988;150:717–722.

19. Maróti Z, Katona M, Orvos H, et al. Heme oxygenase-1 expression in premature and mature neonates during the first week of life. *Eur J Pediatr*. 2007;166: 1033–1038.

20. Yachie A, Niida Y, Wada T, et al. Oxidative stress causes enhanced endothelial cell injury in human heme oxygenase-1 deficiency. *J Clin Invest*. 1999;103:129–135.

21. Yoshiki N, Kubota T, Aso T. Expression and localization of heme oxygenase in human placental villi. *Biochem Biophys Res Commun*. 2000;276:1136–1142.

22. Brodersen R. Binding of bilirubin to albumin. *Crit Rev Clin Lab Sci*. 1980;11:305–399.

23. Brodersen R. Bilirubin. Solubility and interaction with albumin and phospholipids. *J Biol Chem*. 1979;254:2364–2369.

24. Jacobsen J, Wennberg RP. Determination of unbound bilirubin in the serum of newborns. *Clin Chem*. 1974;20:783–789.

25. Cashore WJ. Free bilirubin concentrations and bilirubin-binding affinity in term and preterm infants. *J Pediatr*. 1980;96:521–527.

26. Wong RJ, Stevenson DK, Ahlfors CE, Vreman HJ. Neonatal jaundice: bilirubin physiology and clinical chemistry. *NeoReviews*. 2007;8:e58–e67.

27. Ebbesen F, Foged N, Brodersen R. Reduced albumin binding of MADDS—a measure of bilirubin binding in sick children. *Acta Paediatr Scand*. 1986;75:550–554.

28. Bender GJ, Cashore WJ, Oh W. Ontogeny of bilirubin-binding capacity and the effect of clinical status in premature infants born at less than 1300 grams. *Pediatrics*. 2007;120:1067–1073.

29. Bratlid D. Pharmacologic aspects of neonatal hyperbilirubinemia. *Birth Defects Orig Artic Ser*. 1976;12:184–189.

30. Blanc WA, Johnson L. Studies on kernicterus. Relationship with sulfonamide intoxication, report on kernicterus in rats with glucuronyl transferase deficiency, and review of pathogenesis. *J Neuropathol Exp Neurol*. 1959;18:165–189.

31. Blauer G. Complexes of bilirubin with proteins. *Biochim Biophys Acta*. 1986;884:602–604.

32. Suzuki N, Yamaguchi T, Nakajima H. Role of high-density lipoprotein in transport of circulating bilirubin in rats. *J Biol Chem*. 1988;263:5037–5043.

33. Bratlid D. Bilirubin binding by human erythrocytes. *Scand J Clin Lab Invest*. 1972;29:91–97.

34. Bratlid D. The effect of pH on bilirubin binding by human erythrocytes. *Scand J Clin Lab Invest*. 1972;29:453–459.

35. Berk PD, Potter BJ, Stremmel W. Role of plasma membrane ligand-binding proteins in the hepatocellular uptake of albumin-bound organic anions. *Hepatology*. 1987;7:165–176.

36. Tiribelli C, Ostrow JD. New concepts in bilirubin chemistry, transport and metabolism: report of the International Bilirubin Workshop, April 6–8, 1989, Trieste, Italy. *Hepatology*. 1990;11:303–313.

37. Wolkoff AW, Goresky CA, Sellin J, Gatmaitan Z, Arias I. Role of ligandin in transfer of bilirubin from plasma to liver. *Am J Physiol*. 1979;236:E638–E648.

38. Di Ilio C, Del Boccio G, Casalone E, Aceto A, Sacchetta P. Activities of enzymes associated with the metabolism of glutathione in fetal rat liver and placenta. *Biol Neonate*. 1986;49:96–101.

39. Faulder CG, Hirrell PA, Hume R, Strange RC. Studies on the development of basic, neutral, and acidic isoenzymes of glutathione S-transferase in human liver, adrenal, kidney, and spleen. *Biochem J*. 1987;241:221–228.

40. Jacobsen C. Chemical modification of the high-affinity bilirubin-binding site of human serum albumin. *Eur J Biochem*. 1972;27:513–519.

41. Jacobsen C. Lysine residue 240 of human serum albumin is involved in high-affinity binding of bilirubin. *Biochem J*. 1978;171:453–459.

42. Hansen TWR, Mathiesen SBW, Walaas SI. Modulation of the effect of bilirubin on protein phosphorylation by lysine-containing peptides. *Pediatr Res*. 1997;42: 615–617.

43. Levi AJ, Gatmaitan Z, Arias IM. Deficiency of hepatic organic anion-binding protein, impaired organic anion uptake by liver and "physiologic" jaundice in newborn monkeys. *N Engl J Med*. 1970;283:1136–1139.

44. McDonagh AF, Palma LA, Schmid R. Reduction of biliverdin and placental transfer of bilirubin and biliverdin in the pregnant guinea pig. *Biochem J*. 1981;194:273–282.

45. Schanker LS. Passage of drugs across body membranes. *Pharmacol Rev*. 1962;14:501–530.

46. Serrano MA, Bayon JE, Pascolo L, et al. Evidence for carrier-mediated transport of unconjugated bilirubin across plasma membrane vesicles from human placental trophoblast. *Placenta.* 2002;23:527–535.

47. Briz O, Macias RIR, Serrano MA, et al. Excretion of fetal bilirubin by the rat placenta–maternal liver tandem. *Placenta.* 2003;24:462–472.

48. Briz O, Serrano MA, Macias RI, Gonzalez-Gallego J, Marin JJ. Role of organic anion-transporting polypeptides, OATP-A, OATP-C and OATP-8, in the human placenta–maternal liver tandem excretory pathway for foetal bilirubin. *Biochem J.* 2003;371:897–905.

49. Vander Jagt DL, Wilson SP, Heidrich JE. Purification and bilirubin binding properties of glutathione *S*-transferase from human placenta. *FEBS Lett.* 1981;136:319–321.

50. St-Pierre MV, Serrano MA, Macias RI, et al. Expression of members of the multidrug resistance protein family in human term placenta. *Am J Physiol Regul Integr Comp Physiol.* 2000;279:R1495–R1503.

51. St-Pierre MV, Stallmach T, Freimoser Grundschober A, et al. Temporal expression profiles of organic anion transport proteins in placenta and fetal liver of the rat. *Am J Physiol Regul Integr Comp Physiol.* 2004;287: R1505–R1516.

52. Serrano MA, Macias RI, Vallejo M, et al. Effect of ursodeoxycholic acid on the impairment induced by maternal cholestasis in the rat placenta–maternal liver tandem excretory pathway. *J Pharmacol Exp Ther.* 2003;305: 515–524.

53. Jedlitschky G, Leier I, Buchholz U, Center M, Keppler D. ATP-dependent transport of bilirubin glucuronides by the multidrug resistance protein MRP1 and its hepatocyte canalicular isoform MRP2. *Biochem J.* 1997;327: 305–310.

54. Briz O, Macias RI, Perez MJ, Serrano MA, Marin JJ. Excretion of fetal biliverdin by the rat placenta–maternal liver tandem. *Am J Physiol Regul Integr Comp Physiol.* 2006;290:R749–R756.

55. Rosenthal P. Human placental bilirubin metabolism. *Pediatr Res.* 1990;27:223A.

56. Monte MJ, Rodriguez-Bravo T, Macias RI, et al. Relationship between bile acid transport gradients and transport across the fetal-facing plasma membrane of the human trophoblast. *Pediatr Res.* 1995;38:156–163.

57. Mandelbaum B, LaCroix GC, Robinson AR. Determination of fetal maturity by spectrophotometric analysis of amniotic fluid. *Obstet Gynecol.* 1967;29:471–474.

58. Bevis DCA. The antenatal prediction of hemolytic disease of the newborn. *Lancet.* 1952;1:395–398.

59. Walker AHC. Liquor amnii studies in the prediction of hemolytic disease of the newborn. *Br Med J.* 1957;2: 376.

60. Sikkel E, Pasman SA, Oepkes D, Kanhai HH, Vandenbussche FP. On the origin of amniotic fluid bilirubin. *Placenta.* 2004;25:463–468.

61. Taylor WG, Walkinshaw SA, Farquharson RG, Fisken RA, Gilmore IT. Pregnancy in Crigler–Najjar syndrome. Case report. *Br J Obstet Gynaecol.* 1991;98:1290–1291.

62. Hannam S, Moriaty P, O'Reilly H, et al. Normal neurological outcome in two infants treated with exchange transfusions born to mothers with Crigler–Najjar type 1 disorder. *Eur J Pediatr.* 2009;168:427–429.

63. Hansen TWR, Nietsch L, Norman E, et al. Apparent reversibility of acute intermediate phase bilirubin encephalopathy. *Acta Paediatr.* 2009;98:1689–1694.

64. Fevery J, Heirwegh KPM. Bilirubin metabolism. In: Javitt NB, ed. *Liver and Biliary Tract Physiology. International Review of Physiology.* Vol. 21. Baltimore: University Park Press; 1980:171–220.

65. Alexander DP, Andrews WHH, Britton HG, Nixon DA. Bilirubin in the foetal sheep. *Biol Neonate.* 1970;15:103–111.

66. Gartner LM, Lee K, Vaisman S, Lane D, Zarufu I. Development of bilirubin in the newborn rhesus monkey. *J Pediatr.* 1977;90:513–531.

67. Muraca M, Blanckaert N, Rubaltelli FF, Fevery J. Unconjugated and conjugated bilirubin pigments during perinatal development. I. Studies on rat serum and intestine. *Biol Neonate.* 1986;49:90–95.

68. Hintz SR, Kwong LK, Vreman HJ, Stevenson DK. Recovery of exogenous heme as carbon monoxide and biliary heme in adult rats after tin protoporphyrin treatment. *J Pediatr Gastroenterol Nutr.* 1987;6:302–306.

69. Royer M, Rodriguez Garay E, Argerich T. Action of biliverdin on biliary elimination of bilirubin and biliverdin in the rat. *Acta Physiol Latinoam.* 1962;12:84–95.

70. Stocker R, Yamamoto Y, McDonagh AF, Glazer AN, Ames BN. Bilirubin is an antioxidant of possible physiological importance. *Science.* 1987;235:1043–1046.

71. Sedlak TW, Snyder SH. Bilirubin benefits: cellular protection by a biliverdin reductase antioxidant cycle. *Pediatrics.* 2004;113:1776–1782.

72. Jansen PLM, Chowdhury JR, Fischberg EB, Arias IM. Enzymatic conversion of bilirubin monoglucuronide to diglucuronide by rat liver plasma membranes. *J Biol Chem.* 1977;252:2710–2716.

73. Munoz ME, González J, Esteller A. Effect of glucose administration on bilirubin excretion in the rabbit. *Experientia.* 1987;43:166–168.

74. Iyanagi T, Emi Y, Ikushiro S. Biochemical and molecular aspects of genetic disorders of bilirubin metabolism. *Biochim Biophys Acta.* 1998;1407:173–184.

75. Keitel V, Nies AT, Brom M, et al. A common Dubin–Johnson syndrome mutation impairs protein

maturation and transport activity of MRP2 (ABCC2). *Am J Physiol Gastrointest Liver Physiol.* 2003;284: G165–G174.

76. Arias IM, Johnson L, Wolfson S. Biliary excretion of injected conjugated and unconjugated bilirubin by normal and Gunn rats. *Am J Physiol.* 1961;200:1091–1094.

77. Natschka JC, Odell GB. The influence of albumin on the distribution and excretion of bilirubin in jaundiced rats. *Pediatrics.* 1966;37:51–61.

78. Gourley GR, Odell GB. Bilirubin metabolism in the fetus and neonate. In: Lebenthal E, ed. *Human Gastrointestinal Development.* New York: Raven Press; 1989:581–621.

79. Kawade N, Onishi S. The prenatal and postnatal development of UDP-glucuronyl transferase activity towards bilirubin and the effect of premature birth on this activity in the human liver. *Biochem J.* 1981;196:257–260.

80. De Wolf-Peeters C, Moens-Bullens AM, Van Assche A, Desmet V. Conjugated bilirubin in foetal liver in erythroblastosis. *Lancet.* 1969;1:471.

81. Blumenthal SG, Stucker T, Rasmussen RD, et al. Changes in bilirubins in human prenatal development. *Biochem J.* 1980;186:693–700.

82. Fevery JM, Van de Vijver M, Michiels R, De Groote J, Heirwegh KPM. Comparison in different species of biliary bilirubin-IXα conjugates with the activities of hepatic and renal bilirubin-IXα uridine diphosphate glycosyltransferases. *Biochem J.* 1977;164:737–746.

83. Muraca M, Rubaltelli FF, Blanckaert N, Fevery J. Unconjugated and conjugated bilirubin pigments during perinatal development. II. Studies on serum of healthy newborns and of neonates with erythroblastosis fetalis. *Biol Neonate.* 1990;57:1–9.

84. Peters WHM, Jansen PLM, Nauta H. The molecular weights of UDP-glucuronyl transferase determined with radiation-inactivation analysis: a molecular model of bilirubin UDP-glucuronyl transferase. *J Biol Chem.* 1984;259:11701–11705.

85. Van Es HH, Bout A, Liu J, et al. Assignment of the human UDP glucuronosyltransferase gene (UGT1A1) to chromosome region 2q37. *Cytogenet Cell Genet.* 1993;63: 114–116.

86. Rayburn W, Donn S, Piehl E, Compton A. Antenatal phenobarbital and bilirubin metabolism in the very low birth weight infant. *Am J Obstet Gynecol.* 1988;159:1491–1493.

87. Valaes T, Petmezaki S, Doxiadis SA. Effect on neonatal hyperbilirubinemia of phenobarbital during pregnancy or after birth: practical value of the treatment in a population with high risk of unexplained severe neonatal jaundice. *Birth Defects Orig Artic Ser.* 1970;6:46–54.

88. Neufeld ND, Corbo L, Brunnerman S, Melmed S. Stimulation of neonatal hepatic UDP-glucuronyl transferase activity with prenatal thyroid analog therapy. *Pediatr Res.* 1985;19:178A.

89. Leaky JEA, Althaus ZR, Bailey JR, Slikker WJ. Dexamethasone increases UDP-glucuronyl transferase activity towards bilirubin, oestradiol and testosterone in foetal liver from rhesus monkey during late gestation. *Biochem J.* 1985;225:183–188.

90. Lindenbaum A, Hernandorena X, Vial M, et al. Traitement curatif de l'ictere du nouveau-ne a terme par le clofibrate. *Arch Fr Pediatr.* 1981;38:867–873.

91. Litwack G, Ketterer B, Arias IM. Ligandin: a hepatic protein which binds steroids, bilirubin, carcinogens and a number of exogenous organic anions. *Nature.* 1971;234:466–467.

92. Bhargava MM, Listowsky I, Arias IM. Ligandin. Bilirubin binding and glutathione-S-transferase activity are independent processes. *J Biol Chem.* 1978;253:4112–4115.

93. Muslu N, Dogruer ZN, Eskandari G, et al. Are glutathione S-transferase gene polymorphisms linked to neonatal jaundice? *Eur J Pediatr.* 2008;167:57–61.

94. Huang MJ, Kua KE, Teng HC, et al. Risk factors for severe hyperbilirubinemia in neonates. *Pediatr Res.* 2004;56:682–689.

95. Gourley GR, Li Z, Kreamer BL, Kosorok MR. A controlled, randomized, double-blind trial of prophylaxis against jaundice among breastfed newborns. *Pediatrics.* 2005;116:385–391.

96. Aziz S, Leroy P, Servaes R, Eggermont E, Fevery J. Bilirubin-IXbeta is a marker of meconium, like zinc coproporphyrin. *J Pediatr Gastroenterol Nutr.* 2001;32:287–292.

97. Bogg TR Jr, Bishop H. Neonatal hyperbilirubinemia associated with high obstruction of the small bowel. *J Pediatr.* 1965;66:349–356.

98. De Carvalho M, Klaus MH, Merkatz RB. Frequency of breast-feeding and serum bilirubin concentration. *Am J Dis Child.* 1982;136:737–738.

99. Odell GB, Gutcher GR, Whitington PF, Yang G. Enteral administration of agar as an effective adjunct to phototherapy in neonatal jaundice. *Pediatr Res.* 1983;17:810–814.

100. Johnson LH, Bhutani VK, Abbasi S, et al. Bilirubin oxidase in addition to intensive phototherapy to eliminate or delay need for exchange. *Pediatr Res.* 1997;41:156A.

101. Weisman LE, Merenstein GB, Digirol M, et al. The effect of early meconium evacuation on early-onset hyperbilirubinemia. *Am J Dis Child.* 1983;137:666–668.

102. Chen JY, Ling UP, Chen JH. Early meconium evacuation: effect on neonatal hyperbilirubinemia. *Am J Perinatol.* 1995;12:232–234.

103. Weisman LE, Merenstein GB, Digirol M, et al. Epidemiology of neonatal hyperbilirubinemia. *Pediatrics.* 1985;75:770–774.

104. Kramer LI. Advancement of dermal icterus in the jaundiced newborn. *Am J Dis Child.* 1969;118:454–458.

105. Bhutani VK, Gourley GR, Adler S, et al. Noninvasive measurement of total serum bilirubin in a multiracial predischarge newborn population to assess the risk of severe hyperbilirubinemia. *Pediatrics.* 2000;106;e17.

106. With TK. *Bile Pigments. Chemical, Biological and Clinical Aspects.* New York: Academic Press; 1968.

107. AAP Subcommittee on Hyperbilirubinemia. Management of hyperbilirubinemia in the newborn infant 35 or more weeks of gestation. *Pediatrics.* 2004;114:297–316.

108. Maisels MJ, Bhutani VK, Bogen D, et al. Hyperbilirubinemia in the newborn infant > or =35 weeks' gestation: an update with clarifications. *Pediatrics.* 2009;124:1193–1198.

109. Maisels MJ, Deridder JM, Kring EA, Balasubramaniam M. Routine transcutaneous bilirubin measurements combined with clinical risk factors improve the prediction of subsequent hyperbilirubinemia. *J Perinatol.* 2009;29:612–617.

110. Riskin A, Tamir A, Kugelman A, Hemo M, Bader D. Is visual assessment of jaundice reliable as a screening tool to detect significant neonatal hyperbilirubinemia? *J Pediatr.* 2008;152:782–787.

111. Newman TB. Data suggest visual assessment of jaundice in newborns is helpful. *J Pediatr.* 2009;153:466.

112. Keren R, Tremont K, Luan X, Cnaan A. Visual assessment of jaundice in term and late preterm infants. *Arch Dis Child Fetal Neonatal Ed.* 2009;94:F317–F322.

113. Hansen TWR. Management of jaundice in the newborn nurseries—measuring, predicting and avoiding sequelae. *Acta Paediatr.* 2009;98:1866–1868.

114. Macsic B, Trollebo AK, Bratlid D. Hyperbilirubinemia in a corhort of infants in a normal newborn nursery (NNN). Proceedings of the 3rd Congress of the European Academy of Pediatric Societies (EAPS), Copenhagen, October 23–26, 2010.

115. Kirk JM. Neonatal jaundice: a critical review of the role and practice of bilirubin analysis. *Ann Clin Biochem.* 2008;45:452–462.

116. Lo SF, Jendrzejczak B, Doumas BT. Laboratory performance in neonatal bilirubin testing using communicable specimens: a progress report on a College of American Pathologists study. *Arch Pathol Lab Med.* 2008;132:1781–1785.

117. Bratlid D, Nakstad B, Hansen TWR. National guidelines for treatment of jaundice in the newborn. *Acta Paediatr.* 2011;100:499–505.

118. Winsnes A, Bratlid D. Unconjugated and conjugated bilirubin in plasma from patients with erythroblastosis and neonatal hyperbilirubinemia. *Acta Paediatr Scand.* 1972;61:405–412.

119. Wu TW. Bilirubin analysis—the state of the art and future prospects. *Clin Biochem.* 1984;17:221–229.

120. Doumas BT, Wu TW. Measurement of bilirubin fractions in serum. *Crit Rev Clin Lab Sci.* 1991;28: 415–445.

121. Bratlid D. The effect of free fatty acids, bile acids, and hematin on bilirubin binding by human erythrocytes. *Scand J Clin Lab Invest.* 1972;30:107–112.

122. Lee Y-K, Daito Y, Katayama Y, Minami H, Negishi H. The significance of measurement of serum unbound bilirubin concentrations in high-risk infants. *Pediatr Int.* 2009;51:795–799.

123. Oh W, Stevenson DK, Tyson JE, et al. Influence of clinical status on the association between plasma total and unbound bilirubin and death or adverse neurodevelopmental outcomes in extremely low birth weight infants. *Acta Paediatr.* 2010;99:673–678.

124. Meberg A, Johansen KB. Screening for neonatal hyperbilirubinemia and ABO alloimmunization at the time of testing for phenylketonuria and congenital hypothyreosis. *Acta Paediatr.* 1998;87:1269–1274.

125. Gartner LM, Herschel M. Jaundice and breastfeeding. *Pediatr Clin North Am.* 2001;48:389–399.

126. Watchko JF, Daood MJ, Biniwale M. Understanding neonatal hyperbilirubinemia in the era of genomics. *Semin Neonatol.* 2002;7:143–152.

127. Silverman WA, Andersen DH, Blanc WA, et al. A difference in mortality rate and incidence of kernicterus among premature infants allotted to two prophylactic antibacterial regimens. *Pediatrics.* 1956;18:614–624.

128. Maruyama K, Harada S, Nishigori H, Iwatsuru M. Classification of drugs on the basis of bilirubin-displacing effect on human serum albumin. *Chem Pharm Bull.* 1984;32:2414–2420.

129. Walker PC. Neonatal bilirubin toxicity. A review of kernicterus and the implications of drug-induced bilirubin displacement. *Clin Pharmacokinet.* 1987;13:25–50.

130. Bratlid D, Langslet A. Displacement of albumin-bound bilirubin by injectable diazepam preparations in vitro. *Acta Paediatr Scand.* 1973;62:510–512.

131. Ballowitz L. Displacement of bilirubin from albumin by drugs. *J Pediatr.* 1978;92:166.

132. Cooper-Peel C, Brodersen R, Robertson A. Does ibuprofen affect bilirubin–albumin binding in newborn infant serum? *Pharmacol Toxicol.* 1996;79:297–299.

133. Ahlfors CE. Effect of ibuprofen on bilirubin–albumin binding. *J Pediatr.* 2004;144:386–388.

134. Soligard HT, Nilsen OG, Bratlid D. Displacement of bilirubin from albumin by ibuprofen in vitro. *Pediatr Res.* 2010;67:614–618.

135. Amin SB. Effect of free fatty acids on bilirubin–albumin binding affinity and unbound bilirubin in premature

infants. *JPEN J Parenter Enteral Nutr.* 2010;34: 414–420.

136. Brans YW, Ritter DA, Kenny JD, et al. Influence of intravenous fat emulsion on serum bilirubin in very low birthweight neonates. *Arch Dis Child.* 1987;62:156–160.

137. Malhotra V, Greenberg JW, Dunn LL, Ennever JF. Fatty acid enhancement of the quantum yield for the formation of lumirubin from bilirubin bound to human albumin. *Pediatr Res.* 1987;21:530–533.

138. Hankø E, Tommarello S, Watchko JF, Hansen TWR. Administration of drugs known to inhibit P-glycoprotein increases brain bilirubin and alters the regional distribution of bilirubin in rat brain. *Pediatr Res.* 2003;54:441–445.

139. Watchko JF, Daood MJ, Hansen TWR. Brain bilirubin content is increased in P-glycoprotein deficient transgenic null mutant mice. *Pediatr Res.* 1998;44:763–766.

140. Tsai CE, Daood MJ, Lane RH, et al. P-glycoprotein expression in mouse brain increases with maturation. *Biol Neonate.* 2002;81:58–64.

141. Schinkel AH. The physiological function of drug-transporting P-glycoproteins. *Semin Cancer Biol.* 1997;8:161–170.

142. Bellamy WT. P-glycoproteins and multidrug resistance. *Annu Rev Pharmacol Toxicol.* 1996;36:161–183.

143. Bellarosa C, Bortolussi G, Tiribelli C. The role of ABC transporters in protecting cells from bilirubin toxicity. *Curr Pharm Des.* 2009;15: 2884–2892.

144. Liu YH, Di YM, Zhou ZW, Mo SL, Zhou SF. Multidrug resistance-associated proteins and implications in drug development. *Clin Exp Pharmacol Physiol.* 2010;37:115–120.

145. Yin J, Wennberg RP, Miller M. Induction of hepatic bilirubin and drug metabolizing enzymes by individual herbs present in the traditional Chinese medicine, yin zhi huang. *Dev Pharmacol Ther.* 1993;20:186–194.

146. Yeung CY, Lee FT, Wong HN. Effect of a popular Chinese herb on neonatal bilirubin protein binding. *Biol Neonate.* 1990;58:98–103.

147. Soligard HT, Bratlid D, Cao C, Liang A, Nilsen OG. Displacement of bilirubin from albumin in plasma from jaundiced newborns. An in vitro study of purified Chinese herbal constituents and sulfisoxazole. *Phytother Res.* 2011. doi:10.1002/ptr.3402.

148. Costalos C, Russell G, Bistarakis L, Pangali A, Philippidou A. Effects of jaundice and phototherapy on gastric emptying in the newborn. *Biol Neonate.* 1984;46: 57–60.

149. De Curtis M, Guandalini S, Fasano A, Saitta F, Ciccimarra F. Diarrhoea in jaundiced neonates treated with phototherapy: role of intestinal secretion. *Arch Dis Child.* 1989;64:1161–1164.

150. Yao AC, Martinussen M, Johansen OJ, Brubakk AM. Phototherapy-associated changes in mesenteric blood flow response to feeding in term neonates. *J Pediatr.* 1994;24:309–312.

151. Hansen TWR. The pathophysiology of bilirubin toxicity. In: Maisels MJ, Watchko JF, eds. *Neonatal Jaundice.* London: Harwood Academic Publishers; 2000:89–104.

152. McDonagh AF. Controversies in bilirubin biochemistry and their clinical relevance. *Semin Fetal Neonatal Med.* 2010;15:141–147.

153. Silberberg DH, Johnson L, Schutta H, Ritter L. Effects of photodegradation products of bilirubin on myelinating cerebellum cultures. *J Pediatr.* 1970;77:613–618.

154. Thaler MM. Toxic effects of bilirubin and its photo-decomposition products. *Birth Defects Orig Artic Ser.* 1970;6:128–130.

155. Brodersen R. Bilirubin transport in the newborn infant, reviewed with relation to kernicterus. *J Pediatr.* 1980;96:349–356.

156. Whitmer DI, Russell PE, Gollan JL. Membrane–membrane interactions associated with rapid transfer of liposomal bilirubin to microsomal UDP-glucuronyltransferase. Relevance to hepatocellular transport and biotransformation of hydrophobic substrates. *Biochem J.* 1987;244:41–47.

157. Ives NK, Brewster F, Gardiner RM. Bilirubin transport at the blood–brain barrier investigated using the Oldendorf technique. *Acta Neurol Scand.* 1985;72:94.

158. Hansen TWR, Cashore WJ. Rates of bilirubin clearance from rat brain regions. *Biol Neonate.* 1995;68:135–140.

159. Hansen TWR. Bilirubin entry into and clearance from rat brain during hypercarbia and hyperosmolality. *Pediatr Res.* 1996;39:72–76.

160. Hansen TWR, Øyasæter S, Stiris T, Bratlid D. Effects of sulfisoxazole, hypercarbia, and hyperosmolality on entry of bilirubin and albumin into young rat brain regions. *Biol Neonate.* 1989;56:22–30.

161. Bratlid D. How bilirubin gets into the brain. *Clin Perinatol.* 1990;17:449–465.

162. Wennberg RP, Ahlfors CE, Rasmussen LF. The pathochemistry of kernicterus. *Early Hum Dev.* 1979;3:353–372.

163. Cashore WJ, Horwich A, Laterra J, Oh W. Effect of postnatal age and clinical status of newborn infants on bilirubin-binding capacity. *Biol Neonate.* 1977;32:304–309.

164. Lee C, Oh W, Stonestreet BS, Cashore WJ. Permeability of the blood brain barrier for 125I-albumin-bound bilirubin in newborn piglets. *Pediatr Res.* 1989;25: 452–456.

165. Roger C, Koziel V, Vert P, Nehlig A. Autoradiographic mapping of local cerebral permeability to bilirubin in immature rats: effect of hyperbilirubinemia. *Pediatr Res.* 1996;39:64–71.

166. Bratlid D, Cashore WJ, Oh W. Effect of acidosis on bilirubin deposition in rat brain. *Pediatrics*. 1984;73:431–434.

167. Mayor F Jr, Pagés M, Díez-Guerra J, Valdivieso F, Major F. Effect of postnatal anoxia on bilirubin levels in rat brain. *Pediatr Res*. 1985;19:231–236.

168. Hansen TWR, Odden JP, Bratlid D. Effects of hyperoxia on entry of bilirubin and albumin into rat brain. *J Perinatol*. 1987;7:217–220.

169. Cowger ML. Mechanism of bilirubin toxicity on tissue culture cells: factors that affect toxicity, reversibility by albumin, and comparison with other respiratory poisons and surfactants. *Biochem Med*. 1971;5:1–16.

170. Mayor F Jr, Díez-Guerra J, Valdivieso F, Mayor F. Effect of bilirubin on the membrane potential of rat brain synaptosomes. *J Neurochem*. 1986;47:363–369.

171. Sugita K, Sato T, Nakajima H. Effects of pH and hypoglycemia on bilirubin cytotoxicity in vitro. *Biol Neonate*. 1987;52:22–25.

172. Brites D, Fernandes A, Falcão AS, et al. Biological risks for neurological abnormalities associated with hyperbilirubinemia. *J Perinatol*. 2009;29(suppl 1):S8–S13.

173. Gulati A, Mahesh AK, Misra PK. Blood brain barrier permeability studies in control and icteric neonates. *Pediatr Res*. 1990;27:206A.

174. Burgess GH, Oh W, Bratlid D, et al. The effects of brain blood flow on brain bilirubin deposition in newborn piglets. *Pediatr Res*. 1985;19:691–696.

175. Hansen NB, Brubakk A-M, Bratlid D, Oh W, Stonestreet BS. The effects of variations in PaCO2 on brain blood flow and cardiac output in the newborn piglet. *Pediatr Res*. 1984;18:1132–1136.

176. Levine RL, Fredricks WR, Rapoport SI. Clearance of bilirubin from rat brain after reversible osmotic opening of the blood–brain barrier. *Pediatr Res*. 1985;19:1040–1043.

177. Hansen TWR, Allen JW. Hemolytic anemia does not increase entry into, nor alter rate of clearance of bilirubin from rat brain. *Biol Neonate*. 1996;69:268–274.

178. Brodersen R, Bartels P. Enzymatic oxidation of bilirubin. *Eur J Biochem*. 1969;10:468–473.

179. Hansen TWR. Bilirubin oxidation in brain. *Mol Genet Metab*. 2000;71:411–417.

180. Hansen TWR. Therapeutic practices in neonatal jaundice: an international survey. *Clin Pediatr*. 1996;35:309–316.

181. Dawodu AH, Owa JA, Familusi JB. A prospective study of the role of bacterial infection and G6PD deficiency in severe neonatal jaundice in Nigeria. *Trop Geogr Med*. 1984;36:127–132.

182. Fernandes A, Brites D. Contribution of inflammatory processes to nerve cell toxicity by bilirubin and efficacy of potential therapeutic agents. *Curr Pharm Des*. 2009;15:2915–2926.

183. Hansen TWR, Maynard EC, Cashore WJ, Oh W. Endotoxemia and brain bilirubin in the rat. *Biol Neonate*. 1993;63:171–176.

184. Hankø E, Lindemann R, Hansen TWR. Spectrum of outcome in infants with extreme neonatal jaundice. *Acta Paediatr*. 2001;90:782–785.

185. Hansen TWR. Acute management of extreme neonatal jaundice—the potential benefits of intensified phototherapy and interruption of enterohepatic bilirubin circulation. *Acta Paediatr*. 1997;86:843–846.

186. Ebbesen F. Recurrence of kernicterus in term and near term infants in Denmark. *Acta Paediatr*. 2001;89:1213–1217.

187. MacDonald MG. Hidden risks: early discharge and bilirubin toxicity due to glucose 6-phosphate dehydrogenase deficiency. *Pediatrics*. 1995;96:734–738.

188. Maisels MJ, Newman TB. Kernicterus in otherwise healthy, breast-fed term newborns. *Pediatrics*. 1995;96:730–733.

189. Hansen TWR, Cashore WJ, Oh W. Changes in piglet auditory brainstem response amplitudes without increases in serum or cerebrospinal fluid neuron-specific enolase. *Pediatr Res*. 1992;32:524–529.

190. Nwaesei CG, Van Aerde J, Boyden M, et al. Changes in auditory brainstem responses in hyperbilirubinemic infants before and after exchange transfusion. *Pediatrics*. 1984;74:800–803.

191. Volpe JJ. *Neurology of the Newborn*. 5th ed. Philadelphia: Elsevier; 2008.

192. Shapiro SM. Definition of the clinical spectrum of kernicterus and bilirubin-induced neurologic dysfunction (BIND). *J Perinatol*. 2005;25:54–59.

193. Kikuchi G, Yoshida T. Function and induction of the microsomal heme oxygenase. *Mol Cell Biochem*. 1983;53–54:163–183.

194. Gemsa D, Woo CH, Fudenberg HH, Schmid R. Stimulation of heme oxygenase in macrophages and liver by endotoxin. *J Clin Invest*. 1974;53:647–651.

195. Beer H, Bernhard K. The effect of bilirubin and vitamin E on the oxidation of unsaturated fatty acids by ultraviolet irradiation [in German]. *Chimia*. 1959;13:291–292.

196. Belanger S, Lavoie JC, Chessex P. Influence of bilirubin on the antioxidant capacity of plasma in newborn infants. *Biol Neonate*. 1997;71:233–238.

197. Doré S, Takahashi HM, Ferris CD, et al. Bilirubin, formed by activation of heme oxygenase-2, protects neurons against oxidative stress injury. *Proc Natl Acad Sci U S A*. 1999;96:2445–2450.

198. McDonagh AF. The biliverdin–bilirubin antioxidant cycle of cellular protection: missing a wheel? *Free Radic Biol Med*. 2010;49:814–820.

199. Temme EH, Zhang J, Schouten EG, Kesteloot H. Serum bilirubin and 10-year mortality risk in a Belgian population. *Cancer Causes Control.* 2001;12:887–894.

200. Breimer LH, Wannamethee G, Ebrahim S, Shaper AG. Serum bilirubin and risk of ischemic heart disease in middle-aged British men. *Clin Chem.* 1995;41:1504–1508.

201. Djoussé L, Levy D, Cupples LA, et al. Total serum bilirubin and risk of cardiovascular disease in the Framingham Offspring Study. *Am J Cardiol.* 2001;87:1196–1200.

202. Lingenhel A, Kollerits B, Schwaiger JP, et al. Serum bilirubin levels, UGT1A1 polymorphisms and risk for coronary artery disease. *Exp Gerontol.* 2008;43:1102–1107.

203. Ekblom K, Marklund SL, Jansson JH, et al. Plasma bilirubin and UGT1A1*28 are not protective factors against first-time myocardial infarction in a prospective, nested case-referent setting. *Circ Cardiovasc Genet.* 2010;3:340–347.

204. Benaron DA, Bowen FW. Variation of initial serum bilirubin rise in newborn infants with type of illness. *Lancet.* 1991;338:78–81.

205. Gaton DD, Gold J, Axer-Siegel R, et al. Evaluation of bilirubin as possible protective factor in the prevention of retinopathy of prematurity. *Br J Ophthalmol.* 1991;75:532–534.

206. Fauchere JC, Meier-Gibbons FE, Koerner F, Bossi E. Retinopathy of prematurity and bilirubin—no clinical evidence for a beneficial role of bilirubin as a physiological anti-oxidant. *Eur J Pediatr.*1994;153:358–362.

207. Hosono S, Ohno T, Kimoto H, et al. No clinical correlation between bilirubin levels and severity of retinopathy of prematurity. *J Pediatr Ophthalmol Strabismus.* 2002;39:151–156.

208. Milner JD, Aly HZ, Ward LB, El-Mohandes A. Does elevated peak bilirubin protect from retinopathy of prematurity in very low birthweight infants. *J Perinatol.* 2003;23:208–211.

209. Heyman E, Ohlsson A, Girschek P. Retinopathy of prematurity and bilirubin. *N Engl J Med.* 1989;320:256.

210. Yeo KL, Perlman M, Hao Y, Mullaney P. Outcomes of extremely premature infants related to their peak serum bilirubin concentrations and exposure to phototherapy. *Pediatrics.* 1998;102:1426–1431.

211. Kao JS, Dawson JD, Murray JC, et al. Possible roles of bilirubin and breast milk in protection against retinopathy of prematurity. *Acta Paediatr.* 2011;100:347–351.

212. Fladmark E, Haram G, Bratlid D. Hyperbilirubinemia in a national cohort of extremely premature infants. Proceedings of the 3rd Congress of the European Academy of Pediatric Societies (EAPS), Copenhagen, October 23–26, 2010.

213. Gartner LM, Snyder RN, Chabon RS, Bernstein J. Kernicterus: high incidence in premature infants with low serum bilirubin concentration. *Pediatrics.* 1970;45:906–917.

214. Watchko JF, Maisels MJ. Jaundice in low birth weight infants: pathobiology and outcome. *Arch Dis Child Fetal Neonatal Ed.* 2003;88:F455–F458.

215. Oh W, Tyson JE, Fanaroff AA, et al. Association between peak serum bilirubin and neurodevelopmental outcomes in extremely low birthweight infants. *Pediatrics.* 2003;112:773–779.

216. Morris BH, Oh W, Tyson JE, et al. Aggressive vs. conservative phototherapy for infants with extremely low birth weight. *N Engl J Med.* 2008;359:1885–1896.

217. Dani C, Poggi C, Barp J, Romagnoli C, Buonocore G. Current Italian practices regarding the management of hyperbilirubinemia in preterm infants. *Acta Paediatr.* 2011;100:666–669.

218. Murray NA, Roberts IA. Haemolytic disease of the newborn. *Arch Dis Child Fetal Neonatal Ed.* 2007;92:F83–F88.

219. Bakkeheim E, Bergerud U, Schmidt-Melbye AC, et al. Maternal IgG anti-A and anti-B titres predict outcome in ABO-incompatibility in the neonate. *Acta Paediatr.* 2009;98:1896–1901.

220. Rubarth LB. Blood types and ABO incompatibility. *Neonatal Netw.* 2011;30:50–53.

221. Kaplan M, Hammerman C. The need for neonatal-glucose-6-phosphate dehydrogenase screening: a global perspective. *J Perinatol.* 2009;29(suppl 1):S46–S52.

222. Christensen RD, Henry E. Hereditary spherocytosis in neonates with hyperbilirubinemia. *Pediatrics.* 2010;125:120–125.

223. Yoshida T, Biro P, Cohen T, Müller RM, Shibahara S. Human heme oxygenase cDNA and induction of its mRNA by hemin. *Eur J Biochem.* 1988;171:457–461.

224. Applegate LA, Luscher P, Tyrrell RM. Induction of heme oxygenase: a general response to oxidant stress in cultured mammalian cells. *Cancer Res.* 1991:51:974–978.

225. Bae JW, Kim MJ, Jang CG, Lee SY. Protective effect of heme oxyganse-1 against MPP(+)-induced cytotoxicity in PC-12 cells. *Neurol Sci.* 2010;31:307–313.

226. Lehmann E, El-Tantawy WH, Ocker M, et al. The heme oxygenase 1 product biliverdin interferes with hepatitis C virus replication by increasing antiviral interferon response. *Hepatology.* 2010;51:398–404.

227. Ulgenalp A, Duman N, Schaefer FV, et al. Analyses of polymorphism for UGT1*1 exon promoter in neonates with pathologic and prolonged jaundice. *Biol Neonate.* 2003;83:258–262.

228. Kadakol A, Ghosh SS, Sappal BS, et al. Genetic lesions of bilirubin uridine-diphosphoglucuronate glucuronosyl-transferase (UGT1A1) causing Crigler–Najjar and Gilbert syndrome: correlation of genotype to phenotype. *Hum Mutat.* 2000;16:297–306.

229. Kaplan M, Renbaum P, Levy-Lahad E, et al. Gilbert syndrome and glucose-6-phosphate dehydrogenase deficiency: a dose-dependent genetic interaction crucial to neonatal hyperbilirubinemia. *Proc Natl Acad Sci U S A.* 1997;94:12128–12132.

230. Beutler E, Gelbart T, Demina A. Racial variability in the UDP-glucuronosyltransferase 1 (UGT1A1) promoter: a balanced poly morphism for regulation of bilirubin metabolism. *Proc Natl Acad Sci U S A.* 1998;95:8170–8174.

231. Maruo Y, Nishizawa K, Sato H, Sawa H, Shimada M. Prolonged unconjugated hyperbilirubinemia associated with breast milk and mutations of the bilirubin uridine diphosphate-glucuronosyltransferase gene. *Pediatrics.* 2000;106:E59.

232. MacGillivray MH, Crawford JD, Robey JS. Congenital hypothyroidism and prolonged neonatal hyperbilirubinemia. *Pediatrics.* 1967;40:283–286.

233. Tiker F, Gurakan B, Tarcan A, Kinik S. Congenital hypothyroidism and early severe hyperbilirubinemia. *Clin Pediatr (Phila).* 2003;42:365–366.

234. Venigalla S, Gourley GR. Neonatal cholestasis. *Semin Perinatol.* 2004;28:348–355.

235. Kopelman AE, Brown RS, Odell GB. The "bronze" baby syndrome: a complication of phototherapy. *J Pediatr.* 1972;81:466–472.

236. Tufano M, Nicastro E, Giliberti P, et al. Cholestasis in neonatal intensive care unit: incidence, aetiology and management. *Acta Paediatr.* 2009;98:1756–1761.

237. Raimondi F, Crivaro V, Capasso L, et al. Unconjugated bilirubin modulates the intestinal epithelial barrier function in a human-derived in vitro model. *Pediatr Res.* 2006;60:30–33.

238. Jährig K, Balke EH, Koenig A, Meisel P. Transepithelial electric potential difference in newborns undergoing phototherapy. *Pediatr Res.* 1987;21:283–284.

239. Indrio F, Raimondi F, Laforgia N, et al. Effect of hyperbilirubinemia on intestinal permeability in healthy term newborns. *Acta Paediatr.* 2007;96:73–75.

240. Söderholm JD, Olaison G, Peterson KH, et al. Augmented increase in tight junction permeability by luminal stimuli in the non-inflamed ileum of Crohn's disease. *Gut.* 2002;50;307–313.

241. Kalach N, Rocchiccioli F, de Boissieu D, Benhamo P-H, Dupont C. Intestinal permeability in children: variation with age and reliability in the diagnosis of cow's milk allergy. *Acta Paediatr.* 2001;90:499–504.

242. Bosi E, Molteni L, Radaelli MG, et al. Increased intestinal permeability precedes clinical onset of type 1 diabetes. *Diabetologica.* 2006;49:2824–2827.

243. Hijazi Z, Molla AM, Al-Habashi H, et al. Intestinal permeability is increased in bronchial asthma. *Arch Dis Child.* 2004;89:227–229.

244. D'Eufemia P, Celli M, Finocchiaro R, et al. Abnormal intestinal permeability in children with autism. *Acta Paediatr.* 1996;85:1076–1079.

245. de Magistris L, Familiari V, Pascotto A, et al. Alterations in the intestinal barrier in patients with autism spectrum disorders and their first-degree relatives. *J Pediatr Gastroenterol Nutr.* 2010;51:418–424.

246. Raimondi F, Indrio F, Crivaro V, et al. Neonatal hyperbilirubinemia increases intestinal protein permeability and the prevalence of cow's milk protein intolerance. *Acta Paediatr.* 2008;97:751–753.

247. Dahlquist G, Källén B. Indications that phototherapy is a risk factor for insulin-dependent diabetes. *Diabetes Care.* 2003;26:247–248.

248. Robertson L, Harrild K. Maternal and neonatal risk factors for childhood type 1 diabetes: a matched case–control study. *BMC Public Health.* 2010;10:281.

249. Aspberg S, Dahlquist G, Kahan T, Källén B. Confirmed association between neonatal phototherapy or neonatal icterus and risk of childhood asthma. *Pediatr Allergy Immunol.* 2010;21:e733–e739.

250. Rubin RA, Balow B, Fisch RO. Neonatal serum bilirubin levels related to cognitive development at ages 4 through 7 years. *J Pediatr.* 1979;94:601–604.

251. Nilsen ST, Finne PH, Bergsjø P, Stamnes O. Males with neonatal hyperbilirubinemia examined at 18 years of age. *Acta Paediatr Scand.* 1984;73:176–180.

252. Seidman DS, Paz I, Stevenson DK, et al. Neonatal hyperbilirubinemia and physical and cognitive performance at 17 years of age. *Pediatrics.* 1991;88:828–833.

253. Newman TB, Klebanoff MA. Neonatal hyperbilirubinemia and long term outcome: another look at the Collaborative Perinatal Project. *Pediatrics.* 1993;92:651–657.

254. Newman TB, Liljestrand P, Jeremy RJ, et al. Outcomes among newborns with total serum bilirubin levels of 25 mg per decilitre or more. *N Engl J Med.* 2006;354:1889–1900.

255. Jangaard KA, Fell DB, Dodds L, Allen AC. Outcomes in a population of healthy term and near term infants with serum bilirubin levels of ≥325 micromol/L (≥19 mg/dl) who were born in Nova Scotia, Canada between 1994 and 2000. *Pediatrics.* 2008;122:119–124.

256. Ebbesen F, Ehrenstein V, Traeger M, Nielsen GL. Neonatal non-hemolytic hyperbilirubinemia: a prevalence study of adult neuropsychiatric disability and cognitive

function in 463 male Danish conscripts. *Arch Dis Child.* 2010;95:583–587.

257. Croen LA, Yoshida CK, Odouli R, Newman TB. Neonatal hyperbilirubinemia and risk of autism spectrum disorders. *Pediatrics.* 2005;115:e135–e138.

258. Maimburg RD, Vaeth M, Schendel DE, et al. Neonatal jaundice: a risk factor for infantile autism? *Paediatr Perinat Epidemiol.* 2008;26:562–568.

259. Maimburg RD, Bech BH, Vaeth M, Møller-Madsen B, Olsen J. Neonatal jaundice, autism and other disorders of psychological development. *Pediatrics.* 2010;126:872.

260. Newman TB, Croen LA. Jaundice–autism link unconvincing. *Pediatrics.* 2011;127:e858–e859.

261. Gardener H, Spiegelman D, Buka SL. Perinatal and neonatal risk factors for autism: a comprehensive meta-analysis. *Pediatrics.* 2011;128:e1–e12.

The Epidemiology of Neonatal Hyperbilirubinemia

M. Jeffrey Maisels and Thomas B. Newman

■ INTRODUCTION

In order to develop an approach to the diagnosis and management of the jaundiced newborn, it is necessary to understand the nonpathologic factors that can affect bilirubin levels in the normal newborn infant as well as the natural history of neonatal bilirubinemia. Many factors have been identified in large epidemiologic studies as having some effect on neonatal bilirubin levels,[1] but their clinical relevance is often questionable. Those that have been shown in recent studies to have an important influence on total serum bilirubin (TSB) levels are listed in Table 6-1.

■ ETHNIC AND FAMILIAL FACTORS

Mean maximum TSB concentrations in East Asian, Native American, and some Hispanic infants (primarily those of Mexican descent) are significantly higher than those in white infants.[2–6] In a study of Hispanic infants, 31% had peak TSB levels >15 mg/dL[6] compared with 3–10% of infants in other US populations.[7,8] The mechanisms responsible for these differences are unknown, although there is some evidence that in the Native American population, increased bilirubin production plays a role.[5] Black infants in the United States and Great Britain have lower TSB levels than white infants.[3,9–11]

Neonatal jaundice runs in families. Khoury et al.[12] studied a population of 3301 newborns born to male US army veterans between 1966 and 1986. If one or more previous siblings had a TSB >12 mg/dL, the subsequent

sibling was three times more likely than controls (10.3% vs. 3.6%) to develop a TSB >12 mg/dL, and if a prior sibling had a TSB level >15 mg/dL, the risk in the subsequent sibling was increased 12.5-fold (10.5% vs. 0.9%). These relationships applied whether or not the siblings were breastfed or formula fed. The familial nature of hyperbilirubinemia has also been documented in Chinese and Danish infants.[13,14]

■ GENETIC FACTORS

The genetics of neonatal jaundice and the inborn errors of hepatic bilirubin uridine diphosphate glucuronosyltransferase (UGT) expression are discussed in detail in Chapter 1. Gilbert's syndrome is not generally classified as a pathologic entity in a newborn, but newborn infants who are heterozygous or homozygous for Gilbert's syndrome (i.e., they have the variant UGT genotype) have significantly elevated bilirubin levels in the first 2–4 days, compared with homozygous normal infants.[15,16] In addition to a decreased ability to conjugate bilirubin, infants with Gilbert's syndrome also appear to have an increase in red cell turnover and therefore bilirubin production.[16] In a population of Scottish, primarily breastfed newborns, with TSB levels of >5.8 mg/dL after 14 days of life, 31% were homozygous for the 7/7 Gilbert's syndrome promoter genotype compared with only 6% of a control group that did not have prolonged hyperbilirubinemia.[17] By itself, the presence of Gilbert's syndrome has a relatively modest effect on TSB levels in the neonate[15] but, when combined with other icterogenic

■ **TABLE 6-1.** Risk Factors for the Development of Hyperbilirubinemia in Infants of 35 or More Weeks Gestation

Elevated predischarge TSB or TcB level[11,57,70,75,118,119]

Jaundice observed in the first 24 h[117] or prior to discharge[71,116]

Blood group incompatibility with positive direct antiglobulin test, other known hemolytic disease (e.g., G6PD deficiency, hereditary spherocytosis) (see Chapters 1 and 8)

Decreasing gestational age[11,69–71]

Previous sibling with jaundice or who received phototherapy[12,13]

Vacuum extraction delivery, cephalhematoma, or significant bruising[11,57–59]

Exclusive breastfeeding, particularly if nursing is not going well and weight loss is excessive[11,22,71,94]

East Asian race[3,11]

Macrosomic infant of a diabetic mother[29,31]

Maternal age ≥25 years[11]

Male gender[11,80]

factors, Gilbert's syndrome plays a ubiquitous role in the pathogenesis of neonatal hyperbilirubinemia. When the Gilbert's genotype is combined with other icterogenic factors such as breastfeeding,[17,18] G6PD deficiency,[19] ABO incompatibility,[20] and pyloric stenosis,[21] there is a dramatic increase in the newborn's risk for hyperbilirubinemia. In a striking example of the contribution of genetic mutations to hyperbilirubinemia in otherwise healthy infants, Huang et al.[22] studied 72 Taiwanese infants with TSB levels ≥20 mg/dL. The factors identified as contributing to hyperbilirubinemia in this study included a genetic polymorphism of the organic anion transporter protein *OATP-2*, a coding sequence gene polymorphism for the hepatic bilirubin conjugating enzyme uridine diphosphate glucuronosyltransferase 1A1 (*UGT1A1*), and breastfeeding. By itself, breastfeeding was associated with an odds ratio (OR) of 4.6 for the risk of developing a TSB ≥20 mg/dL. The combination of the *OATP-2* gene polymorphism with a variant *UGT1A1* gene at nucleotide 211 increased the OR to 22, and when these two genetic variants were combined with breastfeeding, the OR was 88.[22] As genetic testing is not routinely performed in jaundiced newborns, it is difficult to know what, if any, contribution these polymorphisms make to the individual jaundiced infant.

Nevertheless, it is clear that in the presence of a certain genotype, breastfeeding will contribute to the development of marked hyperbilirubinemia.[23]

■ MATERNAL FACTORS

Smoking

Some studies suggest that infants of mothers who smoke during pregnancy have lower TSB levels than infants of nonsmokers,[9,24] but others have not found this.[25,26] These data are confounded by the fact that women who smoke during pregnancy are less likely to breastfeed their infants (OR 0.45, 95% CI 0.31–0.64).[27]

Diabetes

Infants of insulin-dependent diabetic mothers (IDM) are more likely to become jaundiced than are control infants[28–32] and hyperbilirubinemia appears to be most prominent in macrosomic newborns[29] and those with an increased birth weight/length ratio.[31] With better diabetic control, as is currently the norm in developed countries, the risk of hyperbilirubinemia in this population should decrease.[29] The hyperbilirubinemia in these infants is most likely the result of an increase in bilirubin production, which is directly related to the degree of macrosomia.[33] Mean carboxyhemoglobin levels (an index of heme catabolism and bilirubin production) were $1.5 \pm 0.19\%$ (SD) in IDMs who were large for gestation (LGA) compared with $1.10 \pm 0.27\%$ in those who were appropriate for gestation (AGA) and $1.19 \pm 0.33\%$ ($P < .05$) in control infants.[33] IDMs also tend to have higher hematocrits[30,31] and increased erythropoietin levels in cord blood.[34] Diabetic mothers have three times more β-glucuronidase in their breast milk than nondiabetic mothers.[32] This enzyme enhances the enterohepatic reabsorption of bilirubin[35] (see section "Breastfeeding and Jaundice").

■ EVENTS DURING LABOR AND DELIVERY

Drugs

Induction and Augmentation of Labor by Oxytocin

Multiple studies and several controlled trials have shown an association between the use of oxytocin to induce or augment labor and an increased incidence of neonatal hyperbilirubinemia,[36] although the mechanism for this is unclear. An association has also been found between the total dose of oxytocin used for induction and the incidence of neonatal hyperbilirubinemia.[37]

Anesthesia and Analgesia

Anesthetic and analgesic agents readily cross the placenta and produce measurable levels in the newborn[38] and the use of bupivacaine in epidural anesthesia has been associated with neonatal jaundice.[26] Bupivacaine reduces red blood cell filterability in vitro and red cell survival in the rat so that increased bilirubin production could be the explanation for the described association between neonatal jaundice and maternal bupivacaine administration.[39]

Phenobarbital

Phenobarbital is a potent inducer of microsomal enzymes and increases bilirubin conjugation and excretion as well as bile flow.[40] When given in sufficient doses to the mother, the infant, or both, phenobarbital is effective in lowering serum bilirubin levels in term and preterm infants in the first week of life,[40–42] but concerns about long-term toxicity in the infant and even adults militate against the use of phenobarbital in pregnant women for this purpose.[43,44]

Other Drugs

The TSB concentrations at 48 and 72 hours are lower in infants of mothers who have received narcotic agents, barbiturates, aspirin, chloral hydrate, reserpine, and phenytoin, while diazepam and oxytocin lead to higher levels.[45] Infants of heroin-addicted mothers[46] have lower bilirubin levels as do the infants of mothers who received the analgesic and antipyretic, antipyrine, before delivery.[47] Antenatal betamethasone, when used to accelerate lung maturation, did not increase neonatal TSB levels[48] but antenatal dexamethasone was associated with an increased incidence of TSB levels >15 mg/dL in a group of preterm infants.[49]

Beta-agonists used for tocolysis do not affect carbon monoxide (CO) production in preterm neonates of mothers who receive these drugs[50,51] and were not associated with higher bilirubin levels.[51–53]

Delivery Mode

In one study, breastfed, vaginally delivered, term newborns had higher TSB and transcutaneous bilirubin (TcB) levels than those delivered by cesarean section (c-section),[54] although this difference was not found in

■ TABLE 6-2. Mean Breast Milk Transfer (mL/kg) (SD) in Infants Delivered Vaginally and by Cesarean Section

Day	Vaginal	C-Section	P (Adjusted)[a]
1	6 (7.1)	4 (2.9)	.03
2	25 (20.6)	13 (10.8)	<.001
3	66 (33.8)	44 (19.7)	.001
4	106 (36.6)	82 (34.4)	<.001
5	123 (42.2)	111 (32.5)	.046
6	138 (36.6)	129 (31.5)	.118
Total	450 (285)	358 (218)	.001

SD, standard deviation.

[a]Adjusted for breastfeeding experience, parity, and time to first breastfeed.

Data from Evans KC, Evans RG, Royal R, Esterman AJ, James SL. Effect of caesarean section on breast milk transfer to the normal term newborn over the first week of life. *Arch Dis Child Fetal Neonatal Ed.* 2003;88:F380–F382.

a controlled trial of delivery route for very low birth weight (VLBW) infants.[55] Breastfed infants delivered by c-section take in significantly fewer calories in the first 6 days than those delivered vaginally (Table 6-2).[56] Thus, one would except TSB levels to be higher in infants delivered by c-section (see section "Breastfeeding and Jaundice"). The average cumulative intake in a vaginally delivered infant in the first 6 days of life is 450 ± 285 mL (SD) versus 358 ± 218 mL (SD) in c-section infants (P = .001).[56] Infants delivered by c-section have lower hematocrits on day 6 than those delivered vaginally.[54]

Vacuum Extraction

Infants delivered by vacuum extraction[26,57,58] are more likely to have a cephalhematoma and/or bruising of the scalp and, therefore, more likely to develop hyperbilirubinemia. Because the catabolism of 1 g of hemoglobin yields 35 mg of bilirubin, bruising and cephalhematomas can contribute significantly to the infant's bilirubin load.[11,59,60]

Placental Transfusion and the Timing of Umbilical Cord Clamping

A *Cochrane* database review of 11 trials of 2989 mothers[61] and their infants found that in those whose cords were clamped early, significantly fewer required phototherapy for jaundice (RR 0.59, 95% CI 0.38–0.92).

■ **TABLE 6-3.** Effect of Gestation on the Risk of Subsequent Hyperbilirubinemia

Study	Outcome Variable	Gestation (Weeks)	Odds Ratio (95% CI) for Risk of Subsequent Hyperbilirubinemia
Maisels and Kring[71]	Readmission for phototherapy[a]	35 (0/7)–36 (0/7)	13.2 (2.7–64.6)[b]
		36 (1/7)–37 (0/7)	7.7 (2.7–22.0)[b]
Newman et al.[11]	TSB ≥25 mg/dL	36 (0/7)–42 (6/7)	1.7 (1.4–2.5) per week of gestation below 40 weeks
Keren et al.[70]	Within 1 mg/dL of hour-specific AAP phototherapy level (or higher)[a]	35 (0/7)–37 (6/7)	9.2 (4.4–19.0) bivariate
Maisels et al.[94]	TSB ≥17 mg/dL	35 (0/7)–36 (6/7)	20.8 (2.3–184.7)[b]
		37 (0/7)–37 (6/7)	14.9 (1.91–115.4)[b]

[a]Association partly due to lower treatment threshold in less mature infants.
[b]Compared with 40 weeks gestation.

The late clamped group also had a significant increase in hemoglobin levels. The blood volume of term and preterm newborns is increased when there is a delay in cord clamping.[62] In a study of infants 28–36 weeks of gestation, Saigal et al. found that if cord clamping was delayed, the mean TSB level at 72 hours was 7.7 mg/dL compared with 3.2 mg/dL in the early clamped group.[63] On the other hand, in a recent study of late preterm infants, although the late cord clamped group showed higher hemoglobin levels, there was no relationship between delayed clamping and pathologic jaundice or polycythemia and the need for phototherapy.[64]

Umbilical Cord Bilirubin Levels

The association between TSB levels in the cord blood and subsequent peak TSB concentrations was described more than 50 years ago[65] and has since been confirmed in infants with and without hemolytic disease.[66–68]

■ NEONATAL FACTORS

Gestation

In term and late preterm newborns, by far the most important single clinical factor associated with the subsequent risk of hyperbilirubinemia is the infant's gestational age.[11,69–71] This association has been confirmed consistently in multiple studies, although the magnitude of this risk has only recently been quantified (Table 6-3).[11,69–71] How decreasing gestation and other factors contribute to the risk of subsequent hyperbilirubinemia is discussed in detail in Chapter 9.

Birth Weight

Because birth weight is generally a direct reflection of gestational age, it has long been known that decreasing birth weight is associated with an increased risk of hyperbilirubinemia. Currently, it is impossible to determine the natural history of bilirubinemia in the VLBW (<1500 g) or extremely low birth weight (ELBW <1000 g) infant because a large proportion of these infants receive phototherapy. Small studies in the 1950s[72,73] showed a direct correlation between decreasing birth weight and maximum TSB concentrations and also showed that achievement of the peak TSB concentration occurs later in preterm infants than in term infants. In those days, kernicterus in LBW (<2500 g) infants was not uncommon.[74]

Given the association described above between decreasing birth weight and TSB levels, it is a surprise to find that in term and late preterm infants, after controlling for gestational age, there is a positive association between *increasing* birth weight and significant hyperbilirubinemia.[57,75,76] IDMs who are macrocosmic[29] and have an increased birth weight/length ratio[31] are more likely to develop hyperbilirubinemia than those who are AGA and some larger infants could be undiagnosed IDMs. Other potential explanations for the increase in TSB associated with larger birth weight are the need for vacuum extraction delivery[57] and scalp injury during delivery[11,69,76] and the fact that physicians may be less concerned about jaundice in larger babies and use higher TSB levels for initiating phototherapy.[76] Flaherman et al.[76] evaluated 111,009 infants born between 1995 and 1998. They used logistic regression to control for gestational age, scalp injury diagnosis, maternal diabetes, method of delivery, and other confounders, and found that higher birth weight was associated with TSB levels >20 mg/dL in 36–38 weeks gestation infants, but not in infants ≥39 weeks. Birth weight had a small but significant effect on hyperbilirubinemia only for less mature babies. The relationship between increasing birth weight and hyperbilirubinemia is intriguing and requires further investigation to elucidate its pathophysiology.[76]

Gender

As a group, male infants have higher bilirubin levels than females,[11,26,71,77,78] although occasional studies have not found this relationship.[70] In the reported cases of kernicterus, there is a striking preponderance of males.[79,80]

Caloric Intake and Weight Loss

There is a consistent association between hyperbilirubinemia and weight loss in the first few days after birth.[26,70,71,77,78,81] Caloric deprivation is associated with increases in TSB in animals and humans[82] and there is a reciprocal relationship between caloric intake and the degree of hyperbilirubinemia in Gilbert's syndrome.[83] In adults, caloric deprivation is also associated with increased hemolysis.[84] In a randomized controlled trial, infants with birth weights between 1250 and 2000 g were assigned to be fed within 2 hours of birth or 24–36 hours after birth. The earlier fed infants had significantly lower TSB levels between 96 and 144 hours.[85] The primary mechanism responsible for the lower TSB appears to be a decrease in the enterohepatic circulation of bilirubin.[82,86]

Type of Diet

Infants fed a casein hydrolysate formula had significantly lower TSB levels from days 10 to 18 than those in infants fed standard casein or whey-predominant

formulas.[87,88] The cumulative stool output of infants fed a casein hydrolysate formula was lower than that in infants fed the other formulas,[87] suggesting that factors other than stool output and its effect on the enterohepatic circulation must explain these observations. The casein hydrolysate formula (Nutramigen) contains an inhibitor of β-glucuronidase,[89] an enzyme that acts on the hydrolysis of bilirubin glucuronide and therefore facilitates the enterohepatic absorption of unconjugated bilirubin.[35] When fed saccharolactone, an inhibitor of β-glucuronidase, rats excrete less bilirubin in their bile suggesting that inhibition of β-glucuronidase decreased intestinal absorption of bilirubin.[90]

Breastfeeding and Jaundice

The vast majority of studies in the last 30 years have found a strong association between breastfeeding, elevated TSB levels in the first few days, and an increased risk of subsequent significant hyperbilirubinemia (Figure 6-1).[11,22,71,75,91–94] A pooled analysis of 12 studies of more than 8000 newborns showed that breastfed infants were about three times more likely to develop TSB levels of ≥12 mg/dL and six times more likely to develop levels of ≥15 mg/dL than formula-fed infants (Figure 6-1).[93] Table 6-4 lists some recent studies that have quantified the risk of hyperbilirubinemia in exclusively breastfed infants.

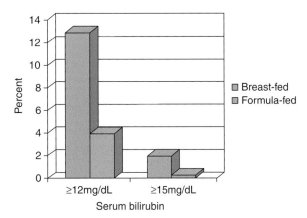

FIGURE 6-1. Pooled analysis of 12 studies showing the percent of breastfed and formula-fed newborns with serum bilirubin levels ≥12 mg/dL and, in 6 of the 12 studies, the percent of newborns with serum bilirubin levels ≥15 mg/dL. (Data from Schneider AP. Breast milk jaundice in the newborn. A real entity. *JAMA*. 1986;255:3270–3274.)

■ TABLE 6-4. Effect of Exclusive Breastfeeding on Risk of Subsequent Hyperbilirubinemia in Newborns ≥35 Weeks of Gestation

Study	N	Outcome Variable Bilirubin (mg/dL)	N with Outcome	OR (95% CI) versus Formula or Partially Breastfed
Maisels and Kring[71]	29,934	19.3 ± 2.7	127 (0.4%)	4.2 (1.8–9.9)
Newman et al.[11]	51,387	≥25	73 (0.14%)	5.7 (2.1–15.5)
Maisels et al.[94]	11,456	≥17	75 (0.65%)	10.75 (2.37–48.8)
Huang et al.[22]	a	≥20	72	4.6 (2.40–8.81)

[a]No denominator provided.

Two broad categories of the association between breastfeeding and jaundice have been described. That which occurs in the first week has been termed "breast-feeding jaundice" or "breastfeeding-associated jaundice," and that which appears later and is associated with prolonged jaundice has been called the "breast milk jaundice syndrome,"[95] but there is considerable overlap between these two entities. As a group, breastfed infants have TSB levels that are higher than those in formula-fed infants for at least 3–6 weeks following birth,[87,96] but these are the same infants who have higher TSB levels in the first week, so it is unclear whether or not those who are still jaundiced at age 3–4 weeks represent a distinct group.

Prolonged indirect-reacting hyperbilirubinemia (beyond 2–3 weeks) occurs in 20–30% of breastfeeding infants[97] and, in some infants, may persist for up to 3 months.[95] In 282 healthy, breastfed Turkish infants ≥37 weeks gestation, TSB at age 28–33 days was >5 mg/dL in 20.2% and >10 mg/dL in 6% of these infants.[98] Of 125 Taiwanese, breastfed infants, 35 (28%) had TSB levels >5.9 mg/dL after age 28 days.[97] Recent evidence suggests that mutations of the *UGT1A1* gene (Gilbert's syndrome) can play a significant role in the pathogenesis of prolonged hyperbilirubinemia[17,18,97] (see section "Genetic Factors").

The Pathogenesis of Jaundice Associated with Breastfeeding

Table 6-5 lists the factors that are thought to play a role in the pathophysiology of jaundice associated with breastfeeding.

Caloric Intake

The association between poor caloric intake and the development of hyperbilirubinemia has led some experts to categorize the jaundice associated with breastfeeding in the first few days after birth as "starvation jaundice" or "breast-nonfeeding jaundice."[95] The implication is that if breastfed infants were nursed effectively from birth, they would not be more jaundiced than formula-fed infants and there is some evidence to support this view.[81,99,100] Bertini et al. studied 2174 well newborns ≥37 weeks gestation.[81] All infants had continuous rooming in with their mothers and TSB levels were measured in jaundiced infants twice daily until there was a decrease in the TSB. Breastfed infants were exclusively breastfed 6–12 times per day and these infants were routinely supplemented with formula if the infant's birth weight was ≤2500 g, or if there was a weight loss of ≥4% at 24 hours, ≥8% at 48 hours, and ≥10% at 72 hours. Formula-fed infants received no breast milk. One hundred and twelve infants (5.1%) developed TSB levels >12 mg/dL and in these infants a positive correlation was found with

■ TABLE 6-5. Pathogenesis of Jaundice Associated with Breastfeeding

Increased enterohepatic circulation of bilirubin
- Decreased caloric intake
- Less cumulative stool output and stools contain less bilirubin (compared with formula-fed infants)
- Increased intestinal fat absorption
- Less formation of urobilin in gastrointestinal tract
- Increased activity of β-glucuronidase in breast milk

Decreased bilirubin conjugation
- Mutations of the *UGT1A1* gene (Gilbert's syndrome)— prolonged breast milk jaundice

■ **TABLE 6-6.** Comparison of Weight Loss and Intake in Breastfed and Formula-Fed Newborns (Mean ± SD)

	Breastfed (n = 15)	Formula Fed (n = 28)	P
Birth weight (kg)	3.26 ± 0.41	3.35 ± 0.35	ns
Gestation (weeks)	39.6 ± 0.9	39.7 ± 1.2	ns
Parity	2.3 ± 1.3	2.4 ± 0.9	ns
Weight loss, day 1 (g)	149 ± 96	130 ± 56	ns
Weight loss, day 2 (g)	67 ± 58	21 ± 46	.015
Intake, day 1 (mL/kg)	9.6 ± 10.3	18.5 ± 9.6	.011
Intake, day 2 (mL/kg)	13.0 ± 11.3	42.2 ± 14.2	<.001

Reproduced from Dollberg S, Lahav S, Mimouni FB. A comparison of intakes of breast-fed and bottle-fed infants during the first two days of life. *J Am Coll Nutr.* 2001;20:209–211, with permission.

formula supplementation (in 22%) and an increased weight loss at age 72 hours. Neither breastfeeding nor c-section was correlated with hyperbilirubinemia. The authors concluded that there is no increase in TSB levels in those infants who are breastfed effectively and who do not lose excess weight, while those who received formula supplementation because of excess weight loss were more likely to be jaundiced. These data support the view that it is less effective breastfeeding, rather than breastfeeding or breast milk per se, that is responsible for the association of breastfeeding and hyperbilirubinemia. In normal adults and those with Gilbert's syndrome, caloric deprivation increases hemolysis and bilirubin production[84] so that, in addition to its effect on the enterohepatic circulation, poor caloric intake in infants might also produce an increase in bilirubin production due to hemolysis.

Intestinal Reabsorption of Bilirubin

Intestinal reabsorption of bilirubin (the enterohepatic circulation) appears to be an important mechanism responsible for the jaundice associated with breast-feeding.[92] In the first few days after birth, breastfed infants take in significantly less volume and, therefore, fewer calories than formula-fed infants[101] (Table 6-6), and there is a relationship between decreased caloric intake and an increase in the enterohepatic circulation of bilirubin.[82,86] Further evidence for the role of the enterohepatic circulation can be found in the data of De Carvalho et al.[102] and Gourley et al.[87,103] Figure 6-2 shows that although breastfed and formula-fed infants passed the same number of stools in the first 3 days of life, formula-fed infants passed significantly more stool

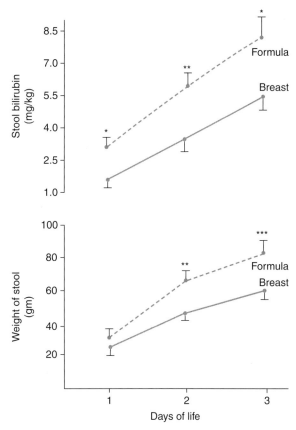

FIGURE 6-2. Mean ± SEM cumulative weight of stools and fecal bilirubin excretion in breastfed and formula-fed infants. (Reproduced from De Carvalho M, Robertson S, Klaus M. Fecal bilirubin excretion and serum bilirubin concentration in breast-fed and bottle-fed infants. *J Pediatr.* 1985;107:786–790. Copyright 1985, with permission from Elsevier.)

(w/w), and the bilirubin content of that stool was significantly greater than that of breastfed infants.[102] The rate of bilirubin production is similar in breastfed and formula-fed infants,[104] which indicates that, in addition to receiving more calories,[101] formula-fed infants have significantly less enterohepatic reabsorption of bilirubin than breastfed infants.

The relationship between fecal bilirubin excretion and TSB levels may also be related to the fecal excretion of unabsorbed fat.[105] The breast milk received by infants who developed TSB levels of more than 15 mg/dL contained significantly more fat than the milk fed to breastfed control infants.[106] Thus, the presence of increased fat in the intestine appears to facilitate the reabsorption of unconjugated bilirubin. In Gunn rats fed orlistat, a lipase inhibitor, the intestinal absorption of fat is inhibited, fecal fat excretion increases significantly, the enterohepatic circulation of unconjugated bilirubin is interrupted, and there is a significant decrease in unconjugated bilirubin levels.[105,107] This suggests that a substance that increases fecal excretion of fat will decrease the enterohepatic absorption of unconjugated bilirubin and facilitate bilirubin excretion in the gut. Breastfed infants absorb fat more efficiently than formula-fed infants, possibly related to the presence of bile salt–stimulated lipase in human milk,[108] and it is possible that neonatal hyperbilirubinemia could be prevented or mitigated by giving orlistat to newborns,[105,107] although it is unlikely that the resulting decrease in caloric intake would justify this. All of these findings support a major role for the enterohepatic circulation in the jaundice associated with breastfeeding.

Urobilinogen Formation

In adults, bilirubin in the gut is reduced rapidly by the action of colonic bacteria to urobilinogen and urobilin. At birth, the fetal gut is sterile, and although there is an increase in the bacterial content of the gut after delivery, the neonatal intestinal flora does not convert conjugated bilirubin to urobilin. This leaves conjugated bilirubin in the bowel and allows it to be deconjugated and thus available for reabsorption. Formula-fed infants excrete urobilin in their stools sooner than breastfed infants do, perhaps as a consequence of the effect of formula feeding on the intestinal flora.[109] Thus, the effect of breast milk on intestinal flora, by slowing the formation of urobilin, further enhances the possibility of intestinal reabsorption of bilirubin.

β-Glucuronidase

This is an enzyme that cleaves the ester linkage of bilirubin glucuronide, producing unconjugated bilirubin, which can then be reabsorbed through the gut. Significant concentrations of β-glucuronidase are found in the neonatal intestine, and its activity is higher in human milk than in infant formulas.[87] Gourley and Arend[35] found a positive relation between TSB levels and breast milk β-glucuronidase activity in the first 3–4 days after birth, but other investigators have not been able to confirm these findings.[110,111]

Meconium Passage

Because the enterohepatic circulation of bilirubin is an important contributor to neonatal hyperbilirubinemia, increasing the rate of bilirubin evacuation from the bowel should decrease the incidence of neonatal jaundice. Randomized studies have yielded conflicting results. In two studies, the early passage of meconium (stimulated by a rectal thermometer or a suppository) reduced peak TSB levels by about 1 mg/dL when compared with control groups[112,113] while in two other randomized trials, the use of glycerin enemas or glycerin suppositories following birth did not affect the number of infants who had a TSB level ≥15 mg/dL[114] or the mean TSB levels at age 48 hours (6.5 ± 1.3 mg/dL vs. 7.0 ± 2.3 mg/dL).[115] Male neonates who received glycerin suppositories had lower bilirubin levels than male controls (6.1 ± 2.8 mg/dL vs. 7.5 ± 2.4 mg/dL, $P = .02$).[115] The effect, if any, of early meconium evacuation on TSB levels is modest.

Other Factors

Jaundice and the Predischarge Bilirubin Level

Infants who are clinically jaundiced in the first few days[71,116] and particularly those jaundiced in the first 24 hours[117] are much more likely to subsequently develop significant hyperbilirubinemia and a measurement of a TSB or TcB level prior to discharge is a powerful predictor of the risk of subsequent hyperbilirubinemia.[11,57,70,75,118,119] These are dealt with in detail in a subsequent chapter 9.

Extravascular Blood

Cephalhematoma, bruising, intracranial or pulmonary hemorrhage, or any occult bleeding can lead to an elevated TSB level from the breakdown of extravascular erythrocytes.[11,120–122] Severe hyperbilirubinemia followed delayed absorption of intraperitoneal blood in infants who received intraperitoneal fetal transfusions before birth.[122] In the VLBW infant, the presence of intraventricular or periventricular hemorrhage was associated with an increase in TSB levels in some studies[123,124] but not in others.[125]

Polycythemia

It is often assumed that a high hematocrit is a risk factor for neonatal jaundice, because an increase in the erythrocyte mass should increase the bilirubin load presented to the liver. Nevertheless, mean bilirubin levels and the incidence of hyperbilirubinemia were similar in polycythemic infants randomly assigned to receive either partial exchange transfusions or symptomatic treatment.[126–128] As noted above (see section "Placental Transfusion and the Timing of Umbilical Cord Clamping"), when cord clamping was delayed the mean TSB level at 72 hours was 7.7 mg/dL compared with 3.2 mg/dL in the early clamped group.[63] On the other hand, in a study of late preterm infants, although the late clamped group showed higher hemoglobin levels, there was no relationship between delayed clamping and pathologic jaundice or polycythemia and the need for phototherapy.[64]

Phenolic Detergents

The use of phenolic detergents to disinfect incubators and other nursery surfaces was associated with an epidemic of neonatal hyperbilirubinemia in two hospitals.[129,130] These detergents should not be used in the nursery.

Altitude

Thirty-nine percent of infants born at an altitude of 3100 m had a TSB ≥12 mg/dL versus 13–16% of those born at 1600 m.[131,132] Possible mechanisms for these observations include an increase in bilirubin load because of increased red cell turnover as well as high hematocrits.[132]

Drugs Administered to the Infant

The use of pancuronium and chloral hydrate in the neonate is associated with an increase risk of hyperbilirubinemia.[133–135] Chloral hydrate is metabolized to trichloroacetic acid and the toxic trichloroethanol, both of which accumulate in the tissues of compromised infants. The administration of chloral hydrate is associated with both indirect-reacting and direct-reacting hyperbilirubinemia.[134]

Free Radical Production

Bilirubin appears to have an important physiologic function as an antioxidant and may play a role in the prevention of oxidative membrane damage in vivo.[136] Infants with circulatory failure, sepsis, aspiration syndromes, and asphyxia—conditions believed to enhance free radical production—had a significantly lower daily rise in mean TSB levels than control infants.[136] These findings are consistent with the hypothesis that bilirubin is a free radical scavenger and is consumed as an antioxidant.[137–140]

■ NORMAL BILIRUBIN VALUES

Defining what represents "a normal bilirubin level" in the term and late preterm infant has long represented a challenge. Hour-specific TSB levels vary considerably depending on the racial composition of the population, the prevalence of breastfeeding, the mean gestational age of the infants evaluated, and other genetic and epidemiologic factors. In addition, the method used by the clinical laboratory to measure TSB adds its own variation to the data.[141,142]

Since the advent of phototherapy, it has been difficult to obtain a true picture of the natural history of neonatal bilirubinemia because we treat some infants with rising bilirubin levels in the first 24–72 hours, even though many have no defined pathologic or other known cause for the rising bilirubin level. Thus, what we generally see is a "damped" picture of the natural history, and whether infants who have received phototherapy but do not have a clear diagnosis should be omitted from studies that attempt to define a "normal" population is worthy of debate.

The age of the population studied also affects our definition of normal values, particularly the upper limits, as infants who develop higher bilirubin levels may not be seen until they are 6–10 days old. These infants are usually not included in studies restricted to hospitalized populations.

Data from the Collaborative Perinatal Project (CPP) conducted from 1955 to 1961 (when 30% or fewer mothers breastfed their infants and phototherapy was not available) showed that approximately 95% of all infants had TSB concentrations that did not exceed 12.9 mg/dL and this value became accepted as the upper limit of "physiologic jaundice."[10] More recent studies

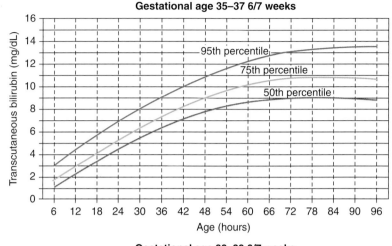

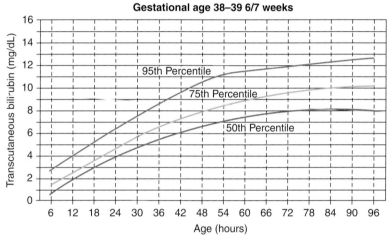

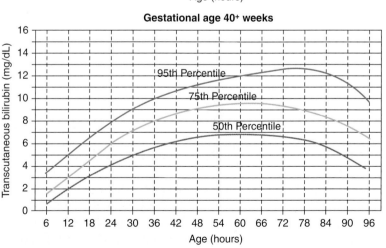

FIGURE 6-3. Transcutaneous bilirubin levels in the first 96 hours in a normal newborn population of ≥35 weeks gestation. Effect of gestational age on transcutaneous bilirubin levels and on the time course of bilirubinemia. Smoothed curves of the 50th, 75th, and 95th percentiles. Data from 9397 TcB measurements on 3984 healthy newborns. Infants who required phototherapy prior to discharge were excluded (*n* = 139). (Reproduced from Maisels MJ, Kring E. Transcutaneous bilirubin levels in the first 96 hours in a normal newborn population of 35 or more weeks' of gestation. *Pediatrics.* 2006;117:1169–1173, with permission. Copyright 2006 by the American Association of Pediatrics.)

that have included readmitted infants have defined the 95th percentile as a level of 17.5 mg/dL.[7,119] Newman et al. studied 51,387 infants born between 1995 and 1996, ≥36 weeks gestation and ≥2000 g birth weight in 11 Northern California Kaiser Permanente hospitals.[7] TSB ≥15 mg/dL occurred in 9.3% of all births (compared with 2% of those >2500 g in the CPP) and levels of 20 mg/dL or more in 2% (vs. 0.95% in the CPP). One in 700 infants had a maximum TSB of 25 mg/dL or more, and ~1 in 10,000 had maximum levels ≥30 mg/dL.

In the international multicenter study referenced above[75] a value of 17 mg/dL was 2 standard deviations above the mean and the 95th percentile was 15.5 mg/dL.[143] In a Greek population[144] the 95th percentile at 108 hours was a TSB level of 15.1 mg/dL. Recognizing that there will be significant differences in different populations, these data suggest, at least in US populations where approximately 70% of mothers initiate breastfeeding in the hospital,[145] that peak TSB levels are normally 17–18 mg/dL or less.

From the clinician's point of view, this implies that a 4- to 5-day-old breastfed infant, whose TSB level is 15 mg/dL, does not require any laboratory investigation to find out *why* the infant is jaundiced, although follow-up is necessary to ensure that the bilirubin levels do not become excessive.[146,147] In the international multicenter study, the mean TSB level at 96 ± 6.5 hours was 8.9 ± 4.4 (SD) mg/dL in breastfed infants and 7.6 ± 3.58 (SD) mg/dL in those fed formula ($P < .0001$).[75] Because so many LBW, VLBW, and ELBW infants receive phototherapy, it is not possible to provide reference values for these infants.

■ THE NATURAL HISTORY OF NEONATAL BILIRUBINEMIA

The availability of electronic TcB measurements has made it possible to obtain frequent measurements (as often as every 6–12 hours), and to study the natural history of bilirubinemia and bilirubin kinetics in large contemporary populations.[144,148–152] TcB nomograms for newborn populations have been developed in the United States,[148,149] Canada,[153] Italy,[150] Greece,[144,154] Thailand,[152] China,[155] Japan,[156] and other parts of the world. These studies provide normative data for different populations and the nomograms have been used to identify unusually

elevated levels and trends in the rate of rise of TcB, and for assessment of risk for the subsequent development of severe hyperbilirubinemia (discussed in detail in Chapter 9).

Short hospital stays in the United States have made it necessary to restrict the study of the natural history of neonatal bilirubinemia to measurements in the first 96 hours and, after 72 hours, to include only infants delivered by c-section. In Calgary, follow-up at home by public health nurses has permitted the development of a nomogram that extends out to 144 hours.[157] De Luca et al.[151] compared four published TcB nomograms and analyzed the differences in TcB levels and kinetics in these populations. The weighted mean TcB value at 73–96 hours was 8.6 ± 3.3 mg/dL with a range of 6.9–10.4 mg/dL. The data of Maisels and Kring[148] demonstrate clearly the differences in natural history between infants of gestational age ≥40 weeks and those <40 weeks, showing how much earlier the TcB values peak and then decline in the more mature infants (Figure 6-3). Perhaps the most complete data to date have been provided by Fouzas et al.[144,154] who gathered data on large populations of term and late preterm infants in the first 120 postnatal hours. Infants with a positive DAT and those who required phototherapy in the first 24 hours were excluded in these studies, so all of the percentiles are lower than if they reflected the true natural history. Because of the tendency to use more phototherapy in less mature infants, exclusion of infants receiving phototherapy may also have attenuated the association between lower gestational age and higher bilirubin percentiles at each age.

REFERENCES

1. Maisels MJ. Jaundice. In: MacDonald MG, Seshia MMK, Mullett MD, eds. *Avery's Neonatology*. Philadelphia, PA: Lippincott Co; 2005:768–846.
2. Horiguchi T, Bauer C. Ethnic differences in neonatal jaundice: comparison of Japanese and Caucasian newborn infants. *Am J Obstet Gynecol.* 1975;121:71–74.
3. Newman TB, Easterling MJ, Goldman ES, Stevenson DK. Laboratory evaluation of jaundiced newborns: frequency, cost and yield. *Am J Dis Child.* 1990;144:364–368.
4. Munroe M, Shah CP, Badgley R, Bain HW. Birthweight, length, head circumference and bilirubin level in Indian newborns in the Sioux Lookout Zone, Northwestern Ontario. *Can Med Assoc J.* 1984;131:453–456.

5. Johnson JD, Angelus P, Aldrich M, Skipper BJ. Exaggerated jaundice in Navajo neonates: the role of bilirubin production. *Am J Dis Child.* 1986;140:889–890.

6. Engle WD, Jackson GL, Sendelbach D, Manning D, Frawley W. Assessment of a transcutaneous device in the evaluation of neonatal hyperbilirubinemia in a primarily Hispanic population. *Pediatrics.* 2002;110:61–67.

7. Newman TB, Escobar GJ, Gonzales VM, et al. Frequency of neonatal bilirubin testing and hyperbilirubinemia in a large health maintenance organization. *Pediatrics.* 1999;104:1198–1203.

8. Maisels MJ, Ostrea E Jr, Touch S, et al. Evaluation of a new transcutaneous bilirubinometer. *Pediatrics.* 2004;113: 1628–1635.

9. Linn S, Schoenbaum SC, Monson RR, et al. Epidemiology of neonatal hyperbilirubinemia. *Pediatrics.* 1985;75:770–774.

10. Hardy JB, Drage JS, Jackson EC. *The First Year of Life: The Collaborative Perinatal Project of the National Institutes of Neurological and Communicative Disorders and Stroke.* Baltimore, MD: Johns Hopkins University Press; 1979.

11. Newman TB, Xiong B, Gonzales VM, Escobar GJ. Prediction and prevention of extreme neonatal hyperbilirubinemia in a mature health maintenance organization. *Arch Pediatr Adolesc Med.* 2000;154:1140–1147.

12. Khoury MJ, Calle EE, Joesoef RM. Recurrence risk of neonatal hyperbilirubinemia in siblings. *Am J Dis Child.* 1988;142:1065–1069.

13. Nielsen HE, Haase P, Blaabjerg J, et al. Risk factors and sib correlation in physiological neonatal jaundice. *Acta Paediatr Scand.* 1987;76:504–511.

14. Fok TF, Lau SP, Hui CW. Neonatal jaundice: its prevalence in Chinese babies and associating factors. *Aust Paediatr J.* 1986;22(3):215–219.

15. Roy-Chowdhury N, Deocharan B, Bejjanki HR, et al. Presence of the genetic marker for Gilbert syndrome is associated with increased level and duration of neonatal jaundice. *Acta Paediatr.* 2002;91:100–101.

16. Kaplan M, Hammerman C, Rubaltelli F, et al. Hemolysis and bilirubin conjugation in association with UDP-glucuronosyltransferase 1A1 promoter polymorphism. *Hepatology.* 2002;35:905–911.

17. Monaghan G, McLellan A, McGeehan A, et al. Gilbert's syndrome is a contributory factor in prolonged unconjugated hyperbilirubinemia of the newborn. *J Pediatr.* 1999;134:441–446.

18. Maruo Y, Nishizawa K, Sato H, Sawa H, Shimada M. Prolonged unconjugated hyperbilirubinemia associated with breast milk and mutations of the bilirubin uridine diphosphate glucuronosyltransferase gene. *Pediatrics.* 2000;106:E59. Available at: http://www.pediatrics.org/cgi/content/full/106/5/e59:e59.

19. Kaplan M, Renbaum P, Levi-Lahad E, et al. Gilbert syndrome and glucose-6-phosphate dehydrogenase deficiency: a dose-dependent genetic interaction crucial to neonatal hyperbilirubinemia. *Proc Natl Acad Sci U S A.* 1997;94:12128–12132.

20. Kaplan M, Hammerman C, Renbaum P, Klein G, Levy-Lahad E. Gilbert's syndrome and hyperbilirubinaemia in ABO-incompatible neonates. *Lancet.* 2000;356: 652–653.

21. Trioche P, Chalas J, Francoual J, et al. Jaundice with hypertrophic pyloric stenosis as an early manifestation of Gilbert syndrome. *Arch Dis Child.* 1999;81: 301–303.

22. Huang M-J, Kua K-E, Teng H-C, Tang K-S, Weng H-W, Huang C-S. Risk factors for severe hyperbilirubinemia in neonates. *Pediatr Res.* 2004;56:682–689.

23. Watchko JF. Genetics and the risk of neonatal hyperbilirubinemia. *Pediatr Res.* 2004;56:677–678.

24. Diwan VK, Vaughan TL, Yang CY. Maternal smoking in relation to the incidence of early neonatal jaundice. *Gynecol Obstet Invest.* 1989;27:22–25.

25. Knudsen A. Maternal smoking and the bilirubin concentration in the first three days of life. *Eur J Obstet Gynecol Reprod Biol.* 1991;25:37–41.

26. Gale R, Seidman DS, Dollberg S, Stevenson DK. Epidemiology of neonatal jaundice in the Jerusalem population. *J Pediatr Gastroenterol Nutr.* 1990;10:82–86.

27. van Rossem L, Oenema A, Steegers EA, et al. Are starting and continuing breastfeeding related to educational background? The generation R study. *Pediatrics.* 2009;123(6):e1017–e1027.

28. Ballard JL, Rosenn B, Khoury J, Miodovnik M. Diabetic fetal macrosomia: significance of disproportionate growth. *J Pediatr.* 1993;122:115–119.

29. Peevy KJ, Landaw SA, Gross SJ. Hyperbilirubinemia in infants of diabetic mothers. *Pediatrics.* 1980;66: 417–419.

30. Berk MA, Mimouni F, Miodovnik M, Hertzberg V, Valuck J. Macrosomia in infants of insulin-dependent diabetic mothers. *Pediatrics.* 1989;83:1029–1034.

31. Jährig D, Jährig K, Striet S, et al. Neonatal jaundice in infants of diabetic mothers. *Acta Paediatr Scand (Suppl).* 1989;360:101–107.

32. Sirota L, Ferrera M, Lerer N, Dulitzky F. Beta-glucuronidase and hyperbilirubinaemia in breast fed infants of diabetic mothers. *Arch Dis Child.* 1992;67:120–121.

33. Stevenson DK, Bartoletti AL, Johnson JD. Pulmonary excretion of carbon monoxide in the human infant as an index of bilirubin production. II. Infants of diabetic mothers. *J Pediatr.* 1979;94:956–958.

34. Widness JA, Susa JB, Garcia JF, et al. Increased erythropoiesis and elevated erythropoietin in infants born

to diabetic mothers and in hyperinsulinemic rhesus fetuses. *J Clin Invest.* 1981;67:637–642.

35. Gourley GR, Arend RA. Beta-glucuronidase and hyperbilirubinemia in breast-fed and formula-fed babies. *Lancet.* 1986;1:644–646.

36. Maisels MJ. Neonatal jaundice. In: Sinclair JC, Bracken MB, eds. *Effective Care of the Newborn Infant.* Oxford: Oxford University Press; 1992:507–561.

37. Beazley JM, Alderman B. Neonatal hyperbilirubinemia following use of oxytocin in labor. *Br J Obstet Gynaecol.* 1975;82:265–271.

38. Pedersen H, Morishima HO, Finster M. Uptake and effects of local anesthetics in mother and fetus. *Int Anesthesiol Clin.* 1978;16:73–89.

39. Clark DA, Landaw SA. Bupivacaine alters red blood cell properties: a possible explanation for neonatal jaundice associated with maternal anesthesia. *Pediatr Res.* 1985;19:341–343.

40. Valaes T, Harvey-Wilkes K. Pharmacologic approaches to the prevention and treatment of neonatal hyperbilirubinemia. *Clin Perinatol.* 1990;17:245–274.

41. Valaes T. Pharmacological approaches to the prevention and treatment of neonatal hyperbilirubinemia. In: Maisels MJ, Watchko JF, eds. *Neonatal Jaundice.* London, UK: Harwood Academic Publishers; 2000: 205–214.

42. Chavla D, Parmar V. Phenobarbitone for prevention and treatment of unconjugated hyperbilirubinemia in preterm neonates: a systematic review and meta-analysis. *Indian Pediatr.* 2010;47(5):401–407.

43. Yaffe SJ, Dorn LD. Effects of prenatal treatment with phenobarbital. *Dev Pharmacol Ther.* 1990;15:215.

44. Reinisch JM, Sanders SA, Mortensen EL, Rubin DB. In utero exposure to phenobarbital and intelligence deficits in adult men. *JAMA.* 1995;15:18–25.

45. Drew JH, Kitchen WH. The effect of maternally administered drugs on bilirubin concentrations in the newborn infant. *J Pediatr.* 1976;89:657–661.

46. Nathenson G, Cohen MI, Litt IF, McNamara H. The effect of maternal heroin addition on neonatal jaundice. *J Pediatr.* 1972;81:899–903.

47. Lewis PJ, Friedman LA. Prophylaxis of neonatal jaundice with maternal antipyrine treatment. *Lancet.* 1979;1:300–302.

48. Liggins GC, Howie RN. A controlled trial of antepartum glucocortioid treatment for prevention of the respiratory distress syndrome in premature infants. *Pediatrics.* 1972;50:515.

49. Nemeth I, Szeleczki T, Boda D. Hyperbilirubinemia and urinary D-glucose and excretion in premature infants following antepartum dexamethasone treatment. *J Perinat Med.* 1981;9:35–39.

50. Hopper AO, Cohen RS, Ostrander CR, Brackman FS, Uekand K, Stevenson DK. Maternal adrenergic tocolysis and neonatal bilirubin production. *Am J Dis Child.* 1983;137:58–60.

51. Ferguson JE II, Schutz TE, Stevenson DK. Neonatal bilirubin production after preterm labor tocolysis with nifedipine. *Dev Pharmacol Ther.* 1989;12: 113–117.

52. Hancock DJ, Setzer ES, Beydown SN. Physiologic and biochemical effects of ritodrine therapy on the mother and perinate. *Am J Perinatol.* 1985;2:1–6.

53. Caritis SN, Toig G, Heddinger LA, Ashmead G. A double-blind study comparing ritodrine and terbutaline in the treatment of preterm labor. *Am J Obstet Gynecol.* 1984;150:7–14.

54. Yamauchi Y, Yamanouchi I. Difference in TcB readings between full term newborn infants born vaginally and by cesarean section. *Acta Paediatr Scand.* 1989;78: 824–828.

55. Wallace RL, Schifrin BS, Paul RH. The delivery route for very-low-birth-weight infants. A preliminary report of a randomized, prospective study. *J Reprod Med.* 1984;29:736–740.

56. Evans KC, Evans RG, Royal R, Esterman AJ, James SL. Effect of caesarean section on breast milk transfer to the normal term newborn over the first week of life. *Arch Dis Child Fetal Neonatal Ed.* 2003;88: F380–F382.

57. Keren R, Bhutani VK, Luan X, Nihtianova S, Cnaan A, Schwartz JS. Identifying newborns at risk of significant hyperbilirubinaemia: a comparison of two recommended approaches. *Arch Dis Child.* 2005;90: 415–421.

58. Arad I, Fainmesser P, Birkenfeld A, Gulaiev B, Sadovsky E. Vacuum extraction and neonatal jaundice. *J Perinat Med.* 1982;10(6):273–278.

59. Maisels MJ, Gifford K, Antle CE, Leib GR. Jaundice in the healthy newborn infant: a new approach to an old problem. *Pediatrics.* 1988;81:505–511.

60. Kuzniewicz MW, Escobar GJ, Wi S, Liljestrand P, McCulloch C, Newman TB. Risk factors for severe hyperbilirubinemia among infants with borderline bilirubin levels: a nested case–control study. *J Pediatr.* 2008;153:234–240.

61. McDonald SJ, Middleton P. Effect of timing of umbilical cord clamping of term infants on maternal and neonatal outcomes. *Cochrane Database Syst Rev.* 2008;16(2):CD004074.

62. Aladangady N, McHugh S, Aitchison TC, Wardrop CAJ, Holland BM. Infants' blood volume in a controlled trial of placental transfusion at preterm delivery. *Pediatrics.* 2006;117(1):93–98.

63. Saigal S, O'Neill A, Surainder Y, Chua LB, Usher R. Placental transfusion and hyperbilirubinemia in the premature. *Pediatrics.* 1972;49:406–419.

64. Ultee CA, van der Deure J, Swart J, Lasham C, van Baar AL. Delayed cord clamping in preterm infants delivered at 34–36 weeks' gestation: a randomised controlled trial. *Arch Dis Child Fetal Neonatal Ed.* 2008;93(1): F20–F23.

65. Dubey AP, Garg A, Bhatia BD. Fetal exposure to maternal hyperbilirubinemia. *Ind Pediatr.* 1983;20: 527–528.

66. Knudsen A, Lebech M. Maternal bilirubin, cord bilirubin and placental function at delivery in the development of jaundice in mature newborns. *Acta Obstet Gynecol Scand.* 1989;68:719–724.

67. Rosenfeld J. Umbilical cord bilirubin levels as a predictor of subsequent hyperbilirubinemia. *J Fam Pract.* 1986;23:556–558.

68. Risemberg HM, Mazzi E, MacDonald MG, et al. Correlation of cord bilirubin levels with hyperbilirubinemia in ABO incompatibility. *Arch Dis Child.* 1977;52: 219–222.

69. Newman T, Liljestrand P, Escobar G. Combining clinical risk factors with bilirubin levels to predict hyperbilirubinemia in newborns. *Arch Pediatr Adolesc Med.* 2005;159:113–119.

70. Keren R, Luan X, Friedman S, Saddlemire S, Cnaan A, Bhutani V. A comparison of alternative risk-assessment strategies for predicting significant neonatal hyperbilirubinemia in term and near-term infants. *Pediatrics.* 2008;121:e170–e179. Available at: http://www.pediatrics.org/cgi/content/full/121/1/e170:e170-e179.

71. Maisels MJ, Kring EA. Length of stay, jaundice and hospital readmission. *Pediatrics.* 1998;101:995–998.

72. Hsia DYY, Allen FH, Diamond LK, Gellis SS. Serum bilirubin levels in the newborn infant. *J Pediatr.* 1953;42:277–285.

73. Billing BH, Cole PG, Lathe GH. Increased plasma bilirubin in newborn infants in relation to birth weight. *BMJ.* 1954;2:1263–1265.

74. Shnier MH, Levin SE. Hyperbilirubinaemia and kernicterus in premature and full-term Bantu newborn infants. *Br Med J.* 1959;1:1004–1007.

75. Stevenson DK, Fanaroff AA, Maisels MJ, et al. Prediction of hyperbilirubinemia in near-term and term infants. *Pediatrics.* 2001;108:31–39.

76. Flaherman VJ, Ferrara A, Newman TB. Predicting significant hyperbilirubinaemia using birth weight. *Arch Dis Child Neonatal Ed.* 2008;93:F307–F309.

77. Wood B, Culley P, Roginski C, Powell J, Waterhouse J. Factors affecting neonatal jaundice. *Arch Dis Child.* 1979;54:111–115.

78. Frishberg Y, Zelicovic I, Merlob P, Reisner SH. Hyperbilirubinemia and influencing factors in term infants. *Isr J Med Sci.* 1989;25:28–31.

79. Ip S, Chung M, Kulig J, et al. An evidence-based review of important issues concerning neonatal hyperbilirubinemia. *Pediatrics.* 2004;114:e130–e153. Available at: www.pediatrics.org/cgi/content/full/114/1/e130:e130-e153.

80. Bhutani VK, Johnson LH, Maisels MJ, et al. Kernicterus: epidemiological strategies for its prevention through systems-based approaches. *J Perinatol.* 2004;24:650–662.

81. Bertini G, Dani C, Trochin M, Rubaltelli F. Is breast feeding really favoring early neonatal jaundice? *Pediatrics.* 2001;107:E41. Available at: http://www.pediatrics.org/cgi/content/full/101/2/e41.

82. Fevery J. Fasting hyperbilirubinemia: unraveling the mechanism involved. *Gastroenterology.* 1997;113:1798–1800.

83. Felsher BF, Rickard D, Redeker AG. The reciprocal relation between caloric intake and the degree of hyperbilirubinemia in Gilbert's syndrome. *N Engl J Med.* 1970;283:170–172.

84. Bensinger TA, Maisels MJ, Carlson DE, Conrad ME. Effect of low caloric diet on endogenous carbon monoxide production: normal adults and Gilbert's syndrome. *Proc Soc Exp Biol Med.* 1973;144:417–419.

85. Wu PYK, Teilmann P, Gabler M, Vaughan M, Metcoff J. "Early" vs. "late" feeding of low birth weight neonates: effect on serum bilirubin, blood sugar and responses to glucagon and epinephrine tolerance tests. *Pediatrics.* 1967;39:733–739.

86. Gärtner U, Goeser T, Wolkoff AW. Effect of fasting on the uptake of bilirubin and sulfobromophthalein by the isolated perfused rat liver. *Gastroenterology.* 1997;113:1707–1713.

87. Gourley GR, Kreamer B, Arend R. The effect of diet on feces and jaundice during the first three weeks of life. *Gastroenterology.* 1992;103:660.

88. Gourley GR, Kreamer B, Cohnen M, Kosorok MR. Neonatal jaundice and diet. *Arch Pediatr Adolesc Med.* 1999;153:184–188.

89. Gourley GR, Li Z, Kreamer BL, Kosorok MR. A controlled, randomized, double-blind trial of prophylaxis against jaundice among breastfed newborns. *Pediatrics.* 2005;116:385–391.

90. Gourley GR, Gourley MF, Arend R, Palta M. The effect of saccharolactone on rat intestinal absorption of bilirubin in the presence of human breast milk. *Pediatr Res.* 1989;25:234–238.

91. Ebbesen F, Brodersen R. Risk of bilirubin acid precipitation in preterm infants with respiratory distress syndrome: considerations of blood/brain bilirubin transfer equilibrium. *Early Hum Dev.* 1982;6:341–355.

92. Gourley GR. Breast-feeding, neonatal jaundice and kernicterus. *Semin Neonatol.* 2002;7:135–141.

93. Schneider AP. Breast milk jaundice in the newborn. A real entity. *JAMA.* 1986;255:3270–3274.

94. Maisels MJ, DeRidder JM, Kring EA, Balasubramaniam M. Routine transcutaneous bilirubin measurements combined with clinical risk factors improve the prediction of subsequent hyperbilirubinemia. *J Perinatol.* 2009;29:612–617.

95. Gartner L. Breastfeeding and jaundice. *J Perinatol.* 2001;21:S25–S29.

96. Kivlahan C, James EJP. The natural history of neonatal jaundice. *Pediatrics.* 1984;74:364–370.

97. Chang P-F, Lin Y-C, Liu K, Yeh S-J, Ni T-H. Prolonged unconjugated hyperbilirubinemia in breast-fed male infants with a mutation of uridine diphosphate-glucuronosyl transferase. *J Pediatr.* 2009;155:860–863.

98. Tiker F, Gurakan B, Tarcan A, Kinik S. Serum bilirubin levels in 1-month-old, healthy, term infants from southern Turkey. *Ann Trop Paediatr.* 2002;22:225–228.

99. De Carvalho M, Klaus MH, Merkatz RB. Frequency of breastfeeding and serum bilirubin concentration. *Am J Dis Child.* 1982;136:737–738.

100. Yamauchi Y, Yamanouchi I. Breast-feeding frequency during the first 24 hours after birth in full-term neonates. *Pediatrics.* 1990;86:171–175.

101. Dollberg S, Lahav S, Mimouni FB. A comparison of intakes of breast-fed and bottle-fed infants during the first two days of life. *J Am Coll Nutr.* 2001;20(3):209–211.

102. De Carvalho M, Robertson S, Klaus M. Fecal bilirubin excretion and serum bilirubin concentration in breast-fed and bottle-fed infants. *J Pediatr.* 1985;107:786–790.

103. Gourley GR. Pathophysiology of breast-milk jaundice. In: Polin RA, Fox WW, eds. *Fetal and Neonatal Physiology.* Philadelphia, PA: WB Saunders Co; 1998:1499.

104. Stevenson DK, Vreman HJ, Oh W, et al. Bilirubin production in healthy term infants as measured by carbon monoxide in breath. *Clin Chem.* 1994;40:1934–1939.

105. Verkade HJ. A novel hypothesis on the pathophysiology of neonatal jaundice. *J Pediatr.* 2002;141:594–595.

106. Amato M, Berthet G, von Muralt G. Influence of fatty diet on neonatal jaundice in breast-fed infants. *Acta Paediatr Jpn.* 1988;30(4):492–496.

107. Nishioka T, Hafkamp AM, Havinga R, Van Lierop PPE, Velvis H, Verkade HJ. Orlistat treatment increases fecal bilirubin excretion and decreases plasma bilirubin concentrations in hyperbilirubinemic Gunn rats. *J Pediatr.* 2003;143:327–334.

108. Hamosh M. Digestion in the newborn. *Clin Perinatol.* 1996;23:191–209.

109. Yoshioka H. Development and differences of intestinal flora in the neonatal period in breast-fed and bottle-fed infants. *Pediatrics.* 1983;72:317–321.

110. Alonso EM, Whitington PF, Whitington SH, Rivard WA, Given G. Enterohepatic circulation of non-conjugated bilirubin in rats fed with human milk. *J Pediatr.* 1991;118:425–430.

111. Wilson DC, Afrasiabi M, Reid MM. Breast-milk beta-glucuronidase and exaggerated jaundice in the early neonatal period. *Biol Neonate.* 1992;61:232–234.

112. Cottrell BH, Anderson GC. Rectal or axillary temperature measurement: effect on plasma bilirubin and intestinal transit of meconium. *J Pediatr Gastroenterol Nutr.* 1984;3:734–739.

113. Weisman LE, Merenstein GB, Digirol M, Collins J, Frank G, Hudgins C. The effect of early meconium evacuation on early-onset hyperbilirubinemia. *Am J Dis Child.* 1983;137:666–668.

114. Chen J-Y, Ling U-P, Chen J-H. Early meconium evacuation: effect on neonatal hyperbilirubinemia. *Am J Perinatol.* 1995;12(4):232–234.

115. Bader D, Yanir Y, Kuglman A, Wilhelm-Kafil M, Riskin A. Induction of early meconium evacuation: is it effective in reducing the level of neonatal hyperbilirubinemia? *Am J Perinatol.* 2005;22:329–333.

116. Soskolne EI, Schumacher R, Fyock C, Young ML, Schork A. The effect of early discharge and other factors on readmission rates of newborns. *Arch Pediatr Adolesc Med.* 1996;150:373–379.

117. Newman TB, Liljestrand P, Escobar GJ. Jaundice noted in the first 24 hours after birth in a managed care organization. *Arch Pediatr Adolesc Med.* 2002;156:1244–1250.

118. Kaplan M, Hammerman C, Feldman R, Brisk R. Pre-discharge bilirubin screening in glucose-6-phosphate dehydrogenase-deficient neonates. *Pediatrics.* 2000;105:533–537.

119. Bhutani VK, Johnson L, Sivieri EM. Predictive ability of a predischarge hour-specific serum bilirubin for subsequent significant hyperbilirubinemia in healthy-term and near-term newborns. *Pediatrics.* 1999;103:6–14.

120. Rajagopalan I, Katz BZ. Hyperbilirubinemia secondary to hemolysis of intrauterine intraperitoneal blood transfusion. *Clin Pediatr.* 1984;23:511–512.

121. Rose J, Berdon WE, Sullivan T, Baker DH. Prolonged jaundice as presenting sign of massive adrenal hemorrhage in newborn. *Radiology.* 1971;98:263–272.

122. Wright K, Tarr PI, Hickman RO, Guthrie RD. Hyperbilirubinemia secondary to delayed absorption of intraperitoneal blood following intrauterine transfusion. *J Pediatr.* 1982;100:302–304.

123. Epstein MF, Leviton A, Kuban KC, et al. Bilirubin intraventricular hemorrhage and phenobarbital in very low birth weight babies. *Pediatrics.* 1988;82:350.

124. Pasnick M, Lucey JF. Serum bilirubin in preterm infants following intracranial hemorrhage. *Pediatr Res.* 1983;17:329A.

125. Amato M, Fouchere JC, von Muralt G. Relationship between peri-intraventricular hemorrhage and neonatal hyperbilirubinemia in very low birth weight infants. *Am J Perinatol.* 1987;4:275–278.

126. Black VD, Lubchenco LO, Luckey DW, et al. Developmental and neurologic sequelae in the neonatal hyperviscosity syndrome. *Pediatrics.* 1982;69:426–431.

127. Black VD, Lubchenco LO, Koops BL, Poland RL, Powell DP. Neonatal hyperviscosity: randomized study of effect of partial plasma exchange transfusion on long-term outcome. *Pediatrics.* 1985;75:1048–1053.

128. Goldberg K, Wirth FH, Hathaway WE, et al. Neonatal hyperviscosity II. Effect of partial plasma exchange transfusion. *Pediatrics.* 1982;69:419–425.

129. Daum F, Cohen MI, McNamara H. Experimental toxicologic studies on a phenol detergent associated with neonatal hyperbilirubinemia. *J Pediatr.* 1976;89:853.

130. Wysowski DK, Flynt JW, Goldfield M, et al. Epidemic neonatal hyperbilirubinemia and use of a phenolic disinfectant detergent. *Pediatrics.* 1978;61:165.

131. Moore LG, Newberry MA, Freeby GM, Crnic LS. Increased incidence of neonatal hyperbilirubinemia at 3,100 m in Colorado. *Am J Dis Child.* 1984;138:157–161.

132. Leibson C, Brown M, Thibodeau S, et al. Neonatal hyperbilirubinemia at high altitude. *Am J Dis Child.* 1989;143(8):983–987.

133. Freeman J, Lesko S, Mitchell AA, Epstein MF, Shapiro S. Hyperbilirubinemia following exposure to pancuronium bromide in newborns. *Dev Pharmacol Ther.* 1990;14:209–215.

134. Lambert GH, Muraskas J, Anderson CL, Myers TF. Direct hyperbilirubinemia associated with chloral hydrate administration in the newborn. *Pediatrics.* 1990;86:277–281.

135. Reimche LD, Sankaran K, Hindmarsh KW, Kasian GF, Gorecki DKJ, Tan L. Chloral hydrate sedation in neonates and infants—clinical and pharmacologic considerations. *Dev Pharmacol Ther.* 1989;12:57–64.

136. Benaron DA, Bowen FW. Variation of initial serum bilirubin rise in newborn infants with type of illness. *Lancet.* 1991;338:78–81.

137. Gopinathan V, Miller NJ, Milner AD, Rice-Evans CA. Bilirubin and ascorbate antioxidant activity in neonatal plasma. *FEBS Lett.* 1994;349:197–200.

138. Hegyi T, Goldie E, Hiatt M. The protective role of bilirubin in oxygen radical disease of the preterm infant. *J Perinatol.* 1994;14:296–300.

139. Sedlak TW, Snyder SH. Bilirubin benefits: cellular protection by a biliverdin reductase antioxidant cycle. *Pediatrics.* 2004;113:1776–1782.

140. Stocker R, Yamamoto Y, McDonagh AF, et al. Bilirubin as an antioxidant of possible physiological importance. *Science.* 1987;235:1043–1046.

141. Lo SF. Total or neonatal bilirubin assays in the Vitros 5,1 FS: hemoglobin interference, hemolysis, icterus index. *Clin Chem.* 2007;53:799.

142. Lo SF, Jendrzejczak BA, Doumas BT. Laboratory performance in neonatal bilirubin testing using commutable specimens. *Arch Pathol Lab Med.* 2008;132:1781–1785.

143. Maisels MJ, Fanaroff AA, Stevenson DK, et al. Serum bilirubin levels in an international, multiracial newborn population. *Pediatr Res.* 1999;45:167A.

144. Fouzas S, Mantagou L, Skylogianni E, Mantagos S, Varvarigou A. Transcutaneous bilirubin levels for the first 120 postnatal hours in healthy neonates. *Pediatrics.* 2010;125:e52–e57.

145. Ryan AS, Wenjun MS, Acosta A. Breastfeeding continues to increase into the new millennium. *Pediatrics.* 2002;110:1103–1109.

146. American Academy of Pediatrics, Subcommittee on Hyperbilirubinemia. Clinical practice guideline: management of hyperbilirubinemia in the newborn infant 35 or more weeks of gestation. *Pediatrics.* 2004;114:297–316.

147. Maisels MJ, Bhutani VK, Bogen D, Newman TB, Stark AR, Watchko JF. Hyperbilirubinemia in the newborn infant ≥t35 weeks' gestation: an update with clarifications. *Pediatrics.* 2009;124(4):1193–1198.

148. Maisels MJ, Kring E. Transcutaneous bilirubin levels in the first 96 hours in a normal newborn population of 35 or more weeks' of gestation. *Pediatrics.* 2006;117:1169–1173.

149. Engle WD, Lai S, Ahmad N, Manning MD, Jackson GL. An hour-specific nomogram for transcutaneous bilirubin values in term and late preterm Hispanic neonates. *Am J Perinatol.* 2009;26(6):425–430.

150. De Luca D, Romagnoli C, Tiberi E, Zuppa AA, Zecca E. Skin bilirubin nomogram for the first 96 h of life in a European normal healthy newborn population, obtained with multiwavelength transcutaneous bilirubinometry. *Acta Paediatr.* 2008;97:146–150.

151. De Luca D, Jackson GL, Tridente A, Carnielli VP, Engle W. Transcutaneous bilirubin nomograms: a systematic

review of population differences and analysis of bilirubin kinetics. *Arch Pediatr Adolesc Med*. 2009;163(11): 1054–1059.

152. Sanpavat S, Nuchprayoon I, Smathakanee C, Hansuebsai R. Nomogram for prediction of the risk of neonatal hyperbilirubinemia, using transcutaneous bilirubin. *J Med Assoc Thai*. 2005;88:1187–1193.

153. Wainer S, Rabi Y, Parmar SM, Allegro D, Lyon M. Impact of skin tone on the performance of a transcutaneous jaundice meter. *Acta Paediatr*. 2009;98:1909–1915.

154. Fouzas S, Karatza AA, Skylogianni E, Mantagou L, Varvarigou A. Transcutaneous bilirubin levels in late preterm neonates. *J Pediatr*. 2010;157:762–766.

155. Yu Z-B, Dong X-Y, Han S-P, et al. Transcutaneous bilirubin nomogram for predicting neonatal hyperbilirubinemia in healthy term and late-preterm Chinese infants. *Eur J Pediatr*. 2011;170:185–191.

156. Yamauchi Y, Yamanouchi I. Transcutaneous bilirubinometry in normal Japanese infants. *Acta Paediatr Jpn*. 1989;31:65–72.

157. Wainer S, Parmar S, Allegro D, Rabi Y, Lyon M. Impact of a transcutaneous bilirubinometry program on resource utilization and incidence of severe neonatal hyperbilirubinemia. *Pediatrics*. 2011. In press.

Bilirubin Toxicity

Dora Brites and Maria Alexandra Brito

■ INTRODUCTION

For many years, unconjugated bilirubin (UCB) was thought to be a useless waste product of heme catabolism, with no physiological function, but with potential toxicity. Toxicity resulting from unconjugated hyperbilirubinemia has been known for more than a century, since the landmark study of Schmorl describing autopsy findings from 120 jaundiced infants, as cited by Hansen.[1]

Interestingly, evidence obtained in the last decade revealed a beneficial role of the molecule. Indeed, physiological or modestly elevated serum levels of UCB have been shown to have a protective effect in several disorders, ironically even including neurodegenerative diseases.[2] Protective effects of UCB rely on its antioxidant properties.

Above a certain threshold, toxic effects of UCB become evident. In this circumstance, prolonged exposure and accumulation of UCB can lead to reversible or irreversible cell damage, or even cell death.[3] In fact, severe neonatal hyperbilirubinemia can lead to acute bilirubin encephalopathy (ABE) and kernicterus,[4–6] underscoring the need for models to enhance our understanding of how hyperbilirubinemia causes permanent brain damage in some infants.

UCB binding to human serum albumin (HSA) provides UCB solubility and thus facilitates its transport to the liver. Decreased levels of HSA and lower capacity for UCB binding, usually found in neonates, especially in preterm babies, may contribute to higher tissue UCB levels. Under such conditions, there is an increase in the unbound (free) UCB (Bf) fraction, increased cellular uptake, and greater likelihood of bilirubin-induced neurological dysfunction (BIND).[7–9] Bf is able to enter the cells by passive or facilitated diffusion and usually represents less than 0.1% of serum UCB.[10]

In neonates, serum UCB is usually elevated for the first 2 weeks of postnatal life due to increased breakdown of fetal erythrocytes, deficient HSA transport to the liver, and decreased conjugation.[11] The central nervous system (CNS) is the most vulnerable site to UCB toxicity in the neonatal period, resulting in a wide array of neurological deficits collectively known as BIND.[12]

Despite the number of studies performed in patients and animal models, as well as in tissues and in different cellular systems, the molecular mechanisms underlying or contributing to UCB cytotoxicity are not completely understood. The disruption of several cellular functions rather than a single death-signaling pathway suggests that UCB toxicity is mediated by multifaceted mechanisms. On the other hand, there is difficulty in the extrapolation of in vitro observations to infants, namely because many studies are of doubtful relevance due to the use of nonphysiological concentrations of UCB, binding proteins, or improper experimental conditions.[3]

Here, we will summarize the most recent and relevant information on the widespread effects of UCB toxicity.

■ EXPERIMENTAL MODELS TO EVALUATE BILIRUBIN TOXICITY

Experimental in vitro and in vivo models have been developed to study UCB toxicity and valuable data have been obtained by both. Nevertheless, each approach has its advantages and disadvantages. While animal models are believed to better mimic BIND, in vitro models are important to isolate specific pathways and mechanisms of injury.[13]

Monocultures of specific cell types are suitable for evaluation of acute toxicities, while co-cultures of different cell types and slices of explanted tissue that survive up to months may be used to assess chronic damage. Most important, the robustness of any finding, independent of the model used, will be enhanced when tested across other models. Combinations of both in vitro and in vivo models may then lead to a better understanding of the pathophysiology of BIND and, therefore, to effective preventive and therapeutic measures. However, a good, reproducible, integrated model that reproduces unconjugated hyperbilirubinemia and its acute toxicity and long-lasting sequelae is still needed.

In this section, we will address the strengths and weaknesses of different experimental BIND model systems that have been used to dissect the molecular mechanisms and to test the efficacy of potential drugs for prevention or treatment of BIND.

In Vitro Models

The principal hypotheses proposed to explain the mechanisms of BIND have been studied mostly in models in vitro, such as primary cell cultures or immortalized cell lines. In vitro systems offer ease of manipulation and are particularly suitable for dissecting interacting intracellular signaling cascades that ultimately lead to cell dysfunction and death. Nevertheless, pure neuronal cultures do not fully take into account the interplay between neurons and glia. Therefore, a growing number of studies have been conducted over the past two decades on the development and optimization of acute and organotypic brain slice models, which allow the realistic interaction of neurons with glia.

Cell Lines and Primary Cultures

Cell lines are the less complex systems and are easy to obtain, but often are derived from tumors or from transformed cells, and hence resemble less the in vivo circumstance. As such, neuroblastoma cell lines often display morphological, developmental, and signaling characteristics that differ from isolated neurons.[14] Advantages of using cell lines reside in the unlimited number of cells available for studies and the guarantee of a single cell type. Cell lines have also significant disadvantages. Because they have a high proliferation rate, they retain some degree of plasticity, and their properties can change with the number of passages over time.[15] The mouse hepatoma Hepa

1c1c7,[16] human neuroblastoma SH-SY5Y,[17,18] NT2-N neurons,[19] and murine lymphoma L5178Y-R[20] cell lines were used in the last 5 years to study the cytotoxic effects of UCB.

Dissociated primary cell cultures are also a simplified model that allows the evaluation of cell response, reactivity, and demise on UCB exposure in a very pure and particular cell type. Thus, a major advantage of this culture technique relates to the possible evaluation of how different cell types respond to a UCB stimulus. Interestingly, it seems that the development of neural cells in vivo corresponds to their development in vitro, thus allowing the study of age-related vulnerabilities to UCB.[21] Another benefit, in contrast to cell lines, is that the neural cells used for the cultures, derived from late embryonic (E18 for neurons) or early postnatal days (1–2 days for glial cells), are quite immature and better represent the conditions that might be associated with neonatal jaundice. However, if the cells are maintained in vitro, adult cell characteristics will be expressed. Another interesting aspect of such culture systems is the possibility to study regional susceptibilities to UCB when isolating cells from different brain regions, such as the cortex, hippocampus, or cerebellum. Primary cultures of dissociated neurons are the most commonly used in vitro preparations to evaluate UCB-induced neurodegeneration[22,23] and for testing compounds with either protective[24–26] or detrimental[27] effects.

Co-cultures, where neurons are cultivated on the top of astrocytes or the glial cells seeded onto culture plates with neurons, produce more stable cultures and provide the means to directly evaluate the cross-talk between two different cell types.

Organotypic Slice Cultures

Compared with the culture of dissociated neuronal cells, organotypic cultures made from slices of explanted tissue (e.g., hippocampus) represent a complex multicellular in vitro environment and have the advantage of preserving in vivo cell-to-cell interactions.[28] Fresh (acute) slice preparations are used mostly for electrophysiological measurements. Organotypic slice preparations are maintained in vitro for weeks to months and routinely used to evaluate the pathophysiology of neuronal dysfunction and to screen novel therapies, replicating many aspects of the in vivo system. For review, the reader is referred to Lein et al.[29] Slices are obtained from brains of neonatal pups at postnatal days 3–9 (P3–P9) and chopped into

400-μm thick sections.[30,31] Advantages to be considered over animal models are the easy access, the control of the extracellular environment, and the possibility to evaluate both short- and long-term alterations.[31]

Recently, Chang et al.,[32] by using rat organotypic hippocampal slice cultures, have shown that 24-hour incubations with UCB impairs long-term synaptic plasticity. Presynaptic damage by UCB was later observed in acute brain slices of the auditory brainstem from P16–P18 Gunn rats at 18 hours after intraperitoneal (IP) administration of sulfadimethoxine.[33] These findings add to the understanding of UCB-induced deafness and temporary or permanent impairment of mental function by hyperbilirubinemia.

In Vivo Animal Models

Given the complexities of living organisms, in vivo animal models of BIND would appear to offer the best systems to evaluate the pathophysiological mechanisms of UCB neurotoxicity and for testing therapeutic strategies, provided that they closely mimic the symptoms and temporal progression of UCB encephalopathy in human neonates. The existence of redundant compensatory and adaptive systems in transgenic mouse models may limit their usefulness as the sole approach to test specific biochemical hypotheses.

Gunn Rat

The Gunn rat, a mutant jaundiced rat of the Wistar rat strain, has provided the opportunity to study kernicterus and the mechanisms that underlie BIND. Jaundice in the Gunn rat derives from the rat's inability to conjugate bilirubin and, like the human Crigler–Najjar Syndrome Type I, results from a mutation in the *UDP-glucuronosyltransferase (UGT) 1A1 gene*. Nonetheless, hyperbilirubinemia in the Gunn rat is milder (~7 mg/dL)[34] and usually not severe enough by itself to cause kernicterus or to produce neonatal morbidity. Therefore, to trigger a sudden elevation of the Bf fraction and produce UCB encephalopathy, either sulfadimethoxine[9] (a displacer of UCB from albumin) or phenylhydrazine[35] (an inducer of hemolysis) has been used. A limitation of the model resides in the occurrence of maximal hyperbilirubinemia only at P16, instead of the particularly vulnerable first week in human newborns.[36] Nonetheless, this model is without doubt the most used by several authors to evaluate mechanisms that mediate BIND,[37,38] regional

brain susceptibilities to UCB,[39] hearing loss,[33,40] and neuroprotective therapeutic approaches to BIND.[26,41–45]

Murine Models

The *Ugt1*-null mouse phenotype[34] mimics the irreversible damage produced by UCB in severely ill infants and in Crigler–Najjar Type I patients, leading to kernicterus. Jaundice in the range of 7–10 mg/dL at P5 is present as a phenotypical orange skin color in the first 8 hours of postnatal life and all *Ugt1*-null mice develop kernicterus and die within 11 days following birth. Although only showing a difference of 2 mg/dL in total serum bilirubin (TSB) from that observed in the Gunn rat, its earlier presentation seems to be sufficient to initiate CNS toxicity and lethal encephalopathy in mice neonates. Nevertheless, experiments to examine the impact of BIND in these mice have not yet been performed.

Mild to moderate hyperbilirubinemia is observed in another form of inheritable condition known as Gilbert syndrome[46] associated, but not exclusively, with an additional TA insertion into the UGT1A1 promoter, generating the *UGT1A1*28* allele instead of the normal *UGT1A1*1* allele.[47] The generation of humanized UGT1 mice expressing the *UGT1A1*28* allele (h*UGT1A1*28*)[36] may represent a better model to evaluate the mechanisms leading to more subtle CNS abnormalities. These mice have TSB levels that may exceed 15 mg/dL at P7–P14 and 10% of these animals show CNS toxicity, seizures, and death. In survivors, TSB concentrations decrease to 0.8–1.2 mg/dL at P14–P21. It seems that resistance to BIND is developed as mice mature and become capable of combating the impact of high levels of UCB. The h*UGT1A1*28* mouse model offers an interesting approach to establish valid in vivo correlations between cellular alterations and harmful outcomes.

■ TREATMENT OF CELL AND TISSUE CULTURES WITH BILIRUBIN

UCB has been widely reported as a beneficial molecule mainly due to its antioxidant properties at low nanomolar concentrations of Bf. Elevated levels of UCB and Bf, however, can have harmful pro-oxidant effects as well, under some conditions.

Studies dealing with the mechanisms of UCB toxicity should use UCB to HSA molar ratios (UCB:HSA) or Bf levels considered clinically relevant.[48] To experimentally evaluate UCB toxicity, incubations should be prepared with a molar excess of albumin over UCB to obtain stable solutions and avoid aggregation. The most frequently used UCB:HSA are between 0.5 and 1.0.[32,49] An alternative to this is to work with a concentration of Bf equal to or slightly higher than 70 nM,[50–52] which is the limit of bilirubin aqueous solubility in the absence of albumin.[53] Nevertheless, Bf values below or equal to 1000 nM (1 μM) are still considered clinically relevant.[54] Neurotoxic effects of even purified UCB can be observed at Bf levels ranging from 71 to 770 nM in in vitro studies.[55] Similar values by calculated Bf were obtained in Gunn rats treated with sulfadimethoxine[56] and a considerable overlap was observed between those and the predicted values in human neonates with a TSB of 35 mg/dL.[9]

UCB is unstable and readily oxidized when exposed to extreme pH values or to even traces of oxygen.[57,58] The rate of UCB decomposition increases with exposure to light.[59] Thus, experiments should be performed under light-limited conditions to avoid or minimize photodegradation,[58,60] as these photoproducts may be less toxic than UCB.[61]

■ BILIRUBIN INTERACTION WITH PLASMA AND INTRACELLULAR MEMBRANES

General cellular injury by UCB appears to start at the cell membrane, considered one of the first, if not the primary or the initiating, targets of UCB toxicity,[62] which is followed by interaction with the intracellular membranes that surround various organelles. First studies in erythrocytes exposed to UCB pointed to morphological alterations and perturbation in phospholipid distribution with the translocation of the inner aminophospholipid phosphatidylserine to the outer leaflet of the membrane.[63] This feature is a sign of cell senescence and is recognized by macrophages. Interestingly, in a recent study on the effects of UCB in immature neurons, increased apoptosis based on the interaction between annexin V and phosphatidylserine was observed,[64] thus supporting this finding.

Damage to membranes increases with the UCB concentration, bilirubin-displacing drugs, time of exposure, and acidic pH. Inhibition of cell endocytosis and glutamate uptake, alterations in membrane potential, inefficiency of membrane receptors, as well as transporters and enzymes are some of the toxic effects produced by UCB at the membrane level.[11,65] Most of these effects culminate in cell death and may lead to hemolysis of erythrocytes, thus contributing to the production of UCB.[63] Although

in vitro studies have shown that increases in heme catabolism directly relate to the hyperbilirubinemia observed in the first 4 days after birth[66] and that increased photohemolysis occurs in spherocytes treated with UCB,[67] stronger evidence is needed to support its clinical significance.[68]

Direct effects of UCB in synaptosomal membrane systems have been observed through the production of reactive oxygen species (ROS), protein oxidation, and lipid peroxidation,[69] which were later confirmed to also occur in other cells, mainly in neurons.[25,70] Reduced activity of membrane-bound Na^+/K^+-ATPase and Mg^{2+}-ATPase (aminophospholipid translocase, flippase), which selectively pumps the phosphatidylserine from the outer to the inner monolayer, also occurred in neocortical synaptosomes.[69]

Studies by electron paramagnetic resonance spectroscopy have indicated that UCB intercalates superficially in the C-5 hydrocarbon of the membrane bilayer, disrupting protein order and rendering inner regions more fluid and more permeable to water diffusion, with a maximum expression at the C-7 level.[11,71]

■ TOXICITY OF BILIRUBIN AT DIFFERENT SUBCELLULAR COMPARTMENTS

Membrane dynamic properties may be changed by UCB but do not appear to be a significant obstacle to the entry of UCB into cells. In fact, UCB passage across cellular membranes appears to involve passive diffusion through the hydrophobic lipid core.[72] Therefore, UCB effects have been observed in several intracellular organelles.

Mitochondria

Although it is not known whether the cell membranes or mitochondria are the primary target for the toxic effects of UCB, mitochondria are particularly vulnerable. Similar to the erythrocyte membrane, it seems that UCB is preferentially accommodated at the C-5 level in mitochondrial membranes, despite having the maximum effect at the C-7 level, indicating that perturbation of membrane dynamics by UCB has common features regardless of the type of membrane model.[11] Physical perturbation of mitochondrial membrane results from protein order disruption, oxidative injury, mitochondria swelling, and release of cytochrome c. This latter event and the activation of caspase-9 and -3 (Figure 7-1) further suggest

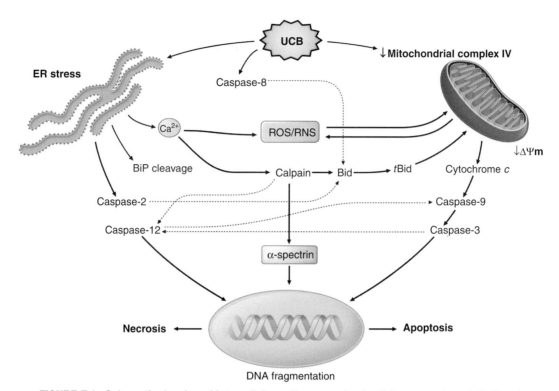

FIGURE 7-1. Schematic drawing of intracellular pathways and subcellular compartments believed to be involved in cell damage by unconjugated bilirubin (UCB). UCB causes mitochondrial dysfunction with collapse of inner mitochondrial membrane potential ($\Delta\psi$m), a diminished activity of complex IV (cytochrome c oxidase), and the release of cytochrome c to the cytosol, where it activates caspase-9, which in turn activates caspase-3, triggering the initiation of apoptosis (mitochondrial intrinsic pathway). UCB can also induce apoptosis by the extrinsic pathway, whereby activation of caspase-8 is involved. The caspase-8 signal may be enhanced by the cleavage of BH3-only protein (Bid) into the truncated form (tBid) that is translocated to mitochondria, thus propagating the apoptotic signal. Another relevant mechanism of cell damage involves endoplasmic reticulum (ER) stress, which leads to an intracellular overload of Ca^{2+} and interferes with Ca^{2+}-binding proteins, as calpain. In addition, it leads to the dissociation of an ER luminal chaperone, the immunoglobulin heavy chain binding protein (Bip), as well as to the activation of caspase-2 and -12, which also trigger apoptosis. While caspase-12 is activated by caspase-3 and, in turn, activates caspase-9, caspase-2 cleaves Bid into tBid. Production of reactive oxygen species (ROS) and reactive nitrogen species (RNS) appears as a common denominator in the mechanisms of cell death, being related to both mitochondrial disruption and ER stress. Oxidation of cellular components interferes with cytoskeleton proteins, as α-spectrin, thus disrupting its normal assembly. Moreover, oxidation of nucleic acid bases compromises DNA integrity, leading to its fragmentation. All these events can culminate in cell death by both apoptosis and necrosis.

that UCB-induced apoptosis is mediated at least in part by mitochondria.[53] Inhibition of cytochrome c oxidase (complex IV), the terminal component of the mitochondrial respiratory chain, by UCB was verified in brain and liver mitochondria,[50] as well as in immature neurons.[64] Reductions in the rates of oxygen consumption and inner mitochondrial membrane potential further compromise cell viability.

Endoplasmic Reticulum and Golgi Complex

The endoplasmic reticulum (ER) regulates protein synthesis, protein folding and trafficking, cellular responses to stress, and intracellular calcium (iCa^{2+}) levels. Alterations of the Golgi complex by UCB include the presence of enlarged vacuoles and increased vesicles in animals with kernicterus.[73] Hypertrophy and hyperplasia of the ER with unusual prominences of the Golgi apparatus were noticed in the liver of Crigler–Najjar Type II patients, a less severe syndrome than the Type I.[74] Similar ER alterations and mitochondria abnormalities were induced in astrocytes after exposure to UCB.[75] Accumulation of UCB within the cell provokes ER stress[76] and many related genes have been shown to be upregulated by UCB.[16] ER stress can either initiate or contribute to apoptotic cell death[77] by the ER-resident caspase-2 and -12 (Figure 7-1). While caspase-2 was identified as the premitochondrial protease,[78] caspase-12 was shown to be activated by calpain and caspase-3, thus activating caspase-9.[79] Cleavage of proapoptotic BH3-only protein (Bid) into truncated Bid (tBid) may occur either via caspase-2 or via calpain and caspase-8 activation,[80] and immunoglobulin heavy chain binding protein (Bip) derives from ER stress.[81] Activation of caspase-8 and cleavage of Bid into tBid by UCB in immature cortical neurons[23] and the decrease in the caspase-12 pro-form in Hepa 1c1c7 cells[16] corroborate the existence of a mitochondrial- and ER-stress-mediated apoptotic pathway. Upregulated BiP in SH-SY5Y cells further reflects an ER stress response to UCB.[76] Some UCB-induced genes also suggest a role for autophagy, which is believed to be implicated in cell growth inhibition.[82,83]

Nucleus

UCB-induced cell demise is in part due to oxidative stress, which causes a signal blockade on cell cycle progression and leads to subsequent DNA damage.[17] Interestingly, cell cycle arrest was shown to be induced by UCB through activation of extracellular signal-regulated kinases 1 and 2 (ERK1/2) in colon cancer,[84] and genes linked to cell cycle dependence are repressed in Ugt-null mice.[34] High TSB levels were considered to be genotoxic in an in vivo study performed with jaundiced newborns.[85] In accordance, autopsy analysis of cases of BIND revealed immunostaining for markers of DNA oxidation.[86] This DNA oxidation causes S-phase progression delay and triggers apoptosis,[17] which is recognized when cells show condensed and fragmented nuclei (Figure 7-2), thus revealing DNA as a potential target of UCB toxicity. Considering the potential carcinogenic and mutagenic consequences of DNA strand breaks,[87] it can be hypothesized that potential side effects of a carcinogenic or genetic nature may ensue later in life, as a result of DNA damage caused by neonatal hyperbilirubinemia.

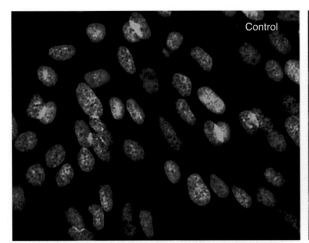 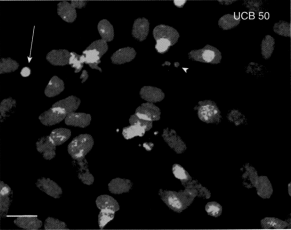

FIGURE 7-2. Morphological assessment of cell death by apoptosis in astrocytes incubated with unconjugated bilirubin (UCB). Astrocytes were isolated from brain cortices of 2-day-old rats and cultured for 10 days in vitro. Cells were incubated with 100 µM human serum albumin (HSA) in the absence (control) or in the presence of 50 µM UCB. Coverslips with adherent astrocytes were collected after 4 hours of incubation and then washed. Cells were fixed with 4% paraformaldehyde and stained with Hoechst 33258 dye. Alterations in nuclei morphology were observed by fluorescence microscopy. Apoptotic cells show condensed chromatin uniformly stained (stronger blue fluorescence nuclei, arrow) and nuclear fragmentation (bright fluorescent spherical beads, arrowhead). Scale bar equals 25 µm.

■ OVERVIEW ON THE POTENTIAL MECHANISMS

High concentrations of UCB disrupt several cell functions, not only via a single cell-death pathway but also involving effects in different intracellular organelles as noted above. Despite decades of study, the determinants of damage, vulnerability, and reversibility, as well as the underlying mechanisms of BIND, still remain unclear. Icteric brain sections have revealed that UCB accumulates within neurons, neuronal processes, and microglia,[88] but cell-dependent sensitivity to UCB toxicity and the role of each cell type are still not fully understood. In vitro assays have shown that UCB leads to oxidative stress, exerts immunomodulatory effects, determines an increase in iCa^{2+}, induces the release of glutamate, and leads to cell death. Structural–functional relationship studies might help in the understanding of the pathological processes and developmental difficulties experienced by jaundiced babies.

Oxidative Stress

The brain is particularly vulnerable to ROS, especially the developing brain,[89] and low antioxidant defenses will favor mitochondria senescence and cell demise. Increased production of ROS, protein oxidation, lipid peroxidation, and cell death in neurons, as compared with astrocytes, may be due to the reduced stores of total glutathione.[70] Recently, it was demonstrated that UCB determines glutathione depletion in neurons,[90] as well as in splenocytes,[91] by decreasing the reduced glutathione (GSH) and increasing the oxidized disulfide form (GSSG).

Although the precise molecular mechanisms by which UCB exerts toxicity remain unknown, generation of ROS is surely involved and an initial event in the UCB-mediated cell death in neurons.[70,90] Increased production of superoxide radical anion has also been observed with the exposure of neutrophils to UCB.[92] Thus, N-acetylcysteine (NAC), a glutathione precursor, N-ω-nitro-L-arginine methyl ester hydrochloride (L-NAME) that prevents the formation of excessive amounts of nitric oxide (NO) by inhibiting the NO synthase (NOS), and glycoursodeoxycholic acid (GUDCA),[25] a bile acid with antiapoptotic, anti-inflammatory, and antioxidant properties, have been shown to counteract the disruption of the redox status by UCB in neurons.

Production of lipid peroxides, hydrogen peroxide, and hydroxyl radical, as well as a decrease in glutathione content and reduction of the mitochondrial membrane potential by UCB, was also shown to induce caspase-3 activation and apoptosis.[93] Recently, it has been demonstrated that UCB differentially regulates several genes and determines a consistent downregulation of several antioxidant enzymes.[16] Thus, it is not surprising that the increased production of ROS by UCB has been observed in HeLa cells, mouse embryonic fibroblasts, astrocytes, and neurons, among other cells.[25,51,70] The ability of UCB to upregulate DJ-1,[17] a redox-sensitive chaperone,[94] was identified as a cell defense mechanism in the human neuroblastoma cell line. Although similar results were achieved in neurons acutely exposed to UCB, increased incubation times effected the downregulation of DJ-1,[90] appearing to negatively influence the adaptive cell response mechanism of neuroprotection.

Increased Cytoplasmic Calcium

Signaling cascades initiated or regulated by iCa^{2+}, ROS, and reactive nitrogen species (RNS) are essential to diverse physiological and pathological processes. Mitochondria are central to energy metabolism and a hub for Ca^{2+}, which is in a delicate balance with ROS generated by mitochondria and ER; yet iCa^{2+} and ROS overload can lead to oxidative stress, mitochondrial dysfunction, and cell death.[95] Elevated iCa^{2+} and ROS production were obtained in synaptosomes treated with UCB, which may in turn engender more production of ROS (Figure 7-1).[11] Increased iCa^{2+} perturbs intracellular homeostasis and may cause ER stress. In a hyperbilirubinemic newborn mouse model, it was found that UCB-induced neurotoxicity was associated with augmented iCa^{2+} concentrations and activation of caspase-3 in the brain.[96] Autopsy analysis of several cases of BIND revealed a decrease in the immunoreactivity for Ca^{2+}-binding proteins,[86] which are implicated in Ca^{2+} homeostasis.[97] Furthermore, downregulation of these proteins was observed after treatment of Hepa 1c1c7 cells with UCB,[16] thus leading to elevated iCa^{2+}. Therefore, it is not surprising that taurine has been shown to limit BIND by inhibiting iCa^{2+} overload.[96]

Immunostimulation and Immunotoxicity

Several studies suggest that UCB possesses multiple biological activities, which differ accordingly with the use of low/normal levels or, in opposite, of pathophysiological concentrations of UCB. Therefore, when, low concentrations of UCB having antioxidant properties are assayed, inhibition of transendothelial migration of murine splenic lymphocytes across endothelial cells is observed. These levels of UCB[98] block the vascular cell adhesion molecule-1 (VCAM-1) signaling and the consequent activation of the matrix metalloproteinases (MMPs)-2 and -9 as well as suppress Th2 cytokine-mediated airway inflammation in response to an allergen challenge. In contrast, higher concentrations of UCB have been shown to be toxic to murine splenocytes and human peripheral blood mononuclear cells.[91] UCB was shown to arrest the cell cycle at a pre-G1 phase and cause DNA fragmentation and caspase-3 activation in splenocytes. UCB-induced apoptosis was observed to involve either the extrinsic (upregulation of CD95 expression and increase in caspase-8) or the intrinsic apoptotic pathways (activated Bax, caspase-9 activation, increased cytoplasmic calcium, and loss of MMPs) in these cells (Figure 7-1). Similar to what has been previously obtained in primary cultures of rat cortical astrocytes,[99] p38 mitogen-activated protein kinase (MAPK) activation was also demonstrated to have a key role in UCB-induced apoptosis and be related to cell depletion of glutathione.[91] More important, p38 MAPK activation was associated with alterations produced by UCB in the host immune response in vivo. In fact, IP injection of UCB (25–50 mg/kg body weight [BW]) to mice triggered a significant decrease in the number of erythrocytes and leukocytes, including variations in the percentage of lymphocytes and monocytes, hemoglobin levels, spleen weight, and viability of spleen and bone marrow cells, which was attenuated by the administration of SB203580, a p38 MAPK inhibitor. This is not without precedent since MAPK transduction pathways have been identified as key players in the UCB-induced secretion of proinflammatory cytokines, such as tumor necrosis factor-α (TNF-α) and interleukin (IL)-1β and -6, as well as in cell death of UCB-treated astrocytes.[99,100] The activation of the nuclear factor-kappa B (NF-κB) signal transduction pathway, one of the most important regulators of inflammatory gene expression mediating the synthesis of cytokines, may also contribute to the inflammatory response.[101,102]

Recent work by Loftspring et al.[92,103] established that UCB is associated with increased edema, neutrophil infiltration, and intercellular adhesion molecule-1 (ICAM-1) expression, as well as with perihematomal neutrophils in an intracerebral hemorrhage (ICH) mouse model. This interacting cascade of chemical, cellular, and cytokine events may result from the degradation of heme to UCB and UCB-derived oxidative products, which further may activate the release of cytokines by microglia and astrocytes, and determine the potent and delayed inflammatory response that follows ICH. In vitro studies with microglia have shown that the initial activation by UCB is followed by a later cell death.[104,105] Therefore, the reduced perihematomal microglial-immunoreactivity observed in the ICH mouse model[92] may be explained on the basis of a hyperacute microglial activation ending in cell senescence.

Accumulation of Extracellular Glutamate and Excitotoxicity

Glutamate is the primary excitatory amino acid neurotransmitter in the CNS and a potent neurotoxin that may lead to the death of nerve cells. Extracellular accumulation of glutamate overstimulates glutamatergic receptors and increases the production of reactive and excitotoxic oxygen/nitrogen species triggering oxidative/nitrosative stress and neuronal death. Glutamate transporters, which are mainly expressed in astroglial cells, are responsible for 90% of total glutamate uptake.[106] When astrocytes were incubated with UCB, accumulation of extracellular glutamate was associated with a decreased uptake and an increased and fast efflux from astrocytes.[71] Release of glutamate by neurons, although lower than that produced by UCB in microglia or astrocytes, was also significant[107] and may play a role in the mediation of neurotoxicity by UCB. The protective effect of L-carnitine may involve inhibition of the glutamate and/or N-methyl-D-aspartate (NMDA) receptor, preventing Ca^{2+} influx and causing an antioxidant effect.[108]

Overstimulation of NMDA receptors was initially indicated to be involved in UCB-induced apoptosis in developing rat brain neurons[109] and later to be associated with increased neuronal NOS (nNOS).[110] When the NMDA receptor antagonist MK-801 was used, neuronal apoptosis,[111] nNOS expression, NO release, and 3′,5′-cyclic guanosine monophosphate (cGMP) production, as well as cell dysfunction and demise, were abrogated.[110] Intriguingly, other studies showed that MK-801 was unable to protect neuronal viability in the presence of UCB or from abnormalities in brainstem auditory-evoked potentials (BAEPs) in Gunn rat pups.[37] Nevertheless, further data obtained by gramicidin-perforated patch clamp techniques indicated that UCB facilitates presynaptic glutamate release and activates both α-amino-3-hydroxy-5-methyl-4-isoxazole propionic acid (AMPA) and NMDA receptors to produce neuronal hyperexcitation.[112]

■ HARMFUL EFFECTS OF BILIRUBIN ON CELL-TO-CELL ADHESION

The blood–brain and the intestinal barriers are dynamic and complex interfaces that strictly control and provide protection against many toxic compounds and pathogens. Epithelial permeability and polarization are determined by the apical junctional complex consisting of tight junctions (TJ) and *adherens* junctions, and inflammatory conditions are known to compromise the barrier function.

UCB was shown to increase the paracellular permeability in Caco-2 monolayers, widely used to mimic the intestinal epithelia, by triggering the redistribution of the TJ protein occludin.[113] Disruption of intestinal integrity by UCB was shown to also involve disassembly of other TJ proteins, such as claudins and zonula occludens.[114] Increased intestinal permeability by hyperbilirubinemia was also observed in neonates on the third day of life.[115] Similar to the Caco-2 monolayers,[113] loss of cell viability caused by UCB was observed in confluent monolayers of human brain microvascular endothelial cells, together with an increase in caspase-3 activation. Elevated levels of UCB and longer exposure times determined the release of IL-6, IL-8, and vascular endothelial growth factor, as well as the disruption of the redox status, which may contribute to the observed increased permeability.[49] This deleterious action by high levels of UCB in the cerebral microvascular integrity may act synergistically with cytokines in facilitating immune cell trafficking into the CNS.

■ BILIRUBIN INJURY TO NEURONS AND GLIAL CELLS

Newborns are particularly susceptible to BIND, especially if born prematurely, probably related to a greater susceptibility to toxic stimuli. This is why most of the cases of kernicterus, still reported today in the literature, have occurred in premature infants with or without associated sepsis and/or glucose-6-phosphate dehydrogenase deficiency.[6,116,117]

The primary concern with respect to unconjugated hyperbilirubinemia is its potential for neurotoxic effects causing irreversible and/or long-lasting neurological sequelae. Response to insult will depend on the cell type,

intensity and duration of insult, neurodevelopmental maturity differences, brain regional vulnerabilities, and interactions between cells in the tissue.

Glial cells, including astrocytes, microglia, and oligodendrocytes (OLGs), have acquired recently a special relevance in brain injuries. Astrocytes are the most abundant type of glia[118] and like microglia have supportive and immune functions (with a neuroprotective or a neurotoxic role), express neurotransmitter receptors, and modulate neuronal activity and synaptic plasticity. This implies that neurons depend on glia for survival, which are highly vulnerable to neurotoxic compounds that they may release. OLGs do not seem to play a role in promoting inflammation, although, like neurons, they may be damaged by inflammatory processes and oxidative stress. Therefore, besides UCB neurotoxicity, glial cells also have been the subject of intensive research. In the following sections we will address neurons and glial cells, highlighting their interplay, and how they sense and respond to UCB.

Neurons

Neurons perform a diversity of functions in different parts of the CNS and are highly specialized for the processing and transmission of cellular signals. Glial cells, the other cell types present in the CNS are now considered essential to the maintenance of the neuronal network, to neuronal migration during development, and to the generation of myelin. Damage to the CNS usually involves the loss of axonal connections and leads to neuronal dysfunction and cell death. In neurons, the transport of mitochondria to specific locations where they are needed allows appropriate nerve cell function.[119] Overall, the most difficult thing to identify is the first site of injury, location, and cell type, as injury can differ in time, severity, and site between one cell and another.[120] Despite the differential vulnerability of neuron subpopulations,[121] they generally produce higher levels of ROS, suffer greater protein oxidation and lipid peroxidation than astrocytes, and are more susceptible to UCB-induced demise, probably as a result of lower glutathione stores.[70]

Neurogenesis, Neuritogenesis, and Synaptogenesis
During development, elongation of several short processes in neurons gives rise to neurites (neuritogenesis) approximately equal in length (Figure 7-3A).[122,123] One will extend more rapidly and give rise to the axon (axonogenesis), while the others elongate a few days later and become

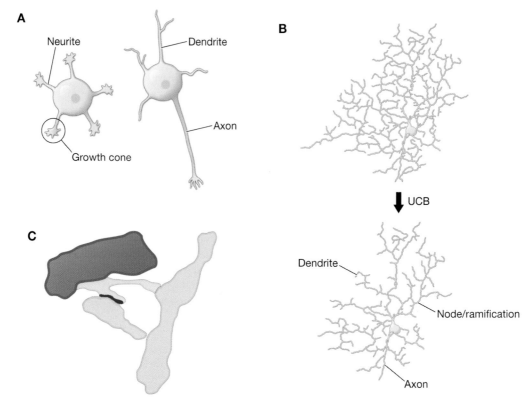

FIGURE 7-3. Representative images of (A) neuronal development showing minor processes called neurites, from which one becomes the axon and the remaining develop into dendrites; (B) alterations in the arborization in a "healthy" neuron caused by unconjugated bilirubin (UCB) as evidenced by a reduced dendritic and axonal arborization that may lead to aberrations in neuronal connectivity; and (C) partial reconstruction of an axonal bouton synapsing with one head of a branched spine arising from a dendrite, where the dendrite is dark blue, spines are lighter blues, axon segments are gray, and one postsynaptic density visible on branch is red. (Panel C: Redrawn from http://synapses.clm.utexas.edu/anatomy/axon/reconh.stm. SynapseWeb, Kristen M. Harris, PI. http://synapses.clm.utexas.edu/)

branched dendrites (dendritogenesis).[122] Neural stem cells have the potential to generate most of the different types of neurons and glia found in the brain. The discovery of continuous neurogenesis in the hippocampus and in the subventricular zone of the lateral ventricle throughout life provides new insight into the possible treatment of neurological and psychiatric disorders despite the lack of effective regeneration after injury of neurons.[124] A recent study has demonstrated that UCB decreases the viability of neural stem cells and mitochondrial function during differentiation.[125] Moreover, UCB has been shown to decrease neurogenesis without affecting astrogliogenesis. UCB also has evidenced to impair dendritic arborization and spinogenesis. When immature hippocampal neurons were exposed to UCB, the number of dendritic and axonal branches, as well as of growth cone areas, was decreased (Figure 7-3B).[125] Moreover, a reduction in neurite extension and number of nodes was revealed to be particularly marked in immature neurons incubated with UCB,[22] and preferentially in those from the hippocampus as compared to those from the cortex or cerebellum.[90] These neurite changes and apparent hippocampal susceptibility are consistent with the specific regional deposition of UCB in BIND, as found in a follow-up period ranging from 2 to 9 years.[126] UCB also decreased the density of dendritic spines and synapses (Figure 7-3C), and caused a change in spine development, thus impairing proper formation of neuronal circuits in the brain.[125]

Synaptic Plasticity

UCB alters synaptic plasticity,[32] as it was demonstrated by the exposure of organotypic hippocampal slice cultures to UCB for 24 hours, impairing the induction of long-term potentiation (LTP) and long-term depression (LTD). In prior studies, acute application of UCB potentiated inhibitory synaptic transmission.[127] UCB causes an increase in presynaptic iCa^{2+} and a decrease in the expression of the presynaptic proteins synaptophysin and SNAP-25,[127,128] which participate in synapse establishment and neurotransmitter release.[129] This finding is consistent with the presynaptic degeneration observed by Haustein et al.[33] in the Gunn rat. Electrophysiological data and electron microscopy confirmed presynaptic failure of synaptic transmission and supported evidence for healthy postsynaptic neurons.

Cytoskeleton Dynamics

Tau is the major microtubule-associated protein (MAP) of a mature neuron. The other two neuronal MAPs are MAP1 and MAP2. Tau is localized in the axon and MAP2 somatodendritically compartmentalized, as represented in Figure 7-4 (control). Exposure of immature hippocampal neurons to UCB induced an increased axonal entry of MAP2 (Figure 7-4).[130,131] When neurons degenerate or an axonal injury occurs, tau is released into the extracellular space where it is proteolytically

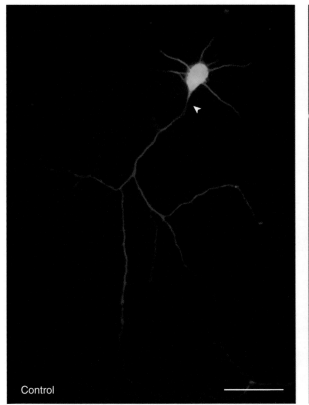
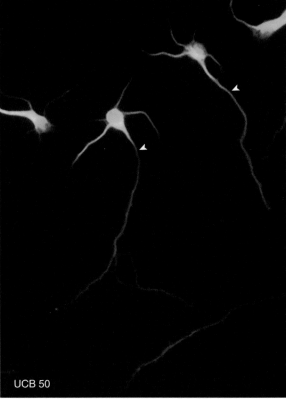

FIGURE 7-4. Exposure of immature hippocampal neurons to unconjugated bilirubin (UCB) induces microtubule-associated protein 2 (MAP2) axonal entry. Embryonic hippocampal neurons were treated with 100 μM human serum albumin (HSA) in the absence (control) or in the presence of 50 μM UCB (UCB/HSA = 0.5) for 24 hours at 1 day in vitro and fixed at 3 days in vitro. Hippocampal neurons were immunostained with MAP2 (green) to identify the cell body and dendrites, and tau1 (red) to identify the axon. White arrows indicate the entry limit of MAP2 into the axon. Scale bar equals 20 μm. (Used with permission from Adelaide Fernandes, PhD.)

cleaved and diffuses into the cerebrospinal fluid and plasma.[132,133] Interestingly, serum levels of tau in jaundiced term newborns have been correlated with TSB levels and early phase bilirubin encephalopathy,[133] and tau levels were demonstrated to be predictive of neurodegeneration.[134,135] Moreover, UCB was found to induce changes in motor proteins (dynein and kinesin), which transport mitochondria along the axon.[122] This may result in the formation of stationary and aggregated mitochondria (Figure 7-5), which could be the basis of several neurological diseases.[119] This may be more important than synapse loss in that it can precipitate

irreversible cell and axon death,[121] thus contributing to subtle kernicterus or BIND.

Cell Failure: Determinants and Modulators

UCB induces the release of glutamate from neurons, mainly from immature ones (Figure 7-6A),[136] overstimulating NMDA receptors (as indicated in section "Accumulation of Extracellular Glutamate and Excitotoxicity"), and leading to the increase of nNOS expression and neurotoxicity.[110] Oxidative stress is a very important player in neuronal dysfunction, apoptosis, and demise as indicated in section "Oxidative Stress." Inhibition of cytochrome *c* oxidase

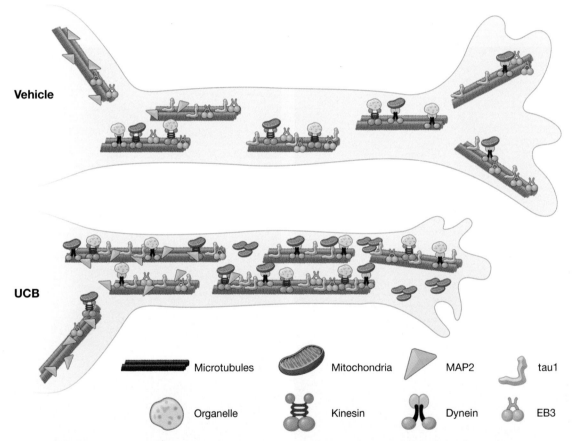

FIGURE 7-5. Schematic drawing of the cytoskeletal alterations produced by unconjugated bilirubin (UCB) in axons of immature hippocampal neurons. UCB has been shown to impair neuronal network formation by reducing axonal elongation and microtubule polymerization at the apical portion of the axon, under the regulation of microtubule plus end-associated proteins as EB3. UCB increases microtubule-associated protein 2 (MAP2) axonal entry and tau1 expression and their binding to microtubules, together with alterations in transport-related proteins, such as kinesin (anterograde transport) and dynein (retrograde transport), contributing to the accumulation of mitochondria in certain regions of the axons. (Used with permission from Eduarda Coutinho.)

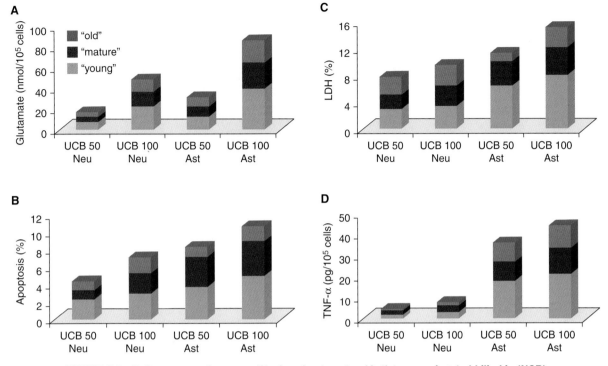

FIGURE 7-6. Cell response of neurons (Neu) and astrocytes (Ast) to unconjugated bilirubin (UCB) is mainly increased in immature cells. To mimic "young," "mature," and "old" cells, and to have the cells in the same stage of differentiation, rat cortical astrocytes and neurons were cultured for 5, 10, and 20 days in vitro or 4, 8, and 18 days in vitro, respectively. Cells were incubated with 50 or 100 μM UCB, or no addition (control), in the presence of 100 μM human serum albumin, at pH 7.4, for 4 hours, at 37°C. **A.** Release of glutamate to the incubation medium was assessed by an enzymatic assay. **B.** Apoptosis was estimated by analysis of nuclear morphology following staining with Hoechst 33258 dye. **C.** Lactate dehydrogenase (LDH) release by nonviable cells was determined using a commercial kit and results expressed as percent cell death relative to total cell lysis. **D.** The proinflammatory cytokine tumor necrosis factor-α (TNF-α) released to the culture medium was determined by an enzyme-linked immunosorbent assay (ELISA). Mean values are differences from the respective control. (Data from Falcão AS, Fernandes A, Brito MA, Silva RF, Brites D. Bilirubin-induced immunostimulant effects and toxicity vary with neural cell type and maturation state. *Acta Neuropathol.* 2006;112(1):95–105.)

activity by UCB in isolated mitochondria from brain, liver, and immature neurons was recently documented.[50,64] The bioenergetic and oxidative crises are accompanied by an increased glycolytic activity, superoxide radical anion production, and GSSG and adenosine-5'-triphosphate (ATP) release,[64] with all of these events counteracted by coincubation of the cells with GUDCA. All these players are direct participants in neuronal cytolysis and apoptosis,[107] which, similar to glutamate, are more evident in young cells (Figure 7-6B and C).[136] Collapse of inner mitochondrial membrane potential and activation of the executioner caspase-3, together with both mitochondrial-dependent caspase-9 and mitochondrial-independent caspase-8

pathways, as well as of JNK1/2, are implicated, and both L-NAME and the selective JNK1/2 inhibitor SP600125 abolish the activation of these cascades.[23] Neuronal death by UCB also occurs independently of apoptosis,[19] and apoptosis also arises from caspase-independent pathways.[23]

The presence of sepsis and inflammation can increase the susceptibility of immature neurons to UCB in vitro, where the slight release of TNF-α on incubation with UCB (Figure 7-6D) increased to values of ~5 and 10 pg × 10^5 cells by cotreatment with lipopolysaccharide (LPS),[136] and coincubation with TNF-α + IL-1β intensified the activation of NO/NOS, JNK1/2, and caspase-signaling pathways by UCB (Figure 7-7).[23]

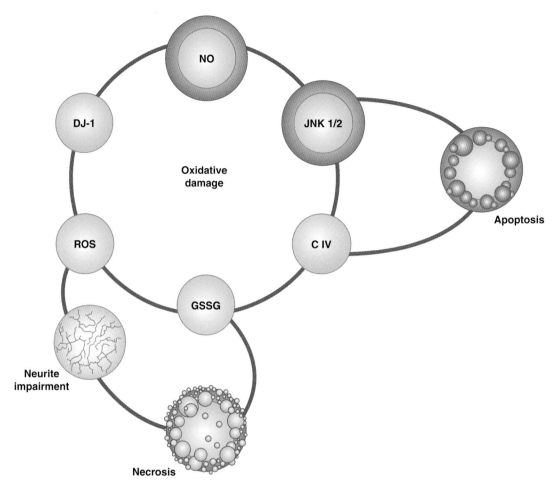

FIGURE 7-7. Schematic drawing of the key players in oxidative damage by unconjugated bilirubin (UCB), and aggravating effects produced by tumor necrosis factor (TNF)-α and interleukin (IL)-1β. Rat neurons exposed to UCB in conditions mimicking neonatal hyperbilirubinemia (50 μM UCB, 100 μM human serum albumin [HSA]) in immature cells (3 days in vitro neurons) suffered oxidative and nitrosative stress, as shown by reactive oxygen species (ROS) and nitric oxide (NO) production, together with a disruption of the antioxidant system, as revealed by the elevation of oxidized glutathione (GSSG) and the decrease in the redox-sensitive protein DJ-1 after a transient initial increase. In parallel, mitochondrial dysfunction occurs in association with an energetic crisis, reflected by the decrease of complex IV (C IV) activity. c-Jun N-terminal kinases 1 and 2 (JNK1/2) are activated and intervene in apoptotic- and necrotic-"like" cell death. All these events are represented by green circles. Oxidative injury also impacts on neurite arborization and ultimately leads to neuronal death. TNF-α and IL-1β, used to mimic neuroinflammation, intensified all the assayed parameters that include nitrosative stress, JNK1/2 activation, necrosis, and cell death by apoptosis (outside circle in brown).

Immature neurons from different brain origins have diverse responses to the UCB stimulus, with hippocampal neurons showing the highest vulnerability to UCB-induced toxicity mediated by enhanced nNOS and transient DJ-1 expression, cGMP, NO, and ROS production, as well as GSSG formation and caspase-3 activity, together with diminished cell viability and neurite outgrowth and branching as compared with those from cortex or cerebellum.[90] Increased expression of DJ-1 by UCB was observed in the SH-SY5Y cells and its overexpression, counteracted by NAC,[90] resulted in reduced cell death.[17] Nevertheless, DJ-1 expression in cerebellar and hippocampal neurons decreased in UCB extended incubations.[90] Curiously, while suppression of DJ-1 promotes NMDA-induced neuronal death, a neuroprotective effect is simultaneously exerted by suppression of DJ-1 dysfunction-mediated neuronal death.[137] This complexity of differentially regulated cell function and dysfunction cascades may then limit the efficacy of compounds intended to augment DJ-1 activity.

Astrocytes

Astrocytes contribute to the plasticity of CNS synapses and to the dynamic regulation of local cerebral blood flow,[138–140] and can release transmitters such as glutamate and ATP.[141] By participating in the uptake of glutamate, they may counteract its effects as a potential neurotoxin[118,139] and are able to prevent microglial overactivation,[142] and also may enhance immune responses and inhibit myelin repair.[142] Because astrocyte dysfunction has acquired a special relevance in the pathogenesis of CNS disorders,[143] therapeutic strategies are considering astrocytes as potential targets for prevention and therapy. Although the contribution of astrocytes to the process of BIND has not been clearly defined, an abundance of data highlights the importance of astrocytes in both the initiation and propagation of neuronal injury.

Signaling, Reactivity, and Immunosuppression

Elevation of extracellular glutamate that follows incubation of astrocytes with UCB is higher than that observed with neurons (Figure 7-6A), occurs 5 minutes after exposure (R. F. M. Silva, personal communication), increases from old and mature cells to immature ones,[136] and is insensitive to LPS or TNF-α treatments.[71] Neither IL-10 nor GUDCA was able to decrease the release of glutamate.[144]

The first evidence that astrocytes release IL-6, TNF-α, and IL-1β appeared in 2004[100] and later it was shown that immature astrocytes were the most responsive in releasing TNF-α and IL-1β on UCB exposure as compared with more differentiated cells (Figure 7-6D), and that coincubation with LPS further enhanced its secretion.[71]

The UCB-stimulation pathway involves increased TNF-α and IL-1β mRNA expression together with the activation of TNF-α-converting enzyme (TACE) and IL-1β-converting enzyme (ICE), known as caspase-1, leading to the conversion of the cytokine pro-forms into active forms (Figure 7-8).[144] This activated intracellular signaling is inhibited by GUDCA and IL-10.[144]

By first interacting with the cytoplasmic membrane of astrocytes, UCB upregulates both the TNF-α and IL-1β receptors (TNFR1 and IL-1R1, respectively),[145] which triggers the recruitment of the receptors' molecular adaptors TRAF2 and TRAF6, respectively (Figure 7-8), and then activates all three MAPK pathways, p38, JNK1/2, and ERK1/2, determining the release of IL-6, TNF-α, and IL-1β.[99,102] In parallel, UCB induces the translocation of NF-κB to the nucleus that was shown to be prevented by the suppression of TNF-α/TNFR1 and IL-1β/IL-1R1 cascades.[145] Activation of NF-κB by UCB was blocked by IL-10[144] and increased in immature astrocytes and in those exposed to associated hypoxia or oxygen–glucose deprivation preconditioning.[136,146]

Altogether, the relevance of UCB-induced activation of inflammatory pathways substantiates the use of anti-inflammatory compounds as preventive strategies. Administration of minocycline in Gunn rats was shown to protect from UCB-induced central auditory dysfunction[42] and to abrogate acute BAEP abnormalities.[45]

Cell Death and Role of Efflux Pumps

Two transmembrane proteins belonging to the ATP-binding cassette (ABC) family have been identified as potential cellular UCB exporters. While P-glycoprotein (Pgp) displays a low affinity for UCB, the multidrug resistance-associated protein-1 (Mrp1) possesses a very high affinity for UCB.[38] Both proteins are present in astrocytes[147,148] and their expression parallels astrocyte maturation.[71] Decreased expression in immature astrocytes may account for their increased loss of cell viability on UCB treatment, which is followed by a gradual tolerance (Figure 7-6B and C).[136] Inhibition of Mrp1 by MK571 further increased the release of glutamate by UCB, together with that of TNF-α and IL-1β, and enhanced cell demise[147] suggesting that Mrp1 is a key player in protecting astrocytes from UCB toxicity. Decreased expression in neurons also accounted for increased susceptibility to UCB injury.

Death of astrocytes by both necrosis and apoptosis increased with the time of exposure,[101] associated hypoxia or oxygen–glucose deprivation,[146] and UCB concentration.[107,136] Cotreatment with LPS aggravated astrocyte damage.[136] Because astrocytes are closely associated with neurons, degeneration of astrocytes in the brain parenchyma may compromise neuronal survival and functional recovery after BIND.

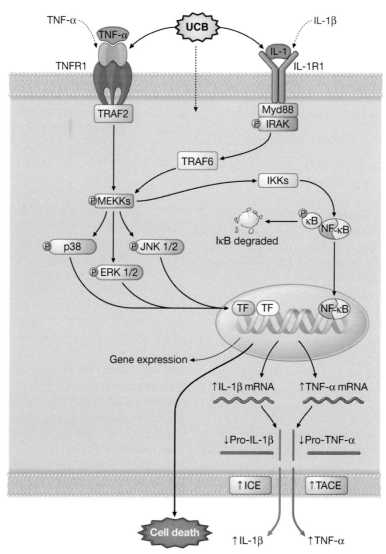

FIGURE 7-8. Schematic drawing of the inflammatory signaling pathways involved in tumor necrosis factor (TNF)-α and interleukin (IL)-1β release following astroglial activation by unconjugated bilirubin (UCB). UCB either diffuses across the plasma membrane or interacts with the cell-surface TNF receptor 1 (TNFR1) and IL-1 receptor 1 (IL-1R1) as a ligand, similarly to TNF-α and IL-1β. IL-1R1 activation triggers the recruitment of myeloid differentiation factor 88 (Myd88) that associates with IL-1R1-associated kinase (IRAK) and subsequently activates TRAF6. TNFR1 activation leads to the binding of the receptor molecular adaptor TRAF2. These events activate the members of mitogen-activated protein kinase (MAPK) family (MEKKs) with subsequent phosphorylation of MAPKs, namely, p38, extracellular signal-regulated kinases 1 and 2 (ERK1/2), and c-Jun N-terminal kinases 1 and 2 (JNK1/2) that activate downstream transcription factors (TF). Phosphorylation of ERK1/2 and JNK1/2 showed to be directly involved in the activation of the nuclear factor-kappa B (NF-κB) and translocation to the nucleus. Stimulation of the NF-κB pathway is initiated by the phosphorylation of the inhibitor of NF-κB (IκB) kinase complex (IKK), which is crucial for the degradation of IκB allowing NF-κB to translocate into the nucleus favoring gene transcription and even cell death. Exposure of astrocytes to UCB also stimulates both TNF-α and IL-1β mRNA expressions, as well as the activation of TNF-α and IL-1β-converting cell-surface enzymes (TACE and ICE, respectively), which are responsible for the conversion of the cytokine pro-forms into the active forms, thus decreasing their intracellular content. The activation of this signaling pathway determines an increased secretion of both TNF-α and IL-1β that will bind to their receptors, TNFR1 and IL-1R1, respectively, and will initiate the same intracellular cascade. (Adapted, with permission, from Fernandes and Brites.[101])

Microglia

Microglia constitute about 10–20% of the total glial cell population[149] and have a higher density within the hippocampus, basal ganglia, and substantia nigra.[150] Microglial cells are characterized by a very low threshold of activation by injury, altering their morphology and phenotype[151] according to the functional states that may change from surveillance to phagocytosis, activation, overactivation, and senescence. Microglial activation occurs within minutes, but can be long-lasting.[152]

The role of microglia in neonatal jaundice was nearly forgotten and the subtle balance between its protective and harmful effects scarcely explored or recognized. Microglia were first recognized to be activated by UCB in 2006,[104] changing from an elongated to an amoeboid appearance, with the release of glutamate and proinflammatory cytokines when exposed to UCB. Recently, it was observed that microglia become dystrophic and senescent showing fragmented cytoplasmic processes or condensation after prolonged exposure to UCB (Figure 7-9A), before degenerating.[105] These features were recognized in other conditions as well,[153,154] and may underlie a loss of microglial functionality and support.

Surprisingly, early microglial activation by UCB increases their phagocytic properties, which is followed by an inflammatory phenotype (Figure 7-9B). Thus, microglia seem to first respond to UCB by removing defunct axon terminals and by preserving neuronal connections, before dying by both apoptosis and necrosis (Figure 7-9C and D). Nevertheless, microglial phagocytosis also contributes to the loss of neurons, release of inflammatory cytokines, and perpetuation of damage.[152,155,156]

UCB-induced secretion of proinflammatory cytokines by microglia occurs before that of astrocytes, but both processes are preceded by the activation of MAPKs and NF-κB.[105] Coexistence of different phenotypes, indicating activation as a shift between different activity states and not a simultaneous process,[157,158] may explain the activation of caspase-3, -8, and -9, and cell death in the meantime (Figure 7-9C and D).

In some cases, BAEP abnormalities disappear or improve after phototherapy or exchange transfusion, but it may require several months to normalize, indicating the importance of plasticity of the developing injured brain and the potential for "reversibility" of some UCB toxicity.[159] Microglia may have an important role in this process.

Oligodendrocytes

OLGs are mature glial cells that myelinate axons in the brain and spinal cord. They arise from oligodendrocyte precursor cells (OPCs) that proliferate and differentiate just before and after birth.[71] Damage to OPCs and OLGs causes loss of myelin synthesis and interruption of proper axonal function.[160]

Cytotoxicity of UCB to rat OLGs in vitro was initially documented by Genc et al.,[161] who observed decreased OLGs viability, as well as increased apoptotic cell death and NO production. In fact, areas affected by kernicterus generally show demyelination.[12,126,162] Moreover, it seems that UCB preferentially binds to myelin[71,163] and that white matter abnormalities precede gray matter damage in severely jaundiced neonates.[164]

Recently, OPCs were shown to be particularly vulnerable to UCB, evidencing a rapid increase in features of ER stress, with the consequent release of Ca^{2+}, activation of JNK1/2 and calpain, mitochondrial dysfunction, and generation of ROS, apoptosis, and necrosis (Figures 7-1 and 7-10).[165] Moreover, UCB also delays differentiation of OPCs enhancing the number of progenitors chondroitin sulfate proteoglycan NG2-expressing (i.e., NG2) cells and reducing OLGs (myelin basic protein positive cells) when compared with vehicle-treated OPCs (Figure 7-10). These findings indicate that UCB, besides compromising OPC proliferation, may also delay myelination. Therefore, hyperbilirubinemia during the early phase of developmental myelination, when an unusual synthesis rate of myelin structural proteins is necessary,[166] may impair differentiation of OPCs into OLGs and trigger a defective myelination that will contribute to the emergence of neurological damage. This may have relevance in BIND once neuroinflammation and dysfunction of OLGs provide high risk for axonal loss.[167]

Bilirubin in the Interplay Between Neurons and Glia

Until today, little has been known about the interplay between microglia, astrocytes, and neurons in response to UCB, especially in early postnatal development. Moreover, communication between neurons, astrocytes, and OLGs may have strong and diverse influences on the cascades of astrocytic and microglial responses, leading to beneficial or detrimental outcomes. Studies with co-cultures and organotypic slice cultures focused on identifying the role of astrocytes and microglia may add relevant information to our understanding of the mechanisms of BIND.

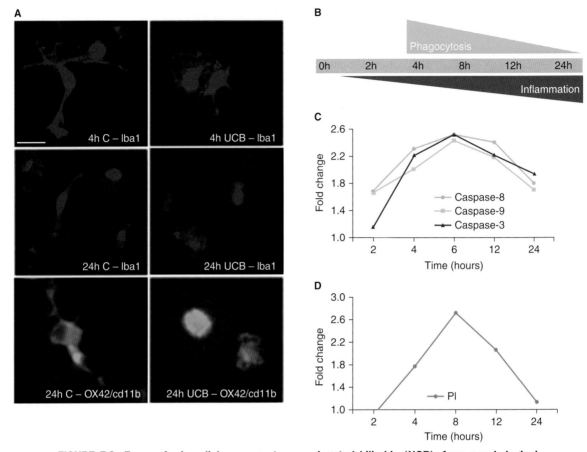

FIGURE 7-9. Faces of microglial response to unconjugated bilirubin (UCB): from morphological changes to reactive phenotypes and cell death. Rat cortical microglia were exposed to 50 μM UCB (UCB/human serum albumin [HSA] = 0.5) or to HSA (control - C) for the indicated time periods. **A.** Representative morphologies for elongated microglia (control, 4-hour incubation) and amoeboid/ dystrophic phenotypes from 4 to 24 hours incubation with UCB after immunostaining for Iba1 (red) and OX42/cd11b (green). **B.** Schematic drawing of the temporal profile of microglial activation by UCB, showing that phagocytosis precedes inflammation. **C.** Activities of caspase-3, -8, and -9 (determined in cell lysates by enzymatic cleavage of chromophore pNA) are increased from 4 to 12 hours. **D.** Microglial death, assessed as propidium iodide (PI)–positive cells and expressed as fold versus respective control, is elevated from 4 to 12 hours. Scale bar equals 20 μm. (Panels with Iba1-stained microglia in A and data in B–C images are reprinted and adapted from Silva SL, Vaz AR, Barateiro A, et al. Features of bilirubin-induced reactive microglia: from phagocytosis to inflammation. *Neurobiol Dis.* 2010;40(3):663–675, with permission from Elsevier.)

By investigating dysfunction of neurons caused by UCB when co-cultured with astrocytes in the absence of any direct cell-to-cell contact, but sharing the same culture medium, an increased neuritic atrophy was observed, as well as apoptosis and loss of cell viability, relative to pure neuron cultures. These findings indicate that pathological neuron-to-astrocyte interactions may be involved in neuronal derangement and contribute to injury.[168] Once again, GUDCA was shown to counteract the neurotoxic effects

by UCB (AS Falcão, personal communication). A most interesting finding was the increased extracellular levels of S100B in these neuron–astrocyte co-cultures treated with UCB, which was not produced in pure neuronal cultures. S100B is considered a protein biomarker that reflects CNS injury.[169] This corroborates previous data relating increased serum levels of S100B and tau with TSB levels from 5.3 to 37.3 mg/dL in jaundiced neonates.[133] These data are unique in corroborating UCB damage to both neurons (tau) and

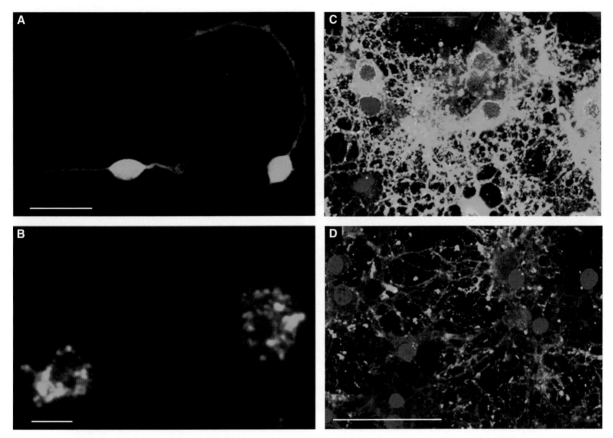

FIGURE 7-10. Unconjugated bilirubin (UCB) impairs oligodendrocyte precursor cells (OPCs) survival and delays oligodendrocyte (OLG) differentiation in vitro. Primary cultures of OPCs were isolated from mixed glial cultures. OPCs were treated with human serum albumin (HSA) alone (**A** and **C**) or with 50 μM UCB plus 100 μM HSA (**B** and **D**) for 24 hours. In cells labeled for A2B5 + O4 (preoligodendrocytes, in green), we may see the normal bipolar morphology of HSA-treated cells (**A**) and dying cells after treatment with UCB (**B**). Myelination capacity (**C** and **D**) was evaluated by chondroitin sulfate proteoglycan NG2 expressing density for OLG progenitors (red) and myelin basic protein (MBP) for differentiated cells (green). Nuclei were stained with Hoechst 33258 dye (blue). UCB showed to impair OPC differentiation into OLG, thus delaying myelination by reducing the number of MBP⁺ cells and increasing that of NG2⁺ cells as compared with HSA treated OPCs. Scale bar equals 20 μm (**A** and **B**) and 50 μm (**D**). C has the same magnification as D. (Used with permission from Andreia Barateiro.)

astrocytes (S100B) and suggest that S100B and tau could be used as biomarkers of BIND, as a strong correlation of S100B with abnormal BAEPs and with auditory neuropathy has been observed.[133]

The interplay between CNS cells may influence microglial responses. Using conditioned media from neurons treated with UCB, microglial activation with increased production of IL-6 and NO, as well as increased microglial demise, was observed, when compared with the direct action of UCB on microglia.[170] Moreover, soluble factors released by UCB-

treated neurons have been shown to further stimulate the UCB-induced phagocytic role of microglia (Figure 7-11). Taking a look at the effects of UCB-reactive microglia on neurons (1:10, microglia:neurons), the reduction of neurite extension and ramification by UCB treatment was not seen in these mixed cultures.[170] These findings are probably a result of microglial phagocytosis of damaged neurons, similarly to that observed by others.[171–173] Accordingly, fewer propidium iodide–positive nuclei were seen in pure neuron cultures after UCB treatment. Hence, UCB-injured

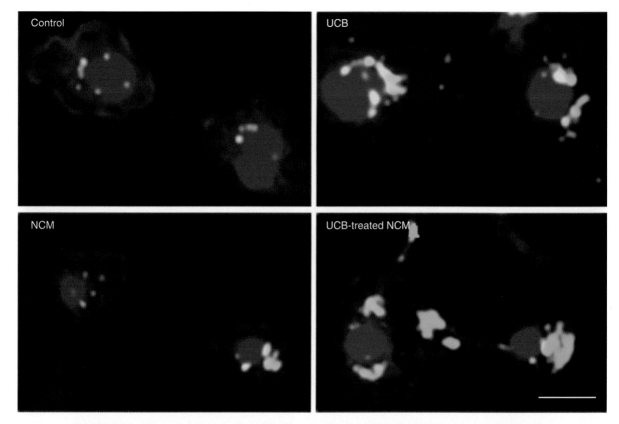

FIGURE 7-11. Microglial phagocytic ability that revealed to increase on exposure to unconjugated bilirubin (UCB) is further enhanced if incubated with neuronal conditioned media (NCM) from UCB-treated neurons. Microglia were incubated for 4 hours with human serum albumin (HSA) alone (Control) or with 50 μM UCB in the presence of 100 μM HSA (UCB/HSA = 0.5). In parallel experiments, microglia was similarly treated with NCM collected from HSA-treated neurons or from UCB-treated neurons (UCB-treated NCM), after 12 hours of incubation. Microglial cells were counterstained with an antibody raised against Iba-1 (red). Cells were incubated with green fluorescent latex beads to evaluate microglial phagocytic ability by the number of ingested beads per cell. Low phagocytosis in control and in NCM experiments contrasts with enhanced microglial phagocytosis on exposure to UCB or to UCB-treated NCM. Scale bar equals 20 μm. (Partly reproduced, with permission, from Silva SL, Osório C, Vaz AR, et al. Dynamics of neuron-glia interplay upon exposure to unconjugated bilirubin. *J Neurochem.* 2011;117(3):412–424.)

neurons might be signaling functional microglia to engage in phagocytosis.

When organotypic-cultured hippocampal slices were exposed to UCB, the noxious effects were clearly observed by a generalized neural cell death[128] (Figure 7-12). To better assess the signaling produced by microglia in this complex cell interplay system, depleted and nondepleted slices in microglia[174] were treated with UCB, revealing that the presence of microglia increased NO release and cell death.

Therefore, instead of inducing defensive cell actions and diminishing UCB toxic effects, microglia aggravated the UCB-induced nitrosative stress and increased the number of cells that lost viability.[128] As mentioned previously, relative to other UCB-induced cytotoxic effects, here again GUDCA was able to abrogate hippocampal NO production and cell death. Whether modulation of microglial activation will be considered a therapeutic goal to prevent BIND is presently unknown.

Collectively, we may assume that the wide range of harmful effects in neural cells includes glia activation and neurodegeneration, and that the close proximity between the cells makes them more susceptible to UCB injury (Figure 7-13).

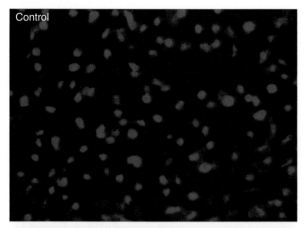

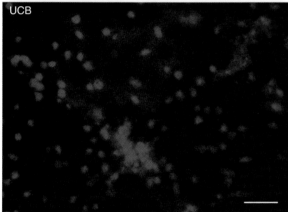

FIGURE 7-12. Unconjugated bilirubin (UCB) triggers cell death in organotypic-cultured hippocampal slices. Organo-typic-cultured hippocampal slices were prepared from P8–P10 Wistar rat brains (400 μm coronal sections) and placed on the top of a Transwell tissue insert. Hippocampal slices cultured for 3 days in vitro were exposed to 100 μM human serum albumin (HSA) in the absence (control) or in the presence of 50 μM UCB for 24 hours, and further incubated with propidium iodide (PI). Enhancement of PI-positive cells by UCB is shown in pink. Scale bar equals 20 μm. (Used with permission from Sandra Silva, Dora Brites lab.)

■ BILIRUBIN TOXICITY: INFLAMMATION AND NEURODEVELOPMENT STAGE AS RISK FACTORS

Areas classically damaged by UCB include the cerebellum, particularly the Purkinje cells, and the hippocampus. Besides this kernicterus spectrum, less severe injury, including mild neurological abnormalities, and isolated neural hearing loss are now comprised in the BIND classification.[12] As previously mentioned in sections "Neurons" and "Astrocytes," immature neurons, as well as astrocytes, show a higher susceptibility to UCB toxicity than more differentiated ones.[136] This is in line with the concept that injury to the developing brain is associated with increased risk for potential lifelong consequences, which seems to depend more on the age of the neonate than on the type of adverse event.[175,176]

The wider spectrum of MRI findings in both preterm and term infants[164] highlights the need for further study of the effects of the stage of neurodevelopment on BIND sequelae, as well as the rate of rise and duration of hyperbilirubinemia. In fact, differences in neurological sequelae encountered between the *Ugt1*-null and the h*UGT1A1*28* mice[34,36] indicate the existence of temporal windows of neurodevelopment that may account for the higher susceptibility of the first model to BIND. In the Gunn rat, the neuropathological damage by UCB is at first auditory and then motor at later stages of neurodevelopment.[12] There is no doubt about the particular susceptibility of preterm neonates and the prevalence of kernicterus cases in this at-risk cohort,[6,177] in the absence of acute neurological signs.[178] Thus, temporal windows of susceptibility depend on the developmental stage of the CNS at the time of insult.

The presence of inflammatory features was observed during or following moderate to severe hyperbilirubinemia, and neonatal sepsis is believed to contribute to neurodevelopmental sequelae and to UCB encephalopathy.[71] As indicated in section "Neurons," when immature neurons were incubated with UCB and LPS, further decreased cell viability and increased TNF-α production were observed, as compared with those treated with UCB alone. Co-incubation with TNF-α plus IL-1β also produced increased nitrosative stress, JNK1/2 MAPK activation, cell demise, and apoptosis by both mitochondrial-dependent and -independent apoptotic pathways. Therefore, the association of inflammation and hyperbilirubinemia may increase functional deregulation and even degeneration of neurons, with the consequent disruption of nerve terminal activity and loss of synapses. Moreover, inflammatory cytokines may increase blood–brain barrier permeability by acting on endothelial cells and TJ,[118] facilitating UCB passage across the barrier and further exacerbating its accumulation in brain parenchyma. These findings indicate inflammation as a risk factor for BIND and open new avenues for further studies aimed to clearly demonstrate its damaging effects.

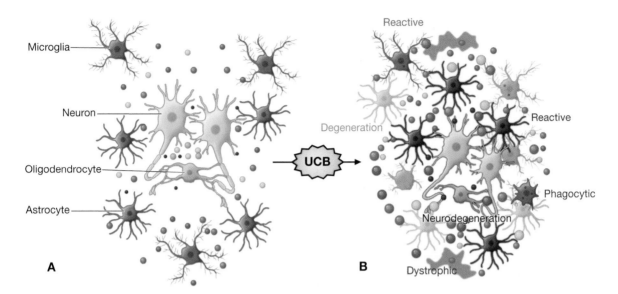

FIGURE 7-13. Interplay between neurons and glial cells. A. In physiological conditions, neurons and glia (astrocytes, microglia, and oligodendrocytes) are extensively linked and have profound effects on each other's function. Neurons release gliotransmitters (yellow circles) and oligodendrocyte signaling molecules (blue circles). Glutamate (red circles) and soluble factors (e.g., cytokines, trophic factors) from astrocytes (purple circles) and microglia (orange circles) provide endogenous neuroprotection. **B.** In unconjugated hyperbilirubinemia, nitrosative and oxidative stress, neuroinflammation, and excitotoxicity determine: (i) microglial migration to the injury and astrogliosis; (ii) different phenotypes on microglia, from reactive to phagocytic and dystrophic microglia (senescent); (iii) reactivity of astrocytes followed by degeneration; (iv) disruption of synaptic plasticity and reduced neurite arborization, as well as loss of connectivity and function preceding neuronal death; and (v) deficient oligodendrocyte precursor proliferation and decreased myelin biogenesis. Thus, therapeutic strategies directed at controlling the activation of microglia and astrocytes, and the excessive production of proinflammatory and pro-oxidant factors, may add on the prevention and recovery of neurological sequelae resulting from unconjugated hyperbilirubinemia.

■ CONCLUDING REMARKS

Early lesions in the first and second postnatal weeks of life probably determine sequelae that may be diverse in nature, severity, and enduring effects. Nevertheless, most of the knowledge has been acquired by examining "end stage" or post-lesions. Therefore, the current knowledge on the cellular mechanisms of neonatal brain injury caused by UCB was presented from the perspective of temporal windows of susceptibility dependence. Time of exposure and UCB concentration, as well as associated conditions such as acidosis, sepsis, and hypoxia or oxygen–glucose deprivation, are contributors to BIND, at least in in vitro studies.

Immature nerve cells are prone to mitochondria dysfunction, ER stress, bioenergetic crisis, oxidative stress, apoptosis, and long-lasting neurological sequelae caused by UCB, probably due to low levels of Pgp and Mrp1. Brain region susceptibility to BIND appears to relate to low levels of the redox-sensitive protein DJ-1 and greater disruption of the cellular redox status. Nevertheless, future studies are necessary to understand how variable protein expression can influence cell survival in the presence of high levels of UCB, and to better clarify the cascade of events and the intervening mediators that lead to long-term adverse neurodevelopment effects. Potential harmful effects of UCB in myelinogenesis also deserve to be evaluated. Whether modulation of astrocytic and microglial reactivity will help to sustain BIND deserves continued investigation inasmuch as glial cells are now believed to provide more to neurons than structural and nutritional support.[152] Another critical point is to define whether the enhanced plasticity of the developing brain will have negative or positive effects on recovery after early life brain injury by UCB.

These studies will open new perspectives for therapeutic approaches where cells can be specifically targeted for preserving their function and/or survival, and will renew interest in strategies aimed at circumventing enduring injurious effects of neonatal brain insults by UCB.

■ ACKNOWLEDGMENTS

Due to space limitations, we would like to apologize in advance to all our colleagues whose research was not cited in this chapter, but whose work has certainly advanced our understanding in this field of research. Moreover, we express our gratitude to the coauthors of the publications cited in this chapter, in particular our team members: Rui Silva, Adelaide Fernandes, Ana Sofia Falcão and Ana Rita Vaz. We also thank our colleagues: Rolf Brodersen, François Trivin, and Claudio Tiribelli in the bilirubin field; Allan Butterfield in biomembranes; and Lorene Lanier in neurosciences for sharing their expertise with us.

We acknowledge our funding support from Fundação para a Ciência e a Tecnologia (FCT), Lisbon, Portugal, through the grants POCI/SAU-MMO/55955/2004, PTDC/SAU-NEU/64385/2006, PEst-OE/SAU/UI4013/2011 and PTDC/SAU-FCF/68819/2006, as well as FEDER.

REFERENCES

1. Hansen TWR. Pioneers in the scientific study of neonatal jaundice and kernicterus. *Pediatrics.* 2000;106(2):E15.
2. Cuadrado A, Rojo AI. Heme oxygenase-1 as a therapeutic target in neurodegenerative diseases and brain infections. *Curr Pharm Des.* 2008;14(5):429–442.
3. McDonagh AF. Controversies in bilirubin biochemistry and their clinical relevance. *Semin Fetal Neonatal Med.* 2010;15(3):141–147.
4. Bhutani VK, Johnson L. Kernicterus in late preterm infants cared for as term healthy infants. *Semin Perinatol.* 2006;30(2):89–97.
5. Bhutani VK, Johnson L. Kernicterus in the 21st century: frequently asked questions. *J Perinatol.* 2009;29(suppl 1):S20–S24.
6. Okumura A, Kidokoro H, Shoji H, et al. Kernicterus in preterm infants. *Pediatrics.* 2009;123(6):e1052–e1058.
7. Calligaris SD, Bellarosa C, Giraudi P, et al. Cytotoxicity is predicted by unbound and not total bilirubin concentration. *Pediatr Res.* 2007;62(5):576–580.
8. Ahlfors CE, Wennberg RP, Ostrow JD, Tiribelli C. Unbound (free) bilirubin: improving the paradigm for evaluating neonatal jaundice. *Clin Chem.* 2009;55(7):1288–1299.
9. Daood MJ, McDonagh AF, Watchko JF. Calculated free bilirubin levels and neurotoxicity. *J Perinatol.* 2009;29(suppl 1):S14–S19.
10. Ostrow JD, Tiribelli C. Bilirubin, a curse and a boon. *Gut.* 2003;52(12):1668–1670.
11. Brito MA, Silva RFM, Brites D. Cell response to hyperbilirubinemia: a journey along key molecular events. In: Chen FJ, ed. *New Trends in Brain Research.* New York: Nova Science Publishers Inc; 2006:1–38.
12. Shapiro SM. Chronic bilirubin encephalopathy: diagnosis and outcome. *Semin Fetal Neonatal Med.* 2010; 15(3):157–163.
13. Bar PR. Motor neuron disease in vitro: the use of cultured motor neurons to study amyotrophic lateral sclerosis. *Eur J Pharmacol.* 2000;405(1–3):285–295.
14. LePage KT, Dickey RW, Gerwick WH, Jester EL, Murray TF. On the use of neuro-2a neuroblastoma cells versus intact neurons in primary culture for neurotoxicity studies. *Crit Rev Neurobiol.* 2005;17(1):27–50.
15. De Vries GH, Boullerne AI. Glial cell lines: an overview. *Neurochem Res.* 2010;35(12):1978–2000.
16. Oakes GH, Bend JR. Global changes in gene regulation demonstrate that unconjugated bilirubin is able to upregulate and activate select components of the endoplasmic reticulum stress response pathway. *J Biochem Mol Toxicol.* 2010;24(2):73–88.
17. Deganuto M, Cesaratto L, Bellarosa C, et al. A proteomic approach to the bilirubin-induced toxicity in neuronal cells reveals a protective function of DJ-1 protein. *Proteomics.* 2010;10(8):1645–1657.
18. Corich L, Aranda A, Carrassa L, et al. The cytotoxic effect of unconjugated bilirubin in human neuroblastoma SH-SY5Y cells is modulated by the expression level of MRP1 but not MDR1. *Biochem J.* 2009;417(1):305–312.
19. Hankø E, Hansen TWR, Almaas R, Rootwelt T. Recovery after short-term bilirubin exposure in human NT2-N neurons. *Brain Res.* 2006;1103(1):56–64.
20. Roll EB. Bilirubin-induced cell death during continuous and intermittent phototherapy and in the dark. *Acta Paediatr.* 2005;94(10):1437–1442.
21. Silva RFM, Falcão AS, Fernandes A, et al. Dissociated primary nerve cell cultures as models for assessment of neurotoxicity. *Toxicol Lett.* 2006;163(1):1–9.
22. Falcão AS, Silva RFM, Pancadas S, et al. Apoptosis and impairment of neurite network by short exposure of immature rat cortical neurons to unconjugated bilirubin increase with cell differentiation and are additionally enhanced by an inflammatory stimulus. *J Neurosci Res.* 2007;85(6):1229–1239.

23. Vaz AR, Silva SL, Barateiro A, et al. Pro-inflammatory cytokines intensify the activation of NO/NOS, JNK1/2 and caspase cascades in immature neurons exposed to elevated levels of unconjugated bilirubin. *Exp Neurol.* 2011;229(2):381–390.

24. Zhang B, Yang X, Gao X. Taurine protects against bilirubin-induced neurotoxicity in vitro. *Brain Res.* 2010;1320:159–167.

25. Brito MA, Lima S, Fernandes A, et al. Bilirubin injury to neurons: contribution of oxidative stress and rescue by glycoursodeoxycholic acid. *Neurotoxicology.* 2008;29(2):259–269.

26. Lin S, Wei X, Bales KR, et al. Minocycline blocks bilirubin neurotoxicity and prevents hyperbilirubinemia-induced cerebellar hypoplasia in the Gunn rat. *Eur J Neurosci.* 2005;22(1):21–27.

27. Berns M, Toennessen M, Koehne P, Altmann R, Obladen M. Ibuprofen augments bilirubin toxicity in rat cortical neuronal culture. *Pediatr Res.* 2009;65(4):392–396.

28. Su T, Paradiso B, Long YS, Liao WP, Simonato M. Evaluation of cell damage in organotypic hippocampal slice culture from adult mouse: a potential model system to study neuroprotection. *Brain Res.* 2011;1385:68–76.

29. Lein PJ, Barnhart CD, Pessah IN. Acute hippocampal slice preparation and hippocampal slice cultures. *Methods Mol Biol.* 2011;758:115–134.

30. Tovar YRLB, Santa-Cruz LD, Tapia R. Experimental models for the study of neurodegeneration in amyotrophic lateral sclerosis. *Mol Neurodegener.* 2009;4:31.

31. Cho S, Wood A, Bowlby MR. Brain slices as models for neurodegenerative disease and screening platforms to identify novel therapeutics. *Curr Neuropharmacol.* 2007;5(1):19–33.

32. Chang FY, Lee CC, Huang CC, Hsu KS. Unconjugated bilirubin exposure impairs hippocampal long-term synaptic plasticity. *PLoS One.* 2009;4(6):e5876.

33. Haustein MD, Read DJ, Steinert JR, et al. Acute hyperbilirubinaemia induces presynaptic neurodegeneration at a central glutamatergic synapse. *J Physiol.* 2010;588(pt 23):4683–4693.

34. Nguyen N, Bonzo JA, Chen S, et al. Disruption of the *Ugt1* locus in mice resembles human Crigler–Najjar type I disease. *J Biol Chem.* 2008;283(12):7901–7911.

35. Rice AC, Shapiro SM. A new animal model of hemolytic hyperbilirubinemia-induced bilirubin encephalopathy (kernicterus). *Pediatr Res.* 2008;64(3):265–269.

36. Fujiwara R, Nguyen N, Chen S, Tukey RH. Developmental hyperbilirubinemia and CNS toxicity in mice humanized with the UDP glucuronosyltransferase 1 (*UGT1*) locus. *Proc Natl Acad Sci U S A.* 2010;107(11):5024–5029.

37. Shapiro SM, Sombati S, Geiger A, Rice AC. NMDA channel antagonist MK-801 does not protect against bilirubin neurotoxicity. *Neonatology.* 2007;92(4):248–257.

38. Gazzin S, Berengeno AL, Strazielle N, et al. Modulation of Mrp1 (ABCc1) and Pgp (ABCb1) by bilirubin at the blood–CSF and blood–brain barriers in the Gunn rat. *PLoS One.* 2011;6(1):e16165.

39. Cannon C, Daood MJ, O'Day TL, Watchko JF. Sex-specific regional brain bilirubin content in hyperbilirubinemic Gunn rat pups. *Biol Neonate.* 2006;90(1):40–45.

40. Shaia WT, Shapiro SM, Spencer RF. The jaundiced Gunn rat model of auditory neuropathy/dyssynchrony. *Laryngoscope.* 2005;115(12):2167–2173.

41. Hafkamp AM, Havinga R, Sinaasappel M, Verkade HJ. Effective oral treatment of unconjugated hyperbilirubinemia in Gunn rats. *Hepatology.* 2005;41(3):526–534.

42. Geiger AS, Rice AC, Shapiro SM. Minocycline blocks acute bilirubin-induced neurological dysfunction in jaundiced Gunn rats. *Neonatology.* 2007;92(4):219–226.

43. Cuperus FJ, Hafkamp AM, Havinga R, et al. Effective treatment of unconjugated hyperbilirubinemia with oral bile salts in Gunn rats. *Gastroenterology.* 2009;136(2):673–682.e1.

44. Cuperus FJ, Iemhoff AA, van der Wulp M, Havinga R, Verkade HJ. Acceleration of the gastrointestinal transit by polyethylene glycol effectively treats unconjugated hyperbilirubinaemia in Gunn rats. *Gut.* 2010;59(3):373–380.

45. Rice AC, Chiou VL, Zuckoff SB, Shapiro SM. Profile of minocycline neuroprotection in bilirubin-induced auditory system dysfunction. *Brain Res.* 2011;1368:290–298.

46. Strassburg CP. Pharmacogenetics of Gilbert's syndrome. *Pharmacogenomics.* 2008;9(6):703–715.

47. Bosma PJ. Inherited disorders of bilirubin metabolism. *J Hepatol.* 2003;38(1):107–117.

48. Ostrow JD, Pascolo L, Shapiro SM, Tiribelli C. New concepts in bilirubin encephalopathy. *Eur J Clin Invest.* 2003;33(11):988–997.

49. Palmela I, Cardoso FL, Bernas M, et al. Elevated levels of bilirubin and long-term exposure impair human brain microvascular endothelial cell integrity. *Curr Neurovasc Res.* 2011;8(2):153–169.

50. Malik SG, Irwanto KA, Ostrow JD, Tiribelli C. Effect of bilirubin on cytochrome *c* oxidase activity of mitochondria from mouse brain and liver. *BMC Res Notes.* 2010;3:162.

51. Cesaratto L, Calligaris SD, Vascotto C, et al. Bilirubin-induced cell toxicity involves PTEN activation through an APE1/Ref-1-dependent pathway. *J Mol Med.* 2007;85(10):1099–1112.

52. Calligaris S, Cekic D, Roca-Burgos L, et al. Multidrug resistance associated protein 1 protects against bilirubin-induced cytotoxicity. *FEBS Lett.* 2006;580(5):1355–1359.

53. Ostrow JD, Pascolo L, Brites D, Tiribelli C. Molecular basis of bilirubin-induced neurotoxicity. *Trends Mol Med.* 2004;10(2):65–70.

54. Ostrow JD, Pascolo L, Tiribelli C. Reassessment of the unbound concentrations of unconjugated bilirubin in relation to neurotoxicity *in vitro*. *Pediatr Res*. 2003;54(1):98–104.

55. Ostrow JD, Pascolo L, Tiribelli C. Reassessment of the unbound concentrations of unconjugated bilirubin in relation to neurotoxicity in vitro. *Pediatr Res*. 2003;54(6):926.

56. Daood MJ, Watchko JF. Calculated *in vivo* free bilirubin levels in the central nervous system of Gunn rat pups. *Pediatr Res*. 2006;60(1):44–49.

57. Vitek L, Ostrow JD. Bilirubin chemistry and metabolism; harmful and protective aspects. *Curr Pharm Des*. 2009;15(25):2869–2883.

58. Ostrow JD, Mukerjee P. Solvent partition of ^{14}C-unconjugated bilirubin to remove labeled polar contaminants. *Transl Res*. 2007;149(1):37–45.

59. McDonagh AF. Ex uno plures: the concealed complexity of bilirubin species in neonatal blood samples. *Pediatrics*. 2006;118(3):1185–1187.

60. Weisiger RA, Ostrow JD, Koehler RK, et al. Affinity of human serum albumin for bilirubin varies with albumin concentration and buffer composition: results of a novel ultrafiltration method. *J Biol Chem*. 2001;276(32):29953–29960.

61. Hansen TWR. Phototherapy for neonatal jaundice—therapeutic effects on more than one level? *Semin Perinatol*. 2010;34(3):231–234.

62. Watchko JF. Kernicterus and the molecular mechanisms of bilirubin-induced CNS injury in newborns. *Neuromol Med*. 2006;8(4):513–529.

63. Brito MA, Silva RFM, Brites D. Bilirubin toxicity to human erythrocytes: a review. *Clin Chim Acta*. 2006;374(1–2):46–56.

64. Vaz AR, Delgado-Esteban M, Brito MA, et al. Bilirubin selectively inhibits cytochrome *c* oxidase activity and induces apoptosis in immature cortical neurons: assessment of the protective effects of glycoursodeoxycholic acid. *J Neurochem*. 2010;112(1):56–65.

65. Brito MA, Rosa AI, Silva RFM, et al. Oxidative stress and disruption of the nervous cell. In: Resch CJ, ed. *Focus on Brain Research*. New York: Nova Science Publishers Inc; 2007:1–33.

66. Maisels MJ, Kring E. The contribution of hemolysis to early jaundice in normal newborns. *Pediatrics*. 2006;118(1):276–279.

67. Roll EB, Christensen T, Gederaas OA. Effects of bilirubin and phototherapy on osmotic fragility and haematoporphyrin-induced photohaemolysis of normal erythrocytes and spherocytes. *Acta Paediatr*. 2005;94(10):1443–1447.

68. McDonagh AF. Bilirubin toxicity to human erythrocytes: a more sanguine view. *Pediatrics*. 2007;120(1):175–178.

69. Brito MA, Brites D, Butterfield DA. A link between hyperbilirubinemia, oxidative stress and injury to neocortical synaptosomes. *Brain Res*. 2004;1026(1):33–43.

70. Brito MA, Rosa AI, Falcão AS, et al. Unconjugated bilirubin differentially affects the redox status of neuronal and astroglial cells. *Neurobiol Dis*. 2008;29(1):30–40.

71. Brites D. Bilirubin injury to neurons and glial cells: new players, novel targets and newer insights. *Semin Perinatol*. 2011;35(3):114–120.

72. Zucker SD, Goessling W, Hoppin AG. Unconjugated bilirubin exhibits spontaneous diffusion through model lipid bilayers and native hepatocyte membranes. *J Biol Chem*. 1999;274(16):10852–10862.

73. Chen HC, Wang CH, Tsan KW, Chen YC. An electron microscopic and radioautographic study on experimental kernicterus. II. Bilirubin movement within neurons and release of waste products via astroglia. *Am J Pathol*. 1971;64(1):45–66.

74. Gollan JL, Huang SN, Billing B, Sherlock S. Prolonged survival in three brothers with severe type 2 Crigler–Najjar syndrome. Ultrastructural and metabolic studies. *Gastroenterology*. 1975;68(6):1543–1555.

75. Silva RFM, Mata LM, Gulbenkian S, Brites D. Endocytosis in rat cultured astrocytes is inhibited by unconjugated bilirubin. *Neurochem Res*. 2001;26(7):793–800.

76. Calligaris R, Bellarosa C, Foti R, et al. A transcriptome analysis identifies molecular effectors of unconjugated bilirubin in human neuroblastoma SH-SY5Y cells. *BMC Genomics*. 2009;10:543.

77. Lai E, Teodoro T, Volchuk A. Endoplasmic reticulum stress: signaling the unfolded protein response. *Physiology (Bethesda)*. 2007;22:193–201.

78. Upton JP, Austgen K, Nishino M, et al. Caspase-2 cleavage of BID is a critical apoptotic signal downstream of endoplasmic reticulum stress. *Mol Cell Biol*. 2008;28(12):3943–3951.

79. Martinez JA, Zhang Z, Svetlov SI, et al. Calpain and caspase processing of caspase-12 contribute to the ER stress-induced cell death pathway in differentiated PC12 cells. *Apoptosis*. 2010;15(12):1480–1493.

80. Billen LP, Shamas-Din A, Andrews DW. Bid: a Bax-like BH3 protein. *Oncogene*. 2008;27(suppl 1):S93–S104.

81. Naidoo N. Cellular stress/the unfolded protein response: relevance to sleep and sleep disorders. *Sleep Med Rev*. 2009;13(3):195–204.

82. Matus S, Lisbona F, Torres M, et al. The stress rheostat: an interplay between the unfolded protein response (UPR) and autophagy in neurodegeneration. *Curr Mol Med*. 2008;8(3):157–172.

83. Rubinsztein DC. The roles of intracellular protein-degradation pathways in neurodegeneration. *Nature*. 2006;443(7113):780–786.

84. Ollinger R, Kogler P, Troppmair J, et al. Bilirubin inhibits tumor cell growth via activation of ERK. *Cell Cycle.* 2007;6(24):3078–3085.

85. Karakukcu C, Ustdal M, Ozturk A, Baskol G, Saraymen R. Assessment of DNA damage and plasma catalase activity in healthy term hyperbilirubinemic infants receiving phototherapy. *Mutat Res.* 2009;680(1–2):12–16.

86. Hachiya Y, Hayashi M. Bilirubin encephalopathy: a study of neuronal subpopulations and neurodegenerative mechanisms in 12 autopsy cases. *Brain Dev.* 2008;30(4):269–278.

87. Kryston TB, Georgiev AB, Pissis P, Georgakilas AG. Role of oxidative stress and DNA damage in human carcinogenesis. *Mutat Res.* 2011;711(1–2):193–201.

88. Martich-Kriss V, Kollias SS, Ball WS Jr. MR findings in kernicterus. *AJNR Am J Neuroradiol.* 1995;16 (4 suppl):819–821.

89. Ikonomidou C, Kaindl AM. Neuronal death and oxidative stress in the developing brain. *Antioxid Redox Signal.* 2011;14(8):1535–1550.

90. Vaz AR, Silva SL, Barateiro A, et al. Selective vulnerability of rat brain regions to unconjugated bilirubin. *Mol Cell Neurosci.* 2011;48(1):82–93.

91. Khan NM, Poduval TB. Immunomodulatory and immunotoxic effects of bilirubin: molecular mechanisms. *J Leukoc Biol.* 2011;90(5):997–1015.

92. Loftspring MC, Johnson HL, Feng R, Johnson AJ, Clark JF. Unconjugated bilirubin contributes to early inflammation and edema after intracerebral hemorrhage. *J Cereb Blood Flow Metab.* 2011;31(4): 1133–1142.

93. Kumar S, Guha M, Choubey V, et al. Bilirubin inhibits *Plasmodium falciparum* growth through the generation of reactive oxygen species. *Free Radic Biol Med.* 2008;44(4):602–613.

94. Kahle PJ, Waak J, Gasser T. DJ-1 and prevention of oxidative stress in Parkinson's disease and other age-related disorders. *Free Radic Biol Med.* 2009;47(10): 1354–1361.

95. Feissner RF, Skalska J, Gaum WE, Sheu SS. Crosstalk signaling between mitochondrial Ca^{2+} and ROS. *Front Biosci.* 2009;14:1197–1218.

96. Gao X, Yang X, Zhang B. Neuroprotection of taurine against bilirubin-induced elevation of apoptosis and intracellular free calcium ion *in vivo. Toxicol Mech Methods.* 2011;21(5):383–387.

97. Schwaller B. Cytosolic Ca^{2+} buffers. *Cold Spring Harb Perspect Biol.* 2010;2(11):a004051.

98. Keshavan P, Deem TL, Schwemberger SJ, et al. Unconjugated bilirubin inhibits VCAM-1-mediated transendothelial leukocyte migration. *J Immunol.* 2005;174(6):3709–3718.

99. Fernandes A, Falcão AS, Silva RFM, Brito MA, Brites D. MAPKs are key players in mediating cytokine release and cell death induced by unconjugated bilirubin in cultured rat cortical astrocytes. *Eur J Neurosci.* 2007;25(4):1058–1068.

100. Fernandes A, Silva RFM, Falcão AS, Brito MA, Brites D. Cytokine production, glutamate release and cell death in rat cultured astrocytes treated with unconjugated bilirubin and LPS. *J Neuroimmunol.* 2004;153(1–2): 64–75.

101. Fernandes A, Brites D. Contribution of inflammatory processes to nerve cell toxicity by bilirubin and efficacy of potential therapeutic agents. *Curr Pharm Des.* 2009;15(25):2915–2926.

102. Fernandes A, Falcão AS, Silva RFM, et al. Inflammatory signalling pathways involved in astroglial activation by unconjugated bilirubin. *J Neurochem.* 2006; 96(6):1667–1679.

103. Loftspring MC, Hansen C, Clark JF. A novel brain injury mechanism after intracerebral hemorrhage: the interaction between heme products and the immune system. *Med Hypotheses.* 2010;74(1):63–66.

104. Gordo AC, Falcão AS, Fernandes A, et al. Unconjugated bilirubin activates and damages microglia. *J Neurosci Res.* 2006;84(1):194–201.

105. Silva SL, Vaz AR, Barateiro A, et al. Features of bilirubin-induced reactive microglia: from phagocytosis to inflammation. *Neurobiol Dis.* 2010;40(3):663–675.

106. Kim K, Lee SG, Kegelman TP, et al. Role of excitatory amino acid transporter-2 (EAAT2) and glutamate in neurodegeneration: opportunities for developing novel therapeutics. *J Cell Physiol.* 2011;226(10):2484–2493.

107. Brites D, Fernandes A, Falcão AS, et al. Biological risks for neurological abnormalities associated with hyperbilirubinemia. *J Perinatol.* 2009;29(suppl 1):S8–S13.

108. Tastekin A, Gepdiremen A, Ors R, Buyukokuroglu ME, Halici Z. Protective effect of L-carnitine against bilirubin-induced neuronal cell death. *Brain Dev.* 2006;28(7): 436–439.

109. Grojean S, Koziel V, Vert P, Daval JL. Bilirubin induces apoptosis via activation of NMDA receptors in developing rat brain neurons. *Exp Neurol.* 2000;166(2): 334–341.

110. Brito MA, Vaz AR, Silva SL, et al. N-Methyl-D-aspartate receptor and neuronal nitric oxide synthase activation mediate bilirubin-induced neurotoxicity. *Mol Med.* 2010;16(9–10):372–380.

111. Hankø E, Hansen TWR, Almaas R, Paulsen R, Rootwelt T. Synergistic protection of a general caspase inhibitor and MK-801 in bilirubin-induced cell death in human NT2-N neurons. *Pediatr Res.* 2006;59(1): 72–77.

112. Li CY, Shi HB, Wang J, et al. Bilirubin facilitates depolarizing GABA/glycinergic synaptic transmission in the ventral cochlear nucleus of rats. *Eur J Pharmacol.* 2011;660(2–3):310–317.

113. Raimondi F, Crivaro V, Capasso L, et al. Unconjugated bilirubin modulates the intestinal epithelial barrier function in a human-derived in vitro model. *Pediatr Res.* 2006;60(1):30–33.

114. Zhou Y, Qin H, Zhang M, et al. *Lactobacillus plantarum* inhibits intestinal epithelial barrier dysfunction induced by unconjugated bilirubin. *Br J Nutr.* 2010;104(3):390–401.

115. Indrio F, Raimondi F, Laforgia N, et al. Effect of hyperbilirubinemia on intestinal permeability in healthy term newborns. *Acta Paediatr.* 2007;96(1):73–75.

116. Memon S, Memon AM. Spectrum and immediate outcome of seizures in neonates. *J Coll Physicians Surg Pak.* 2006;16(11):717–720.

117. Zangen S, Kidron D, Gelbart T, et al. Fatal kernicterus in a girl deficient in glucose-6-phosphate dehydrogenase: a paradigm of synergistic heterozygosity. *J Pediatr.* 2009;154(4):616–619.

118. Nair A, Frederick TJ, Miller SD. Astrocytes in multiple sclerosis: a product of their environment. *Cell Mol Life Sci.* 2008;65(17):2702–2720.

119. MacAskill AF, Kittler JT. Control of mitochondrial transport and localization in neurons. *Trends Cell Biol.* 2010;20(2):102–112.

120. Muramatsu R, Ueno M, Yamashita T. Intrinsic regenerative mechanisms of central nervous system neurons. *Biosci Trends.* 2009;3(5):179–183.

121. Conforti L, Adalbert R, Coleman MP. Neuronal death: where does the end begin? *Trends Neurosci.* 2007;30(4):159–166.

122. Poulain FE, Sobel A. The microtubule network and neuronal morphogenesis: dynamic and coordinated orchestration through multiple players. *Mol Cell Neurosci.* 2010;43(1):15–32.

123. Yoshimura T, Arimura N, Kaibuchi K. Signaling networks in neuronal polarization. *J Neurosci.* 2006;26(42):10626–10630.

124. Ming GL, Song H. Adult neurogenesis in the mammalian brain: significant answers and significant questions. *Neuron.* 26 2011;70(4):687–702.

125. Fernandes A, Falcão AS, Abranches E, et al. Bilirubin as a determinant for altered neurogenesis, neuritogenesis, and synaptogenesis. *Dev Neurobiol.* 2009;69(9):568–582.

126. Jangaard KA, Fell DB, Dodds L, Allen AC. Outcomes in a population of healthy term and near-term infants with serum bilirubin levels of ≥325 micromol/L (≥19 mg/dL) who were born in Nova Scotia, Canada, between 1994 and 2000. *Pediatrics.* 2008;122(1):119–124.

127. Shi HB, Kakazu Y, Shibata S, Matsumoto N, Nakagawa T, Komune S. Bilirubin potentiates inhibitory synaptic transmission in lateral superior olive neurons of the rat. *Neurosci Res.* 2006;55(2):161–170.

128. Silva SL. *Molecular Mechanisms of Microglia Reactivity to Bilirubin: Evaluation of Potential Neurological Effects* [PhD thesis]. Portugal: University of Lisbon; 2010. Available at: http://repositorio.ul.pt/bitstream/10451/2477/1/ulsd059482_td_Sandra_Silva.pdf.

129. Wang Y, Tang BL. SNAREs in neurons—beyond synaptic vesicle exocytosis [review]. *Mol Membr Biol.* 2006;23(5):377–384.

130. Fernandes A, Coutinho E, Lanier LM, Brites D. Bilirubin-induced changes at neuronal cytoskeletal dynamics: novel cues for reduced axonal arborization. *Glia.* 2009;57(13):S102–S102.

131. Fernandes A, Coutinho E, Lanier LM, Brites D. Exploring neuronal cytoskeleton defects by unconjugated bilirubin. *Int J Dev Neurosci.* 2010;28(8 special issue: Sp. Iss. SI):715–716.

132. Avila J. Intracellular and extracellular tau. *Front Neurosci.* 2010;4:49.

133. Okumus N, Turkyilmaz C, Onal EE, et al. Tau and S100B proteins as biochemical markers of bilirubin-induced neurotoxicity in term neonates. *Pediatr Neurol.* 2008;39(4):245–252.

134. Wang JZ, Liu F. Microtubule-associated protein tau in development, degeneration and protection of neurons. *Prog Neurobiol.* 2008;85(2):148–175.

135. Noguchi-Shinohara M, Hamaguchi T, Nozaki I, Sakai K, Yamada M. Serum tau protein as a marker for the diagnosis of Creutzfeldt–Jakob disease. *J Neurol.* 2011;258(8):1464–1468.

136. Falcão AS, Fernandes A, Brito MA, Silva RF, Brites D. Bilirubin-induced immunostimulant effects and toxicity vary with neural cell type and maturation state. *Acta Neuropathol.* 2006;112(1):95–105.

137. Chang N, Li L, Hu R, et al. Differential regulation of NMDA receptor function by DJ-1 and PINK1. *Aging Cell.* 2010;9(5):837–850.

138. Koehler RC, Roman RJ, Harder DR. Astrocytes and the regulation of cerebral blood flow. *Trends Neurosci.* 2009;32(3):160–169.

139. Yang CZ, Zhao R, Dong Y, Chen XQ, Yu AC. Astrocyte and neuron intone through glutamate. *Neurochem Res.* 2008;33(12):2480–2486.

140. Faissner A, Pyka M, Geissler M, et al. Contributions of astrocytes to synapse formation and maturation—potential functions of the perisynaptic extracellular matrix. *Brain Res Rev.* 2010;63(1–2):26–38.

141. Takano T, Oberheim N, Cotrina ML, Nedergaard M. Astrocytes and ischemic injury. *Stroke.* 2009;40(3 suppl):S8–S12.

142. Renault-Mihara F, Okada S, Shibata S, Nakamura M, Toyama Y, Okano H. Spinal cord injury: emerging beneficial role of reactive astrocytes' migration. *Int J Biochem Cell Biol.* 2008;40(9):1649–1653.

143. De Keyser J, Mostert JP, Koch MW. Dysfunctional astrocytes as key players in the pathogenesis of central nervous system disorders. *J Neurol Sci.* 2008;267(1–2): 3–16.

144. Fernandes A, Vaz AR, Falcão AS, et al. Glycoursodeoxycholic acid and interleukin-10 modulate the reactivity of rat cortical astrocytes to unconjugated bilirubin. *J Neuropathol Exp Neurol.* 2007;66(9):789–798.

145. Fernandes A, Barateiro A, Falcão AS, et al. Astrocyte reactivity to unconjugated bilirubin requires TNF-α and IL-1β receptor signaling pathways. *Glia.* 2011;59(1):14–25.

146. Falcão AS, Silva RFM, Fernandes A, Brito MA, Brites D. Influence of hypoxia and ischemia preconditioning on bilirubin damage to astrocytes. *Brain Res.* 2007;1149:191–199.

147. Falcão AS, Bellarosa C, Fernandes A, et al. Role of multidrug resistance-associated protein 1 expression in the *in vitro* susceptibility of rat nerve cell to unconjugated bilirubin. *Neuroscience.* 2007;144(3):878–888.

148. Sequeira D, Watchko JF, Daood MJ, O'Day TL, Mahmood B. Unconjugated bilirubin efflux by bovine brain microvascular endothelial cells in vitro. *Pediatr Crit Care Med.* 2007;8(6):570–575.

149. Chew LJ, Takanohashi A, Bell M. Microglia and inflammation: impact on developmental brain injuries. *Ment Retard Dev Disabil Res Rev.* 2006;12(2):105–112.

150. Walter L, Neumann H. Role of microglia in neuronal degeneration and regeneration. *Semin Immunopathol.* 2009;31(4):513–525.

151. Semmler A, Hermann S, Mormann F, et al. Sepsis causes neuroinflammation and concomitant decrease of cerebral metabolism. *J Neuroinflamm.* 2008;5:38.

152. Graeber MB. Changing face of microglia. *Science.* 2010;330(6005):783–788.

153. Streit WJ, Braak H, Xue QS, Bechmann I. Dystrophic (senescent) rather than activated microglial cells are associated with tau pathology and likely precede neurodegeneration in Alzheimer's disease. *Acta Neuropathol.* 2009;118(4):475–485.

154. Fendrick SE, Xue QS, Streit WJ. Formation of multinucleated giant cells and microglial degeneration in rats expressing a mutant Cu/Zn superoxide dismutase gene. *J Neuroinflamm.* 2007;4:9.

155. Mandolesi G, Grasselli G, Musumeci G, Centonze D. Cognitive deficits in experimental autoimmune encephalomyelitis: neuroinflammation and synaptic degeneration. *Neurol Sci.* 2010;31(suppl 2):S255–S259.

156. Brown GC, Neher JJ. Inflammatory neurodegeneration and mechanisms of microglial killing of neurons. *Mol Neurobiol.* 2010;41(2–3):242–247.

157. Carson MJ, Bilousova TV, Puntambekar SS, et al. A rose by any other name? The potential consequences of microglial heterogeneity during CNS health and disease. *Neurotherapeutics.* 2007;4(4):571–579.

158. Hanisch UK, Kettenmann H. Microglia: active sensor and versatile effector cells in the normal and pathologic brain. *Nat Neurosci.* 2007;10(11):1387–1394.

159. Wennberg RP, Ahlfors CE, Bhutani VK, Johnson LH, Shapiro SM. Toward understanding kernicterus: a challenge to improve the management of jaundiced newborns. *Pediatrics.* 2006;117(2):474–485.

160. Arai K, Lo EH. Experimental models for analysis of oligodendrocyte pathophysiology in stroke. *Exp Transl Stroke Med.* 2009;1:6.

161. Genc S, Genc K, Kumral A, Baskin H, Ozkan H. Bilirubin is cytotoxic to rat oligodendrocytes in vitro. *Brain Res.* 2003;985(2):135–141.

162. Brito MA, Zurolo E, Pereira P, et al. Cerebellar axon/myelin loss, angiogenic sprouting and neuronal increase of vascular endothelial growth factor in a preterm infant with kernicterus. *J Child Neurol.* 2011. (Epub ahead of print.)

163. Hansen TWR, Tommarello S, Allen J. Subcellular localization of bilirubin in rat brain after *in vivo* i.v. administration of [³H]bilirubin. *Pediatr Res.* 2001;49(2):203–207.

164. Gkoltsiou K, Tzoufi M, Counsell S, Rutherford M, Cowan F. Serial brain MRI and ultrasound findings: relation to gestational age, bilirubin level, neonatal neurologic status and neurodevelopmental outcome in infants at risk of kernicterus. *Early Hum Dev.* 2008;84(12): 829–838.

165. Barateiro A, Vaz AR, Silva SL, Fernandes A, Brites D. Unconjugated bilirubin induces oligodendrocyte progenitor cell death following a programmed course of intracellular events. *J Neuroimmunol.* 2010;228(1–2):27.

166. Nave KA. Oligodendrocytes and the "micro brake" of progenitor cell proliferation. *Neuron.* 2011;65(5):577–579.

167. Edgar JM, McCulloch MC, Montague P, et al. Demyelination and axonal preservation in a transgenic mouse model of Pelizaeus–Merzbacher disease. *EMBO Mol Med.* 2010;2(2):42–50.

168. Falcão A, Fernandes A, Silva S, et al. Alterations in neurodevelopment occur by moderated levels of unconjugated bilirubin and increase when neurons are co-cultured with astrocytes. *Acta Paediatr.* 2009;98(suppl 460):130–131.

169. Bloomfield SM, McKinney J, Smith L, Brisman J. Reliability of S100B in predicting severity of central nervous system injury. *Neurocrit Care.* 2007;6(2):121–138.

170. Silva SL, Osório C, Vaz AR, et al. Dynamics of neuron–glia interplay upon exposure to unconjugated bilirubin. *J Neurochem.* 2011;117(3):412–424.

171. Napoli I, Neumann H. Microglial clearance function in health and disease. *Neuroscience.* 2009;158(3):1030–1038.

172. Neumann H, Kotter MR, Franklin RJ. Debris clearance by microglia: an essential link between degeneration and regeneration. *Brain.* 2009;132(pt 2):288–295.

173. Tanaka T, Ueno M, Yamashita T. Engulfment of axon debris by microglia requires p38 MAPK activity. *J Biol Chem.* 2009;284(32):21626–21636.

174. Markovic DS, Glass R, Synowitz M, Rooijen N, Kettenmann H. Microglia stimulate the invasiveness of glioma cells by increasing the activity of metalloprotease-2. *J Neuropathol Exp Neurol.* 2005;64(9):754–762.

175. Limperopoulos C. Advanced neuroimaging techniques: their role in the development of future fetal and neonatal neuroprotection. *Semin Perinatol.* 2010;34(1):93–101.

176. Staudt M. Brain plasticity following early life brain injury: insights from neuroimaging. *Semin Perinatol.* 2010;34(1):87–92.

177. Morris BH, Oh W, Tyson JE, et al. Aggressive vs. conservative phototherapy for infants with extremely low birth weight. *N Engl J Med.* 2008;359(18):1885–1896.

178. Watchko JF, Jeffrey Maisels M. Enduring controversies in the management of hyperbilirubinemia in preterm neonates. *Semin Fetal Neonatal Med.* 2010;15(3):136–140.

Hemolytic Disorders and Their Management

Michael Kaplan and Cathy Hammerman

■ ROLE OF HEMOLYSIS IN NEONATAL JAUNDICE AND IN BILIRUBIN-INDUCED NEUROTOXICITY

Imbalance Between Bilirubin Production and Elimination

The total serum bilirubin (TSB) concentration at any point in time reflects a multiplicity of interactions leading to two major processes contributing to this value: bilirubin production and bilirubin elimination.[1] As long as these processes remain in equilibrium, the TSB should remain within normal limits. During the first days of life, because of physiologically increased heme catabolism in combination with diminished activity of the bilirubin conjugating enzyme, UDP-glucuronosyltransferase 1A1 (UGT1A1), there is an imbalance between these processes and bilirubin levels increase. In the majority of cases, this imbalance should remain mild or moderate, and TSB concentrations should not exceed the 95th percentile on the hour-of-life-specific bilirubin nomogram.[2] When the rate of bilirubin production exceeds elimination (the latter process dependent primarily on conjugation), hyperbilirubinemia occurs. Although in many (perhaps most) cases, hyperbilirubinemia is associated with some degree of increased heme catabolism, severe hemolysis is not essential to the process. More important is the concept of lack of equilibrium between bilirubin production and conjugation. Thus, a baby may be hemolyzing and producing large amounts of bilirubin, but because hepatic bilirubin conjugating capacity

is mature, the infant may not develop an increased TSB. On the other hand, a baby with minimally increased hemolysis, but with immature bilirubin conjugating capacity (due to late prematurity or the presence of the $(TA)_7$ repeat UGT1A1 gene promoter polymorphism, associated with Gilbert syndrome), may develop hyperbilirubinemia. This concept of equilibrium, or lack thereof, between bilirubin production and conjugation has been demonstrated mathematically. Kaplan et al. studied the individual contributions of bilirubin production and conjugation to the TSB concentration, as well as the combined effects of these processes in healthy, term neonates on the third day of life.[3] The rate of heme catabolism was indexed by measurements of blood carboxyhemoglobin (COHb) determinations, corrected for ambient carbon monoxide (COHbc), while bilirubin conjugation was assessed by total serum conjugated bilirubin (TCB) expressed as a percentage of TSB (TCB(%)). Over the range of TSB concentrations observed, TSB correlated with both increasing COHbc levels and diminishing TCB(%) values (Figure 8-1A and B). The COHbc and TCB(%) values were then used to construct an index or ratio, COHbc/TCB(%), to reflect the combined forces of these processes. The correlation of this "production–conjugation index" with increasing TSB concentrations was higher than that for either COHbc or TCB(%), independently (Figure 8-2). Thus, the concept of imbalance and interaction between bilirubin production and conjugation, rather than individual or independent processes, in the mechanism of

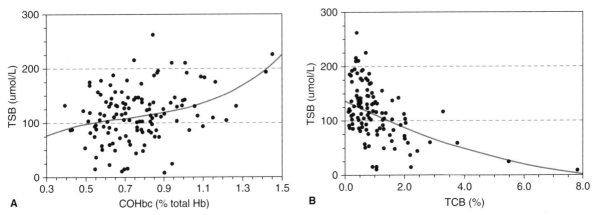

FIGURE 8-1. A. Curvilinear regression analysis between total serum bilirubin (TSB) and carboxyhemoglobin corrected for ambient carbon monoxide (COHbc) values. Increasing TSB values correlated positively with COHbc ($r = 0.38$; $s = 46.1$; $y = 9.36 + 323.5x - 378.4x^2 + 172.5x^3$). **B. Curvilinear regression analysis between TSB values and total conjugated bilirubin (TCB), expressed as a percentage of TSB (TCB(%)).** Increasing TSB values were inversely proportional to TCB(%) ratio ($r = 0.40$; $s = 45.8$; $y = 136.5 - 27.0x + 1.3x^2$). (Reproduced from Kaplan et al.,[3] with permission.)

neonatal bilirubinemia was confirmed. Although the relationship between the index and TSB tended to plateau with increasing index values, at the lower end of the index scale, which included the majority of readings,

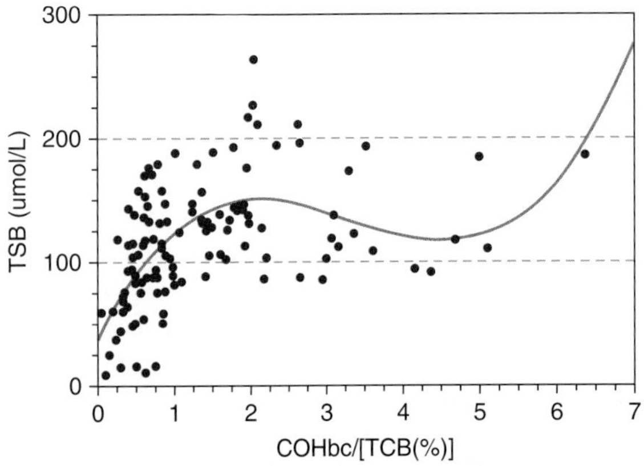

FIGURE 8-2. Curvilinear regression analysis between TSB values and the combined effect of bilirubin production and conjugation, reflected by the bilirubin production/conjugation index COHbc/(TCB(%)). Increasing values of TSB correlated positively to this index ($r = 0.61$; $s = 39.1$; $y = 32.1 + 132.1x - 45.8x^2 + 4.6x^3$). (Reproduced with permission from Kaplan M, Muraca M, Hammerman C, et al. Imbalance between production and conjugation of bilirubin: a fundamental concept in the mechanism of neonatal jaundice. *Pediatrics.* 2002;110:e47. Copyright © 2002 by the American Academy of Pediatrics.)

small increases in the index were associated with large increases in TSB.

Possible Increased Risk Associated with Hemolysis

It is generally believed that neonates with hemolytic disease are at a higher risk of developing bilirubin-induced neurotoxicity than those whose hyperbilirubinemia is not the result of hemolysis.[4–6] Data emanating from a few studies are supportive of this concept. In a Turkish study, a positive direct antiglobulin test (DAT or direct Coombs' test), due to Rh isoimmunization or ABO incompatibility, was used as a presumed marker of hemolysis.[7] Of 102 children aged 8–13 years with indirect hyperbilirubinemia ranging from 17 to 48 mg/dL, DAT positivity was associated with lower IQ scores and a higher incidence of neurologic abnormalities than in controls without a positive test. The incidence of detected neurologic abnormalities also increased with increasing duration of exposure to high TSB levels. In DAT-positive Norwegian males born in the early 1960s who had TSB levels >15 mg/dL for longer than 5 days, IQ scores were significantly lower than average for that population.[8] In the Jaundice and Infant Feeding Study, 5-year outcomes of infants with TSB >25 mg/dL were not significantly different from randomly selected controls. However, in the subgroup ($n = 9$) of infants with TSB >25 mg/dL as well as a positive DAT, IQ values were significantly lower than their counterparts with a negative DAT (−17.8 IQ points, 95% confidence interval [CI] −26.8 to −8.8).[9] In a reanalysis of the data from the Collaborative Perinatal Project, Kuzniewicz et al. found no relationship between maximum TSB levels and IQ scores.[10] But in the presence of a positive DAT, a TSB of ≥25 mg/dL was associated with a 6.7 point decrease in IQ scores. An increase in the duration of exposure to high TSB levels was also associated with an increase in neurologic abnormalities. Finally, in a recent study of 249 newborns admitted to a children's hospital in Cairo, Egypt, with TSB values ≥25 mg/dL, Gamaleldin et al. documented little relationship to the admission TSB and the presence or severity of acute bilirubin encephalopathy.[11] However, there was a marked difference in the development of bilirubin encephalopathy between those with additional risk factors, including Rh incompatibility, ABO incompatibility, and sepsis, compared with those without evidence of risk factors. The threshold TSB in identifying 90% of babies with bilirubin encephalopathy was 25.4 mg/dL in the presence of risk factors, but as high as 31.5 mg/dL in those without risk factors. Furthermore, the neurotoxicity-producing effect was higher in those with Rh incompatibility (odds ratio [OR] 48.6, 95% CI 14, 168) than in those with ABO incompatibility (OR 1.8, 95% CI 0.8, 4.5). Although the DAT testing in that situation was unreliable, the results do suggest that it is not simply the presence of hemolysis but also the etiology of the hemolysis that mediates the neurotoxicity.

The exact mechanism of the effect of hemolysis in increasing the risk of bilirubin neurotoxicity is unknown. The unbound bilirubin fraction, thought to be capable of crossing the blood brain barrier and entering the basal ganglia, correlates better than TSB with neurotoxicity.[12–14] If hemolysis was instrumental in increasing the risk of neurotoxicity, babies exhibiting hemolysis should have a higher unbound bilirubin fraction, but to date this has not been demonstrated.

While anti-D Rh isoimmunized babies are nowadays rarely encountered, DAT-positive neonates, primarily due to ABO incompatibility, as well as other blood antibodies, such as anti-c, anti-E, and others, are still seen. Glucose-6-phosphate dehydrogenase (G6PD) deficiency is a major cause of nonimmune severe hemolytic hyperbilirubinemia. The importance of hemolytic conditions in the pathophysiology of bilirubin encephalopathy can be seen in the report of the US-based Pilot Kernicterus Registry.[15] Of 125 newborns, 31 (25%) were blood group A or B infants born to O mothers. The expected incidence of these blood group combinations is only 15%

(see section "Hemolytic Disease of the Newborn Caused by ABO Heterospecificity"). Eight (6.4%) of these 31 had a positive DAT test, but this figure may be an underestimation as the status in 7 (5.6%) was unknown. The incidence of G6PD deficiency was also overrepresented in the Registry: while 26 (20.8%) of the Kernicterus Registry newborns were G6PD deficient, the expected male incidence in the United States is only 4–7%.[16] Whereas a TSB concentration of 20–24 mg/dL may be associated with kernicterus in a neonate with Rh isoimmunization, in the absence of a hemolytic condition, a healthy, term infant will rarely be endangered by TSB concentrations in this range.

Are We Missing Hemolyzing Babies?

Because hemolytic conditions appear to contribute to the development of bilirubin neurotoxicity to a greater extent than those not overtly hemolytic, the American Academy of Pediatrics (AAP) emphasizes the identification of the hemolyzing newborn.[17] Some authors have used the term "nonhemolytic jaundice" to differentiate newborns with no apparent hemolytic cause for the jaundice from those with a hemolytic etiology, but this may be an oversimplification of the issue.[18–23] Just as presence of a hemolytic condition, such as G6PD deficiency or DAT-positive ABO blood group heterospecificity, does not categorically imply that the jaundice or hyperbilirubinemia is necessarily due to this condition, absence of an identifiable etiology does not necessarily imply that increased hemolysis is not integral to the pathophysiology of the jaundice. Unfortunately, there is no readily available bedside clinical tool to determine the rate of hemolysis. Blood count indices such as decreasing hemoglobin or hematocrit values, or increased reticulocyte count, which may be useful to identify hemolysis in adults, often display overlap between hemolytic and nonhemolytic states in the newborn and may be unreliable indicators of hemolysis.[24] Clearly, in some newborns the hepatic component may be the primary contributor to hyperbilirubinemia and there may be very little increased hemolysis. However, studies utilizing the endogenous production of CO, an accurate index of heme catabolism, have demonstrated that many jaundiced babies do, in fact, have a hemolytic component to their jaundice, even in the absence of a defined hemolytic condition.

In a multicenter, multinational study, an automated device that sampled end-tidal expired air via a nasal catheter to determine the CO concentration corrected for ambient CO (ETCOc) was used.[25] Measurements of both ETCOc and TSB were performed at 30 ± 6 hours of life; TSB also was measured at 96 ± 12 hours, and subsequently if determined according to a flow diagram. Mean (±SD) ETCOc value for 1370 infants who completed the study was 1.48 ± 0.49 ppm. The 120 newborns who developed any TSB concentration >95th percentile for hour of life (hyperbilirubinemia) had significantly higher ETCOc values than those who did not (1.81 ± 0.59 ppm vs. 1.45 ± 0.47 ppm, $P < .0001$). However, high bilirubin production was not a prerequisite for the development of hyperbilirubinemia: some babies with low bilirubin production did, nevertheless, develop hyperbilirubinemia, while others with high production rates did not, confirming the *combined*, rather than individual, contribution of bilirubin production and elimination to the TSB. Using the identical technology, Maisels and Kring found that in 108 newborns ≥36 weeks gestational age who had TSB concentrations >75th percentile, ETCOc values were significantly higher through the first 4 days of life than in 164 neonates with lower TSB levels. Furthermore, while ETCOc values decreased progressively during the study period in the control infants, values increased in those with TSB values >75th percentile.[26] While the increase in ETCOc values in the study infants could not be explained, these authors concluded that increased hemolysis was an important mechanism in the production of jaundice in the first 4 days of life even in the absence of a specific diagnosis of a condition associated with increased hemolysis (Figure 8-3). In a group of African American neonates who were not G6PD deficient, ETCOc values of 27 newborns who developed a TSB concentration >95th hour-specific percentile were significantly higher than 335 neonates whose TSB did not exceed that value (2.6 [2.33–3.45] ppm vs. 2.00 [1.70–2.40] ppm) (median [interquartile range]).[27] Similarly, in another group of newborns, from which both G6PD-deficient and DAT-positive, ABO blood group–incompatible infants had been excluded, higher COHbc values (0.75 ± 0.18%) were noted in newborns who developed any TSB value >15.0 mg/dL during the first week of life than counterparts with lower TSB values (0.53 ± 0.13%, $P < .05$).[28]

Based on the above, it does appear that many hyperbilirubinemic newborns, even in the absence of an obvious hemolytic condition, have some degree of increased heme catabolism. Because universal blood typing with DAT determination and G6PD screening are not universally recommended, and ETCOc testing is currently

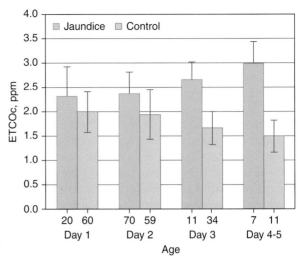

FIGURE 8-3. ETCOc values for jaundiced and control infants. Values shown are the mean ±SD for each age group. The numbers below the bars are the number of infants studied in each group. ("Jaundiced" refers to any TSB value >75th percentile for age in hours.) (Reproduced with permission from Maisels MJ, Kring E. The contribution of hemolysis to early jaundice in normal newborns. *Pediatrics.* 2006;118:276–279. Copyright © 2006 by the American Academy of Pediatrics.)

unavailable as a clinical tool, it is possible that some infants not actually identified as having a hemolytic condition may, in fact, be actively hemolyzing. The term "nonhemolytic jaundice" may not be valid in all cases to which it has been attributed and the increased risk for hyperbilirubinemia and bilirubin encephalopathy attributed to increased hemolysis may go unrecognized in some. Absence of documented hemolysis or presence of an obvious hemolytic etiology should not exclude the potential danger of bilirubin neurotoxicity.

AAP Recommendations Regarding Hemolyzing Babies

The Subcommittee on Hyperbilirubinemia of the AAP includes jaundice developing within the first 24 hours, blood group incompatibility with a positive DAT, and other known hemolytic disease including G6PD deficiency as major risk factors for the development of severe hyperbilirubinemia.[29] The Subcommittee recommends a more aggressive approach to hyperbilirubinemia, by initiating phototherapy or performing exchange transfusions at lower levels of TSB in neonates with neurotoxicity risk factors including isoimmune hemolytic disease and G6PD deficiency.

■ SPECIFIC HEMOLYTIC CONDITIONS

In broad terms, hemolytic conditions encountered in neonates may be divided into two major pathophysiologic groups: immune and nonimmune. A classification of these disorders appears in Table 8-1. The former group includes Rh isoimmunization, which, nowadays, is largely preventable and only occasionally encountered in the western world. The condition will, nevertheless, be discussed in some detail, as much of our knowledge regarding the development of kernicterus derives from the study of babies with this condition. As ABO immune disease (mother blood group O, baby group A or B) is the most common immune condition currently encountered, it will also be discussed in detail. Of the nonimmune causes, G6PD deficiency is by far the most important from a public health standpoint, and is associated with

■ **TABLE 8-1.** Classification of Hemolytic Disorders Encountered in the Newborn

(A) Immune conditions
    Rh isoimmunization
        Including anti-D, anti-c, anti-e
    ABO immunization
    Some rarer immune conditions
        Anti-C
        Anti-E
        Anti-Kell
        Anti-Duffy
        Anti-Kidd
(B) Nonimmune conditions
    Red cell enzyme deficiencies
        G6PD deficiency
        Pyruvate kinase deficiency
        Other rare RBC enzyme deficiencies
    Red cell membrane defects
        Hereditary spherocytosis
        Elliptocytosis
        Ovalocytosis
        Stomatocytosis
        Pyknocytosis
    Hemoglobinopathies
        Unstable hemoglobinopathies
    General conditions
        Sepsis
        Extravasated blood (cephalhematoma, ecchymosis, adrenal hemorrhage, subdural hemorrhage)

the development of unpredictable, extreme hyperbilirubinemia, and acute bilirubin encephalopathy.

Immune Hemolytic Conditions

The Direct Antiglobulin (Agglutination) Test

The DAT, otherwise known as the direct Coombs' test, is the hallmark of isoimmunization.[30] A positive DAT test is indicative of maternally derived IgG antibody directed against and bound to the fetal (and subsequently newborn) RBC antigenic sites, the result of incompatibility between maternal and fetal blood types. The antiglobulin reaches the fetal tissues via the placenta. In the direct form of the test, the antiglobulin is attached to the fetal or newborn erythrocyte, whereas an indirect test relates to the antibody being found in the serum. The DAT detects the presence of an antibody, but is nonspecific and does not identify the specific type of antibody present: for this purpose, further identifying tests are required. DAT is measured by incubating a newborn's blood sample with anti-IgG antiserum. If the RBCs are coated with IgG, these cells will agglutinate. The clumps may be identified visually or microscopically. The DAT is usually measured qualitatively, a stronger test (i.e., the more positive) suggesting a greater amount of antibody present. While a positive DAT is associated with increased hemolysis and hyperbilirubinemia, this may not always be the case. Herschel et al., using a 12-hour ETCOc value ≥95th percentile as a reference for increased hemolysis, found the sensitivity of the DAT in a group of primarily ABO blood group–incompatible newborns to be 38.5% and the specificity 98.5% for the detection of significant hemolysis, while the positive predictive value (PPV) of the DAT for significant hemolysis was 58.8%. In other words, a neonate with a positive DAT had about a 59% chance of having significant hemolysis.[31] Neither, in this study, was a positive DAT universally predictive of clinically significant hyperbilirubinemia: only 9/61 (14.8%) of the DAT-positive neonates developed a TSB ≥75th percentile for age in hours. Ozolek et al. found the same general relationship between DAT and hyperbilirubinemia/jaundice in a large cohort of ABO heterospecific mother–infant pairs.[32]

Rh Isoimmune Hemolytic Disease

Rh disease in pregnancy may lead to intrauterine hemolysis, which if untreated may result in severe intrauterine anemia, hydrops fetalis, and intrauterine death.

Continuation of the hemolytic process following delivery may result in severe hemolytic disease of the newborn (HDN) with the rapid development of anemia and hyperbilirubinemia with the potential of developing bilirubin encephalopathy early in neonatal life.

Background: The Immunization Process

The Rh group comprises the C, c, D, E, and e antigens, one transmitted from each parent to determine the Rh type. While each of these antigens may result in isoimmunization and hemolysis, RhD isoimmunization is the most common, encountered in 90% of Rh group cases, and is therefore of major clinical significance.

The distribution of Rh negativity and isoimmunization varies with racial background and paternal heterozygosity. While in white populations about 13–15% of individuals are Rh negative, only about half that number are encountered in African Americans, and Rh negativity is very unusual in Asian individuals. Because 55% of fathers are heterozygous (D/d), an Rh-negative mother may have an Rh-negative fetus in about 50% of pregnancies. Additional factors influencing the incidence of Rh disease include nonuniversal fetomaternal transmission of fetal blood and variable maternal immune responses. Therefore, in mothers who did not receive immune prophylaxis, the overall incidence of Rh isoimmunization is actually infrequent and reported to be 6.8 cases per 1000 live births.[33]

The Rh D immunization process begins when a D-negative woman is exposed to the D antigen. Antepartum or intrapartum exposure occurs as a result of transplacental, fetomaternal passage of fetal RBCs containing the D antigen. Because most transfer of fetal blood occurs late in pregnancy or during delivery, in first pregnancies the process usually begins too late to allow for sufficient maternal IgG antibody to be produced and transferred across the placenta. Nevertheless, immunization during the first pregnancy is a well-documented phenomenon[34] and not as uncommon as generally believed.[35] Isoimmunization during the first pregnancy and/or in multiparous Rh D-negative women who begin a pregnancy without detectable Rh antibodies occurs in ~1.8% of such women[35] and infants from such pregnancies can be affected; about one in five such babies will require treatment including possible need for exchange transfusion.[34] Transfusion of Rh-positive RBCs may also occur during abortion, blood administration, amniocentesis, chorionic villus sampling, or fetal blood sampling. In response to the antigen exposure, the mother's immune system may respond by the formation of anti-D IgG antibodies. This antiglobulin may then cross the placenta to the fetus, adhere to the D antigen sites of the fetal RBCs, result in an antigen–antibody response, and culminate in hemolysis and anemia. The mother's immune system is now primed and with subsequent pregnancies the immune response may become progressively more severe and have a more rapid onset. Should the anemia be prolonged and sufficiently severe, the bone marrow may be stimulated to release increased numbers of circulating immature RBCs (erythroblastosis). With further progression of the process, extramedullary hematopoiesis with hepatomegaly and splenomegaly may ensue. In its most severe stages, fetal hydrops, which may include generalized tissue edema and pleural, pericardial, and peritoneal effusions, may result. The pathogenesis of this extravascular fluid includes hypoproteinemia, tissue hypoxia, and capillary leak, combined with congestive cardiac failure. The latter may develop due to anemia and venous congestion, the result of poor myocardial function and diminished cardiac output.[36]

Management of the Pregnancy

Hydrops fetalis is associated with a high mortality rate and major efforts should be made to prevent its occurrence by appropriate intervention prior to its appearance. Pregnancies complicated by Rh isoimmunization require active surveillance to detect fetal anemia. Should the fetus become anemic, the option to perform intrauterine transfusion must be weighed against delivery. This decision will depend primarily on the gestational age: with increasing maturity, the potential for inherent complications involved in preterm delivery will decrease relative to the dangers involved in performing intrauterine transfusion. Until recently, amniocentesis was the primary method of fetal monitoring.[37] The degree of hemolysis was assessed by determining the amount of bilirubin in the amniotic fluid by measuring the deviation from linearity at 450 nm, the wavelength at which bilirubin absorbs light. Measurements were divided into three zones and plotted on the Liley chart. Readings in zone III indicated a high level of danger and were indicative of severe hemolysis with a high likelihood of fetal death. Queenan et al. improved on the Liley chart by developing the Queenan curve.[38] This amniocentesis-based regimen, however, has been largely replaced by a combination of advancing ultrasonographic techniques and developing genetic technologies, as described below.

In the absence of prophylaxis, 14% of RhD-negative women who deliver an Rh-positive baby can be expected to develop anti-D antibodies within 6 months of delivery or during the following pregnancy.[39] In the preprophylaxis days, 14% of affected pregnancies could be expected to result in stillbirths and 30% of those live-born to have severe hemolytic disease.[40] An additional 30% may have more moderate disease but, if untreated, may progress to severe hyperbilirubinemia and encephalopathy. The introduction of postpartum prophylaxis reduced the isoimmunization rate to 1.8%.[41,42] Subsequently, it was found that administration of rhesus immune globulin during pregnancy to all nonimmunized, RhD-negative women reduced the incidence of antenatal immunization to 0.1%.[43] Prophylaxis with anti-D globulin is now routine and all pregnant women should have an antibody screen early in pregnancy. Should the woman be RhD-negative with no evidence of anti-D alloimmunization, rhesus immune globulin should be administered at 28 weeks gestation.[36] The globulin should also be administered following spontaneous or elective abortion, amniocentesis, chorionic villus sampling, or fetal blood sampling. Should the woman deliver an RhD-positive infant, a repeat dose should be administered within 72 hours of delivery. As a result of this prophylactic regimen, in most industrialized countries, hemolytic disease due to RhD immunization has been almost completely eradicated. This situation should not be taken for granted in developing countries with underdeveloped health systems. Zipursky and Paul estimated that in India, Pakistan, and Nigeria where the majority of RhD-negative women do not receive postpartum anti-D prophylaxis, thousands of women annually will develop anti-RhD antibodies, and about half the babies born to these women will develop Rh hemolytic disease.[39] This scenario is most likely encountered in many other developing countries where it is likely that as many as 100,000 children may be born annually with RhD hemolytic disease.[39]

Should a pregnant woman be found to be Rh immunized, because this condition is nowadays rare and therapeutic technologies are advancing at a rapid rate, she should be managed in a tertiary center capable of adequately managing a severely affected fetus as well as the newborn infant.

Advances in RhD gene technology have allowed for fetuses either at high or low risk to be identified. The RhD gene is located on the short arm of chromosome 1.[44] Approximately 55% of individuals are heterozygous at the RhD locus and 50% of their fetuses will be RhD positive. Should a fetus be RhD negative, no further testing will be required. In the past, gene frequency tables, combined with the history of RhD-positive or -negative infants fathered by any individual, were used to estimate the likelihood of a specific father being heterozygous. Modern advances in DNA technologies, however, allow for accurate determination of whether the father is heterozygous or homozygous for the RhD gene.[45,46] Should the father be heterozygous, steps should be taken to determine the Rh type of the fetus by retrieving fetal DNA via amniocentesis.[42] A major technological development that may enable the noninvasive determination of the fetal RhD type includes cell-free fetal DNA determination in a maternal blood sample.[45,47,48]

Determination of the maternal anti-D titer is an important step in the monitoring of an RhD-sensitized woman. A critical titer is that which is associated with a high risk of severe hydrops. The critical titer varies from center to center and ranges from 8 to 32 are usually used to predict disease.[36]

Doppler assessment of the blood flow velocity in the fetus' middle cerebral artery is replacing amniocentesis in the detection of fetal anemia. Fetal anemia results in increased blood flow velocity due to decreased blood viscosity and increased cardiac output. In one study, a value of more than 1.5 multiples of the median identified all cases of moderate to severe anemia.[49] In a study comparing diagnostic amniocentesis with middle cerebral artery flow in the detection of anemia, Doppler measurements improved on optical density determinations by 9%.[50] If the results of either of these techniques suggest anemia, fetal blood is sampled by cordocentesis and the hematocrit, DAT, blood type, reticulocyte count, and TSB determined. If the hematocrit is <30% and the fetus <35 weeks gestation, intrauterine transfusion is considered. If the pregnancy has reached 35 weeks gestation or more, the advantages of delivery will generally outweigh the dangers of an intrauterine transfusion. Repeated intrauterine transfusion may cause fetal bone marrow suppression, and in a repeatedly transfused fetus, the RBC mass at the time of delivery may be composed almost entirely of donor cells. In this situation, hemolysis will be minimal and exchange transfusion may be unnecessary, although "top-up" transfusions for subsequent anemia may be required.[51] In experienced hands, the outcome of intrauterine transfusion should be good. In the Netherlands, the survival rate in 254 fetuses was 89%.[52]

Postnatal Management of the Newborn

The clinical manifestations of erythroblastosis fetalis in the neonate range from an asymptomatic infant with laboratory evidence of anemia to severe hydrops, extreme anemia, and cardiac decompensation. Management of a hydropic, severely anemic neonate, especially if complicated by respiratory and other problems of prematurity, is a major neonatal challenge requiring a degree of expertise available only at a tertiary center.[53] Hydropic infants have generalized edema and fluid collections in the pleural, pericardial, and peritoneal spaces. Intubation may be challenging because of oral soft tissue swelling. Pleural and pericardial fluid collections impair ventilation and may require emergency drainage to facilitate adequate respiratory gas exchange. Respiratory support may have to be complemented by surfactant, nitric oxide, and high-frequency ventilation, while anoxic myocardial damage may necessitate use of inotropes. Metabolic acidosis may further complicate the situation[54] and hypoglycemia is common.[53]

A cord blood sample should be obtained immediately after delivery. Hemoglobin values <10 g/dL and TSB >5 mg/dL suggest severe hemolysis. Many of these babies will subsequently require exchange transfusion. Because of the potential of circulatory system overload in combination with poor myocardial function, it may be preferable to correct the anemia isovolumetrically, using a partial exchange transfusion technique via umbilical venous or arterial catheter rather than by simple blood transfusion. Small amounts of anemic blood should be drawn from the newborn and replaced with packed cell donor blood. The hematocrit may be "titrated" until the desired concentration is obtained. Phlebotomy should not be performed routinely on these infants because they are usually normovolemic and may even be hypovolemic[55–57] and their blood volume should not be manipulated without appropriate measurements of central venous pressure (CVP) and arterial blood pressure. In order to measure CVP accurately, the umbilical venous catheter must enter the inferior vena cava via the ductus venosus. If the catheter is in a portal vein or the umbilical vein, the pressures so measured are meaningless and preclude interpretation of the infant's circulatory status. In addition, before making therapeutic decisions based on measurements of CVP, acidosis, hypercarbia, hypoxia, and anemia (all of which can affect the measured CVP) must be corrected. Serum glucose levels must be monitored carefully because hypoglycemia is common.

In the fetus, most bilirubin formed from the hemolytic process will be eliminated via the placenta and severe intrauterine hyperbilirubinemia is rarely a problem, although the cord blood bilirubin level may be elevated to 3–5 mg/dL. Once delivered, however, the placenta no longer participates in the bilirubin elimination process. Continued hemolysis combined with immature conjugative and excretory function may potentiate rapidly rising TSB values with the danger, if untreated, of developing extreme hyperbilirubinemia. As soon as the baby has been stabilized, the TSB is measured and intensive phototherapy started. Should the TSB continue to rise despite intensive phototherapy, exchange transfusion will be necessary according to the thresholds recommended by the 2004 AAP guideline.

Randomized controlled trials (RCT) have shown that the administration of intravenous immune globulin (IVIG) is effective in preventing or limiting the number of exchange transfusions in Rh disease.[58–62] The 2004 AAP guideline also recommends the use of IVIG in order to prevent exchange transfusion in cases of failing phototherapy.[29] Most recently, however, a Dutch RCT found no benefit from the prophylactic administration of IVIG to infants with Rh hemolytic disease[63] and a *Cochrane* report concluded that more information, based on well-designed studies, was needed before IVIG could be recommended for the treatment of isoimmune hemolytic disease.[64] The reason for these conflicting results is not clear but could be related to the type of IVIG used. Even if an exchange transfusion will ultimately be necessary, delay of this procedure by IVIG can be useful in gaining time for stabilization of the patient.

The AAP guideline provides clear criteria for the use of phototherapy and exchange transfusion in these infants.[29]

There is limited information on the long-term neurodevelopmental outcome of fetuses treated with intrauterine transfusion, although, in general, the results to date are encouraging.[54,65] A system for surveillance of children for long-term neurodevelopment outcome following intrauterine transfusion has been established in Holland and should provide relevant data within the next few years.[66]

Hemolytic Disease of the Newborn Caused by ABO Heterospecificity

Definition of ABO Blood Group Heterospecificity

By the term "ABO setup," we refer to a blood group A or B baby born to a group O mother. This combination is seen in about 15% of pregnancies. About one third of these pregnancies (5%) will have a positive DAT, indicative of anti-A or -B antibodies attached to RBCs.[32]

ABO Blood Group Heterospecificity: The Most Frequent Cause of Immune Hemolytic Disease in the Neonate

In the past, the high incidence and severity of hemolytic disease due to Rh isoimmunization obscured the clinical manifestations of DAT-positive ABO heterospecificity. Because Rh hemolytic disease is currently seen only occasionally in the western world, ABO incompatibility has become the most frequent cause of immune hemolytic disease in the neonate. Although ABO heterospecific disease is usually milder than that encountered in Rh-immunized fetuses and newborns, the hyperbilirubinemia may at times be severe and associated with bilirubin encephalopathy. Of 125 babies reported in the US Kernicterus Registry, 31 (25%) were of blood group A or B born to group O mothers.[15] The expected incidence of these combinations in the United States is only about 15%. Eight (6.5%) were DAT positive, but this figure may be an underestimate since in some of the infants, the DAT status was not identified. Between 2002 and 2004, the Canadian Paediatric Surveillance Program identified 258 jaundiced newborns who had either a TSB ≥25 mg/dL or undergone exchange transfusion. A cause for the jaundice was found in 93 (36%). ABO heterospecificity was the most frequent diagnosis among these infants, occurring in 32 of the 93 (34.4%).[67] In the United Kingdom and Ireland, from 2003 to 2005, 108 newborns were identified with a TSB concentration ≥30 mg/dL. Thirty-three (30.6%) were ABO incompatible, of whom 16 (15%) were DAT positive.[68] Similarly, in Denmark, between 2002 and 2005, 113 infants ≥35 weeks gestation were identified with a TSB value ≥26 mg/dL. Fifty-two (48.2%) comprised blood group A or B infants born to group O mothers of whom 16 (31%) were DAT positive (14% of total).[69] In Nigeria, of 115 babies affected with bilirubin encephalopathy between 2001 and 2005, 42 (36.5%) died. Twenty-two (19.1%) were ABO incompatible (DAT status not provided).[70] In a Swiss nationwide study conducted between 2007 and 2008 and encompassing 146,288 infants ≥35 weeks gestation, 60 newborns exceeded the Swiss indications for exchange transfusion.[71] In 31 of these, a diagnosis was determined and the majority (17 [54.8%]) were ABO incompatible.

Unlike Rh disease, hydrops fetalis in ABO immune disease is rare, although a few cases have been reported.[72-74]

The milder disease that characterizes ABO hemolysis might occur because, in the fetus, A and B antigens are not limited to the RBCs, but are found in other fetal tissues including the placenta and in body fluids. These antigens neutralize and dilute transferred maternal antibody, thereby reducing the number of antibodies available to attach to the fetal RBCs. Furthermore, the newborn RBC has fewer A or B reactive sites than the adult RBC that explains the weakly reactive DAT seen in ABO hemolytic disease.[75]

Background: Blood Group Incompatibility and DAT Positivity

The connection between ABO heterospecificity and neonatal jaundice was established in the 1940s. Of infants who were jaundiced in the first 24 hours postdelivery, and excluding cases of Rh hemolytic disease, ABO incompatibility was found in 95%.[76] Shortened RBC survival was demonstrated in affected infants compared with survival of transfused group O cells[77,78] and in 1961, Kochwa et al. demonstrated that anti-A and -B antibodies found in maternal or fetal serum were IgG antibodies and capable of crossing the placenta.[79]

Pathophysiology of ABO Hemolytic Disease

The pathophysiology of ABO hemolytic disease differs from that of Rh isoimmunization. In Rh disease, following the initial pregnancy-related immunization, the antibody titer generally increases with each subsequent pregnancy. ABO disease does not follow an initial immunizing pregnancy. In contrast, some women with type O blood have an inherently high titer of anti-A or -B antibodies that is unrelated to the fetomaternal passage of blood and can be found before their first pregnancy (or even in young girls).[80] Furthermore, group O individuals differ from their blood group A or B counterparts in that their anti-A or -B antibodies comprise IgG molecules, able to cross the placenta, whereas the respective antibodies of blood group A or B individuals are predominantly IgM, larger, and therefore prevented from placental passage. When an affected woman becomes pregnant, the IgG molecules may cross the placenta and attach to the corresponding A or B antigens on the fetal RBCs. This process of isoimmunization then precipitates hemolysis in utero. Extravascular hemolysis of the IgG-coated RBCs is probably mediated by Fc-receptor-bearing cells within the reticuloendothelial system. There is little danger of severe hyperbilirubinemia occurring prior to delivery as the immune process is not usually sufficiently strong and the placenta is able to clear most of the resulting bilirubin. Some infants are born with moderate anemia and continuation of the hemolytic process following delivery can produce severe hyperbilirubinemia.

ABO Setup Versus ABO Hemolytic Disease

ABO heterospecificity, even if the DAT is positive, does not necessarily indicate the presence of ABO *hemolytic disease*. Many of these neonates may have no evidence of ongoing hemolysis and may not develop early jaundice or significant hyperbilirubinemia. Some or all of the following criteria are necessary to support the diagnosis of ABO hemolytic disease:

1. Mother blood group O and baby group A or B
2. Positive DAT
3. Indirect hyperbilirubinemia, especially during the first 24 hours of life
4. Microspherocytosis on peripheral blood smear
5. Increased reticulocyte count

Measurement of the endogenous production of CO will help to quantify hemolysis, but, unfortunately, the instrument for determining end-tidal CO levels is no longer available.

Studies of Hemolysis Incorporating Endogenous Formation of Carbon Monoxide

Measurements of endogenous formation of CO, an index of heme catabolism, have demonstrated an increased rate of heme catabolism in DAT-positive, ABO-incompatible neonates compared with controls, confirming the role of increased hemolysis in the pathophysiology of hyperbilirubinemia in these neonates. Fällström and Bjure found that in 48/62 ABO-incompatible infants with significant jaundice, COHb values exceeded the mean + 2SD for values in healthy, nonicteric newborns.[81] Uetani et al. found that in DAT-positive, ABO-incompatible neonates with TSB values >15 mg/dL, COHb values were higher than those in nonhyperbilirubinemic controls, and that, in the hyperbilirubinemic newborns, COHb levels remained high during the first 5 days of testing.[82] Interestingly, not all DAT-positive neonates had increased COHb levels. In a multinational, multicenter study in which ETCOc was used to detect hemolysis at 30 ± 6 hours, values were higher in 54 DAT-positive babies compared with the total number (1370) of babies studied (1.66 ± 0.55 ppm vs. 1.48 ± 0.49 ppm, $P = .009$).[25] DAT-positive neonates

with TSB >95th percentile had even higher, although not statistically significant, ETCOc values (1.89 ± 0.63). However, only 18.5% of the DAT-positive newborns developed a TSB >95th percentile, implying that, despite the increased hemolysis, many babies were able to handle the increased bilirubin load. Herschel et al., also using ETCOc, documented higher values for DAT-positive, ABO-incompatible neonates (3.4 ± 1.8 ppm, $n = 14$) than for DAT-negative counterparts or ABO-compatible controls (2.2 ± 0.6 ppm, $n = 60$ and 2.1 ± 0.6 ppm, $n = 171$, respectively, $P = .02$).[83] Using COHbc determinations to assess the degree of hemolysis, Kaplan et al. found that overall, DAT-positive neonates had higher COHbc values than previously published for a DAT-negative reference group (1.24 ± 0.40 ppm, $n = 163$ vs. 0.77 ± 0.19 ppm, $n = 131$, $P < .0001$).[84] Furthermore, those who developed hyperbilirubinemia (TSB >95th percentile) had higher COHbc values than the already high values of those whose TSB did not exceed the 95th percentile (1.42 ± 0.39 ppm, $n = 85$ vs. 1.00 ± 0.25 ppm, $n = 78$, $P < .001$). There was a trend for O–B newborns to have higher COHbc values than their O–A counterparts (1.32 ± 0.44 ppm vs. 1.20 ± 0.38 ppm, $P = .07$). Finally, the percentage of newborns who developed hyperbilirubinemia increased in tandem with COHbc, reaching 100% in those with COHbc values >90th percentile (Figure 8-4).

Incidence of Hyperbilirubinemia in ABO Heterospecific Neonates

Despite the increased hemolysis documented in DAT-positive ABO heterospecific newborns and the association with bilirubin encephalopathy, not all affected neonates will develop severe or clinically significant hyperbilirubinemia. In the prephototherapy era (1969–1971), Kanto et al. found that only 26 (11.3%) of 230 ABO-incompatible, DAT-positive newborns born in Augusta, Georgia, developed TSB values >12 mg/dL. In some cases, however, this concentration did reach as high as 23 mg/dL.[85] In Norway, Meberg and Johansen included TSB testing at the time of routine predischarge metabolic screening. Of 17 of 2463 newborns with documented TSB values >20 mg/dL, only 1 was ABO heterospecific.[86] Furthermore, only 19.6% of 92 DAT-positive, ABO heterospecific neonates met the indications for phototherapy. In Pittsburgh, Pennsylvania, of 531 DAT-positive, blood group A or B newborns delivered to group O mothers, only 73 (13.7%) developed TSB concentrations >12.8 mg/dL.[32] Using a recently used definition of hyperbilirubinemia (i.e., any

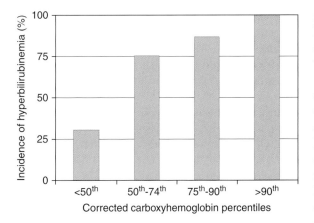

FIGURE 8-4. Incidence of hyperbilirubinemia, defined as any TSB value >95th percentile for hour of life, graded by COHbc percentile value. Note the incidence of hyperbilirubinemia increased in tandem with increasing COHbc percentiles. COHbc percentile ranges (% tHb): <50th percentile, 0.54–1.19; 50th to 74th percentile, 1.20–1.44; 75th to 90th percentile, 1.45–1.76; >90th percentile, 1.79–2.62. COHbc, blood carboxyhemoglobin corrected for ambient CO; tHb: total hemoglobin. (Reprinted from Kaplan M, Hammerman C, Vreman HJ, Wong RJ, Stevenson DK. Hemolysis and hyperbilirubinemia in antiglobulin positive, direct ABO blood group heterospecific neonates. *J Pediatr.* 2010;157:772–777. Copyright 2010, with permission from Elsevier.)

TSB value >95th percentile on the hour-of-life-specific bilirubin nomogram[2,25,87–89]), Kaplan et al. in Jerusalem, Israel, found a high incidence of hyperbilirubinemia, 85 (51.8%) of 164, among DAT-positive, ABO heterospecific neonates.[84] Importantly, 56 newborns (34.1% of the cohort or 66.7% of those with hyperbilirubinemia) had their first TSB >95th percentile documented earlier than 24 hours, while 80 neonates (49%) met the 2004 AAP indications for phototherapy.[29] The incidence of hyperbilirubinemia was substantially higher than that of some other studies, which utilized the identical definition of hyperbilirubinemia,[25,88,89] emphasizing the important role of ABO heterospecificity in the etiology of neonatal hyperbilirubinemia. The fact that all babies responded to phototherapy, none required exchange transfusions, and there were no cases of kernicterus should not detract from the importance of this finding: DAT positivity, TSB values >95th percentile, and hyperbilirubinemia occurring within the first 24 hours are each listed by the AAP as major risk factors for the development of severe hyperbilirubinemia.[29] Any additional process adding to the bilirubin load, such as further hemolysis or immaturity of the bilirubin conjugating system,

may upset the equilibrium and, if untreated, lead to severe hyperbilirubinemia and encephalopathy. These newborns should therefore be vigilantly observed with timely institution of therapy when indicated.

The literature is inconsistent regarding the incidence and severity of hyperbilirubinemia between O–A and O–B groups. Several investigators were unable to show any difference in clinical severity between O–A and O–B HDN.[85,90–94] On the other hand, other authors have reported an increased need for exchange transfusion or IVIG therapy in O–B neonates, compared with O–A counterparts.[95–97] Kaplan et al. reported a trend showing an increased rate of hyperbilirubinemia among O–B infants compared with O–A infants (33/53 [62.3%] vs. 52/111 [46.8%], relative risk [RR] 1.34; 95% CI 0.99–1.77; *P* = .053).[84]

ABO blood group incompatibility with a negative DAT, not usually predictive of hemolysis or hyperbilirubinemia, may sometimes cause early and rapidly progressing jaundice, reminiscent of DAT-positive hemolytic disease. Some of these infants may be displaying a manifestation of coexpression between ABO incompatibility and homozygosity for the $(TA)_7$ UGT1A1 polymorphism.[98] This concept is discussed in section "Genetic Interactions Between Hemolytic Conditions and UGT1A1 Polymorphisms."

Predicting the Severity of Hyperbilirubinemia in ABO Disease

Most blood group A or B neonates born to blood group O mothers will not develop any sign of hemolytic disease. Routine blood group and DAT determination on umbilical cord blood is an option, but not mandatory. It is essential to closely observe any newborn born to a blood group O mother for the development of jaundice and to perform a TSB when indicated. Attempts have been made to predict subsequent hyperbilirubinemia in ABO-incompatible neonates based on TSB concentrations. Sarici et al. found a mean TSB of ≥4 mg/dL at the sixth hour of life had a sensitivity of 86.2%, a negative predictive value (NPV) of 94.5%, and a PPV of 39.7% in the prediction of hyperbilirubinemia. The definition of hyperbilirubinemia varied with the infant's age.[99] Using a mean TSB of 6 mg/dL at age 6 hours improved the prediction, the sensitivity, specificity, NPV, and PPV being 100%, 91.5%, 100%, and 35.3%, respectively, in diagnosing cases of severe ABO hemolytic disease. In the epoch prior to introduction of phototherapy in their unit, Risemberg et al. utilized umbilical cord blood TSB values to predict hyperbilirubinemia in ABO-incompatible neonates. Thirteen of

91 infants (14%) developed a TSB concentration of 16 mg/dL or more at 12–36 hours and underwent exchange transfusion. All newborns except one with severe hyperbilirubinemia had cord TSB >4 mg/dL. Similarly, all 12 newborns with cord TSB >4 mg/dL developed hyperbilirubinemia and required exchange transfusion.[100]

Treatment of ABO Heterospecificity– Associated Neonatal Jaundice

A high degree of vigilance is necessary to detect developing jaundice in newborns born to blood group O mothers. TSB or transcutaneous bilirubin (TcB) should be measured if jaundice is seen in the first 12–24 hours.[2] Phototherapy and exchange transfusions are implemented according to the 2004 AAP guideline.[28] IVIG may be helpful in modifying the rate of rise of bilirubin and is indicated if the TSB is approaching the exchange transfusion threshold despite a trial of intensive phototherapy.[29] In an analysis of 4 randomized trials involving 226 babies affected with Rh and ABO immune disease,[58–61] IVIG in combination with phototherapy significantly reduced the need for exchange transfusions compared with phototherapy alone (RR 0.28; 95% CI 0.17–0.47).[62] In newborns who responded to IVIG administration with a decrease in TSB, COHbc values decreased from baseline in tandem with diminishing TSB concentrations, demonstrating the effect of IVIG on limiting heme catabolism.[101] The effect most likely takes place by blocking Fc receptors in the reticuloendothelial system, IVIG competing with antibody attached to RBCs to prevent further hemolysis.[102] We have occasionally encountered ABO-incompatible newborns with severe, early onset hyperbilirubinemia. Although we have not performed an exchange transfusion in these neonates for many years, we have found IVIG therapy useful in neonates not responding to intense phototherapy and approaching the indications for exchange transfusion.

Tin mesoporphyrin (SnMP), a metalloporphyrin that inhibits HO, produced a 43% reduction in the need for phototherapy and a 42% reduction in its duration in a group of DAT-positive, ABO-incompatible neonates[103] but this drug has not yet been approved by the FDA (see Chapter 9).

Immunization due to Antibodies Other than RhD and ABO

As the number of pregnancies complicated by Rh isoimmunization has decreased, uncommon RBC antigens have become more clinically evident. More than 50 RBC antigens may stimulate antibody formation, thereby causing HDN.[104] The most clinically important antibodies with regard to prenatal hemolysis and the need for intrauterine transfusion include anti-c, -Kell, -Fyᵃ, -Jkᵃ, -C, -E, -Cʷ, -k, and -S.[104–108] Others may also, infrequently, be problematic. Of 55 pregnancies affected by anti-c isoimmunization, 46 had fetuses with a positive DAT. Of these, 12 (26%) had serious HDN, 8 required a fetal transfusion, and the remaining 4 newborns had hemoglobin levels <10 g/dL at delivery. A titer of 1:32 or greater or the presence of hydrops fetalis identified all such fetuses.[105] Of 32 pregnancies in 27 women at risk for hemolytic disease of the fetus or newborn from anti-E isoimmunization, 16 had titers greater than or equal to 1:32. Five (15%) fetuses had hemoglobin levels <10 g/dL, one fetus had hydrops fetalis, and there was one perinatal death, all attributable to anti-E hemolytic disease.[106] Although anti-Cʷ is a relatively commonly occurring antibody, only on rare occasions (11 times in Manitoba, Canada, in 36 years) does anti-Cʷ hemolytic disease occur in newborns. The condition may result in kernicterus unless detected promptly and treated appropriately.[109] Severe fetal anemia requiring in utero fetal blood transfusions has been reported in association with anti-Cʷ.[110] On the other hand, De Young-Owens et al. encountered no cases of severe hemolytic disease among 115 pregnancies affected by anti-M antibody.[111] Anti-Kell isoimmunization warrants special mention. Although the clinical picture is largely due to a hemolytic process, fetal anemia, rather than subsequent hyperbilirubinemia, often predominates.[107] The anemia may be due to erythropoietic suppression in addition to a hemolytic process.[112] Of 156 anti-Kell-positive pregnancies seen in Ohio from 1959 to 1995, 21 fetuses were affected. Eight had severe disease and two fetuses died. All of the severely affected fetuses were associated with maternal serum titers of at least 1:32.[107] On the other hand, Bowman et al. reported cases of hydropic fetuses, including fetal deaths, and concluded that, although rare, Kell hemolytic disease may on occasion be as severe as RhD hemolytic disease.[113]

Fetal surveillance protocols and clinical strategies developed for RhD alloimmunization are useful in monitoring pregnancies alloimmunized by these and other antibodies. Similarly, the postnatal management of affected newborns should be based on the principles outlined above for the management of the RhD-immunized newborn.

■ NONIMMUNE HEMOLYTIC DISEASE

Glucose-6-Phosphate Dehydrogenase Deficiency

G6PD deficiency, a major etiologic factor in the pathogenesis of hyperbilirubinemia, is a well-described cause of extreme hyperbilirubinemia and bilirubin encephalopathy.[114-117] In recent series of neonates with extreme hyperbilirubinemia and/or kernicterus from the United States, Canada, the United Kingdom, and Ireland, G6PD deficiency comprised a major proportion of affected infants and was overrepresented relative to the background frequency of this condition in these populations[15,67,68] (Table 8-2). Because G6PD deficiency has major public health implications with regard to neonatal hyperbilirubinemia, it will be discussed below in some detail.

G6PD deficiency is one of the most common enzyme deficiencies known and is estimated to affect hundreds of millions of people globally.[16,118,123-125] Although the indigenous distribution of this condition includes the Mediterranean basin, Africa, the Middle East, and Asia, immigration patterns and ease of travel have transformed G6PD deficiency into a condition that is now encountered in virtually every part of the globe.

Function of G6PD

G6PD stabilizes the RBC membrane and protects it from oxidative damage.[123-125] The enzyme catalyzes the first step in the hexose monophosphate pathway, oxidizing glucose-6-phosphate to 6-phosphogluconolactone, thereby reducing NAPD to NADPH. NADPH plays a cardinal part in the glutathione antioxidative mechanism and oxidation of reduced glutathione is integral to the body's antioxidative mechanisms. Regeneration of reduced glutathione from oxidized glutathione is dependent on hydrogen ion donation. These ions are contributed by NADPH. The pathway is also instrumental in stimulating catalase, another important antioxidant. If there is a deficiency of G6PD, NADPH will not become available, regeneration of reduced glutathione will be compromised, and cells will be rendered susceptible to oxidative damage. In the steady state, residual G6PD may be sufficient to prevent damaging oxidation but, should an excess of oxygen free radicals be generated, the remaining protective mechanisms may no longer be able to cope and cell damage will occur. In the G6PD deficiency state, the RBC is especially vulnerable as, unlike other body cells, no alternative source of NADPH is available in these cells. Thus, oxidative damage to the RBC membrane occurs and may manifest as hemolysis[125] (Figure 8-5).

Genetics of G6PD Deficiency: Genotype Versus Phenotype

Since G6PD deficiency is an X-linked condition, males may be either normal hemizygotes or deficient hemizygotes depending on whether the maternally derived X

■ **TABLE 8-2.** Overrepresentation of Glucose-6-Phosphate Dehydrogenase (G6PD) Deficiency as a Cause of the Hyperbilirubinemia Among Cases of Kernicterus Relative to the Background Frequency of G6PD Deficiency in Specific Population Groups

	G6PD Deficiency Prevalence	
Country	Background Population (%)[11,112]	Percent of Cases of Kernicterus in which G6PD Deficiency was the Cause of Hyperbilirubinemia
United States	4–7	20.8[15]
Canada	<0.5	21.5[67]
		58[118]
United Kingdom	0–3	21.5[68]
Nigeria	14–22	75[119]
		34[70]
Oman	25	71.5[120]
Singapore	4–7	50[121]
Hong Kong	4–7	55[122]

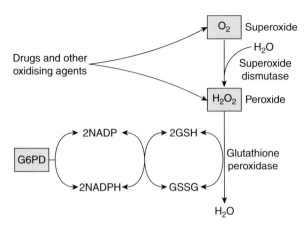

FIGURE 8-5. Diagram demonstrating the role of the enzyme G6PD in regenerating NADPH (reduced form) from NADP, as part of the antioxidant defense mechanism. (Reproduced from WHO Working Group,[125] with permission.)

chromosome carries a mutated G6PD gene or not.[123–125] Phenotypically, there should be no problem in differentiating between the two genotypes in males using either qualitative screening tests or quantitative enzyme assays. Females, on the other hand, because they have one maternally derived and one paternally derived X chromosome, may be normal homozygotes, deficient homozygotes, or heterozygotes depending on whether any of these chromosomes contained a normal or mutated gene (Table 8-3). There should be no problem in categorizing the homozygotes into enzyme-deficient or -normal groups but the heterozygotes are more difficult to classify. By the phenomenon of X chromosome inactivation, only one X chromosome is active in any female cell. The active X chromosome may be either maternally or paternally derived. Usually, 50% of each is active and an enzyme activity test, reflecting

the phenotype, will be intermediate. However, X chromosome inactivation may be nonrandom with varying ratios of mutated chromosomes and therefore varying degrees of enzyme activity. As many as 10% of heterozygotes may be phenotypically G6PD deficient, while another 10% may have normal enzyme activity. Therefore, instead of separating into two groups, as do the males, enzyme activity in females is actually a continuum, with a gradual increase in activity from a low range to normal. As a result, females are difficult to classify by biochemical means, and most studies of the frequency of G6PD deficiency in any population group usually take only the males into account. In the past it was believed that heterozygotes had sufficient residual enzyme activity to protect them from the scourges of G6PD deficiency.[125] In many heterozygotes, however, substantial numbers of G6PD-deficient RBCs may coexist with normal cells[126] (Figure 8-6). Should a hemolytic episode occur, the G6PD-deficient cells may hemolyze and the resultant release of bilirubin may be quite substantial. Extreme hyperbilirubinemia, encephalopathy, and death have been reported.[127]

G6PD Mutations

Many G6PD mutations have been documented[123] and may occur in all exons of the G6PD gene.[128] Some of the most commonly encountered include G6PD A− (202A, 968C, or 680T superimposed on G6PD A+ 376G) and G6PD Mediterranean (563T). The former is indigenously found in Africa and southern Europe, and, because of migration patterns, is today the most common variety encountered in the Americas. G6PD Mediterranean is regarded as the severe type of G6PD deficiency and is indigenous to Mediterranean countries, the Middle East, and India. Another variant encountered primarily in Asia is G6PD

■ TABLE 8-3. Possible G6PD Genotypes (X and Y Chromosomes)		
Males		
Normal hemizygotes	Deficient hemizygotes	
X^{nl} Y	X^{def} Y	
Females		
Normal homozygotes	Heterozygotes	Deficient homozygotes
X^{nl} X^{nl}	X^{nl} X^{def}	X^{def} X^{def}
Normal: G6PD normal; deficiency: G6PD deficient.		

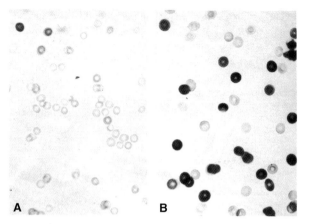

FIGURE 8-6. Erythrocytes stained cytochemically for G6PD activity. A. Patient with homozygous G6PD deficiency. All the cells appear pale. **B.** Patient heterozygous for G6PD deficiency. Pale-staining cells (G6PD deficient) are seen alongside normally staining cells. (Reproduced from Van Noorden and Vogels,[126] with permission from John Wiley & Sons Ltd.)

Canton (1376T). Some frequently encountered mutations include Union, Seattle, and Aures[128] (Table 8-4).

G6PD Deficiency and Hemolysis

Favism   G6PD deficiency is notoriously associated with severe hemolytic episodes with resultant jaundice and anemia, which may occur in both children and adults, following exposure to a hemolytic trigger. Classically, these episodes occur following ingestion of or contact with the fava bean (*Vicia faba*) and this phenomenon is therefore known as favism. These attacks occur more frequently in the spring season when fresh fava beans abound and are more common in young children than in adults. Other chemical triggers such as antimalarials, sulfonamides, and

---

■ **TABLE 8-4.** Some Commonly Encountered G6PD Mutation Types

Mediterranean	Canton
Union	Mahidol
A–(202A, 968C)	Coimbra
Chatarn	Seattle
Kaiping	Taipei
Viangchan	Aures
Santamania	Cosenza

Data from Luzzatto L. Glucose 6-phosphate dehydrogenase deficiency: from genotype to phenotype. *Haematologica.* 2006;91:1303–1306.

---

naphthalene-containing mothballs may be equally dangerous. Beutler[123] has emphasized the role of infections in the pathogenesis of acute hemolysis.

Despite the high frequency with which the condition is encountered, most G6PD-deficient individuals, unless tested for, will for the most part be unaware of their inherited condition. The precautions required by individuals who have been diagnosed with the condition are minimal and allow most affected persons to lead normal lives.

Extreme Neonatal Hyperbilirubinemia   The most extreme and dreaded form of hemolysis associated with G6PD deficiency occurs in neonates. Typically, there is acute, sudden, and unpredictable onset of jaundice. TSB levels may rise exponentially and bilirubin encephalopathy may ensue. Some identifiable substances that may trigger hemolysis in neonates include naphthalene used to store clothes, herbal medicines, henna applications to the skin, or menthol-containing umbilical potions. Frequently, however, no identifiable trigger can be found but, because the hemolytic episodes closely resemble those with an identifiable chemical trigger, it is presumed that these attacks are also trigger induced. Hyperbilirubinemia may progress relentlessly despite phototherapy and exchange transfusion may be the only recourse. Because the jaundice can be extreme and develop suddenly with no prior warning, currently, G6PD deficiency is one reason why kernicterus is not completely preventable.

In spite of the severe hyperbilirubinemia, the typical laboratory findings that suggest hemolysis (decreasing hemoglobin, an elevated reticulocyte count, and changes in the peripheral blood smear), typical of the changes seen in older children and adults, may be absent. This has led some to conclude, erroneously, that these events are not the result of hemolysis.[129] Kaplan et al. recently reported a 35-week gestation G6PD-deficient neonate who was readmitted with a sudden onset of jaundice and TSB of 33 mg/dL.[130] The COHb level was several-fold that of normal, clearly demonstrating the presence of a severe hemolytic process, yet the hemoglobin was slightly higher (15.1 g/dL) than it had been prior to discharge (14.8 g/dL) and the reticulocyte count was only 1.4%.

Other studies of endogenous CO formation, reflective of the rate of heme catabolism, have demonstrated an important role of increased hemolysis in association with this condition.[119,131] Slusher et al. demonstrated significantly higher levels of COHb in Nigerian G6PD-deficient neonates who developed kernicterus, compared with neonates who were hyperbilirubinemic, but did not develop signs of kernicterus.[119]

Moderate Neonatal Hyperbilirubinemia   Most G6PD-deficient neonates manifest a more moderate form of jaundice, although their TSB levels are significantly higher than those of the normal population.[27,28,132,133] Twenty percent of G6PD-deficient black males required phototherapy compared with 6% of controls.[88] The jaundice may resolve spontaneously and usually responds to phototherapy, although exchange transfusion may sometimes be necessary. COHbc and ETCOc studies have demonstrated that G6PD-deficient neonates have consistently, although moderately, increased levels of hemolysis compared with normal controls.[27,28,132] Paradoxically, in contrast to controls, those G6PD-deficient infants in whom hyperbilirubinemia developed did not have higher levels of COHbc or ETCO than those who remained nonhyperbilirubinemic. Furthermore, COHbc concentrations did not correlate with the TSB in the G6PD-deficient newborns as they did in the controls. Increased hemolysis, therefore, could not be implicated as the primary icterogenic factor in this form of jaundice. Consequently, a deficiency in bilirubin conjugation was suspected and, indeed, a predilection for diminished bilirubin conjugation was demonstrated in G6PD-deficient neonates. Decreased serum concentrations of diconjugated bilirubin, reflective of reduced UGT1A1 enzyme activity, were demonstrated in hyperbilirubinemic G6PD-deficient neonates compared with controls.[133] Diminished concentrations of total conjugated bilirubin as well as monoconjugated and diconjugated fractions were also reported in G6PD-deficient neonates who were nonhyperbilirubinemic at the time of sampling but subsequently went on to develop hyperbilirubinemia.[134] The diminished bilirubin conjugation was found to be due to an interaction between G6PD deficiency and the $(TA)_7$ UGT1A1 promoter polymorphism[135] (see section "Genetic Interactions Between Hemolytic Conditions and UGT1A1 Polymorphisms").

Although this moderate form of jaundice is usually benign, it must be realized that the equilibrium between bilirubin production and conjugation may be upset by the inherently increased hemolysis and diminished bilirubin conjugation. These infants may therefore be at high risk for subsequent development of severe hyperbilirubinemia. Should an infant be exposed to additional oxidative stress or should the bilirubin elimination system be further compromised, such as by late

prematurity, further imbalance between bilirubin production and conjugation may ensue with the potential for severe hyperbilirubinemia.[136] In contradistinction to the jaundice that follows the acute and unpredictably severe hemolysis, this milder form of jaundice can be predicted by predischarge serum bilirubin testing. Neonates who had a predischarge TSB concentration below the 50th percentile for hour of life had a very small likelihood of subsequent hyperbilirubinemia. However, as the predischarge TSB increased above the 50th percentile, the chance of subsequent hyperbilirubinemia increased significantly.[137]

Testing for G6PD Deficiency

Biochemical Screening or Testing   Many qualitative or quantitative screening tests are available that should accurately determine the hemizygous state in males or the homozygous state in females. Biochemical tests are based on the oxidation of glucose-6 phosphate by G6PD that results in generation of NADPH, NADPH production reflecting G6PD activity. Fluorescence of NADPH in ultraviolet light is the basis of the fluorescent spot test.[138] Because of its reliability, general usefulness, and lack of disadvantages encountered in other screening tests, the fluorescent spot test is the one recommended by the International Committee for Standardization in Haematology.[139] Spectrophotometric measurement of absorbance at 340 nm reflects NADPH activity and is used in the quantitative measurement of G6PD activity, again, the rate of NADPH generation reflecting actual G6PD activity.

Normal values in adult males range from 7 to 10 IU/g hemoglobin.[128] Because they have many young RBCs with inherently higher G6PD activity than older RBCs, values in neonates are frequently much higher. In African American neonates, who can be presumed to have G6PD A-, male values ranged from 14.5 to 33.8 U/g hemoglobin (mean 21.8 ± 2.2 U/g hemoglobin)[140] and in Sephardic Jewish male newborns, presumably with G6PD Mediterranean, from 10.0 to 21.2 U/g hemoglobin (mean 14.35 ± 2.52 U/g hemoglobin).[141] In male neonates, there should be no problem in differentiating between those with normal values and those with deficient values, as the two groups separate with no overlap.[140] However, in females, because many individuals may be heterozygotes with varying degrees of X chromosome inactivation, the results will be in a continuum, linking the G6PD-deficient and -normal newborns. Based on phenotype, it may therefore be difficult to clearly differentiate between deficient homozygotes, heterozygotes, and normal homozygotes.[136]

Molecular Screening Methods Molecular screening methods have been used.[143] The advantage of such testing is that heterozygotes will be identified. However, for practical purposes, only the mutations commonly encountered in a specific population group can be tested for, and some newborns with mutations not included in the test group may be missed. Furthermore, molecular screening methods are time consuming. In a study by Lin et al., results were available only at the end of the first week. This may be too late for the majority of infants destined to develop kernicterus, as in the Kernicterus Registry report many had already developed kernicterus by age 5 days.[15]

Recent reports suggest that G6PD heterozygotes are not without risk,[127,144–146] and in females of high-risk ethnic groups, close follow-up is necessary to monitor the development of jaundice, a normal-reading screen notwithstanding. Also, during an acute hemolytic episode, biochemical tests may give a falsely normal result, as older RBCs are destroyed, leaving younger cells, with higher enzyme activity, intact.[123,147] A simple solution is to repeat the G6PD testing several weeks after the acute hemolysis has subsided. If a specific mutation is suspected, an alternate method could be to analyze DNA for the specific mutation. If a neonate of a high-risk ethnic group develops severe hyperbilirubinemia, he or she should be treated as if G6PD deficient even if the test is apparently normal.

Screening for G6PD Deficiency Neonatal screening programs for G6PD deficiency may be effective when combined with parental and medical caretaker education.[148,149] For a program to be successful, it is essential for the results to be obtained prior to discharge from the birth hospitalization. This will ensure that the parents can be properly instructed as to which foods and substances to avoid, and to seek medical assistance urgently should they observe jaundice in their infant. Knowledge that an infant is G6PD deficient will not prevent acute attacks of extreme hyperbilirubinemia, but should be instrumental in increasing parental awareness and facilitating access to medical care. Neonatal G6PD screening has been reported in some countries including Greece, Italy (Sardinia), Philippines, Singapore, Hong Kong, Lebanon, Israel (optional), and Pennsylvania/Washington DC.[148–154] There are no randomized, controlled trials demonstrating that screening is actually instrumental in reducing

the incidence of kernicterus. However, some reports have described a decreased incidence of kernicterus following the introduction of screening. These countries include Greece,[150] Saudi Arabia,[151] Asia Pacific area,[152] Hong Kong, Singapore,[153] and Taiwan.[154]

In the United States, although there has been a move to attempt to include G6PD screening in the newborn screening panel,[155] to date this condition has not been recommended officially for routine testing.[156,157] Moreover, the Subcommittee on Hyperbilirubinemia of the AAP does not recommend routine screening of asymptomatic newborns for G6PD deficiency.[29] The most recent statement of the Fetus and Newborn Committee of the Canadian Paediatric Society does recommend selected G6PD screening for at-risk infants of Mediterranean, Middle Eastern, African, or Southeast Asian origin. The Committee does realize that in many Canadian centers it may take several days for a G6PD deficiency screening test result to become available.[158] Both the AAP and the Canadian Paediatric Society do emphasize the importance of G6PD deficiency as a risk factor for severe neonatal hyperbilirubinemia, and recommend including a test for the condition in neonates with otherwise unexplained hyperbilirubinemia or jaundice that is not responding to phototherapy.

The treatment of neonatal hyperbilirubinemia associated with G6PD deficiency should follow the guidelines of the AAP for neonates with hemolytic risk factors.[29] In the event an infant presents with extreme hyperbilirubinemia and neurologic signs consistent with bilirubin encephalopathy, a "crash-cart approach" should be adopted.[15] Intensive phototherapy should be immediately instituted and exchange transfusion performed as soon as practically possible. As there have been reports of reversal of early signs of bilirubin encephalopathy with prompt lowering of the TSB, presence of signs of bilirubin encephalopathy at first presentation should be an indication for expediting the exchange transfusion as soon as possible.[159,160]

Pyruvate Kinase Deficiency

Although it occurs less frequently than G6PD deficiency, pyruvate kinase (PK) deficiency is the most common of the glycolytic defects causing nonspherocytic hemolytic anemia.[161] In the United States, its prevalence in the Caucasian population is estimated to be 1:20,000.[162] Following on G6PD deficiency, it is the second most common cause of nonspherocytic, Coombs'-negative, hemolytic neonatal jaundice in the United States.[163]

PK plays an important part in catalyzing the conversion of phosphoenolpyruvate to pyruvate and the formation of adenosine triphosphate (ATP) from adenosine diphosphate in the Embden–Meyerhof pathway. As such, it is crucial to energy production and is responsible for the production of nearly 50% of total ATP. In humans, 4 PK isoenzymes are encoded by 2 separate genes of which 180 mutations have been identified. Erythrocyte PK is synthesized under the control of the PK-LR gene located on chromosome 1. There are strong ethnic and regional differences in the occurrence of some of the mutations. PK deficiency is inherited in an autosomal recessive manner,[164] while most people with the clinical form of the deficiency are in fact compound heterozygotes, having inherited one mutant PK gene from their father and a different PK mutation from their mother.[163]

The main metabolic abnormalities in the deficiency state include ATP depletion and increased content of 2,3-disphosphoglycerate (2,3-DPG). Subsequently, stasis, acidosis, and hypoxia, by further inhibiting the glycolytic activity, contribute to the entrapment and premature destruction of the affected and poorly deformable RBC in the microcirculation of the reticuloendothelial system. Clinical symptoms may be seen in homozygous and compound heterozygous individuals. Although there are both hepatic and RBC forms of the enzyme, in the deficiency state, only the RBC form is affected clinically. The resultant lack of ATP results in hemolysis that, in severe cases, may lead to severe neonatal anemia and early hyperbilirubinemia.[165] In patients with homozygous null mutations, no functional enzyme is formed, and newborns may be born severely anemic or even die in utero.[161] In those born alive, anemia, reticulocytosis, and severe jaundice may ensue in the newborn period. Kernicterus has been reported in association with the enzyme deficiency.[166]

No specific therapy is available, and treatment is supportive, consisting of exchange transfusion or blood transfusions when necessary. Aggressive management of hyperbilirubinemia may be necessary to avoid bilirubin encephalopathy. Iron overload is common and chelation therapy may be required. Diagnosis is determined by enzyme assay. Enzyme-deficient patients have 5–40% of normal enzyme activity. The condition should be suspected in cases of hemolysis and hyperbilirubinemia not

associated with a positive direct Coombs' test or spherocytosis. A high degree of awareness of this condition is important when evaluating a neonate with DAT-negative hemolytic hyperbilirubinemia.[165] Molecular studies may also confirm the diagnosis by identifying mutations in the coding area of the PK gene.[167]

Hereditary Spherocytosis

Of the hereditary RBC membrane defects that can lead to acute hemolysis and hyperbilirubinemia in the newborn, hereditary spherocytosis (HS) is probably the most common.[168–170] The condition occurs in 1:2500–5000 persons of Northern European descent.[171,172] HS is characterized by a deficiency in one or more of RBC membrane proteins. As a result, the RBCs are abnormally shaped, have higher metabolic requirements, and are prematurely trapped and destroyed in the spleen.[173] In 75% of cases, the condition is inherited in an autosomal dominant fashion, and in the remainder as recessive or de novo mutations. Frequently there is a history of hyperbilirubinemia in a sibling or a parent. It is thought that the condition results in protein deficiencies in the RBC membrane, including ankyrin, band 3, α-spectrin, β-spectrin, and protein 4.2, which leave microscopic patches of the lipid bilayer inner surface bare of proteins. At these points microvesiculization occurs rendering the affected RBCs osmotically fragile. Affected RBCs become trapped in the spleen, the microvesicles aspirated by macrophages, and the cell destroyed. Hemolysis may result in jaundice, anemia, and splenomegaly.

Mutations responsible for HS can lie in one of five genes encoding either transmembrane proteins (i.e., band 3) or membrane skeletal proteins (i.e., α- and β-spectrin) or proteins mediating the attachment of the latter to the former (i.e., protein 4.2 and ankyrin). The majority of mutations leading to HS were found in ankyrin and spectrin.[174,175]

Diagnosis of Hereditary Spherocytosis

The diagnosis of HS is almost always based on the combination of a typical clinical picture combined with the presence of spherocytes on a peripheral blood smear, the setting of familial hemolytic anemia, and an abnormal osmotic fragility test.[173] The latter test may be especially important in differentiating babies with HS from those with direct Coombs'-positive ABO isoimmunization, a condition that may also result in microspherocytosis. Christensen and

Henry recently demonstrated that a mean corpuscular hemoglobin concentration of greater than 36.0 g/dL had 82% sensitivity and 98% specificity for identifying HS.[176] Methods utilizing flow cytometric analysis to measure quantity of band 3 on RBC membranes for diagnosis of HS may be more specific than osmotic fragility.[177]

The diagnosis of HS may be difficult in the neonatal period. At this age splenomegaly is infrequently encountered and reticulocytosis may not be severe, only 35% of affected newborns having a reticulocyte count >10%. Many neonates with HS may not have large numbers of spherocytes in their peripheral blood smears; on the other hand, spherocytes are sometimes seen in neonatal blood films in the absence of disease. These hematological findings do frequently appear later in infancy.[178,179] Also, as neonatal RBCs are more osmotically resistant than are adult cells, the osmotic fragility test is less reliable for diagnosis of this disease. Unless there is an urgent need to arrive at a diagnosis, postponement of testing until the infant is about 6 months of age may be prudent.[170,180]

Clinical Features

In its most severe form, HS may result in hydrops fetalis with intrauterine death.[181] In the neonatal period, HS may be associated with hyperbilirubinemia requiring phototherapy or even exchange transfusion. Of 178 affected Italian term, predominantly breastfed newborns, 112 (63%) developed neonatal hyperbilirubinemia requiring phototherapy.[182] Kernicterus has been described.[183] In many affected individuals there may be no clinical manifestations. This variability in the clinical picture may be related to different molecular defects underlying HS and to bone marrow compensation.[173]

Treatment of hyperbilirubinemia in the neonatal period should be guided by the 2004 AAP guideline.[29] Splenectomy may become necessary later during childhood in order to control the anemia resulting from ongoing hemolysis.

Hereditary Elliptocytosis, Hereditary Pyropoikilocytosis, Hereditary Ovalocytosis, and Hereditary Stomatocytosis

These are rare conditions affecting the erythrocyte membrane. The diagnosis is usually made by microscopic examination of the peripheral blood smear. Hemolysis may occur in the neonatal period and result in anemia and hyperbilirubinemia.

Hereditary elliptocytosis is characterized by the presence of elliptical or oval cigar-shaped erythrocytes on peripheral blood smears of affected individuals. In some of these individuals the RBC life span is shortened leading to anemia. Neonatal jaundice, hemolysis, anemia, and hydrops fetalis have been reported.[184,185]

Hereditary pyropoikilocytosis is characterized by the presence of pyknocytes on peripheral blood smear and increased erythrocyte thermal sensitivity. Erythrocyte morphology resembles that seen in patients with severe burns. It is most common in patients of African descent, and may cause severe anemia and hemolysis in the neonatal period.[169,186,187]

Hereditary stomatocytosis is caused by increased levels of intracellular sodium and potassium that cause water to enter the cell, forming stomatocytes. These cell forms can be identified on the peripheral blood smear. Hemolysis, hyperbilirubinemia, anemia, and hydrops fetalis have been described.[187,188]

Unstable Hemoglobinopathies

Hemoglobinopathies are inherited disorders, the result of mutations of the globin genes, which decrease the solubility of hemoglobin.[189,190] These unstable hemoglobins may precipitate and decrease RBC survival time. Primarily, mutations of γ globin genes may become apparent in the neonatal period. Heinz body inclusions may be seen in the RBC, the product of hemoglobin denaturation. Affected RBCs may be destroyed prematurely in the spleen with resultant hemolysis. The γ globin mutations hemoglobin Poole[191] and hemoglobin Hasharon[192] have been reported to cause neonatal hemolysis with jaundice and anemia. Unstable hemoglobinopathies should be sought in cases of unexplained hemolytic anemias where the more common causes have been excluded.

■ GENETIC INTERACTIONS BETWEEN HEMOLYTIC CONDITIONS AND UGT1A1 POLYMORPHISMS

Diminished serum conjugated bilirubin fractions seen in G6PD-deficient neonates, reflective of decreased conjugative ability,[133,134] have been ascribed to an intriguing interaction between G6PD deficiency and $(TA)_7$ promoter polymorphism of the gene *UGT1A1*, also known as *UGT1A1*28*.[135] This polymorphism is associated with Gilbert syndrome.[193,194] The wild type of the gene promoter contains six runs of the (TA) sequence (TA)$_6$. The (TA)$_7$ polymorphism is seen with an allele frequency of about 0.33 in Caucasians,[135,193,194] and about 0.45 in indigenous Africans and persons of African descent.[195,196] Because the polymorphism involves the noncoding area of the *UGT1A1* gene, it results in diminished expression of a normally structured UGT1A1 enzyme isoform.[195] As a result, the ability to conjugate bilirubin is decreased. The incidence of neonatal hyperbilirubinemia, defined as a TSB ≥15.0 mg/dL, increased in a stepwise, dose-dependent fashion, in G6PD Mediterranean-deficient neonates who were both heterozygous and homozygous for (TA)$_7$.[135] This effect was not seen in the G6PD-normal, control group. Furthermore, G6PD deficiency alone, in the absence of the promoter polymorphism, did not increase the incidence of hyperbilirubinemia over and above that of G6PD-normal counterparts (Figure 8-7). Heterozygosity for UGT1A1 (TA)$_7$ promoter polymorphism in combination with heterozygosity for G6PD Mediterranean was reported in a female infant with fatal bilirubin encephalopathy.[127]

In Asians, in contrast, the (TA)$_7$ polymorphism is rare, but the variation rate within the coding region in the *UGT1A1* gene is much higher for Taiwanese compared with whites (29.3% vs. 0.1%).[197] Furthermore, the

G → A variation at nucleotide 211 of the *UGT1A1* gene (Gly71Arg) is related to hyperbilirubinemia in Japanese and Taiwanese newborns.[198–200] An interaction similar to that reported between G6PD Mediterranean and the promoter polymorphism was therefore sought between G6PD deficiency and coding area mutations of the *UGT1A1* gene in Taiwanese neonates. Overall, the Relative Risk (RR) of developing a TSB >15 mg/dL was significantly higher for the G6PD-deficient group (predominantly a single-point mutation at nucleotide 1376 [Arg459Leu]) than for the G6PD-normal controls (RR 2.0, 95% CI 1.5–2.7; *P* = .01, 15.6% vs. 7.8%). However, the increased incidence of hyperbilirubinemia was limited to those homozygous for the *UGT1A1* nucleotide 211 variation (RR 2.6, 95% CI 1.1–6.0; *P* = .01). All 11 G6PD-deficient subjects homozygous for the 211 G → A variation developed neonatal hyperbilirubinemia.[201]

Not only in the hyperbilirubinemic but also in the steady state did the (TA)$_7$ promoter polymorphism play a crucial role in determining the TSB in G6PD-deficient neonates. While the rate of heme catabolism, reflected by COHbc levels, increased minimally and statistically insignificantly between the three UGT1A1 promoter genotypes (wild-type (TA)$_6$/(TA)$_6$ homozygotes, (TA)$_6$/(TA)$_7$ heterozygotes, and (TA)$_7$/(TA)$_7$ homozygotes), TSB concentrations were significantly higher in the (TA)$_7$ homozygotes (11.1 ± 4.0 mg/dL) compared with 9.1 ± 3.2 mg/dL in the (TA)$_6$/(TA)$_7$ heterozygotes (*P* = .03) and 8.8 ± 3.4 mg/dL, *P* = .02, in the (TA)$_6$ homozygotes.[202] Similar rates of hemolysis, but increased TSB in the G6PD-deficient, (TA)$_7$/(TA)$_7$ homozygotes, implied that diminished bilirubin conjugation, most likely due to (TA)$_7$ homozygosity, was central to the increased bilirubin concentrations in these infants. Similar genetic interactions may also be important in determining adult steady-state TSB concentrations. In a genome-wide association scan performed on adult Sardinians, three loci were associated with TSB modulation: *UGT1A1*, *G6PD*, and a locus on chromosome 2p12.2, *SLCO1B3*, a member of the OATP family.[203]

Lin et al. utilized DNA samples obtained from the DNA Polymorphism Discovery Resource of the National Human Genome Research Institute to determine the risk of coexpression between genes modulating the risk for neonatal hyperbilirubinemia in the United States. This resource is composed of DNA obtained from 450 anonymous US residents with ancestry from the major geographic regions of the world and is thought to be representative of the US population in general. While

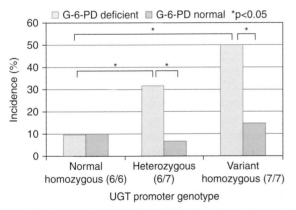

FIGURE 8-7. Incidence of hyperbilirubinemia, defined as TSB ≥15 mg/dL, for G6PD-deficient and control neonates, stratified for the three promoter genotypes of the gene encoding the bilirubin conjugating enzyme UDP glucuronosyltransferase 1A1 (UGT1A1). Note the increasing incidence of hyperbilirubinemia in tandem with progression of the UGT1A1 promoter polymorphism from the wild-type (TA)$_6$ homozygotes to (TA)$_7$ homozygotes, in the G6PD-deficient neonates only. (Reproduced from Kaplan et al.,[135] with permission. Copyright © 1997 National Academy of Sciences, U.S.A.)

no clinical information was available for these individuals, a high rate of gene coexpression of mutations and polymorphisms of *G6PD*, the *UGT1A1* gene promoter, and *OAT1B1* was found. In more than three quarters of the samples, >2 variants were coexpressed. The potential for interaction between these genes suggests an important role for genetic polymorphism coinheritance in the pathogenesis of neonatal hyperbilirubinemia.[204]

Watchko et al. subsequently determined whether the frequency of G6PD deficiency, UGT1A1 polymorphisms, and hepatic solute carrier organic anion transporter 1B1 (*SLCO1B1*) gene variants was greater in neonates who had at least one TSB value >95th percentile compared with those having <40th percentile. While the frequencies of the individual gene variants studied did not vary significantly between case and control subjects, coexpression of the *G6PD* African A− mutation with *UGT1A1* and/or *SLCO1B1* variants was more frequent in the hyperbilirubinemic newborns.[205]

In neonates with HS, Iolascon et al. demonstrated an interaction similar to that described in G6PD-deficient neonates, between their inherent condition and *UGT1A1*.[206] One hundred and seventy-eight newborns affected by HS were studied. Of 30 infants homozygous for (TA)$_7$ promoter polymorphism, 29 (97%) developed a TSB >95th percentile during the first week of life and required phototherapy. In contrast, only 83/148 (56%) of those either homozygous for the wild-type (TA)$_6$ or heterozygous (TA)$_6$/(TA)$_7$ developed hyperbilirubinemia (*P* < .001). Demonstrating the potential of a devastating gene interaction, Berardi et al. described a neonate with HS who developed a TSB of 45.6 mg/dL with resultant kernicterus despite exchange transfusion.[183] *UGT1A1* gene analysis demonstrated that the uncommon (TA)$_7$/ (TA)$_8$ TAA promoter genotype coexisted with HS. As the (TA)$_8$ promoter sequence can be expected to result in gene expression even further diminished than the (TA)$_7$ variant,[196] coexpression of HS with the UGT1A1 promoter sequence was probably responsible for increased bilirubin production combined with diminished bilirubin conjugation and the resultant high TSB.

Finally, Kaplan et al. demonstrated an effect of *UGT1A1* (TA)$_7$ promoter homozygosity, which was crucial to the development of hyperbilirubinemia in DAT-negative, ABO heterospecific neonates.[98] Forty ABO heterospecific and 344 ABO-compatible controls had a combined allele frequency of 0.35 for the variant UGT1A1 (TA)$_7$

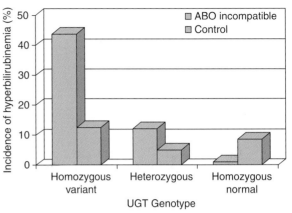

FIGURE 8-8. Incidence of hyperbilirubinemia (TSB value ≥15 mg/dL) for the three UGT1A1 promoter genotypes. ABO-incompatible babies who were also homozygous for the variant (TA)$_7$ UGT1A1 promoter (Gilbert syndrome) had a higher incidence of hyperbilirubinemia than those who were homozygous normal (TA)$_6$. The former subgroup also had a greater incidence of hyperbilirubinemia than any of the three UGT1A1 promoter genotype subgroups in the control (ABO-compatible) infants. (Reprinted from Kaplan M, Hammerman C, Renbaum P, Klein G, Levy-Lahad E. Gilbert's syndrome and hyperbilirubinaemia in ABO-incompatible neonates. *Lancet*. 2000;356:652–653. Copyright 2000, with permission from Elsevier.)

promoter. The incidence of hyperbilirubinemia was significantly higher only in the ABO heterospecific neonates who coexpressed with homozygosity for (TA)$_7$ compared with ABO-incompatible babies homozygous for the wild-type (TA)$_6$ UGT1A1 promoter (43% vs. 0, *P* = .02). The incidence of hyperbilirubinemia in the ABO heterospecific, (TA)$_7$ subgroup was also significantly higher than in the ABO-compatible controls of all UGT genotypes combined (RR 5.65; 95% CI 2.23–14.31) (Figure 8-8).

■ CONCLUSIONS

Hemolytic conditions are highly associated with the development of bilirubin neurotoxicity. Rapid development of hyperbilirubinemia in hemolytic conditions may be due only in part to the increased hemolysis per se: a complexity of interactions between the hemolytic condition itself, the environment, and mutations and polymorphisms of *UGT1A1* may mediate the extraordinary contribution of hemolytic conditions to the development of extreme hyperbilirubinemia and encephalopathy.

REFERENCES

1. Stevenson DK, Dennery PA, Hintz SR. Understanding newborn jaundice. *J Perinatol.* 2001;21(suppl 1): S21–S24.

2. Bhutani VK, Johnson L, Sivieri EM. Predictive ability of a predischarge hour-specific serum bilirubin for subsequent significant hyperbilirubinemia in healthy term and near-term newborns. *Pediatrics.* 1999;103:6–14.

3. Kaplan M, Muraca M, Hammerman C, et al. Imbalance between production and conjugation of bilirubin: a fundamental concept in the mechanism of neonatal jaundice. *Pediatrics.* 2002;110:e47.

4. Newman TB, Maisels MJ. Does hyperbilirubinemia damage the brain of healthy full-term infants? *Clin Perinatol.* 1990;17:331–358.

5. Watchko JF, Oski FA. Bilirubin 20 mg/dL = vigintiphobia. *Pediatrics.* 1983;71:660–663.

6. Newman TB, Maisels MJ. Evaluation and treatment of jaundice in the term newborn: a kinder, gentler approach. *Pediatrics.* 1992;89(5 pt 1):809–818.

7. Ozmert E, Erdem G, Topçu M, et al. Long-term follow-up of indirect hyperbilirubinemia in full-term Turkish infants. *Acta Paediatr.* 1996;85:1440–1444.

8. Nilsen ST, Finne PH, Bergsjø P, Stamnes O. Males with neonatal hyperbilirubinemia examined at 18 years of age. *Acta Paediatr Scand.* 1984;73:176–180.

9. Newman TB, Liljestrand P, Jeremy RJ, et al.; Jaundice and Infant Feeding Study Team. Outcomes among newborns with total serum bilirubin levels of 25 mg per deciliter or more. *N Engl J Med.* 20064;354:1889–1900.

10. Kuzniewicz MW, Escobar GJ, Newman TB. Impact of universal bilirubin screening on severe hyperbilirubinemia and phototherapy use. *Pediatrics.* 2009; 124:1031–1039.

11. Gamaleldin R, Iskander I, Seoud I, et al. An evaluation of risk factors for neurotoxicity in newborns with severe neonatal hyperbilirubinemia. *Pediatrics.* 2011;128:e925–e931.

12. Wennberg RP, Ahlfors CE, Bhutani VK, Johnson LH, Shapiro SM. Toward understanding kernicterus: a challenge to improve the management of jaundiced newborns. *Pediatrics.* 2006;117:474–485.

13. Oh W, Stevenson DK, Tyson JE, et al.; NICHD Neonatal Research Network Bethesda MD. Influence of clinical status on the association between plasma total and unbound bilirubin and death or adverse neurodevelopmental outcomes in extremely low birth weight infants. *Acta Paediatr.* 2010;99:673–678.

14. Ahlfors CE, Wennberg RP, Ostrow JD, Tiribelli C. Unbound (free) bilirubin: improving the paradigm for evaluating neonatal jaundice. *Clin Chem.* 2009;55:1288–1299.

15. Johnson L, Bhutani VK, Karp K, Sivieri EM, Shapiro SM. Clinical report from the pilot USA Kernicterus Registry (1992 to 2004). *J Perinatol.* 2009;29(suppl 1):S25–S45.

16. Nkhoma ET, Poole C, Vannappagari V, Hall SA, Beutler E. The global prevalence of glucose-6-phosphate dehydrogenase deficiency: a systematic review and meta-analysis. *Blood Cells Mol Dis.* 2009;42:267–278.

17. Provisional Committee on Quality Improvement and Subcommittee on Hyperbilirubinemia. Practice parameter: management of hyperbilirubinemia in the healthy, term newborn. *Pediatrics.* 1994;94;558–565.

18. Maisels MJ, Newman TB. Kernicterus in otherwise healthy, breast-fed term newborns. *Pediatrics.* 1995;96(4 pt 1):730–733.

19. Lazar L, Litwin A, Merlob P. Phototherapy for neonatal nonhemolytic hyperbilirubinemia. Analysis of rebound and indications for discontinuing therapy. *Clin Pediatr (Phila).* 1993;32(5):264–267.

20. Ebbesen F, Ehrenstein V, Traeger M, Nielsen GL. Neonatal non-hemolytic hyperbilirubinemia: a prevalence study of adult neuropsychiatric disability and cognitive function in 463 male Danish conscripts. *Arch Dis Child.* 2010;95(8):583–587.

21. Watchko JF. The clinical sequelae of hyperbilirubinemia. In: Maisels MJ, Watchko JF, eds. *Neonatal Jaundice.* Amsterdam: Harwood Academic Publishers; 2000:115–135.

22. de Carvalho M, Mochdece CC, Sá CA, Moreira ME. High-intensity phototherapy for the treatment of severe nonhaemolytic neonatal hyperbilirubinemia. *Acta Paediatr.* 2011;100:620–623. doi: 10.1111/j.1651–2227-.2011.02170.x [Epub ahead of print].

23. Grimmer I, Berger-Jones K, Buhrer C, Brandl U, Obladen M. Late neurological sequelae of non-hemolytic hyperbilirubinemia of healthy term neonates. *Acta Paediatr.* 1999;88:661–663.

24. Blanchette V, Dror Y, Chan A. Hematology. In: MacDonald MG, Mullett MD, Seschia MMK, eds. *Avery's Neonatology: Pathophysiology and Management of the Newborn.* Philadelphia: Lippincott Williams and Wilkins; 2005:1169–1234.

25. Stevenson DK, Fanaroff AA, Maisels MJ, et al. Prediction of hyperbilirubinemia in near-term and term infants. *Pediatrics.* 2001;108:31–39.

26. Maisels MJ, Kring E. The contribution of hemolysis to early jaundice in normal newborns. *Pediatrics.* 2006;118:276–279.

27. Kaplan M, Herschel M, Hammerman C, et al. Studies in hemolysis in glucose-6-phosphate dehydrogenase-deficient African American neonates. *Clin Chim Acta.* 2006;365:177–182.

28. Kaplan M, Vreman HJ, Hammerman C, et al. Contribution of haemolysis to jaundice in Sephardic Jewish

glucose-6-phosphate dehydrogenase deficient neonates. *Br J Haematol.* 1996;93:822–827.

29. American Academy of Pediatrics Subcommittee on Hyperbilirubinemia. Management of hyperbilirubinemia in the newborn infant 35 or more weeks of gestation. *Pediatrics.* 2004;114:297–316.

30. Coombs RR, Mourant AE, Race RR. In-vivo isosensitisation of red cells in babies with haemolytic disease. *Lancet.* 1946;1:264–266.

31. Herschel M, Karrison T, Wen M, Caldarelli L, Baron B. Evaluation of the direct antiglobulin (Coombs') test for identifying newborns at risk for hemolysis as determined by end-tidal carbon monoxide concentration (ETCOc); and comparison of the Coombs' test with ETCOc for detecting significant jaundice. *J Perinatol.* 2002;22:341–347.

32. Ozolek JA, Watchko JF, Mimouni F. Prevalence and lack of clinical significance of blood group incompatibility in mothers with blood type A or B. *J Pediatr.* 1994;125:87–91.

33. Martin JA, Hamilton BE, Sutton PD, et al. Births: final data for 2003. *Natl Vital Stat Rep.* 2005;54:1–116.

34. Goplerud CP, White CA, Bradbury JT, Briggs TL. The first Rh-isoimmunized pregnancy. *Am J Obstet Gynecol.* 1973;115:632–638.

35. Bowman JM, Chown B, Lewis M, Pollock JM. Rh isoimmunization during pregnancy: antenatal prophylaxis. *Can Med Assoc J.* 1978;118:623–627.

36. Moise KJ Jr. Management of rhesus alloimmunization in pregnancy. *Obstet Gynecol.* 2008;112:164–176.

37. Liley AW. Liquor amino analysis in the management of the pregnancy complicated by rhesus sensitization. *Am J Obstet Gynecol.* 1961;82:1359–1370.

38. Queenan JT, Tomai TP, Ural SH, King JC. Deviation in amniotic fluid optical density at a wavelength of 450 nm in Rh-immunized pregnancies from 14 to 40 weeks' gestation: a proposal for clinical management. *Am J Obstet Gynecol.* 1993;168:1370–1376.

39. Zipursky A, Paul VK. The global burden of Rh disease. *Arch Dis Child Fetal Neonatal Ed.* 2011;96: F84–F85.

40. Walker W. Hemolytic disease of the newborn. In Gairdner D, Hull D, eds. *Recent Advances in Pediatrics.* London: JA Churchill; 1971:119–170.

41. Bowman JM, Pollock J. Rh immunization in Manitoba: progress in prevention and management. *Can Med Assoc J.* 1983;129:343–345.

42. Fung Kee Fung K, Eason E, Crane J, et al. Prevention of Rh alloimmunization. *J Obstet Gynaecol Can.* 2003;25:765–773.

43. Bowman JM. The prevention of Rh immunization. *Transfus Med Rev.* 1988;2:129–150.

44. Chérif-Zahar B, Mattéi MG, Le Van Kim C, et al. Localization of the human Rh blood group gene structure to chromosome region 1p34.3–1p36.1 by in situ hybridization. *Hum Genet.* 1991;86:398–400.

45. Lo YM, Hjelm NM, Fidler C, et al. Prenatal diagnosis of fetal RhD status by molecular analysis of maternal plasma. *N Engl J Med.* 1998;339:1734–1738.

46. Van den Veyver IB, Moise KJ Jr. Fetal RhD typing by polymerase chain reaction in pregnancies complicated by rhesus alloimmunization. *Obstet Gynecol.* 1996;88:1061–1067.

47. Kolialexi A, Tounta G, Mavrou A. Noninvasive fetal RhD genotyping from maternal blood. *Expert Rev Mol Diagn.* 2010;10:285–296.

48. Rouillac-Le Sciellour C, Puillandre P, Gillot R, et al. Large-scale pre-diagnosis study of fetal RHD genotyping by PCR on plasma DNA from RhD-negative pregnant women. *Mol Diagn.* 2004;8:23–31.

49. Mari G, Deter RL, Carpenter RL, et al. Noninvasive diagnosis by Doppler ultrasonography of fetal anemia due to maternal red-cell alloimmunization. Collaborative Group for Doppler Assessment of the Blood Velocity in Anemic Fetuses. *N Engl J Med.* 2000;342:9–14.

50. Oepkes D, Seaward PG, Vandenbussche FP, et al. Doppler ultrasonography versus amniocentesis to predict fetal anemia. *N Engl J Med.* 2006;355:156–164.

51. De Boer IP, Zeestraten EC, Lopriore E, et al. Pediatric outcome in Rhesus hemolytic disease treated with and without intrauterine transfusion. *Am J Obstet Gynecol.* 2008;198:54.e1–54.e4

52. Van Kamp IL, Klumper FJ, Oepkes D, et al. Complications of intrauterine intravascular transfusion for fetal anemia due to maternal red-cell alloimmunization. *Am J Obstet Gynecol.* 2005;192:171–177.

53. Greenough A. Rhesus disease: postnatal management and outcome. *Eur J Pediatr.* 1999;158:689–693.

54. Smits-Wintjens VE, Walther FJ, Lopriore E. Rhesus haemolytic disease of the newborn: postnatal management, associated morbidity and long-term outcome. *Semin Fetal Neonatal Med.* 2008;13:265–271.

55. Barss VA, Doubilet PM, St John-Sutton M, Cartier MS, Frigoletto FD. Cardiac output in a fetus with erythroblastosis fetalis: assessment using pulsed Doppler. *Obstet Gynecol.* 1987;70:442–444.

56. Nicolaides KH, Clewell WH, Rodeck CH. Measurement of human fetoplacental blood volume in erythroblastosis fetalis. *Am J Obstet Gynecol.* 1987;157:50–53.

57. Phibbs RH, Johnson P, Tooley WH. Cardiorespiratory status of erythroblastotic newborn infants. II. Blood volume, hematocrit, and serum albumin concentration in relation to hydrops fetalis. *Pediatrics.* 1974;53:13–23.

58. Rübo J, Albrecht K, Lasch P, et al. High-dose intravenous immune globulin therapy for hyperbilirubinemia caused by Rh hemolytic disease. *J Pediatr.* 1992;121: 93–97.

59. Alpay F, Sarici SU, Okutan V, et al. High-dose intravenous immunoglobulin therapy in neonatal immune haemolytic jaundice. *Acta Paediatr.* 1999;88: 216–219.

60. Dağoğlu T, Ovali F, Samanci N, Bengisu E. High-dose intravenous immunoglobulin therapy for rhesus haemolytic disease. *J Int Med Res.* 1995;23:264–271.

61. Voto LS, Sexer H, Ferreiro G, et al. Neonatal administration of high-dose intravenous immunoglobulin in rhesus hemolytic disease. *J Perinat Med.* 1995;23: 443–451.

62. Gottstein R, Cooke RW. Systematic review of intravenous immunoglobulin in haemolytic disease of the newborn. *Arch Dis Child Fetal Neonatal Ed.* 2003;88:F6–F10.

63. Smits-Wintjens VE, Walther FJ, Rath ME, et al. Intravenous immunoglobulin in neonates with rhesus hemolytic disease: a randomized controlled trial. *Pediatrics.* 2011;127:680–686.

64. Alcock GS, Liley H. Immunoglobulin infusion for isoimmune haemolytic jaundice in neonates. *Cochrane Database Syst Rev.* 2002;(3):CD003313. Available at: http://www.nichd.nih.gov/COCHRANE/.

65. Hudon L, Moise KJ Jr, Hegemier SE, et al. Long-term neurodevelopmental outcome after intrauterine transfusion for the treatment of fetal hemolytic disease. *Am J Obstet Gynecol.* 1998;179:858–863.

66. Verduin EP, Lindenburg IT, Smits-Wintjens VE, et al. Long-term follow-up after intrauterine transfusions; the LOTUS study. *BMC Pregnancy Childbirth.* 2010;10:77.

67. Sgro M, Campbell D, Shah V. Incidence and causes of severe neonatal hyperbilirubinemia in Canada. *CMAJ.* 2006;175:587–590.

68. Manning D, Todd P, Maxwell M, Jane Platt M. Prospective surveillance study of severe hyperbilirubinaemia in the newborn in the UK and Ireland. *Arch Dis Child Fetal Neonatal Ed.* 2007;92:F342–F346.

69. Bjerre JV, Petersen JR, Ebbesen F. Surveillance of extreme hyperbilirubinaemia in Denmark. A method to identify the newborn infants. *Acta Paediatr.* 2008;97: 1030–1034.

70. Ogunlesi TA, Dedeke IO, Adekanmbi AF, Fetuga MB, Ogunfowora OB. The incidence and outcome of bilirubin encephalopathy in Nigeria: a bi-centre study. *Niger J Med.* 2007;16:354–359.

71. Zoubir S, Arlettaz Mieth R, Berrut S, Roth-Kleiner M; the Swiss Paediatric Surveillance Unit (SPSU). Incidence of severe hyperbilirubinaemia in Switzerland: a

nationwide population-based prospective study. *Arch Dis Child Fetal Neonatal Ed.* 2011;96:F310–F311 [Epub ahead of print].

72. McDonnell M, Hannam S, Devane SP. Hydrops fetalis due to ABO incompatibility. *Arch Dis Child Fetal Neonatal Ed.* 1998;78:F220–F221.

73. Gilja BK, Shah VP. Hydrops fetalis due to ABO incompatibility. *Clin Pediatr (Phila).* 1988;27:210–212.

74. Sherer DM, Abramowicz JS, Ryan RM, et al. Severe fetal hydrops resulting from ABO incompatibility. *Obstet Gynecol.* 1991;78(5 pt 2):897–899.

75. Voak D, Williams MA. An explanation of the failure of the direct antiglobulin test to detect erythrocyte sensitization in ABO haemolytic disease of the newborn and observations on pinocytosis of IgG anti-A antibodies by infant (cord) red cells. *Br J Haematol.* 1971;20:9–23.

76. Halbrecht I. Role of hemoagglutinins anti-a and anti-b in pathogenesis of jaundice of the newborn (icterus neonatorum precox). *Am J Dis Child.* 1944;68:248–249.

77. Boorman KE, Dodd BE, Trinick RH. Haemolytic disease of the newborn due to anti-A antibodies. *Lancet.* 1949;1(6565):1088–1091.

78. Mollison PL, Cutbush M. Haemolytic disease of the newborn; criteria of severity. *Br Med J.* 1949;1(4594):123–130.

79. Kochwa S, Rosenfield RE, Tallal L, Wasserman LR. Isoagglutinins associated with ABO erythroblastosis. *J Clin Invest.* 1961;40:874–883.

80. Grundbacher FJ. The etiology of ABO hemolytic disease of the newborn. *Transfusion.* 1980;20:563–568.

81. Fällström SP, Bjure J. Endogenous formation of carbon monoxide in newborn infants. 3. ABO incompatibility. *Acta Paediatr Scand.* 1968;57:137–144.

82. Uetani Y, Nakamura H, Okamoto O, et al. Carboxyhemoglobin measurements in the diagnosis of ABO hemolytic disease. *Acta Paediatr Jpn.* 1989;31:171–176.

83. Herschel M, Karrison T, Wen M, Caldarelli L, Baron B. Isoimmunization is unlikely to be the cause of hemolysis in ABO-incompatible but direct antiglobulin test-negative neonates. *Pediatrics.* 2002;110(1 pt 1):127–130.

84. Kaplan M, Hammerman C, Vreman HJ, Wong RJ, Stevenson DK. Hemolysis and hyperbilirubinemia in antiglobulin positive, direct ABO blood group heterospecific neonates. *J Pediatr.* 2010;157:772–777.

85. Kanto WP Jr, Marino B, Godwin AS, Bunyapen C. ABO hemolytic disease: a comparative study of clinical severity and delayed anemia. *Pediatrics.* 1978;62:365–369.

86. Meberg A, Johansen KB. Screening for neonatal hyperbilirubinaemia and ABO alloimmunization at the time of testing for phenylketonuria and congenital hypothyreosis. *Acta Paediatr.* 1998;87:1269–1274.

87. Bhutani VK, Johnson LH, Jeffrey Maisels M, et al. Kernicterus: epidemiological strategies for its

prevention through systems-based approaches. *J Perinatol.* 2004;24:650–662.

88. Kaplan M, Herschel M, Hammerman C, Hoyer JD, Stevenson DK. Hyperbilirubinemia among African American, glucose-6-phosphate dehydrogenase-deficient neonates. *Pediatrics.* 2004;114:e213–e219.

89. Kaplan M, Herschel M, Hammerman C, et al. Neonatal hyperbilirubinemia in African American males: the importance of glucose-6-phosphate dehydrogenase deficiency. *J Pediatr.* 2006;149:83–88.

90. Peevy KJ, Wiseman HJ. ABO hemolytic disease of the newborn: evaluation of management and identification of racial and antigenic factors. *Pediatrics.* 1978;61:475–478.

91. Brink S. A laboratory survey of A-B-O blood-group incompatibility and neonatal jaundice. *S Afr Med J.* 1969;43:1047–1050.

92. Dufour DR, Monoghan WP. ABO hemolytic disease of the newborn. A retrospective analysis of 254 cases. *Am J Clin Pathol.* 1980;73:369–373.

93. Sisson TR. Reply to Pildes RS, Phototherapy in ABO incompatibility. *J Pediatr.* 1972;80:1063–1064.

94. Chan-Shu SY, Blair O. ABO hemolytic disease of the newborn. *Am J Clin Pathol.* 1979;71:677–679.

95. Bakkeheim E, Bergerud U, Schmidt-Melbye AC, et al. Maternal IgG anti-A and anti-B titres predict outcome in ABO-incompatibility in the neonate. *Acta Paediatr.* 2009;98:1896–1901.

96. Clifford JH, Mathews P, Reiquam CW, Palmer HD. Screening for hemolytic disease of the newborn by cord blood Coombs testing—analysis of a five-year experience. *Clin Pediatr (Phila).* 1968;7:465–469.

97. Farrell AG. A-B-O incompatibility and haemolytic disease of the newborn. *S Afr Med J.* 1970;44:211–213.

98. Kaplan M, Hammerman C, Renbaum P, Klein G, Levy-Lahad E. Gilbert's syndrome and hyperbilirubinaemia in ABO-incompatible neonates. *Lancet.* 2000;356:652–653.

99. Sarici SU, Yurdakök M, Serdar MA, et al. An early (sixth-hour) serum bilirubin measurement is useful in predicting the development of significant hyperbilirubinemia and severe ABO hemolytic disease in a selective high-risk population of newborns with ABO incompatibility. *Pediatrics.* 2002;109:e53.

100. Risemberg HM, Mazzi E, MacDonald MG, Peralta M, Heldrich F. Correlation of cord bilirubin levels with hyperbilirubinaemia in ABO incompatibility. *Arch Dis Child.* 1977;52:219–222.

101. Hammerman C, Vreman HJ, Kaplan M, Stevenson DK. Intravenous immune globulin in neonatal immune hemolytic disease: does it reduce hemolysis? *Acta Paediatr.* 1996;85:1351–1353.

102. Urbaniak SJ. ADCC (K-cell) lysis of human erythrocytes sensitized with rhesus alloantibodies. II. Investigation into the mechanism of lysis. *Br J Haematol.* 1979;42:315–325.

103. Kappas A, Drummond GS, Manola T, Petmezaki S, Valaes T. Sn-protoporphyrin use in the management of hyperbilirubinemia in term newborns with direct Coombs-positive ABO incompatibility. *Pediatrics.* 1988;81:485–489.

104. Moise KJ. Red blood cell alloimmunization in pregnancy. *Semin Hematol.* 2005;42:169–178.

105. Hackney DN, Knudtson EJ, Rossi KQ, Krugh D, O'Shaughnessy RW. Management of pregnancies complicated by anti-c isoimmunization. *Obstet Gynecol.* 2004;103:24–30.

106. Joy SD, Rossi KQ, Krugh D, O'Shaughnessy RW. Management of pregnancies complicated by anti-E alloimmunization. *Obstet Gynecol.* 2005;105:24–28.

107. McKenna DS, Nagaraja HN, O'Shaughnessy R. Management of pregnancies complicated by anti-Kell isoimmunization. *Obstet Gynecol.* 1999;93:667–673.

108. Bowman JM. The management of alloimmune fetal hemolytic disease. In: Maisels MJ, Watchko JF, eds. *Neonatal Jaundice.* Amsterdam: Harwood Academic Publishers; 2000:23–33.

109. Bowman JM, Pollock J. Maternal CW alloimmunization. *Vox Sang.* 1993;64:226–230.

110. Byers BD, Gordon MC, Higby K. Severe hemolytic disease of the newborn due to anti-Cw. *Obstet Gynecol.* 2005;106(5 pt 2):1180–1182.

111. De Young-Owens A, Kennedy M, Rose RL, Boyle J, O'Shaughnessy R. Anti-M isoimmunization: management and outcome at the Ohio State University from 1969 to 1995. *Obstet Gynecol.* 1997;90:962–966.

112. Vaughan JI, Warwick R, Letsky E, et al. Erythropoietic suppression in fetal anemia because of Kell alloimmunization. *Am J Obstet Gynecol.* 1994;171:247–252.

113. Bowman JM, Pollock JM, Manning FA, Harman CR, Menticoglou S. Maternal Kell blood group alloimmunization. *Obstet Gynecol.* 1992;79:239–244.

114. Valaes T. Severe neonatal jaundice associated with glucose-6-phosphate dehydrogenase deficiency: pathogenesis and global epidemiology. *Acta Paediatr Suppl.* 1994;394:58–76.

115. Kaplan M, Hammerman C. Severe neonatal hyperbilirubinemia. A potential complication of glucose-6-phosphate dehydrogenase deficiency. *Clin Perinatol.* 1998;25:575–590.

116. Kaplan M, Hammerman C. Glucose-6-phosphate dehydrogenase deficiency: a hidden risk for kernicterus. *Semin Perinatol.* 2004;28:356–364.

117. Kaplan M, Hammerman C. Glucose-6-phosphate dehydrogenase deficiency and severe neonatal

hyperbilirubinemia: a complexity of interactions between genes and environment. *Semin Fetal Neonatal Med.* 2010;15:148–156.

118. AlOtaibi SF, Blaser S, MacGregor DL. Neurological complications of kernicterus. *Can J Neurol Sci.* 2005;32: 311–315.

119. Slusher TM, Vreman HJ, McLaren DW, et al. Glucose-6-phosphate dehydrogenase deficiency and carboxyhemoglobin concentrations associated with bilirubin-related morbidity and death in Nigerian infants. *J Pediatr.* 1995;126:102–108.

120. Nair PAK, Al Khussiby SM. Kernicterus and G6PD deficiency—a case series from Oman. *J Trop Pediatr.* 2003;49:74–77.

121. Wong HB. Singapore kernicterus—the position in 1965. *J Singapore Paediatr Soc.* 1965;7:35–43.

122. Lai HC, Lai MP, Leung KS. Glucose-6-phosphate dehydrogenase deficiency in Chinese. *J Clin Pathol.* 1968;21: 44–47.

123. Beutler E. G6PD deficiency. *Blood.* 1994;84:3613–3636.

124. Cappellini MD, Fiorelli G. Glucose-6-phosphate dehydrogenase deficiency. *Lancet.* 2008;371:64–74.

125. WHO Working Group. Glucose-6-phosphate dehydrogenase deficiency. *Bull World Health Organ.* 1989;67: 601–611.

126. Van Noorden CJ, Vogels IM. A sensitive cytochemical staining method for glucose-6-phosphate dehydrogenase activity in individual erythrocytes. II. Further improvements of the staining procedure and some observations with glucose-6-phosphate dehydrogenase deficiency. *Br J Haematol.* 1985;60:57–63.

127. Zangen S, Kidron D, Gelbart T, et al. Fatal kernicterus in a girl deficient in glucose-6-phosphate dehydrogenase: a paradigm of synergistic heterozygosity. *J Pediatr.* 2009;154:616–619.

128. Luzzatto L. Glucose 6-phosphate dehydrogenase deficiency: from genotype to phenotype. *Haematologica.* 2006;91:1303–1306.

129. Meloni T, Cutillo S, Testa U, Luzzatto L. Neonatal jaundice and severity of glucose-6-phosphate dehydrogenase deficiency in Sardinian babies. *Early Hum Dev.* 1987;15:317–322.

130. Kaplan M, Hammerman C, Vreman HJ, Wong RJ, Stevenson DK. Severe hemolysis with normal blood count in a glucose-6-phosphate dehydrogenase deficient neonate. *J Perinatol.* 2008;28:306–309.

131. Necheles TF, Rai US, Valaes T. The role of haemolysis in neonatal hyperbilirubinaemia as reflected in carboxyhaemoglobin levels. *Acta Paediatr Scand.* 1976;65:361–367.

132. Kaplan M, Vreman HJ, Hammerman C, et al. Combination of ABO blood group incompatibility and glucose-6-phosphate dehydrogenase deficiency: effect on hemolysis and neonatal hyperbilirubinemia. *Acta Paediatr.* 1998;87:455–457.

133. Kaplan M, Rubaltelli FF, Hammerman C, et al. Conjugated bilirubin in neonates with glucose-6-phosphate dehydrogenase deficiency. *J Pediatr.* 1996;128: 695–697.

134. Kaplan M, Muraca M, Hammerman C, et al. Bilirubin conjugation, reflected by conjugated bilirubin fractions, in glucose-6-phosphate dehydrogenase-deficient neonates: a determining factor in the pathogenesis of hyperbilirubinemia. *Pediatrics.* 1998;102:E37.

135. Kaplan M, Renbaum P, Levy-Lahad E, et al. Gilbert syndrome and glucose-6-phosphate dehydrogenase deficiency: a dose-dependent genetic interaction crucial to neonatal hyperbilirubinemia. *Proc Natl Acad Sci U S A.* 1997;94:12128–12132.

136. Kaplan M, Muraca M, Vreman HJ, et al. Neonatal bilirubin production–conjugation imbalance: effect of glucose-6-phosphate dehydrogenase deficiency and borderline prematurity. *Arch Dis Child Fetal Neonatal Ed.* 2005;90:F123–F127.

137. Kaplan M, Hammerman C, Feldman R, Brisk R. Predischarge bilirubin screening in glucose-6-phosphate dehydrogenase-deficient neonates. *Pediatrics.* 2000;105: 533–537.

138. Beutler E. A series of new screening procedures for pyruvate kinase deficiency, glucose-6-phosphate dehydrogenase deficiency, and glutathione reductase deficiency. *Blood.* 1966;28:553–562.

139. Beutler E, Blume KG, Kaplan JC, et al. International Committee for Standardization in Haematology: recommended screening test for glucose-6-phosphate dehydrogenase (G-6-PD) deficiency. *Br J Haematol.* 1979;43:465–467.

140. Kaplan M, Hoyer JD, Herschel M, Hammerman C, Stevenson DK. Glucose-6-phosphate dehydrogenase activity in term and near-term, male African American neonates. *Clin Chim Acta.* 2005;355:113–117.

141. Kaplan M, Leiter C, Hammerman C, Rudensky B. Enzymatic activity in glucose-6-phosphate dehydrogenase-normal and -deficient neonates measured with a commercial kit. *Clin Chem.* 1995;41:1665–1667.

142. Fairbanks VF, Fernandez MN. The identification of metabolic errors associated with hemolytic anemia. *JAMA.* 1969;208:316–320.

143. Lin Z, Fontaine JM, Freer DE, Naylor EW. Alternative DNA-based newborn screening for glucose-6-phosphate dehydrogenase deficiency. *Mol Genet Metab.* 2005;86:212–219.

144. Kaplan M, Beutler E, Vreman HJ, et al. Neonatal hyperbilirubinemia in glucose-6-phosphate dehydrogenase-deficient heterozygotes. *Pediatrics.* 1999;104:68–74.

145. Kaplan M, Hammerman C, Vreman HJ, Stevenson DK, Beutler E. Acute hemolysis and severe neonatal hyperbilirubinemia in glucose-6-phosphate dehydrogenase-deficient heterozygotes. *J Pediatr.* 2001;139: 137–140.

146. Herschel M, Ryan M, Gelbart T, Kaplan M. Hemolysis and hyperbilirubinemia in an African American neonate heterozygous for glucose-6-phosphate dehydrogenase deficiency. *J Perinatol.* 2002;22:577–579.

147. Herschel M, Beutler E. Low glucose-6-phosphate dehydrogenase enzyme activity level at the time of hemolysis in a male neonate with the African type of deficiency. *Blood Cells Mol Dis.* 2001;27:918–923.

148. Kaplan M, Hammerman C. The need for neonatal glucose-6-phosphate dehydrogenase screening: a global perspective. *J Perinatol.* 2009;29(suppl 1):S46–S52.

149. Kaplan M, Hammerman C. Neonatal screening for glucose-6-phosphate dehydrogenase deficiency: biochemical vs. genetic technologies. *Semin Perinatol.* 2011;35:155–161.

150. Missiou-Tsagaraki S. Screening for glucose-6-phosphate dehydrogenase deficiency as a preventive measure: prevalence among 1,286,000 Greek newborn infants. *J Pediatr.* 1991;119:293–299; Missiou-Tsagaraki S. Reply. *J Pediatr.* 1992;12:166.

151. Mallouh AA, Imseeh G, Abu-Osba YK, Hamdan JA. Screening for glucose-6-phosphate dehydrogenase deficiency can prevent severe neonatal jaundice. *Ann Trop Paediatr.* 1992;12:391–395.

152. Padilla CD, Therrell BL. Newborn screening in the Asia Pacific region. *J Inherit Metab Dis.* 2007;30:490–506.

153. Joseph R, Ho LY, Gomez JM, et al. Mass newborn screening for glucose-6-phosphate dehydrogenase deficiency in Singapore. *Southeast Asian J Trop Med Public Health.* 1999;30(suppl 2):70–71.

154. Hsiao K-J, Chiang SH, Chang TT, Liew DG, Chao YY. Experience of neonatal G6PD deficiency screening in Taiwan. In: Wilcken B, Webster D, eds. *Neonatal Screening in the Nineties.* Leura, NSW: The Kelvin Press; 1991:217–218.

155. *A StakeHolders Conference to Determine the Feasibility of G6PD Deficiency Identification for Prevention of Severe Neonatal Hyperbilirubinemia.* Sponsored by the National Newborn Screening and Genetics Resource Center at the University of Texas, Health Science Center, San Antonio; July 2009; Bethesda, MD.

156. American College of Medical Genetics. Newborn screening: towards a uniform screening panel and system. *Genet Med.* 2006;8:S12–S52.

157. American College of Obstetricians and Gynecologists Committee on Genetics. Committee opinion no. 481: newborn screening. *Obstet Gynecol.* 2011;117:762–765.

158. Fetus and Newborn Committee, Canadian Paediatric Society. Guidelines for detection, management and prevention of hyperbilirubinemia in term and late preterm newborn infants (35 or more weeks' gestation)—summary. *Paediatr Child Health.* 2007;12: 401–407.

159. Hansen TW, Nietsch L, Norman E, et al. Reversibility of acute intermediate phase bilirubin encephalopathy. *Acta Paediatr.* 2009;98:1689–1694.

160. Harris MC, Bernbaum JC, Polin JR, Zimmerman R, Polin RA. Developmental follow-up of breastfed term and near-term infants with marked hyperbilirubinemia. *Pediatrics.* 2001;107:1075–1080.

161. Zanella A, Bianchi P, Fermo E. Pyruvate kinase deficiency. *Haematologica.* 2007;92:721–723.

162. Beutler E, Gelbart T. Estimating the prevalence of pyruvate kinase deficiency from the gene frequency in the general white population. *Blood.* 2000;95:3585–3588.

163. Glader B. Hereditary hemolytic anemias due to red blood cell enzyme disorders. In: Greer JP, Foerster J, Rodgers GM, et al., eds. *Wintrobe's Clinical Hematology.* Philadelphia: Lippincott Williams & Wilkins; 2009: 942–944.

164. Mentzer WC. Pyruvate kinase deficiency and disorders of glycolysis. In: Nathan DG, Orkin SH, eds. *Nathan and Oski's Hematology of Infancy and Childhood.* Philadelphia: WB Saunders Company; 1998:665–703.

165. Christensen RD, Eggert LD, Baer VL, Smith KN. Pyruvate kinase deficiency as a cause of extreme hyperbilirubinemia in neonates from a polygamist community. *J Perinatol.* 2010;30:233–236.

166. Oski FA, Nathan DG, Sidel VW, Diamond LK. Extreme hemolysis and red-cell distortion in erythrocyte pyruvate kinase deficiency. *N Engl J Med.* 1964;270: 1023–1030.

167. Bianchi P, Zanella A. Hematologically important mutations: red cell pyruvate kinase (third update). *Blood Cells Mol Dis.* 2000;26:47–53.

168. Iolascon A, Miraglia del Giudice E, Perrotta S, et al. Hereditary spherocytosis: from clinical to molecular defects. *Haematologica.* 1998;83:240–257.

169. Steiner LA, Gallagher PG. Erythrocyte disorders in the perinatal period. *Semin Perinatol.* 2007;31:254–261.

170. Perrotta S, Gallagher PG, Mohandas N. Hereditary spherocytosis. *Lancet.* 2008;372:1411–1426.

171. Eber SW, Pekrun A, Neufeldt A, Schroter W. Prevalence of increased osmotic fragility of erythrocytes in German blood donors: screening using a modified glycerol lysis test. *Ann Hematol.* 1992;64:88–92.

172. Godal HC, Heisto H. High prevalence of increased osmotic fragility of red blood cells among Norwegian blood donors. *Scand J Hematol.* 1981;27:30–34.

173. Iolascon A, Avvisati RA, Piscopo C. Hereditary spherocytosis. *Transfus Clin Biol.* 2010;17:138–142.

174. Del Giudice E, Perrotta S, Nobili B, et al. Coinheritance of Gilbert syndrome increases the risk for developing gallstones in children affected with hereditary spherocytosis. *Blood.* 1999;94:2259–2262.

175. Iolascon A, Avvisati RA. Genotype/phenotype correlation in hereditary spherocytosis. *Haematologica.* 2008;93: 1283–1288.

176. Christensen RD, Henry E. Hereditary spherocytosis in neonates with hyperbilirubinemia. *Pediatrics.* 2010;125: 120–125.

177. King MJ, Behrens J, Rogers C, et al. Rapid flow cytometric test for the diagnosis of membrane cytoskeleton associated haemolytic anaemia. *Br J Haematol.* 2000;111:924–933.

178. Eber SW, Armbrust R, Schröter W. Variable clinical severity of hereditary spherocytosis: relation to erythrocytic spectrin concentration, osmotic fragility, and autohemolysis. *J Pediatr.* 1990;117:409–416.

179. Delhommeau F, Cynober T, Schischmanoff PO, et al. Natural history of hereditary spherocytosis during the first year of life. *Blood.* 2000;95:393–397.

180. Schroter W, Kahsnitz E. Diagnosis of hereditary spherocytosis in newborn infants. *J Pediatr.* 1983;103: 460–463.

181. Whitfield CF, Follweiler JB, Lopresti-Morrow L, Miller BA. Deficiency of alpha-spectrin synthesis in burst-forming units—erythroid in lethal hereditary spherocytosis. *Blood.* 1991;78:3043–3051.

182. Iolascon A, Perrotta S, Stewart GW. Red blood cell membrane defects. *Rev Clin Exp Hematol.* 2003;7:1–35.

183. Berardi A, Lugli L, Ferrari F, et al. Kernicterus associated with hereditary spherocytosis and UGT1A1 promoter polymorphism. *Biol Neonate.* 2006;90:243–246.

184. Gallagher PG, Weed SA, Tse WT, et al. Recurrent fatal hydrops fetalis associated with a nucleotide substitution in the erythrocyte beta-spectrin gene. *J Clin Invest.* 1995;95:1174–1178.

185. Gallagher PG, Petruzzi MJ, Weed SA, et al. Mutation of a highly conserved residue of beta spectrin associated with fatal and near-fatal neonatal hemolytic anemia. *J Clin Invest.* 1997;99:267–277.

186. Zarkowsky HS, Mohandas N, Speaker CB, Shohet SB. A congenital haemolytic anaemia with thermal sensitivity of the erythrocyte membrane. *Br J Haematol.* 1975;4:537–543.

187. Delaunay J, Stewart G, Iolascon A. Hereditary dehydrated and overhydrated stomatocytosis: recent advances. *Curr Opin Hematol.* 1999;6:110–114.

188. Grootenboer-Mignot S, Cretien A, Laurendeau I, et al. Sub-lethal hydrops as a manifestation of dehydrated hereditary stomatocytosis in two consecutive pregnancies. *Prenat Diagn.* 2003;23:380–384.

189. Kutlar F. Diagnostic approach to hemoglobinopathies. *Hemoglobin.* 2007;31:243–250.

190. Murray NA, Roberts IA. Haemolytic disease of the newborn. *Arch Dis Child Fetal Neonatal Ed.* 2007;92: F83–F88.

191. Lee-Potter JP, Deacon-Smith RA, Simpkiss MJ, Kamuzora H, Lehmann H. A new cause of haemolytic anaemia in the newborn. A description of an unstable fetal haemoglobin: F Poole, alpha2-G-gamma2 130 trptophan yeilds glycine. *J Clin Pathol.* 1975;28:317–320.

192. Levine R, Lincoln DR, Buchholz WM, Gribble JT, Schwartz HC. Hemoglobin Hasharon in a premature infant with hemolytic anemia. *Pediatr Res.* 1975;9: 7–11.

193. Bosma PJ, Chowdhury JR, Bakker C, et al. The genetic basis of the reduced expression of bilirubin UDP-glucuronosyltransferase 1 in Gilbert's syndrome. *N Engl J Med.* 1995;333:1171–1175.

194. Monaghan G, Ryan M, Seddon R, Hume R, Burchell B. Genetic variation in bilirubin UPD-glucuronosyltransferase gene promoter and Gilbert's syndrome. *Lancet.* 1996;347:578–581.

195. Beutler E, Gelbart T, Demina A. Racial variability in the UDP-glucuronosyltransferase 1 (UGT1A1) promoter: a balanced polymorphism for regulation of bilirubin metabolism? *Proc Natl Acad Sci U S A.* 1998;95: 8170–8174.

196. Kaplan M, Slusher T, Renbaum P, et al. (TA)n UDP-glucuronosyltransferase 1A1 promoter polymorphism in Nigerian neonates. *Pediatr Res.* 2008;63:109–111.

197. Huang CS, Luo GA, Huang MJ, Yu SC, Yang SS. Variations of the bilirubin uridine-diphosphoglucuronosyl transferase 1A1 gene in healthy Taiwanese. *Pharmacogenetics.* 2000;10:539–544.

198. Maruo Y, Nishizawa K, Sato H, Doida Y, Shimada M. Association of neonatal hyperbilirubinemia with bilirubin UDP-glucuronosyltransferase polymorphism. *Pediatrics.* 1999;103:1224–1227.

199. Maruo Y, Nishizawa K, Sato H, Sawa H, Shimada M. Prolonged unconjugated hyperbilirubinemia associated with breast milk and mutations of the bilirubin uridine diphosphate glucuronosyltransferase gene. *Pediatrics.* 2000;106:1127.

200. Huang CS, Chang PF, Huang MJ, et al. Relationship between bilirubin UDP-glucuronosyl transferase 1A1 gene and neonatal hyperbilirubinemia. *Pediatr Res.* 2002;52:601–605.

201. Huang CS, Chang PF, Huang MJ, Chen ES, Chen WC. Glucose-6-phosphate dehydrogenase deficiency, the UDP-glucuronosyl transferase 1A1 gene, and

neonatal hyperbilirubinemia. *Gastroenterology*. 2002;123: 127–133.

202. Kaplan M, Renbaum P, Vreman HJ, et al. (TA)*n* UGT 1A1 promoter polymorphism: a crucial factor in the pathophysiology of jaundice in G-6-PD deficient neonates. *Pediatr Res*. 2007;61:727–731.

203. Sanna S, Busonero F, Maschio A, et al. Common variants in the SLCO1B3 locus are associated with bilirubin levels and unconjugated hyperbilirubinemia. *Hum Mol Genet*. 2009;18:2711–2718.

204. Lin Z, Fontaine J, Watchko JF. Coexpression of gene polymorphisms involved in bilirubin production and metabolism. *Pediatrics*. 2008;122:e156–e162.

205. Watchko JF, Lin Z, Clark RH, et al. Complex multifactorial nature of significant hyperbilirubinemia in neonates. *Pediatrics*. 2009;124:e868–e877.

206. Iolascon A, Faienza MF, Moretti A, Perrotta S, Miraglia del Giudice E. UGT1 promoter polymorphism accounts for increased neonatal appearance of hereditary spherocytosis. *Blood*. 1998;91:1093.

Prevention, Screening, and Postnatal Management of Neonatal Hyperbilirubinemia

M. Jeffrey Maisels and Thomas B. Newman

■ INTRODUCTION

As noted in several other chapters in this book, bilirubin encephalopathy and kernicterus are still occurring throughout the world with population-based estimates of incidence in North America and Europe ranging from 0.5 to 2.4 cases per 100,000 live births[1] (Table 9-1). In contrast to the early clinical case descriptions, most of the infants who now develop kernicterus are not those with Rh disease and they often have no documented evidence of hemolytic disease.[9] Many are term and late preterm infants who have been discharged from the nursery as "healthy newborns," yet have returned to a pediatrician's office, a clinic, or an emergency department with total serum bilirubin (TSB) levels often exceeding 30 mg/dL[9]—and have gone on to develop the classic neurodevelopmental findings associated with kernicterus.[10] There is also a smaller group of infants, more difficult to identify, who suffer an unanticipated precipitous increase in the TSB while still in the hospital or soon after discharge and present with acute bilirubin encephalopathy.[9,11,12] Glucose-6-phosphate dehydrogenase (G6PD) deficiency is an important cause of the hyperbilirubinemia in some of these infants.[9,12]

The American Academy of Pediatrics (AAP) in 2004[10] and the Canadian Paediatric Society in 2007[13] published guidelines on the management of hyperbilirubinemia in the newborn infant 35 or more weeks of gestation, and

similar, consensus-based guidelines have been published recently in Israel, Norway, and the United Kingdom.[14–16] The key elements of the AAP guideline are listed in Table 9-2 and, although a recent commentary[17] has provided some important modifications to these guidelines, the basic principles still apply.

In this chapter, we describe an approach to newborn infants in the well-baby nursery that is designed to help clinicians identify and manage the jaundiced newborn, intervene when appropriate, and prevent bilirubin-induced brain damage.

■ PHYSIOLOGIC AND PATHOLOGIC JAUNDICE

Because at some point during the first week almost every newborn has a TSB level that exceeds 1 mg/dL—the upper limit of normal for an adult—and approximately four of five newborns are jaundiced to the clinician's eye,[18] this type of transient bilirubinemia has been called "physiologic jaundice." When TSB levels exceed the 95th percentile for the infant's age in hours,[19] the infant is often described as having "hyperbilirubinemia" or "pathologic jaundice," a distinction that is arbitrary and not particularly helpful, as discussed below. Presumably, physiologic jaundice should apply to newborns whose TSB levels fall within a certain range but, as noted in Chapter 6, defining the normal serum bilirubin level in every population

■ TABLE 9-1. Population-Based Estimates of Kernicterus Incidence

Author(s)	Country	Years	Ascertainment Case Definition	No. of Cases	Denominator	Rate
Bjerre and Ebbesen[2]	Denmark	1994–2002	Registry; voluntary reports; ≥35 weeks gestation; TSB ≥31.1 mg/dL; symptoms of chronic bilirubin encephalopathy	8	576,000	1.4/100,000
Bjerre et al.[3]	Denmark	1994–2002	National laboratory information system linked to medical reports; ≥35 weeks gestation and ≤28 days of age; TSB ≥26.5 mg/dL and advanced phase symptoms of bilirubin encephalopathy	1	249,308[a]	0.4/100,000[a]
Manning et al.[4]	United Kingdom	2003–2005	Voluntary reports; ≥35 weeks gestation and <1 month of age; TSB ≥30 mg/dL; death or postmortem examination or typical sequelae at 12-month follow-up	7	1,500,052	0.46/100,000
Sgro et al.[5]	Canada	2002–2004	Surveillance program; voluntary reports; ≥35 weeks gestation and ≤60 days of age TSB ≥25 mg/dL and/or exchange transfusion and clinically important neurologic abnormalities at final discharge	13	640,000	2/100,000
Sgro et al.[6]	Canada	2007–2008	Surveillance program; voluntary reports; any child up to 6 years old; ≥35 weeks gestation at birth; TSB ≥25 mg/dL or exchange transfusion and two or more signs/symptoms of kernicterus; or abnormal MRI with history of hyperbilirubinemia	22	900,000	2.4/100,000
Burke et al.[7]	United States	1988–2005	Hospital discharge abstracts; ≤30 days of age; ICD-9 for kernicterus and CPT for phototherapy or exchange transfusion	436	Not stated	2.7/100,000
Brooks et al.[8]	California	1988–1997	State registry for developmental services; ICD-9 for kernicterus	25	5,697,147	0.49/100,000

Abbreviations: TSB, total serum bilirubin; MRI, magnetic resonance imaging; ICD-9, *International Statistical Classification of Diseases—Ninth Revision*; CPT, Current Procedural Terminology.

[a]Denominator is dependent on whether or not patients lost to follow-up are counted and/or considered to have kernicterus. If only patients followed up are counted in denominator (69,806), calculated incidence would be 1.4/100,000.

Reproduced from Burgos AE, Flaherman VJ, Newman TB. Screening and follow-up for neonatal hyperbilirubinemia: a review. *Clin Pediatr (Phila).* 2012;51(1):7–16. Copyright © 2012. Reprinted by Permission of SAGE Publications.

■ TABLE 9-2. Key Elements in the AAP Guideline on Management of Hyperbilirubinemia in the Newborn Infant 35 or More Weeks of Gestation

1. Promote and support successful breastfeeding
2. Establish nursery protocols for the identification and evaluation of hyperbilirubinemia
3. Measure the total serum bilirubin (TSB) or transcutaneous bilirubin (TcB) level on infants jaundiced in the first 24 h
4. Recognize that visual estimation of the degree of jaundice can lead to errors, particularly in darkly pigmented infants
5. Interpret all bilirubin levels according to the infant's age in hours
6. Recognize that infants at less than 38 weeks gestation, particularly those who are breastfed, are at higher risk of developing hyperbilirubinemia and require closer surveillance and monitoring
7. Perform a systematic assessment on all infants before discharge for the risk of severe hyperbilirubinemia
8. Provide parents with written and verbal information about newborn jaundice
9. Provide appropriate follow-up based on the time of discharge and the risk assessment
10. Treat newborns, when indicated, with phototherapy or exchange transfusion

Reproduced from American Academy of Pediatrics, Subcommittee on Hyperbilirubinemia. Clinical practice guideline: management of hyperbilirubinemia in the newborn infant 35 or more weeks of gestation. *Pediatrics.* 2004;114:297–316. Copyright 2004 by the American Academy of Pediatrics.

---

is not easy. Furthermore, in many infants in whom the bilirubin level clearly exceeds the 95th or even the 99th percentile, a battery of tests yields no identifiable pathology.[20,21] Finally, interpreting bilirubin levels in the newborn provides a unique challenge because these levels change hourly for the first week or more, so that meaningful interpretation of TSB levels can only be made in relationship to the infant's age in hours.[10]

Defining a Normal Bilirubin Value

Sackett et al.[22] discuss the question of how to define the term "normal" and provide six different definitions of this term. The definition depends on why we are asking the question. In term and late preterm newborns, the most practical way of describing normal bilirubin levels is to use hour-specific percentiles,[19,23–25] but this cannot be used in more premature infants. If untreated, low birth weight infants have exaggerated and prolonged hyperbilirubinemia and because this occurs in all preterm infants, it might be considered physiologic. But in these infants, TSB levels well within the "physiologic range" are potentially hazardous[26,27] and are treated with phototherapy (see Chapter 10). Thus, today, the natural history of bilirubinemia in the very low birth weight infant is never observed and population-based norms cannot be applied to these infants. A TSB level of 10 mg/dL on day 4 in a 750-g neonate requires no investigation to identify a cause for the jaundice. Nevertheless, almost all neonatologists

would treat this infant with phototherapy, because it is believed that treatment is much more likely to do good than harm.[15,16,28] The TSB level of 10 mg/dL in this infant can be said to exceed a "therapeutic normal" level, defined by Sackett et al. as a "range of test results beyond which therapy does more good than harm."[22]

The therapeutic normal level is also sometimes defined as an "operational" level for purposes of intervention.[22] The recommendations of the AAP[10] for the use of phototherapy and exchange transfusion in term and late preterm newborns are examples of the use of operational levels. The AAP recommends using phototherapy in a well term infant if the TSB level is ~15 mg/dL at age 48 hours. Although a level of 15 mg/dL poses no imminent threat to the infant's well-being, at that age it is well above the 95th percentile[19] and, if left untreated, might increase to a level that is dangerous to the infant. The suggested intervention, phototherapy, is believed to be safe and effective and, under these circumstances, more likely to do good than harm.

Terminology

We suggest that the terms physiologic and pathologic jaundice should be abandoned and instead "neonatal bilirubinemia" should be used. If we can agree on the terminology, then we should be able to agree on other descriptors for different TSB levels in term and late preterm infants. Others have suggested descriptors that are appropriate for different degrees of hyperbilirubinemia[9] and it would be helpful to develop an approved common terminology so that terms such as "severe hyperbilirubinemia" have the same meaning for all clinicians. In term and late preterm infants, we suggest that hyperbilirubinemia is the appropriate term for a TSB level that exceeds the 95th percentile for the infant's age in hours in that population.[19] After 96 hours, TSB levels >20 mg/dL might be called severe hyperbilirubinemia and those >25 or 30 mg/dL extreme hyperbilirubinemia.

■ PRIMARY PREVENTION

Screening for Isoimmunization

All pregnant women should be tested for ABO and Rh (D) blood type and undergo a serum screen for unusual immune antibodies.[10] If such prenatal testing has not been performed, then a direct antibody test (DAT or direct Coombs), blood group, and Rh (D) type on the infant's cord blood should be done. Identification of Rh-negative mothers is important because they require anti-D gamma-globulin to prevent Rh (D) sensitization. In infants of group O Rh-positive mothers, routine testing for blood type and DAT is optional provided there is appropriate surveillance and risk assessment before discharge and follow-up[10] so that significantly jaundiced infants are not missed.

■ PREVENTING HYPERBILIRUBINEMIA

Ensuring Successful Breastfeeding

The first of 10 key elements in the AAP guidelines (Table 9-2) notes that clinicians should "promote and support successful breastfeeding," although exclusive breastfeeding is associated with an increased risk of hyperbilirubinemia[30–32] (see Chapter 6). In many, but not all, cases of severe hyperbilirubinemia in breastfed infants, poor caloric intake as a result of less effective breastfeeding (and manifested by increased weight loss) appears to play an important role.[20,33–35] Although hypernatremic dehydration associated within inadequate breastfeeding is a well-known phenomenon,[36] by itself, dehydration does not provide a plausible mechanism for severe hyperbilirubinemia. It is much more likely that in breastfed, dehydrated infants, it is the caloric deprivation and its effect on the enterohepatic circulation of bilirubin (see Chapter 6) that is primarily responsible for the hyperbilirubinemia.[37–39]

Currently, the only primary preventive intervention available that can mitigate the development of hyperbilirubinemia in exclusively breastfed infants is to provide appropriate lactation support to ensure that breastfeeding is successful.[40,41] A recommended first step is to ask mothers to nurse their infants at least 8–12 times per day for the first several days[42] because increasing the frequency of nursing significantly decreases the likelihood of subsequent hyperbilirubinemia.[40,41,43] Evidence for adequate intake in the breastfed infant includes four to six wet diapers in 24 hours by day 3 accompanied by changes in stool color.[44] By the fourth to fifth day, stools in an infant who is nursing well should have changed from meconium to mustard-colored, seedy stools.[44,45]

Unsupplemented breastfed infants experience their maximum weight loss by day 3 and, on average, lose $6.1 \pm 2.5\%$ (SD) of their birth weight.[34,40,46–51] Thus, approximately 5–10% of exclusively breastfed infants lose 10% or more of their birth weight by day 3. The adequacy of milk production and transfer should be evaluated and the infant monitored if the weight loss is greater than 7–10%.[44,52]

■ IDENTIFYING THE JAUNDICED NEWBORN

All infants should be monitored clinically for the development of jaundice in the nursery and protocols established for assessing the jaundiced newborn.[10] Detection of jaundice is enhanced by blanching the skin with digital pressure, thus revealing the underlying color of the skin and subcutaneous tissue. It is important for this assessment to be done in a well-lit room and preferably in daylight at a window.

Nursing Protocols

The AAP recommends that protocols for assessing jaundice should include the circumstances in which a nurse can order a TSB measurement without a physician's order.[10] The nurse should order a TSB level in any infant who appears jaundiced before age 24 hours.[53] If routine transcutaneous bilirubin (TcB) monitoring is used, the policy should indicate the TcB level (in relation to the infant's age in hours) that calls for a TSB measurement. Examples include requiring a TSB if the TcB exceeds the 95th percentile on a TcB nomogram[25] or the 75th percentile on the Bhutani nomogram[19] (Figure 9-1).

Visual Estimates of Jaundice

Cephalocaudal Progression of Jaundice
For reasons that are, as yet, unexplained, dermal icterus is usually seen first in the face and then progresses in a

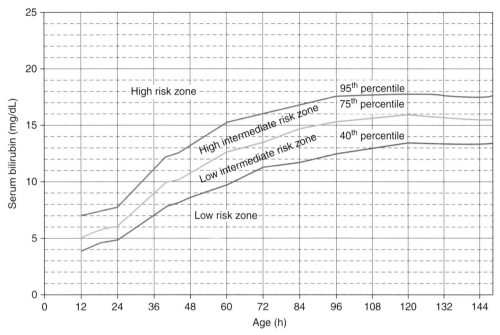

FIGURE 9-1. Nomogram for designation of risk in 2840 well newborns at ≥36 weeks gestational age with birth weight of ≥2000 g or ≥35 weeks gestational age and birth weight of ≥2500 g based on the hour-specific serum bilirubin values. The serum bilirubin level was obtained before discharge and the zone in which the value fell predicted the likelihood of a subsequent bilirubin level exceeding the 95th percentile. Note that because of sampling bias,[109] this nomogram should not be used to represent the natural history of neonatal hyperbilirubinemia. (Reproduced from Bhutani VK, Johnson L, Sivieri EM. Predictive ability of a predischarge hour-specific serum bilirubin for subsequent significant hyperbilirubinemia in healthy-term and near-term newborns. *Pediatrics.* 1999;103:6–14, with permission. Copyright 1999 by the American Academy of Pediatrics.)

caudal manner to the trunk and extremities so that, for a given bilirubin level, the skin of the face will appear more yellow than that of the foot.[54] Although the cephalocaudal progression of jaundice has been confirmed repeatedly with visual assessment as well as by transcutaneous bilirubinometry,[54–61] there is considerable overlap in the ranges of TSB levels corresponding to each of the dermal zones.[54] Nevertheless, several studies suggest that more than 95% of newborns with TSB levels of ≥12 mg/dL will have jaundice below the level of the nipples, although this is also seen in many infants with lower TSB levels.[55,57,62]

On the other hand, an infant might have a TSB of 8 or 9 mg/dL at age 24 hours, a value that is above the 95th percentile[19] (Figure 9-1), yet show no sign of jaundice,[63] producing a false sense of security when further evaluation and early follow-up are required (see sections "Risk Assessment" and "Follow-Up"). Estimates of TSB levels (from physical examination by observers who have had various levels of training) and measured TSB levels have produced

correlation coefficients of 0.4–0.7, but these studies have included mostly newborns with TSB levels of 12–15 mg/dL or less and have not directly addressed how frequently TSB levels high enough to warrant treatment at older ages would be missed.[18,55,62,64,65] Darker skin pigmentation also makes visual assessment of jaundice more difficult.[62,66]

Before infants are discharged from the hospital, the TSB levels that require additional investigation, initiation of phototherapy, or closer follow-up are quite low[10] and visual estimation at these TSB levels is not sufficiently accurate to allow these decisions to be made with confidence. Certainly, any newborn who appears jaundiced in the first 24 hours should have a TSB measured,[10,53] and a recent consensus-based commentary recommends measurement of TcB or TSB in all infants prior to discharge.[17] Some experts, and the recently published NICE guideline,[16] recommend measurement of a TcB or TSB level in all jaundiced infants regardless of age but, in older infants with mild jaundice, we believe there is room for clinical judgment.

■ TRANSCUTANEOUS BILIRUBIN MEASUREMENTS

When light is transmitted to the skin, the yellowness of the reflected light can be measured to provide an objective measurement of skin color, and these principles have been applied to predict TSB levels from skin reflectance[67,68] using easily portable transcutaneous bilirubinometers.[69–71] Currently available devices marketed in the United States include the Draeger JM-103 (Draeger Medical, Hatboro, PA)[69] and the BiliChek (Philips Children's Medical Ventures, Monroeville, PA).[70,71] Although these instruments use different algorithms and measurement techniques, the operating principles are similar. The details of how these bilirubinometers work have been described in Chapter 3 and we will deal here with a few clinically relevant issues.

TcB measurements have been evaluated in hospital nurseries[18,25,72] and outpatient settings.[73,74] They have the advantage of providing instantaneous information as well as reducing the likelihood that a clinically significant TSB will be missed.[75] TcB measurements correlate quite closely with TSB measurements and are generally within 2–3 mg/dL of the TSB,[71,76,77] although they are not a substitute for TSB values. The TcB is a measurement of the yellow color of the blanched skin and subcutaneous tissues, not the serum bilirubin, and should be used as a screening tool to help determine whether the TSB should be measured. TcB measurements can significantly reduce the number of TSB measurements needed in both the term nursery and the NICU.[78–80] They help to estimate the risk of subsequent hyperbilirubinemia[18,30] and they are invaluable in the outpatient setting.[73,74] Because they are noninvasive, TcB measurements can be repeated several times during the birth hospitalization and provide useful information about the rate of rise of the bilirubin. When plotted on a nomogram (Figure 9-1), TcB levels that are crossing percentiles indicate the need for additional observation and evaluation.

Factors Affecting TcB Measurements

Skin Pigmentation and Gestation
Large studies of both the BiliChek and the JM-103 have shown good correlation between TcB and TSB measurements in diverse populations.[25,69,71,81,82] The JM-103 tends to overestimate TSB measurements in darkly pigmented infants. As TcB measurements are used as a screening tool,

this does not increase the risk of missing an elevated TSB, but will increase the number of unnecessary TSB measurements. The effect of skin tone on the performance of the JM-103 has been studied by Wainer et al.[83] The highest precision and lowest bias were observed for medium skin toned infants. There was a tendency to underread the TSB in the lighter skin tone group and to overread it in the darker skin tone group. Nevertheless, the JM-103 performed well as a screening device in all skin tone groups.[83]

Preterm and Low Birth Weight Infants
Although some studies have suggested that TcB measurements in infants <1000 g or 28 weeks of gestation are less reliable,[84] others have not found this to be the case.[80,85,86] Several studies have demonstrated the utility of TcB measurements in both LBW and ELBW infants in the NICU.[77,80,84–88] In all of these studies, screening infants with TcB measurements using different cutoff values identified with appropriate accuracy infants who required a TSB measurement or phototherapy.

Effect of TSB Level
TcB measurements are less accurate and tend to underestimate the TSB at higher TSB levels.[72,80,89–91] Thus, as the TSB increases, the number of false-negative TcBs also increases.[30,83] If appropriate cutoff values are used, however, TcB measurements still work well as a screening device even at TSB levels of >15 mg/dL.[74,83]

Clinical Application of TcB Measurements
Because variation among instruments can occur, the accuracy of the TcB instrument should be compared with laboratory TSB values before it can be relied upon as a screening tool. A TSB level should always be obtained when therapeutic intervention is being considered. Because the TcB tends to underestimate the TSB at higher TSB levels,[75] investigators have adopted various techniques to avoid missing a high TSB level (i.e., a false-negative TSB measurement). These techniques include measuring the TSB if:

- The TcB value is at 70% of the TSB level recommended for the use of phototherapy.[80]
- The TcB value is above the high-intermediate risk line on the Bhutani nomogram (Figure 9-1)[19] or the 95th percentile on a TcB nomogram.[25] In one study, if the TcB was <75th percentile on the Bhutani

nomogram, 0 of 349 infants had a TSB level above the 95th percentile (a negative predictive value of 100%).[71,92]

- At follow-up after discharge, the TcB value is >13 mg/dL.[73,74] In two outpatient studies, no infant who had a TcB value ≤13 mg/dL had a TSB value of >17 mg/dL.[73,74]

TcB measurements are very helpful in the outpatient setting,[73,74] but the price of these instruments has deterred practicing physicians from purchasing them. Ultimately, one might anticipate that TcB measurements will become as indispensable in the care of the jaundiced newborn as pulse oximetry is in assessing oxygen saturation in the newborn infant, or the asthmatic child.

Effect of Phototherapy on TcB Measurements

Because phototherapy bleaches the skin, both visual assessments of jaundice and TcB measurements in infants undergoing phototherapy are not reliable. If an area of the skin is covered during phototherapy, however, TcB measurements in that area can be used to monitor the response to phototherapy.[93,94]

Site of Sampling

Instructions for the use of the BiliChek and JM-103 recommend obtaining TcB measurements from the forehead or the sternum. When JM-103 measurements from the forehead and sternum were compared with TSB measurements in 475 infants, the Pearson correlation coefficients were higher for the sternum (0.953) than those for the forehead (0.914).[80] Because the forehead is exposed to ambient light, both in the nursery and following discharge, while the sternum is almost always covered, measurements from the sternum are probably a better choice. In a study of 31 infants comparing outpatient BiliChek measurements from the brow and sternum, brow readings were 20% lower than TSB values, but chest readings were only 5% lower.[95]

■ RISK ASSESSMENT

Clinical Risk Factors

The risk factors for the development of hyperbilirubinemia have been discussed in Chapter 6. Those that are considered to be most relevant for the practicing clinician are listed in Table 9-3. Almost all of these factors can be identified readily without recourse to the laboratory

TABLE 9-3. Risk Factors for the Development of Hyperbilirubinemia in Infants of 35 or More Weeks Gestation

Elevated predischarge TSB or TcB level[18,19,31,101,110,111]

Jaundice observed in the first 24 h[53] or prior to discharge[106,107]

Blood group incompatibility with positive direct antiglobulin test, other known hemolytic disease (e.g., G6PD deficiency, hereditary spherocytosis) (see Chapter 8)

Decreasing gestational age[18,31,105,106]

Previous sibling with jaundice or who received phototherapy[96,97]

Vacuum extraction delivery, cephalohematoma, or significant bruising[31,33,98,101]

Exclusive breastfeeding, particularly if nursing is not going well and weight loss is excessive[30–32,106]

East Asian race[21,31]

Macrosomic infant of a diabetic mother[99,100]

Maternal age ≥25 years[31]

Male gender[9,31]

but, because these risk factors are common and the risk of severe hyperbilirubinemia is small, individually, these factors are of limited use as predictors of severe hyperbilirubinemia. Nevertheless, the more risk factors that are present, the greater the risk of severe hyperbilirubinemia,[18,31,101] and if no risk factors are present, the risk of severe hyperbilirubinemia is extremely low.[18,30,31] Some factors, such as exclusive breastfeeding (discussed in detail in Chapter 6) and decreasing gestational age, seem to be particularly important.[18,30] It is remarkable, for example, that almost every recently described case of kernicterus occurred in a breastfed infant, even when the infant had underlying G6PD deficiency.[35,102–104]

Cephalocaudal Progression

Keren et al.[18] evaluated the cephalocaudal progression in infants prior to hospital discharge to see whether it might predict the likelihood of the infant subsequently developing a TSB exceeding or within 1 mg/dL of the AAP's recommended phototherapy level.[10] In general, the cephalocaudal progression was not helpful but, at extremes (complete absence of any jaundice, or jaundice in the arms and in the legs below the knees), it had some clinical utility.[18] The complete absence of jaundice had a negative predictive value for the subsequent development of significant hyperbilirubinemia of 98.6%. Jaundice in the arms and legs below the knees was strongly associated with the development of significant hyperbilirubinemia (odds ratio [OR] 6.0; 95% CI 2.1–17.0).[18]

Gestation

The most important single clinical risk factor is the infant's gestational age.[18,31,105,106] The association between decreasing gestation and the risk of hyperbilirubinemia has been confirmed consistently in multiple studies, although the magnitude of this risk has only been quantified recently[18,31,105,106] (see Chapter 6). When combined with a predischarge TcB or TSB level, the effect of gestational age becomes even more significant.[18,30,105]

Newman et al. performed a nested case–control study on a population of 51,387 newborns ≥36 weeks gestation[31] and found that the OR for each increasing week of gestation was 0.6 (95% CI 0.4–0.7) and converted this to a "risk index" for predicting a TSB >25 mg/dL. Looked at another way, for each decreasing week of gestation below 40 weeks, the risk of an infant developing a TSB >25 mg/dL increases by a factor of about 1.6. Thus, a 36-week gestation infant is about $1.6^4 = 6.6$ times more likely to develop a TSB >25 mg/dL than a 40-week gestation infant. In the Beaumont Children's Hospital nursery, infants of 35 weeks gestation are 13 times more likely (95% CI 2.7–64.6) to be readmitted for hyperbilirubinemia following discharge than are 40-week infants.[106]

Predischarge Measurement of the Bilirubin Level

We know that infants who are clinically jaundiced in the first few days,[106,107] and particularly those jaundiced in the first 24 hours,[53] are much more likely to later develop significant hyperbilirubinemia. In a study that has had worldwide impact, Bhutani et al.[19] measured TSB concentrations in 13,003 infants prior to their discharge from the hospital. In 2840 infants additional TSB levels were measured at least once in the 5–6 days following discharge. Infants with ABO incompatibility and a positive DAT were excluded, as were Rh-sensitized infants. The investigators plotted the TSB levels against the infant's age in hours and created a nomogram with percentiles that defined the four risk zones illustrated in Figure 9-1. Of infants whose TSB levels fell in the high-risk zone, 39.5% subsequently had values above the 95th percentile (the positive predictive value), while of 1750 infants whose predischarge TSB level was in the low-risk zone, none was observed to have a TSB >95th percentile. (Some of this apparently perfect negative predictive value is probably due to "double gold standard bias"[108]: subjects with high initial TSB levels were more likely to have a repeat TSB, whereas in those with low initial TSB levels, the level was less likely to be checked again and was assumed never to have gotten high.[109]) TSB values in the low-risk zone[19] could also produce a false sense of security leading to inadequate follow-up or failure to obtain a TSB in a jaundiced infant at follow-up. In a recent study, 3/5727 infants with predischarge TcB levels below the 40th percentile (Figure 9-1) were nevertheless subsequently readmitted with a TSB level >17 mg/dL.[30] It is also important to note that Figure 9-1 does not describe the natural history of bilirubinemia in the newborn. Because only 2840 (21.9%) of the 13,003 infants had subsequent TSB levels measured, there is a sampling bias toward more jaundiced babies (those who were jaundiced were, presumably, more likely to return for follow-up), particularly after 48–72 hours, so that the lower-risk zones are spuriously elevated.[109] This nomogram is also not generalizable to other populations.[23,24] Nevertheless, the utility of the nomogram in helping to predict the risk of subsequent TSB and TcB levels has been amply confirmed in several other studies[18,31,101] including those conducted in other populations.[110,111]

The availability of electronic TcB measurements has made it possible to study the natural history of bilirubinemia in contemporary populations and to improve our understanding of bilirubin kinetics. De Luca et al.[112] analyzed four published studies of populations in the United States (one predominately white and another predominately Mexican/Hispanic), Italy, and Thailand. They calculated the "exaggerated rate of rise" (EROR), which was the rate of increase in the TcB needed to cross the percentile curves at different ages in each study, and provided useful information regarding the rate of rise in the TcB level that might require additional monitoring or testing. In general, a rate of rise in the TSB or TcB of more than 0.2 mg/(dL h) in the first 24 hours, 0.15 mg/(dL h) from 25 to 48 hours, and 0.1 mg/(dL h) thereafter indicates the need for careful assessment, surveillance, and, if necessary, additional laboratory investigation.

Combining Gestation with the Predischarge Bilirubin Level

Although studies using clinical risk factors have a predictive accuracy similar to that of the predischarge bilirubin risk zone,[31,101] combining the predischarge TSB or TcB with clinical risk factors improves the prediction of the risk of subsequent hyperbilirubinemia (Table 9-4).[18,30,105] When the predischarge TSB level was ≥95th percentile on the Bhutani nomogram (Figure 9-1),[19] Newman et al.[105] found that a 40-week gestation infant had about a 10% risk of subsequently developing a TSB level >20 mg/dL, while in a 36-week gestation infant, with a similar predischarge TSB level, the risk was about 42%. To be helpful to the practicing physician, a prediction model should be as parsimonious as possible. Combining the predischarge TSB/TcB with the infant's gestation allows a level of positive and negative prediction that is indistinguishable from models that use additional clinical risk factors.[18]

Keren et al., in a prospective study,[18] analyzed the risk of an infant developing a TSB level within or above 1 mg/dL of the hour-specific AAP threshold for phototherapy.[10] They found that infants ≥40 weeks gestation whose predischarge TSB/TcB levels were below the 95th percentile had about a 0.2% (CI 0.005–1.000) risk of subsequently reaching this TSB level while a 35–37 6/7 week infant whose predischarge TSB/TcB is in the 76th to 95th percentile[19] has a 42% risk (CI 32–52) of reaching a similar bilirubin level[18] (Figure 9-2). There is some bias in this assessment, however, because phototherapy thresholds for 35–37 6/7 weeks gestation infants are about 2.5 mg/dL lower than those of 40 weeks gestation infants.[10]

Based on these data, a group of experts[17] now recommends that a TSB or TcB should be performed on every newborn infant, after age 18 hours and prior to discharge. They developed an algorithm that provides recommendations for management and follow-up according to the predischarge bilirubin measurements, the gestational age, and certain risk factors for subsequent hyperbilirubinemia (Figure 9-3). The authors of this algorithm recognize that the quality of the available evidence for recommending universal predischarge screening and the subsequent management as suggested in Figure 9-4 is limited and, in the absence of better evidence, must be based on expert opinion. It is also important to note that neither the efficacy nor cost efficiency of these recommendations has been established

and that the experience of the authors of this algorithm might lead them to be overly conservative.[116] Most published studies of the predictive value of early (predischarge) bilirubin levels have used much lower TSB levels (17–20 mg/dL) as outcome variables,[116,117] whereas the majority of infants who develop kernicterus have TSB levels of 30 mg/dL or higher. Furthermore, both the US Preventive Services Task Force and the Tufts Evidence-Based Practice Center[118,119] agree that we lack sufficient evidence to conclude that the implementation of these recommendations will reduce the risk of kernicterus or improve clinical outcomes. Nevertheless, recent data suggest that predischarge screening can reduce the incidence of TSB levels ≥25 mg/dL[120–122] (Table 9-5). Some of this effect may be the result of improved surveillance and intervention for inadequate lactation and some from increasing the use of phototherapy prior to discharge.[120]

There are other benefits (but also some risks) associated with obtaining a predischarge TSB or TcB level on every newborn. Knowledge of the hour-specific TSB level can alert the pediatrician to the possibility of a problem that was not previously recognized. A TSB level that is above the 95th percentile, or consecutive measurements that show that the TSB levels are crossing percentiles,[112] suggests the need for increased surveillance, a repeat TSB or TcB level in 4–24 hours, and the possibility of further investigation to establish the cause of this TSB level.[10,17] Documenting the rate of rise of the TSB[112] can be helpful in identifying infants at risk for subsequent hyperbilirubinemia or who require further investigation. The risks of universal bilirubin screening include (unnecessary) additional testing and inappropriate use of phototherapy.[17,116,120]

■ FOLLOW-UP

Figure 9-3 provides current recommendations for follow-up based on the bilirubin risk zone, gestational age, and other risk factors. A general rule is that infants discharged at less than age 72 hours should be seen within 2 days of discharge unless there is a very low risk of subsequent hyperbilirubinemia, in which case a later follow-up is appropriate. This follow-up can be provided in an office, clinic, or home by a physician, physician assistant, or nurse. Both written and oral information should be provided to all parents about newborn jaundice and an excellent example of this is the pamphlet "Jaundice and

TABLE 9-4. Studies Examining the Value of Adding Clinical Risk Factors to Bilirubin Levels for the Prediction of Subsequent Hyperbilirubinemia

Author(s)	Measurement Method	Definition of Subsequent Hyperbilirubinemia	Total N Screened	N with Predischarge Bilirubin in High-Risk Zone	N with Subsequent Hyperbilirubinemia	Prediction Using Total Bilirubin Alone	Prediction Using Total Bilirubin Plus Clinical Risk Factors
Newman et al.[105]	Serum	TSB ≥20 mg/dL	5706	1424	270	C = 0.79 for TSB risk zone; C = 0.83 for TSB z-score	C = 0.86 for TSB z-score plus partial clinical risk index (included race, maternal age ≥25 years, scalp injury diagnosis, male gender, and gestational age but not breastfeeding)
Keren et al.[18]	Serum	TSB exceeded or was within 1 mg/dL of AAP phototherapy treatment threshold	751	82	48	C = 0.88 for TSB risk zone	C = 0.96 for TSB risk zone + gestational age and percent weight loss first 2 days
Maisels et al.[30]	Transcutaneous	TSB ≥17 mg/dL	11,456	574	75	C = 0.77 for TcB percentile group	C = 0.89 for TcB plus gestational age and exclusive breastfeeding

Abbreviations: TSB, total serum bilirubin; C, area under receiver operating characteristic curve; TcB, transcutaneous bilirubin; AAP American Academy of Pediatrics.

Reproduced from Burgos AE, Flaherman VJ, Newman TB. Screening and follow-up for neonatal hyperbilirubinemia: a review. *Clin Pediatr (Phila).* 2012;51(1):7–16. Copyright © 2012. Reprinted by Permission of SAGE Publications.

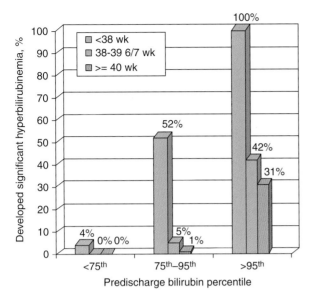

FIGURE 9-2. The probability of an infant developing significant hyperbilirubinemia based on the predischarge TSB or TcB level and the gestational age. Significant hyperbilirubinemia was defined as a TSB level within or above 1 mg/dL of the hour-specific AAP threshold for phototherapy. (Redrawn from data of Keren R, Luan X, Friedman S, Saddlemire S, Cnaan A, Bhutani V. A comparison of alternative risk-assessment strategies for predicting significant neonatal hyperbilirubinemia in term and near-term infants. *Pediatrics.* 2008;121:e170–e179. Available at: http://www.pediatrics.org/cgi/content/full/121/1/e170-e179.)

Your Newborn" published by the AAP (available at www.aap.org/bookstore). The objective is to provide appropriate, balanced information so that parents understand that very high bilirubin levels can be dangerous while they are reassured that the overwhelming majority of jaundiced babies will come to no harm.

It is important to ensure that the provider is contacted if concerning signs arise prior to a scheduled office visit and to ensure that the infant arrives at the scheduled visit. Frequency of breastfeeding, frequency of voiding and stooling, progression of jaundice, and signs of illness can all be monitored by the engaged parent and shared with the provider. At the office visit the provider must assess the percentage change from birth weight and the presence or absence and level of jaundice on examination.

Sunlight Exposure

Exposure of newborns to sunlight will lower the TSB level.[123] Although sunlight provides sufficient irradiance in the 425- to 475-nm band to provide effective phototherapy, the practical difficulties involved in safely exposing a nearly naked newborn to the sun either inside or outside (and avoiding sunburn) preclude the use of sunlight as a reliable therapeutic tool, and it is therefore not recommended by the AAP. On the other hand, in parts of the world where shortages of equipment and electricity preclude consistent and effective use of standard phototherapy devices, the use of sunlight that is filtered to avoid the UV rays is a practical alternative and is currently being investigated in Kenya.[124]

■ HELPING THE PRACTITIONER TO IMPLEMENT GUIDELINES

Effecting change in clinical practice has always been a challenge, but there are a number of tools that have been developed that can assist a practitioner to provide appropriate care for the jaundiced neonate. A Web-based tool, the "BiliTool,"[125] accessible at www.bilitool.org, is a user-friendly, practical (and free) instrument for the management of neonatal jaundice. At the Beaumont Children's Hospital we provide all practitioners with wallet-sized cards that contain the AAP risk factors, the bilirubin nomogram, and the guidelines for the use of phototherapy and exchange transfusion. In addition, the AAP has developed a resource tool kit for both hospitals and physicians to help the practitioner provide appropriate breastfeeding support and manage the jaundiced newborn. This kit, "Safe and Healthy Beginnings," is obtainable from the AAP at www.aap.org.bookstore.

■ PHARMACOLOGIC PREVENTION OF HYPERBILIRUBINEMIA

A number of pharmacologic agents have been investigated for their ability to treat neonatal hyperbilirubinemia but none has yet achieved widespread use[126] (Chapter 10). Tin mesoporphyrin, a potent inhibitor of heme oxygenase, is effective in reducing TSB levels in term and preterm infants and the potential use of this drug to prevent severe hyperbilirubinemia is currently under active investigation.

■ INTERVENTION IN THE BREASTFEEDING JAUNDICED NEWBORN

The practitioner is frequently confronted with a healthy breastfeeding infant whose TSB level is approaching the phototherapy threshold.[10] Two randomized controlled trials have addressed this question.[127,128] In the first, 50 term, breastfed infants, whose TSB levels were ≥15 mg/dL, were randomly assigned to two groups. The first group received phototherapy while breastfeeding was continued and supplemented with 5% glucose water (15 mL/kg per day). In the other group, breastfeeding was discontinued and the infants received formula plus 10% dextrose water instead of phototherapy. There was no difference between the groups in the time it took for the TSB level to fall below 12 mg/dL. In the second study, 125 full-term breastfed infants, whose TSB had reached 17 mg/dL, were randomly assigned to one of four interventions.[129] The outcome variable was the proportion of infants whose TSB levels reached or exceeded 20 mg/dL. The results are shown in Figure 9-4. Discontinuing breastfeeding, temporarily, and using phototherapy was the most effective strategy followed by continuing breastfeeding and using phototherapy.[129] In those not receiving

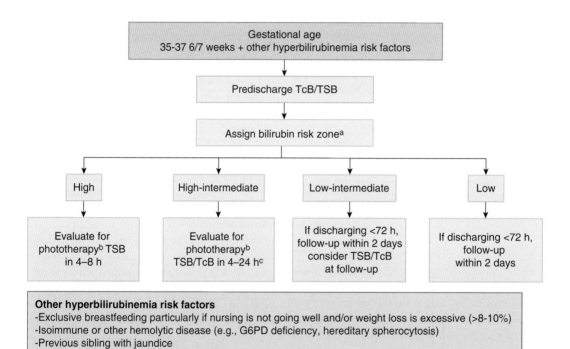

FIGURE 9-3. Algorithm providing recommendations for management and follow-up according to pre-discharge bilirubin measurements, gestation, and risk factors for subsequent hyperbilirubinemia.
[a]Figure 9-1; [b]see Chapter 10; [c]in hospital or as outpatient; [d]follow-up recommendations can be modified according to level of risk for hyperbilirubinemia; depending on the circumstances in infants at low risk, later follow-up can be considered.

- Provide lactation evaluation and support for all breastfeeding mothers.
- Recommendation for timing of repeat TSB measurement depends on age at measurement and how far the TSB level is above the 95th percentile (Figure 9-1). Higher and earlier initial TSB levels require an earlier repeat TSB measurement.
- Perform standard clinical evaluation at all follow-up visits.
- For evaluation of jaundice, see 2004 AAP guideline.[10]

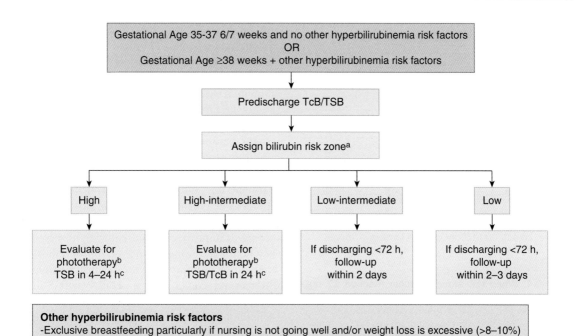

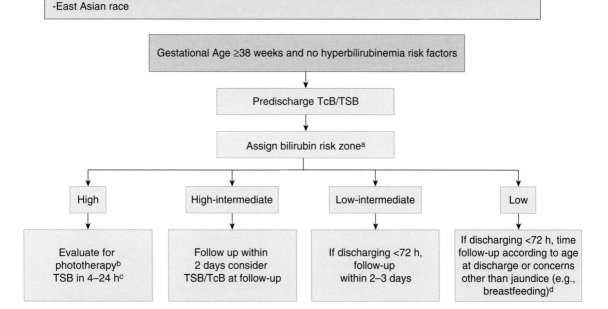

FIGURE 9-3. Continued

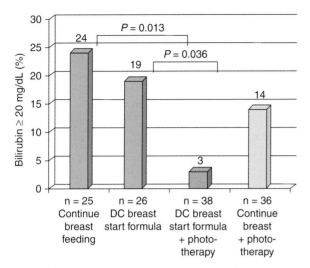

FIGURE 9-4. When the serum bilirubin reached 17 mg/ dL, infants were randomly assigned to one of four interventions. The percentage of infants whose bilirubin levels subsequently reached or exceeded 20 mg/dL is shown. DC, discontinue. Conventional (not intensive) phototherapy was used. (Drawn from the data of Martinez JC, Maisels MJ, Otheguy L, et al. Hyperbilirubinemia in the breast-fed newborn: a controlled trial of four interventions. *Pediatrics.* 1993;91:470–473.)

phototherapy, there was a trend toward lower TSB levels when formula was substituted for breast milk but the effect size was modest (TSB lower by 1 mg/dL at 48 hours, $P = .051$). In the situation where breast milk transfer is clearly inadequate, however, supplementation with expressed breast milk or formula is often necessary. In neither of the above studies was intensive phototherapy used.

In some hospitals it has been a common practice to provide supplemental feedings of water or dextrose water to breastfed infants in the mistaken belief that this will lower their TSB levels. This practice does not decrease TSB levels[48,49] (Figure 9-5) but it can interfere with establishment of effective lactation.[129]

■ CONCLUSIONS

The challenge we face in managing the jaundiced newborn is how to avoid the devastating outcome of kernicterus while minimizing testing and treating in the vast majority of newborns who would do just fine with no interventions for jaundice at all. Because there is

considerable evidence that clinical risk factors (especially gestational age and breastfeeding), and the comparison of TcB or TSB levels with hour-specific norms, can identify most newborns at risk for severe hyperbilirubinemia, we currently have the tools to prevent most cases of kernicterus. Kernicterus is rare in the United States[1,8] and most practitioners will never see a case, perhaps because current follow-up and treatment of jaundiced newborns in the United States prevent most cases. In developing countries, where follow-up and treatment for jaundice are less available, kernicterus appears to be much more common.[130–132]

Auerbach et al. have discussed "the tension between needing to improve care and knowing how to do it."[133] They note that, in the absence of appropriate evidence, "bold efforts at improvement can consume tremendous resources yet confer only a small benefit." Increased attention to neonatal jaundice, including not only predischarge bilirubin screening but also risk assessment, has led to more laboratory testing as well as increases in both appropriate and inappropriate uses of phototherapy.[17,116,120] We believe that predischarge risk assessment (including universal screening) and appropriate follow-up is likely to prevent most cases of kernicterus, although so far, the only positive outcome documented has been a decrease in dangerously high (TSB 25–30 mg/dL) TSB levels.[120–122] Continued research will help to better refine our screening and follow-up recommendations and determine what impact they have on the incidence of kernicterus.

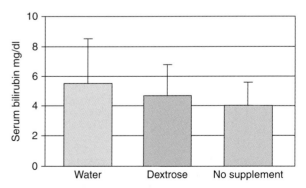

FIGURE 9-5. Effect of supplementary feedings on serum bilirubin levels (mean + 1 SD) in breastfed newborns. (Drawn from the data of Nicoll A, Ginsburg R, Tripp JH. Supplementary feeding and jaundice in newborns. *Acta Paediatr Scand.* 1982;71:759–761.)

■ TABLE 9-5. Studies of the Effect of Universal Bilirubin Screening on Phototherapy Use and Frequency of Hyperbilirubinemia

Author(s); System	N Births Baseline	N Births Screened	Baseline Phototherapy	Change in Phototherapy	Baseline Percentage of Total TSB 20.0–24.9	RRR (%)	Baseline Rate per 1000 TSB 25.0–29.9	RRR (%)	Baseline Rate per 100,000 TSB ≥300	RRR (%)
Eggert et al.[121]; Intermountain Healthcare	48,789	52,483	Not stated; readmissions for jaundice 0.55%	Not stated; 22% decrease in readmissions for jaundice	1.20	−45	0.55	−66	10.3	−44
Kuzniewicz et al.[120]; Northern California Kaiser	38,182	319,904	4.20%	117% increase	2.00	−32	1.20	−74	12.0	−57
Mah et al.[122]; Hospital Corporation of America	129,345	899,472	4.40%	5–16% increase	0.56	−40	0.43	−38	8.5	−65

Abbreviations: TSB, total serum bilirubin; RRR, relative risk reduction.

REFERENCES

1. Burgos AE, Flaherman VJ, Newman TB. Screening and follow-up for neonatal hyperbilirubinemia: a review. *Clin Pediatr (Phila)*. 2012;51(1):7–16.

2. Bjerre JV, Ebbesen F. Incidence of kernicterus in newborn infants in Denmark [in Danish]. *Ugeskr Laeger*. 2006;168:686–691.

3. Bjerre JV, Petersen JR, Ebbesen F. Surveillance of extreme hyperbilirubinaemia in Denmark. A method to identify the newborn infants. *Acta Paediatr*. 2008;97:1030–1034.

4. Manning D, Todd P, Maxwell M, Platt M-J. Prospective surveillance study of severe hyperbilirubinaemia in the newborn in the UK and Ireland. *Arch Dis Child Fetal Neonatal Ed*. 2007;92:342–346.

5. Sgro M, Campbell D, Shah V. Incidence and causes of severe neonatal hyperbilirubinemia in Canada. *CMAJ*. 2006;175:587–590.

6. Sgro M, Campbell DM, Fallah S, Shah V. *Kernicterus—January 2007 to December 2009*. Canadian Paediatric Surveillance Program 2009. Available at: http://www.cps.ca/english/surveillance/CPSP/index.htm.

7. Burke BL, Robbins JM, Bird TM, Hobbs CA, Nesmith C, Tilford JM. Trends in hospitalizations for neonatal jaundice and kernicterus in the United States, 1988–2005. *Pediatrics*. 2009;123:524–532.

8. Brooks JC, Fisher-Owens SA, Wu YW, Strauss DJ, Newman TB. Evidence suggests there was not a "resurgence" of kernicterus in the 1990s. *Pediatrics*. 2011;127:672–679.

9. Bhutani VK, Johnson LH, Maisels MJ, et al. Kernicterus: epidemiological strategies for its prevention through systems-based approaches. *J Perinatol*. 2004;24:650–662.

10. American Academy of Pediatrics, Subcommittee on Hyperbilirubinemia. Clinical practice guideline: management of hyperbilirubinemia in the newborn infant 35 or more weeks of gestation. *Pediatrics*. 2004;114:297–316.

11. Ebbesen F, Andersson C, Verder H, et al. Extreme hyperbilirubinaemia in term and near-term infants in Denmark. *Acta Paediatr*. 2005;94:59–64.

12. Kaplan M, Hammerman C. Glucose-6-phosphate dehydrogenase deficiency: a potential source of severe neonatal hyperbilirubinaemia and kernicterus. *Semin Neonatol*. 2002;7:121–128.

13. Canadian Paediatric Society. Guidelines for detection, management and prevention of hyperbilirubinemia in term and late preterm newborn infants (35 or more weeks' gestation). *Paediatr Child Health*. 2007;12:1B–12B.

14. Kaplan M, Merlob P, Regev R. Israel guidelines for the management of neonatal hyperbilirubinemia and prevention of kernicterus. *J Perinatol*. 2008;28:389–397.

15. Bratlid D, Nakstad B, Hansen TWR. National guidelines for treatment of jaundice in the newborn. *Acta Paediatr*. 2011;100:499–505. doi:10.1111/j.1651–2227.2010.02104.x.

16. National Institute for Health and Clinical Excellence. *Neonatal Jaundice*. London: National Institute for Health and Clinical Excellence; 2010. Available at: www.nice.org.uk/CG98.

17. Maisels MJ, Bhutani VK, Bogen D, Newman TB, Stark AR, Watchko JF. Hyperbilirubinemia in the newborn infant ≥35 weeks' gestation: an update with clarifications. *Pediatrics*. 2009;124(4):1193–1198.

18. Keren R, Luan X, Friedman S, Saddlemire S, Cnaan A, Bhutani V. A comparison of alternative risk-assessment strategies for predicting significant neonatal hyperbilirubinemia in term and near-term infants. *Pediatrics*. 2008;121:e170–e179. Available at: http://www.pediatrics.org/cgi/content/full/121/1/e170:e170-e179.

19. Bhutani VK, Johnson L, Sivieri EM. Predictive ability of a predischarge hour-specific serum bilirubin for subsequent significant hyperbilirubinemia in healthy-term and near-term newborns. *Pediatrics*. 1999;103:6–14.

20. Maisels MJ, Gifford K. Normal serum bilirubin levels in the newborn and the effect of breast feeding. *Pediatrics*. 1986;78:837–843.

21. Newman TB, Easterling MJ, Goldman ES, Stevenson DK. Laboratory evaluation of jaundiced newborns: frequency, cost and yield. *Am J Dis Child*. 1990;144:364–368.

22. Sackett DL, Haynes RB, Guyatt GH, Tugwell P. *Clinical Epidemiology: A Basic Science for Clinical Medicine*. 2nd ed. Boston: Little, Brown and Co; 1991.

23. Fouzas S, Mantagou L, Skylogianni E, Mantagos S, Varvarigou A. Transcutaneous bilirubin levels for the first 120 postnatal hours in healthy neonates. *Pediatrics*. 2010;125:e52–e57.

24. Fouzas S, Karatza AA, Skylogianni E, Mantagou L, Varvarigou A. Transcutaneous bilirubin levels in late preterm neonates. *J Pediatr*. 2010;157:762–766.

25. Maisels MJ, Kring E. Transcutaneous bilirubin levels in the first 96 hours in a normal newborn population of 35 or more weeks' of gestation. *Pediatrics*. 2006;117:1169–1173.

26. Watchko J, Claassen D. Kernicterus in premature infants: current prevalence and relationship to NICHD phototherapy study exchange criteria. *Pediatrics*. 1994;93:996–999.

27. Govaert P, Lequin M, Swarte R, et al. Changes in globus pallidus with (pre) term kernicterus. *Pediatrics*. 2003;112:1256–1263.

28. Maisels MJ, Watchko JF. Treatment of jaundice in low birthweight infants. *Arch Dis Child Neonatal Ed*. 2003;88:F459–F463.

29. Maisels MJ. What's in a name? Physiologic and pathologic jaundice: the conundrum of defining normal bilirubin levels in the newborn. *Pediatrics.* 2006;118:805–807.

30. Maisels MJ, Deridder JM, Kring EA, Balasubramaniam M. Routine transcutaneous bilirubin measurements combined with clinical risk factors improve the prediction of subsequent hyperbilirubinemia. *J Perinatol.* 2009;29:612–617.

31. Newman TB, Xiong B, Gonzales VM, Escobar GJ. Prediction and prevention of extreme neonatal hyperbilirubinemia in a mature health maintenance organization. *Arch Pediatr Adolesc Med.* 2000;154:1140–1147.

32. Huang M-J, Kua K-E, Teng H-C, Tang K-S, Weng H-W, Huang C-S. Risk factors for severe hyperbilirubinemia in neonates. *Pediatr Res.* 2004;56:682–689.

33. Maisels MJ, Gifford K, Antle CE, Leib GR. Jaundice in the healthy newborn infant: a new approach to an old problem. *Pediatrics.* 1988;81:505–511.

34. Bertini G, Dani C, Trochin M, Rubaltelli F. Is breast feeding really favoring early neonatal jaundice? *Pediatrics.* 2001;107:E41. Available at: http://www.pediatrics.org/cgi/content/full/101/2/e41.

35. Maisels MJ, Newman TB. Kernicterus in otherwise healthy, breast-fed term newborns. *Pediatrics.* 1995;96:730–733.

36. Oddie S, Richmond S, Coulthard M. Hypernatraemic dehydration and breast feeding: a population study. *Arch Dis Child.* 2001;85(4):318–320.

37. Gourley GR. Breast-feeding, neonatal jaundice and kernicterus. *Semin Neonatol.* 2002;7:135–141.

38. Fevery J. Fasting hyperbilirubinemia: unraveling the mechanism involved. *Gastroenterology.* 1997;113:1798–1800.

39. Gärtner U, Goeser T, Wolkoff AW. Effect of fasting on the uptake of bilirubin and sulfobromophthalein by the isolated perfused rat liver. *Gastroenterology.* 1997;113:1707–1713.

40. De Carvalho M, Klaus MH, Merkatz RB. Frequency of breastfeeding and serum bilirubin concentration. *Am J Dis Child.* 1982;136:737–738.

41. Yamauchi Y, Yamanouchi I. Breast-feeding frequency during the first 24 hours after birth in full-term neonates. *Pediatrics.* 1990;86:171–175.

42. American Academy of Pediatrics, American College of Obstetricians and Gynecologists. *Guidelines for Perinatal Care.* 5th ed. Elk Grove Village, IL: American Academy of Pediatrics; 2002:220–224.

43. Varimo P, Similä S, Wendt L, Kolvisto M. Frequency of breast feeding and hyperbilirubinemia. *Clin Pediatr.* 1986;25:112.

44. American Academy of Pediatrics, American College of Obstetricians and Gynecologists. *Breastfeeding in the Hospital, the Postpartum Period. Breastfeeding Handbook for Physicians.* Washington, DC: American Academy of Pediatrics, American College of Obstetricians and Gynecologists; 2006:81–99.

45. Lawrence RA. *Management of the Mother–Infant Nursing Couple. A Breastfeeding Guide for the Medical Profession.* 4th ed. St. Louis: Mosby; 1994:215–277.

46. Gourley GR, Kreamer B, Arend R. The effect of diet on feces and jaundice during the first three weeks of life. *Gastroenterology.* 1992;103:660.

47. De Carvalho M, Robertson S, Klaus M. Fecal bilirubin excretion and serum bilirubin concentration in breast-fed and bottle-fed infants. *J Pediatr.* 1985;107:786–790.

48. De Carvalho M, Hall M, Harvey D. Effects of water supplementation on physiological jaundice in breast fed babies. *Arch Dis Child.* 1981;56:568–569.

49. Nicoll A, Ginsburg R, Tripp JH. Supplementary feeding and jaundice in newborns. *Acta Paediatr Scand.* 1982;71:759–761.

50. Butler DA, MacMillan JP. Relationship of breast feeding and weight loss to jaundice in the newborn period: review of the literature and results of a study. *Cleve Clin Q.* 1983;50:263–268.

51. Maisels MJ, Gifford K. Breast feeding, weight loss and jaundice. *J Pediatr.* 1983;102:117–118.

52. Laing IA, Wong CM. Hypernatraemia in the first few days: is the incidence rising? *Arch Dis Child Neonatal Ed.* 2002;87:F158–F162.

53. Newman TB, Liljestrand P, Escobar GJ. Jaundice noted in the first 24 hours after birth in a managed care organization. *Arch Pediatr Adolesc Med.* 2002;156:1244–1250.

54. Kramer LI. Advancement of dermal icterus in the jaundiced newborn. *Am J Dis Child.* 1969;118:454–458.

55. Madlon-Kay DJ. Recognition of the presence and severity of newborn jaundice by parents, nurses, physicians, and icterometer. *Pediatrics.* 1997;100:e3.

56. Tayaba R, Gribetz D, Gribetz I, Holzman IR. Noninvasive estimation of serum bilirubin. *Pediatrics.* 1998;102:e28.

57. Ebbesen F. The relationship between the cephalopedal progress of clinical icterus and the serum bilirubin concentration in newborn infants without blood type sensitization. *Acta Obstet Gynaecol Scand.* 1975;54:329–332.

58. Hegyi T, Hiatt M, Gertner I, et al. Transcutaneous bilirubinometry: the cephalocaudal progression of dermal icterus. *Am J Dis Child.* 1981;135:547.

59. Knudsen A. The cephalocaudal progression of jaundice in newborns in relation to the transfer of bilirubin from plasma to skin. *Early Hum Dev.* 1990;22:23–28.

60. Knudsen A. The influence of the reserve albumin concentration and pH on the cephalocaudal progression of jaundice in newborns. *Early Hum Dev.* 1991;25:37–41.

61. Knudsen A, Broderson R. Skin colour and bilirubin in neonates. *Arch Dis Child*. 1989;64:605.

62. Moyer VA, Ahn C, Sneed S. Accuracy of clinical judgment in neonatal jaundice. *Arch Pediatr Adolesc Med*. 2000;154:391–394.

63. Davidson LT, Merritt KK, Weech AA. Hyperbilirubinemia in the newborn. *Am J Dis Child*. 1941;61: 958–980.

64. Riskin A, Kuglman A, Abend-Weinger M, Green M, Hemo M, Bader D. In the eye of the beholder: how accurate is clinical estimation of jaundice in newborns? *Acta Paediatr*. 2003;92:574–576.

65. Riskin A, Abend-Weinger M, Bader D. How accurate are neonatologists in identifying clinical jaundice in newborns? *Clin Pediatr*. 2003;42:153–158.

66. Hoyt C, Billson FA, Alpins M. The supranuclear disturbances of gaze in kernicterus. *Ann Ophthalmol*. 1978;10:1487.

67. Hannemann RE, DeWitt DP, Hanley EJ, Schreiner RL, Bonderman P. Determination of serum bilirubin by skin reflectance: effect of pigmentation. *Pediatr Res*. 1979;13:1326–1329.

68. Hannemann RE, DeWitt DP, Wiechel JF. Neonatal serum bilirubin from skin reflectance. *Pediatr Res*. 1978;12:207–210.

69. Yasuda S, Itoh S, Isobe K, et al. New transcutaneous jaundice device with two optical paths. *J Perinat Med*. 2003;31:81–88.

70. Rubaltelli F, Gourley GR, Loskamp N, et al. Transcutaneous bilirubin measurement: a multicenter evaluation of a new device. *Pediatrics*. 2001;107:1264–1271.

71. Bhutani V, Gourley GR, Adler S, Kreamer B, Dalman C, Johnson LH. Noninvasive measurement of total serum bilirubin in a multiracial predischarge newborn population to assess the risk of severe hyperbilirubinemia. *Pediatrics*. 2000;106:e17.

72. Engle WD, Jackson GL, Sendelbach D, Manning D, Frawley W. Assessment of a transcutaneous device in the evaluation of neonatal hyperbilirubinemia in a primarily Hispanic population. *Pediatrics*. 2002; 110:61–67.

73. Engle WD, Jackson GL, Stehel EK, Sendelbach D, Manning MD. Evaluation of a transcutaneous jaundice meter following hospital discharge in term and near-term neonates. *J Perinatol*. 2005;25:486–490.

74. Maisels MJ, Engle W, Wainer S, Jackson GL, McManus S, Artinian F. Transcutaneous bilirubin levels in an outpatient and office population. *J Perinatol*. 2011;31:621–624. doi:10.1038/jp.2011.5.

75. Maisels MJ. Transcutaneous bilirubinometry. *NeoReviews*. 2006;7:217–225.

76. Maisels MJ, Ostrea E Jr, Touch S, et al. Evaluation of a new transcutaneous bilirubinometer. *Pediatrics*. 2004;113:1628–1635.

77. De Luca D, Zecca E, De Turrist P, Barbato G, Marras M, Romagnoli C. Using BiliCheck for preterm neonates in a sub-intensive unit: diagnostic usefulness and suitability. *Early Hum Dev*. 2007;83:313–317.

78. Maisels MJ, Kring E. Transcutaneous bilirubinometry decreases the need for serum bilirubin measurements and saves money. *Pediatrics*. 1997;99:599–601.

79. Dai J, Krahn J, Parry DM. Clinical impact of transcutaneous bilirubinometry as an adjunctive screen for hyperbilirubinemia. *Clin Biochem*. 1996;29:581–586.

80. Ebbesen F, Rasmussen LM, Wimberley PD. A new transcutaneous bilirubinometer, BiliCheck, used in the neonatal intensive care unit and the maternity ward. *Acta Paediatr*. 2002;91:203–211.

81. Thomson J, Culley V, Monfrinoli A, Sinha A. Transcutaneous bilirubinometers and ethnicity. *Arch Dis Child Fetal Neonatol Ed*. 2008;93:F474.

82. Ho H, Ng TK, Tsui KC, Lo YC. Evaluation of a new transcutaneous bilirubinometer in Chinese newborns. *Arch Dis Child Fetal Neonatol Ed*. 2006;91:F434–F438.

83. Wainer S, Rabi Y, Parmar SM, Allegro D, Lyon M. Impact of skin tone on the performance of a transcutaneous jaundice meter. *Acta Paediatr*. 2009;98:1909–1915.

84. Namba F, Kitajimi H. Utility of a new transcutaneous jaundice device with two optical paths in premature infants. *Pediatr Int*. 2007;49:497–501.

85. Schmidt ET, Wheeler CA, Jackson GL, Engle WD. Evaluation of transcutaneous bilirubinometry in preterm neonates. *J Perinatol*. 2009;29:564–569.

86. Karolyi L, Pohlandt F, Muche R, Franz AR, Mihatsch WA. Transcutaneous bilirubinometry in very low birthweight infants. *Acta Paediatr*. 2004;93:941–944.

87. Amato M, Huppi P, Markus D. Assessment of neonatal jaundice and low birthweight infants comparing transcutaneous, capillary and arterial bilirubin levels. *Eur J Pediatr*. 1990;150:59–61.

88. Willems WA, van den Berg LM, de Wit H, Molendijk A. Transcutaneous bilirubinometry with the Bilicheck in very premature newborns. *J Matern Fetal Neonatal Med*. 2004;16:209–214.

89. Holland L, Blick K. Implementing and validating transcutaneous bilirubinometry for neonates. *Am J Clin Pathol*. 2009;132:555–561.

90. Kazmierczak SC, Robertson AF, Briley KP, Kreamer B, Gourley GR. Transcutaneous measurement of bilirubin in newborns: comparison with an automated Jendrassik–Grof procedure and HPLC. *Clin Chem*. 2004;50:433–435.

91. Slusher TM, Angyo IA, Bode-Thomas F, et al. Transcutaneous bilirubin measurements and serum total bilirubin levels in indigenous African infants. *Pediatrics.* 2004;113:1636–1641.

92. Arias IM, Gartner IM, Seifter SA, et al. Prolonged neonatal unconjugated hyperbilirubinemia associated with breastfeeding and a steroid, pregnane-3-alpha 20 beta-diol in maternal milk that inhibits glucuronide formation in vitro. *J Clin Invest.* 1964;43:2037.

93. Jangaard KA, Curtis H, Goldbloom RB. Estimation of bilirubin using BiliChek, a transcutaneous bilirubin measurement device: effects of gestational age and use of phototherapy. *Paediatr Child Health.* 2006;11: 79–83.

94. Nanjundaswamy S, Petrova A, Mehta R, Hegyi T. Transcutaneous bilirubinometry in preterm infants receiving phototherapy. *Am J Perinatol.* 2005;22:127–131.

95. Poland RL, Hartenberger C, McHenry H, Hsi A. Comparison of skin sites for estimating serum total bilirubin in in-patients and out-patients: chest is superior to brow. *J Perinatol.* 2004;24:541–543.

96. Khoury MJ, Calle EE, Joesoef RM. Recurrence risk of neonatal hyperbilirubinemia in siblings. *Am J Dis Child.* 1988;142:1065–1069.

97. Nielsen HE, Haase P, Blaabjerg J, et al. Risk factors and sib correlation in physiological neonatal jaundice. *Acta Paediatr Scand.* 1987;76:504–511.

98. Arad I, Fainmesser P, Birkenfeld A, Gulaiev B, Sadovsky E. Vacuum extraction and neonatal jaundice. *J Perinat Med.* 1982;10(6):273–278.

99. Peevy KJ, Landaw SA, Gross SJ. Hyperbilirubinemia in infants of diabetic mothers. *Pediatrics.* 1980;66: 417–419.

100. Jährig D, Jährig K, Striet S, et al. Neonatal jaundice in infants of diabetic mothers. *Acta Paediatr Scand (Suppl).* 1989;360:101–107.

101. Keren R, Bhutani VK, Luan X, Nihtianova S, Cnaan A, Schwartz JS. Identifying newborns at risk of significant hyperbilirubinaemia: a comparison of two recommended approaches. *Arch Dis Child.* 2005;90:415–421.

102. Penn AA, Enzman DR, Hahn JS, Stevenson DK. Kernicterus in a full term infant. *Pediatrics.* 1994;93:1003–1006.

103. MacDonald M. Hidden risks: early discharge and bilirubin toxicity due to glucose-6-phosphate dehydrogenase deficiency. *Pediatrics.* 1995;96:734–738.

104. Johnson L, Bhutani VK, Karp K, Sivieri EM, Shapiro SM. Clinical report from the pilot USA kernicterus registry (1992 to 2004). *J Perinatol.* 2009;29:S25–S45.

105. Newman T, Liljestrand P, Escobar G. Combining clinical risk factors with bilirubin levels to predict hyperbilirubinemia in newborns. *Arch Pediatr Adolesc Med.* 2005;159:113–119.

106. Maisels MJ, Kring EA. Length of stay, jaundice and hospital readmission. *Pediatrics.* 1998;101:995–998.

107. Soskolne EI, Schumacher R, Fyock C, Young ML, Schork A. The effect of early discharge and other factors on readmission rates of newborns. *Arch Pediatr Adolesc Med.* 1996;150:373–379.

108. Newman TB, Kohn MA. Critical appraisal of studies of diagnostic tests. In: *Evidence-Based Diagnosis.* New York, NY: Cambridge University; 2009:94–111.

109. Maisels MJ, Newman TB. Predicting hyperbilirubinemia in newborns: the importance of timing. *Pediatrics.* 1999;103:493–495.

110. Stevenson DK, Fanaroff AA, Maisels MJ, et al. Prediction of hyperbilirubinemia in near-term and term infants. *Pediatrics.* 2001;108:31–39.

111. Kaplan M, Hammerman C, Feldman R, Brisk R. Predischarge bilirubin screening in glucose-6-phosphate dehydrogenase-deficient neonates. *Pediatrics.* 2000;105:533–537.

112. De Luca D, Jackson GL, Tridente A, Carnielli VP, Engle W. Transcutaneous bilirubin nomograms: a systematic review of population differences and analysis of bilirubin kinetics. *Arch Pediatr Adolesc Med.* 2009;163(11):1054–1059.

113. De Luca D, Romagnoli C, Tiberi E, Zuppa AA, Zecca E. Skin bilirubin nomogram for the first 96h of life in a European normal healthy newborn population, obtained with multiwavelength transcutaneous bilirubinometry. *Acta Paediatr.* 2008;97:146–150.

114. Engle WD, Lai S, Ahmad N, Manning MD, Jackson GL. An hour-specific nomogram for transcutaneous bilirubin values in term and late preterm Hispanic neonates. *Am J Perinatol.* 2009;26(6):425–430.

115. Sanpavat S, Nuchprayoon I, Smathakanee C, Hansuebsai R. Nomogram for prediction of the risk of neonatal hyperbilirubinemia, using transcutaneous bilirubin. *J Med Assoc Thai.* 2005;88:1187–1193.

116. Newman TB. Universal bilirubin screening, guidelines, and evidence. *Pediatrics.* 2009;124(4):1199–1201.

117. Newman TB, Maisels MJ. Less aggressive treatment of neonatal jaundice and reports of kernicterus: lessons about practice guidelines. *Pediatrics.* 2000;105:242–245.

118. Trikalinos T, Chung M, Lau J, Ip S. Systematic review of screening for bilirubin encephalopathy in neonates. *Pediatrics.* 2009;124(4):1162–1171.

119. US Preventive Services Task Force. Screening of infants for hyperbilirubinemia to prevent chronic bilirubin encephalopathy: US preventive services task force recommendation statement. *Pediatrics.* 2009;124(4):1172–1177.

120. Kuzniewicz MW, Escobar GJ, Newman TB. Impact of universal bilirubin screening on severe hyper-bilirubinemia and phototherapy use. *Pediatrics.* 2009;124(4):1031–1039.

121. Eggert L, Wiedmeier SE, Wilson J, Christensen R. The effect of instituting a prehospital-discharge newborn bilirubin screening program in an 18-hospital health system. *Pediatrics.* 2006;117:e855–e862.

122. Mah MP, Clark SL, Akhigbe E, et al. Reduction of severe hyperbilirubinemia after institution of predischarge bili-rubin screening. *Pediatrics.* 2010;125:e1143–e1148.

123. Cremer RJ, Perryman PW, Richards DH. Influence of light on the hyperbilirubinemia of infants. *Lancet.* 1958;1:1094–1097.

124. Slusher T, Faber K, Cline B, et al. Selectively filtered sun-light phototherapy: safe and effective for treatment of neonatal jaundice in Nigeria. *E-PAS2011*:2918.254.

125. Longhurst C, Turner S, Burgos AE. Development of a web-based decision support tool to increase use of neo-natal hyperbilirubinemia guidelines. *Jt Comm J Qual Patient Saf.* 2009;35(5):256–262.

126. Dennery P. Pharmacological interventions for the treat-ment of neonatal jaundice. *Semin Neonatol.* 2002;7: 111–119.

127. Amato M, Howald H, von Muralt G. Interruption of breast-feeding vs. phototherapy as treatment of hyper-bilirubinemia in full term infants. *Helv Paediatr Acta.* 1985;40:127–131.

128. Martinez JC, Maisels MJ, Otheguy L, et al. Hyperbiliru-binemia in the breast-fed newborn: a controlled trial of four interventions. *Pediatrics.* 1993;91:470–473.

129. Kuhr M, Paneth N. Feeding practices and early neonatal jaundice. *J Pediatr Gastr Nutr.* 1982;1:485–488.

130. Banerjee TK, Hazra A, Biswas A, et al. Neurological disorders in children and adolescents. *Indian J Pediatr.* 2009;76:139–146.

131. Mezaal MA, Nouri KA, Abdool S, Safar KA, Nadeem ASM. Cerebral palsy in adults consequences of non pro-gressive pathology. *Open Neurol J.* 2009;3:24–26.

132. Slusher TM, Vreman HJ, McLaren D, et al. Glucose-6-phosphate dehydrogenase deficiency and carboxyhemo-globin concentrations associated with bilirubin related morbidity and death in Nigerian infants. *J Pediatr.* 1995;126:102–108.

133. Auerbach AD, Landefeld CS, Shojania K. The tension between needing to improve care and knowing how to do it. *N Engl J Med.* 2007;357:608–613.

Phototherapy and Other Treatments

M. Jeffrey Maisels, David K. Stevenson, Jon F. Watchko, and Antony F. McDonagh

■ PHOTOTHERAPY

We owe the development of clinical phototherapy to an astute observation made, more than 50 years ago, by Sister J. Ward, the nurse in charge of the premature baby unit at the former Rochford General Hospital in Essex, England.[1] As described by Dobbs and Cremer, Sister Ward recognized the value of sunshine and fresh air to all, including premature babies, and she would take the "more delicate infants out into the courtyard, sincerely convinced that the combination of fresh air and sunshine would do them much more good than the stuffy, overheated atmosphere of the incubator."[1] During a ward round in 1956, Sister Ward showed the pediatricians a jaundiced, premature infant who appeared pale yellow except for a triangle of skin that was much yellower than the rest of the body. Apparently, a corner of the sheet had covered this part of the baby and the Sister recognized that the rest of the baby had been "bleached" by the sun. (It was only recognized more than a decade later that the mechanism for the bleaching of yellow serum and skin—photooxidation—probably plays a minor role in the reduction of the serum bilirubin concentration in newborns treated with phototherapy.)[2,3]

A few weeks later, in the same nursery, a tube of blood, inadvertently exposed to sunlight for several hours, showed a total serum bilirubin (TSB) level of 10 mg/dL, much lower than anticipated.[1] This led to the hypothesis that visible light could affect serum bilirubin levels in vivo and the concept of using phototherapy as a clinical tool was born.[4] Cremer et al. then showed that exposing jaundiced infants either to sunlight or to blue fluorescent lights effectively lowered their bilirubin levels.[4] Although the observations of Cremer et al. were published in 1958 and confirmed in multiple subsequent publications in Europe and Central and South America, it was not until Lucey et al. published their findings in 1968[5] that this simple, apparently safe, and effective treatment for hyperbilirubinemia achieved widespread acceptance in the United States and phototherapy is now used worldwide. Although there exists a vast body of literature from human, animal, and laboratory investigation dealing with the mechanism of action, biological effects, complications, and clinical use of phototherapy, there is a need for additional information on how phototherapy works, how its dosage should be measured, and how it should be administered most effectively. Jährig et al. provide a reference source on phototherapy data up to 1993[6] and the recent, remarkably comprehensive and critical review by the National Institute for Health and Clinical Excellence (NICE) in the United Kingdom is an excellent resource for additional reading.[7]

Mechanism of Action

Phototherapy is a mechanism for detoxifying bilirubin and lowering the TSB level. It achieves this by using light energy to change the shape and structure of bilirubin, converting it to molecules that can be excreted even when normal conjugation is deficient (Figures 10-1 and 10-2).[3,8]

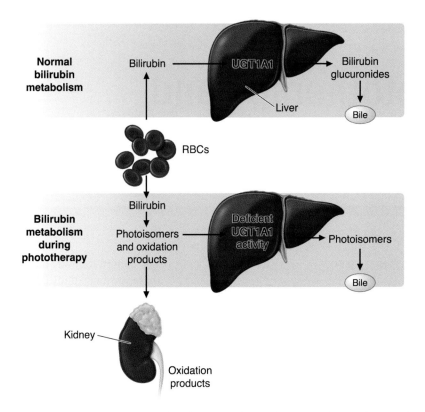

FIGURE 10-1. Normal bilirubin metabolism and bilirubin metabolism during phototherapy. In normal metabolism, lipophilic bilirubin, which results predominantly from the catabolism of red cells, circulates in blood mainly as a noncovalent conjugate with serum albumin. After uptake by the liver, it is converted into two isomeric monoglucuronides and a diglucuronide (direct bilirubin) by the enzyme uridine diphosphoglucuronosyltransferase 1A1 (UGT1A1). The water-soluble glucuronides are excreted in bile with the aid of a canalicular multidrug resistance-associated transport protein, MRP2. Without glucuronidation, bilirubin cannot be excreted in bile or urine. In neonates, hepatic UGT1A1 activity is deficient and the lifetime of red cells is shorter than in adults, leading to accumulation and increased formation of bilirubin, with eventual jaundice. Phototherapy converts bilirubin to yellow photoisomers and colorless oxidation products that are less lipophilic than bilirubin and do not require hepatic conjugation for excretion. Photoisomers are excreted mainly in bile, and oxidation products predominantly in urine. (Reproduced from Maisels MJ, McDonagh AF. Phototherapy for neonatal jaundice. *N Engl J Med.* 2008;358:920–928, with permission.)

Absorption of light by dermal and subcutaneous bilirubin induces a fraction of the pigment to undergo several photochemical reactions that occur at different rates. These reactions generate yellow stereoisomers of bilirubin and colorless derivates of lower molecular weight (Figure 10-2). These products are less lipophilic than bilirubin, they have less internal hydrogen bonding, and, unlike bilirubin, they can be excreted in bile or urine without the need for conjugation. The relative contributions of the various reactions to the overall elimination of bilirubin are unknown, although in vitro and in vivo studies suggest that photoisomerization is more important than photodegradation.[2] Bilirubin elimination depends on the rate of bilirubin formation as well as the rates of clearance of the photoproducts. Photoisomerization occurs rapidly during phototherapy, and some isomers appear in the blood long before the level of plasma bilirubin begins to decline.[8–10]

Configurational (Z → E) Isomerization
There are four possible configurational isomers of bilirubin (Figure 10-3). In infants receiving phototherapy

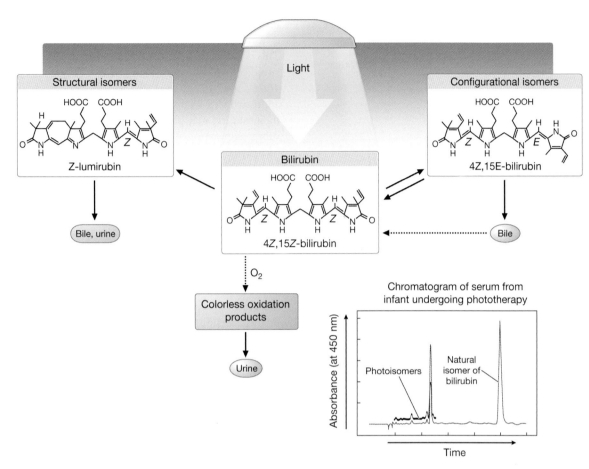

FIGURE 10-2. Mechanism of phototherapy. The absorption of light by the normal form of bilirubin (4Z,15Z-bilirubin) generates transient excited-state bilirubin molecules. These fleeting intermediates can react with oxygen to produce colorless products of lower molecular weight, or they can undergo rearrangement to become structural isomers (lumirubins) or isomers in which the configuration of at least one of the two Z-configuration double bonds has changed to an E configuration. (Z and E, from the German *zusammen* [together] and *entgegen* [opposite], respectively, are prefixes used for designating the stereochemistry around a double bond. The prefixes 4 and 15 designate double-bond positions.) Only the two principal photoisomers formed in humans are shown. Configurational isomerization is reversible and much faster than structural isomerization, which is irreversible. Both occur much more quickly than photooxidation. The photoisomers are less lipophilic than the 4Z,5Z form of bilirubin and can be excreted unchanged in bile without undergoing glucuronidation. Lumirubin isomers can also be excreted in urine. Photooxidation products are excreted mainly in urine. Once in bile, configurational isomers revert spontaneously to the natural 4Z,15Z form of bilirubin. The graph, a high-performance liquid chromatogram of serum from an infant undergoing phototherapy, shows the presence of several photoisomers in addition to the 4Z,15Z isomer. Photoisomers are also detectable in the blood of healthy adults after sunbathing. (Reproduced from Maisels MJ, McDonagh AF. Phototherapy for neonatal jaundice. *N Engl J Med*. 2008;358:920–928, with permission.)

the stable 4Z,15Z isomer is converted predominantly to the 4Z,15E isomer (Figure 10-2) but why this particular isomer is favored is not understood.[8,11] The formation of 4Z,15E-bilirubin is spontaneously reversible in the dark and this occurs rapidly in bile. Thus, the 4Z,15E-bilirubin formed in the skin and excreted by the liver is readily converted back to unconjugated bilirubin, some of which can be reabsorbed through the gut.

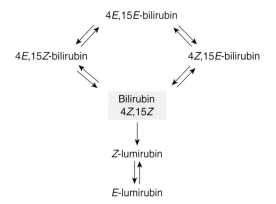

FIGURE 10-3. Configurational and structural isomers of 4Z,15Z-bilirubin in infants undergoing phototherapy.

When phototherapy is initiated, photoisomerization occurs almost instantaneously,[8] and is detectable in the blood of newborns, within 15 minutes[10] (Figure 10-4), but the clearance of the light-generated 4Z,15E isomer is slow ($T_{1/2}$ ~ 15 hours). Although the concentration of this isomer can account for 20–30% of the total unconjugated bilirubin,[10,12] it might play only a minor role in lowering the serum bilirubin concentration.[13] After 2 hours of phototherapy, ~20% of the TSB is in the form of the 4Z,15E photoisomer and small amounts of 4Z,15E-bilirubin are

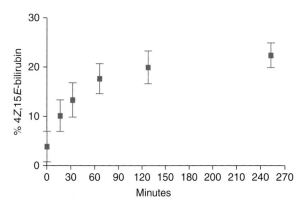

FIGURE 10-4. Formation of 4Z,15E-bilirubin. 4Z,15E-bilirubin is shown as a percentage (mean ± SD) of TSB (4Z,15E + 4Z,15Z) in 20 jaundiced infants treated with phototherapy ($F = 79.06$, $P < .0001$, one-way ANOVA). The difference from time 0 was significant from 15 minutes onward. (Reproduced from Mreihil K, McDonagh A, Nakstad B, Hansen TWR. Early isomerization of bilirubin in phototherapy of neonatal jaundice. *Pediatr Res.* 2010;67:656–659, with permission.)

present even before phototherapy begins, presumably as a result of exposure of the infants to ambient light. This is not surprising, as 4Z,15E-bilirubin is seen in non-jaundiced adults exposed to daylight.[14] Clearance of the 4E,15Z and 4E,15E isomers, which do not accumulate appreciably in serum, is faster than that of 4Z,15E and these isomers may play a greater role in accelerating bilirubin elimination during phototherapy than currently recognized.

Because the products of photoisomerization are less lipophilic than 4Z,15Z-bilirubin, they should be less likely to cross the blood–brain barrier and the fact that phototherapy rapidly converts 20–30% of circulating bilirubin to a less lipophilic and possibly less toxic isomer suggests that a benefit of phototherapy might be the partial detoxification of bilirubin even before it is eliminated.[8,10]

Structural Isomerization

In this reaction (Figures 10-2 and 10-3), intramolecular cyclization of the bilirubin (an irreversible process) occurs in the presence of light to form a substance known as lumirubin that also forms Z and E isomers that can be excreted in bile and in urine.[13] During phototherapy, the serum concentration of lumirubin can reach about 2–6% of the TSB, much lower than the concentration of the configurational isomers that account for approximately 20–30% of the TSB[10,12] but, because lumirubins are cleared from the serum much more rapidly than the 4Z,5E isomer, it has been suggested that lumirubin formation is mainly responsible for the phototherapy-induced decline in serum bilirubin in the human infant.[13] However, the relative contributions of individual photoisomers are not known with any certainty.[15]

Photooxidation

Bilirubin can be photooxidized to water-soluble, colorless products that can be excreted in the urine (Figure 10-2). This is a slow process and is probably only a minor contributor to the overall elimination of bilirubin during phototherapy.

Terminology

Light Spectrum

The spectrum of light delivered by a phototherapy unit is determined by the type of light source and any filters used. Unconjugated bilirubin in tissues absorbs light most strongly in the blue region of the spectrum, near 460 nm,

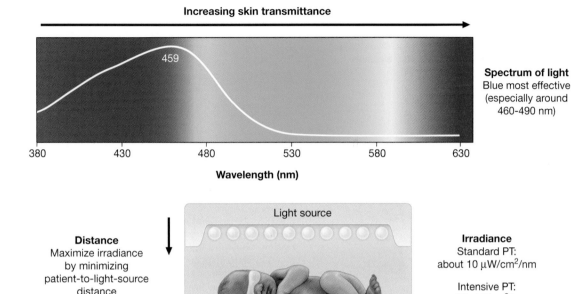

Increasing skin transmittance

459

Spectrum of light
Blue most effective
(especially around
460-490 nm)

380   430   480   530   580   630

Wavelength (nm)

Distance
Maximize irradiance
by minimizing
patient-to-light-source
distance

Light source

Light source

Irradiance
Standard PT:
about 10 μW/cm^2/nm

Intensive PT:
$\geq$ 30 μW/cm^2/nm
(430-490 nm)

Skin area exposed
Maximize for intensive phototherapy
with additional light source below infant

FIGURE 10-5. Important factors in the efficacy of phototherapy. The absorbance spectrum of bilirubin bound to human serum albumin (white line) is shown superimposed on the spectrum of visible light. Clearly, blue light is most effective for phototherapy, but because the transmittance of skin increases with increasing wavelength, the best wavelengths to use are probably in the range of 460–490 nm. Term and near-term infants should be treated in a bassinet, not an incubator, to allow the light source to be brought to within 10–15 cm of the infant (except when halogen or tungsten lights are used), increasing irradiance and efficacy. For intensive phototherapy, an auxiliary light source (light-emitting diode [LED] mattress, LED/fiber-optic pad, or special blue fluorescent tubes) can be placed below the infant or bassinet. If the infant is in an incubator, the light rays should be perpendicular to the surface of the incubator in order to minimize loss of efficacy due to reflectance. (Redrawn from Maisels MJ, McDonagh AF. Phototherapy for neonatal jaundice. *N Engl J Med.* 2008;358:920–928, with permission.)

and the penetration of tissue by light increases markedly with increasing wavelength (Figure 10-5). The rate of formation of bilirubin photoproducts is highly dependent on the light intensity in the wavelengths used—only wavelengths that penetrate tissue and are absorbed by bilirubin have a phototherapeutic effect. There is a common misconception that ultraviolet (UV) light (<400 nm) is used for phototherapy. Phototherapy lights in current use do not emit significant erythemal UV radiation. In addition, the plastic cover of the lamp and, in the case of preterm infants, the incubator all filter out UV light.

Irradiance

Irradiance is the radiant power incident on a surface per unit area of the surface and the irradiance in a specific wavelength band is called the *spectral irradiance* and is expressed as μW/cm^2 per nm (Table 10-1). Although there is generally a direct relationship between the efficacy of phototherapy and the irradiance used[16] (Figure 10-6), the concentration of plasma bilirubin at any given time depends on a number of complex kinetic factors: the rate of formation of bilirubin, the rates of elimination of the photoisomers, the rates of migration of

■ TABLE 10-1. Radiometric Quantities Used

Quantity	Dimensions	Usual Units of Measure
Irradiance (radiant power incident on a surface per unit area of the surface)	W/m^2	W/cm^2
Spectral irradiance (irradiance in a certain wavelength band)	$\mu W/m^2$ per nm	$\mu W/cm^2$ per nm
Spectral power (average spectral irradiance across a surface area)	W/nm	mW/nm

Reproduced from Maisels MJ. Why use homeopathic doses of phototherapy? *Pediatrics.* 1996;98:283–287, with permission. Copyright 1996 by the American Academy of Pediatrics.

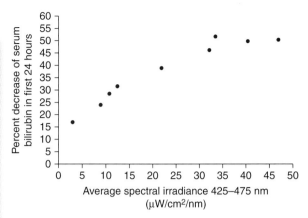

FIGURE 10-6. Relationship between average spectral irradiance and decrease in total serum bilirubin concentration. Full-term infants with nonhemolytic hyperbilirubinemia were exposed to special blue lights (Phillips TL 52/20W) of different intensities. Spectral irradiance was measured as the average of readings at the head, trunk, and knees. Drawn from the data of Tan.[16] (Reproduced from Maisels MJ. Why use homeopathic doses of phototherapy? *Pediatrics.* 1996;98:283–287, with permission. Copyright 1996 by the American Academy of Pediatrics.)

bilirubin and the individual photoisomers into and out of the blood, and the rate of reabsorption of bilirubin from the intestine into the blood. Clearly, some of these rates are independent of the irradiance.

The data in Figure 10-6 suggest that there is a saturation point beyond which an increase in the irradiance produces no added efficacy. However, for technical reasons, the data in Figure 10-6 were obtained not by gradually increasing the intensity of an array of identical light sources, but by switching between different combinations (and configurations?) of two different light sources that, experimentally, can introduce some uncertainty. Presently it is unknown that a saturation point exists. As the conversion of bilirubin to excretable products is partly irreversible and follows first-order kinetics, there may not be a saturation point and we do not know the maximum and safe effective dose of phototherapy.

Spectral Power

This is the product of the skin surface irradiance and spectral irradiance across the surface area. Because both irradiance and the surface area of the infant exposed to phototherapy are key elements in determining the efficacy of phototherapy, the use of spectral power is the only meaningful way

of comparing the dose of phototherapy received by infants under different phototherapy systems.[17]

Effect on Irradiance of the Light Spectrum and the Distance Between the Light and the Subject

Figure 10-7 shows that the light intensity (measured as spectral irradiance) is inversely related to the distance from the source.[17] The relationship between intensity and distance is almost (but not quite) linear, indicating that these data do not obey the law of inverse squares, which states that the light intensity will decrease with the square of the distance. That law only applies to a point source of light and phototherapy units do not provide a point source of light—the light source has features of both a cylindrical and a planar source. Thus, the light intensity is a function of the distance but does not vary with the square of the distance. Figure 10-7 also demonstrates the dramatic difference in the irradiance produced within the 425- to 475-nm band by different types of fluorescent tubes. Table 10-2 lists the factors that affect the dose and efficacy of phototherapy.

Clinical Use and Efficacy of Phototherapy

Since the only effective alternative to phototherapy in infants with significant hyperbilirubinemia is exchange transfusion, one measure of the efficacy of phototherapy

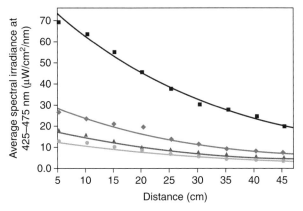

FIGURE 10-7. Effect of light source and distance from the light source to the infant on average spectral irradiance. Measurements were made across the 425- to 475-nm band using a commercial radiometer (Olympic Bilimeter Mark II). The phototherapy unit was fitted with eight 24-in fluorescent tubes. (■) Special blue, General Electric 20-W F20T12/BB tube; (♦) blue, General Electric 20-W F20T12/B tube; (▲) daylight blue, four General Electric 20-W F20T12/B blue tubes and four Sylvania 20-W F20T12/D daylight tubes; and (●) daylight, Sylvania 20-W F20T12/D daylight tube. Curves were plotted using linear curve fitting (True Epistat; Epistat Services, Richardson, TX). The best fit is described by the equation $y = A\,e^{Bx}$. (Reproduced from Maisels MJ. Why use homeopathic doses of phototherapy? *Pediatrics.* 1996;98:283–287, with permission. Copyright 1996 by the American Academy of Pediatrics.)

is the dramatic reduction in the number of exchange transfusions being performed. This effect has been particularly noticeable in very low birth weight (VLBW) infants, for whom exchange transfusions, once common procedures in the neonatal intensive care unit (NICU), are now rare.[18–20] In the first National Institutes of Child Health and Human Development (NICHD) randomized controlled trial of phototherapy,[21] control infants did not receive phototherapy and were subject to exchange transfusions if their bilirubin levels increased sufficiently. In this group, 36% of infants with birth weights <1500 g required an exchange transfusion. When phototherapy was used in a similar population, only 2 of 833 infants (0.24%) received exchange transfusions.[22] In the recent Neonatal Research Network (NRN) study, only 5/1974 (0.25%) infants with birth weights ≤1000 g required an exchange transfusion.[18] In Northern California Kaiser Permanente hospitals, only 1/130 term and late preterm infants with a TSB between 25 and 29.9 mg/dL received an exchange transfusion.[23]

The factors that influence the dose and efficacy of phototherapy are listed in Table 10-2, and illustrated in Figure 10-5. There is a clear dose–response relationship between the irradiance (energy output of the phototherapy device) delivered to the infant and the rate of decline in the TSB (Figure 10-6).[16] It is, therefore, important to perform regular measurements of the irradiance with a radiometer or spectroradiometer. Phototherapy units that deliver between 30–40 µW/cm² per nm in the 430- to 490-nm band have been found to be effective in clinical studies.

Light Sources
In general, none of the light sources used for phototherapy were designed specifically for that purpose, except for special blue fluorescent bulbs for which a modified phosphor was developed. In the first phototherapy unit, the light source was commercially available standard blue fluorescent tubes.[4] Over the next decade, daylight or cool-white fluorescent tubes were frequently used prior to the introduction of tungsten and halogen spotlights. Most of the radiation emitted by tungsten and halogen light sources is not therapeutically effective with respect to phototherapy. Lights that deliver irradiance predominately in the blue spectrum (460–490 nm) are desirable because at these wavelengths there is adequate skin penetration and absorption of the light by dermal and subcutaneous bilirubin (Figure 10-5). Today, there is a wide spectrum of phototherapy units including those that are built-in components of radiant warmer systems. Special blue fluorescent tubes are effective because they provide light predominantly in the blue spectrum. The imprint F20-T12/BB (General Electric, Westinghouse, Sylvania) or TL52/20W (Philips, Eindhoven, the Netherlands) is found on special blue tubes. Note that these are different from regular blue tubes (labeled F20-T12/B),[13] which put out significantly less irradiance than the special blue tubes (Figure 10-7). Special blue tubes do impart a bluish tinge to an infant and there have been concerns that this can induce nausea in caregivers and that it might obscure cyanosis, although we have never encountered these problems in our nursery. Full-term or late preterm hyperbilirubinemic newborns, who are otherwise healthy and require phototherapy, are very unlikely to be cyanotic, and in the NICU, pulse oximetry identifies abnormal oxygen saturations. The blue color of the lights sometimes leads to the misconception that UV light is being used.

A wide variety of new phototherapy devices has been marketed in the last several years,[24,25] and some of the

■ **TABLE 10-2.** Factors That Affect the Dose and Efficacy of Phototherapy (PT)

Factor	Technical Terminology	Rationale	Clinical Application
Type of light source	Spectrum of light (nm)	Blue-green spectrum is most effective at lowering total serum bilirubin (TSB); light at this wavelength penetrates skin well and is absorbed strongly by bilirubin	Use special blue fluorescent tubes or light-emitting diodes (LED) or another light source with output in blue-green spectrum for intensive PT
Distance of light source from patient	Spectral irradiance (a function of both distance and light source) delivered to surface of infant	↑ irradiance leads to ↑ rate of decline in TSB. Standard PT units deliver 8–10 μW/cm² per nm; intensive PT delivers ≥30 μW/cm² per nm	If special blue fluorescent tubes are used, bring tubes as close as possible to infant to increase irradiance. (Do *not* do this with halogen lamps because of danger of burn.) Positioning special blue tubes 10–15 cm above infant will produce an irradiance of at least 35 μW/cm² per nm
Surface area exposed	Spectral power (a function of spectral irradiance and surface area)	↑ surface area exposed leads to ↑ rate of decline in TSB	For intensive PT, expose maximum surface area of infant to PT. Place lights above and below[a] or around[b] the infant. For maximum exposure, line sides of bassinet, warmer bed, or incubator with aluminum foil or white material
Cause of jaundice		PT is likely to be less effective if jaundice is caused by hemolysis or if cholestasis is present (direct bilirubin is increased)	When hemolysis is present, start PT at a lower TSB level and use intensive PT. Failure of PT suggests hemolysis is cause of the jaundice. When direct bilirubin is elevated, watch for bronze baby syndrome or blistering
TSB level at start of PT		The higher the TSB, the more rapid the decline in TSB with PT	Use intensive PT for higher TSB levels. Anticipate a more rapid decrease in TSB with higher TSB levels

Modified from Maisels MJ. Watchko JF. Treatment of hyperbilirubinemia. In: Buonocore G, Bracci R, Weindling M, eds. *Neonatology: A Practical Approach to Neonatal Diseases.* Milan: Springer-Verlag; 2011;629–640, with permission.

[a]Commercially available sources for light below include special blue fluorescent tubes available in the Olympic Bili-Bassinet (Natus Medical, Inc), the BiliSoft fiber-optic/LED mattress (GE Healthcare), and neoBLUE cozy mattress and neoBLUE blanket (Natus Medical, Inc).

[b]The Mediprema Cradle 360 (Mediprema) provides 360° exposure to special blue fluorescent light.

commercial suppliers as well as some irradiance measurements from different devices are provided in Table 10-3 and the footnotes to Table 10-2. Halogen and tungsten lamps have the advantage of being more compact than fluorescent systems but, unlike fluorescent lamps, *they cannot be brought close to the infant (to increase the irradiance) without incurring the risk of a burn.* In addition, the surface area covered by most of these lamps is small[25] and much of the energy output of the lamps is not in an effective region of the spectrum.

Fiber-optic systems have found widespread use and provide a convenient way to deliver home phototherapy or double phototherapy when it is necessary to expose more of the infant's surface area. Earlier halogen/fiber-optic

■ **TABLE 10-3.** Maximum Spectral Irradiance (μW/cm² per nm) of Phototherapy Devices Measured with Commercial Light Meters and Compared with Clear-Sky Sunlight

	Footprint Irradiance (μW/cm² per nm)[b]							
	Halogen/Fiber-Optic			Fluorescent		LED		Sunlight @ Zenith on 8/31/05
		Wallaby (Neo)[c]			Martin/			
Light Meter (Range, Peak[a])	BiliBlanket[b] @ Contact	II[c] @ Contact	III[c] @ Contact	PEP Bed[d] @ 10 cm	Philips BB[e] @ 25 cm	neoBLUE[f] @ 30 cm	PortaBed[g] @ 10 cm	Level Ground
BiliBlanket Meter II[b] (400–520, 450 nm)	34	28	34	40	69	34	76	144
Bili-Meter, Model 22[f] (425–475, 460 nm)	29	16	32	49	100	25	86	65[h]
Joey Dosimeter, JD-100[c] (420–550, 470 nm)	53	51	60	88	174	84	195	304[h]
PMA-2123 Bilirubin Detector[i] (400–520, 460 nm)	24	24	37	35	70	38	73	81
GoldiLux UVA Photometer, GRP-1[j,k] (315–400, 365 nm)	<0.04	<0.04	<0.04	<0.04	<0.04	<0.04	<0.04	2489

Data from Vreman et al.[103] Modified from Bhutani VK, Committee on Fetus and Newborn. Technical report: phototherapy to prevent severe neonatal hyperbilirubinemia in the newborn infant 35 or more weeks of gestation. *Pediatrics.* 2011;128:e1046–e1052.

[a] As reported by the manufacturer.

[b] Ohmeda Medical Inc, Columbia, MD 21046.

[c] Philips Respironics, Inc, Andover, MA 01810.

[d] Physician Engineered Products, Fryeburg, ME 04037.

[e] Floyd Martin, Mifflinburg, PA 17844.

[f] Natus Medical, Inc.

[g] Stanford University, Stanford, CA 94305 and Dutch Crigler–Najjar Association (used by Crigler–Najjar patients).

[h] Irradiance presented to this meter exceeded its range. Measurement was made through a stainless steel screen that attenuated the measured irradiance to 57%, which was subsequently corrected by this factor.

[i] Solar Light Company, Inc, Glenside, PA 19038.

[j] Oriel Instruments, Stratford, CT 06615.

[k] SmartMeter GRP-1 with UV-A probe. GRP-1 measures UV-A light as μW/cm². No artificial light source delivered significant UV-A radiation at the distances measured. (All measurements <0.04 μW/cm².)

systems provided relatively small pads; with a larger pad the light is distributed over a greater surface area, thus reducing the irradiance. This problem has recently been addressed by combining fiber-optic and light-emitting diode (LED) technology (currently marketed as the BiliSoft, GE Healthcare, Wauwatosa, WI, and neoBLUE Blanket, Natus Medical, Inc, San Carlos, CA) in which an LED light source is conducted down a fiber-optic bundle to a pad or blanket. The pad sizes with these newer devices are adequate to cover the full dorsal or ventral surface of a preterm or term infant and the high intensity of the LED light source provides adequate irradiance over an appropriate surface area.

LED light sources are becoming widely used. These high-intensity, gallium nitride LEDs provide a high irradiance, in whichever spectrum is chosen, with virtually no heat generation.[26] A randomized controlled trial comparing LED phototherapy with special blue fluorescent lamps (at similar irradiance levels) showed that the two systems were equally effective in lowering the TSB level.[27]

Using Phototherapy Effectively

Irradiance   In the United States, phototherapy was initially used in low birth weight (LBW) and term infants primarily to prevent slowly rising TSB levels from reaching levels that might require an exchange transfusion[5] and this is how phototherapy is used today in the NICU. But many term and late preterm infants have been discharged and subsequently readmitted for treatment of TSB levels of 20 mg/dL or more. In these infants, therapeutic rather than prophylactic phototherapy is indicated and a full therapeutic dose of phototherapy (now termed *intensive phototherapy*)[28] is recommended to reduce the bilirubin level as soon as possible.[17,29] By choosing the appropriate light spectrum and maximizing the irradiance and the surface area of the infant exposed to phototherapy, the best therapeutic effect can be achieved. If special blue fluorescent tubes are used, the infant should be placed in a bassinette and not an incubator, because the top of the incubator prevents the light from being brought sufficiently close to the infant.[17] In a bassinette it is possible to bring the fluorescent lights within about 10 cm of the infant and achieve a spectral irradiance of more than 50 µW/cm² per nm (Figures 10-5 and 10-7). The small amount of heat produced by the fluorescent lamps maintains a normal body temperature for these infants (naked except for a diaper). One disadvantage of LED lights is that they emit almost no heat so that a naked infant in a bassinette might become cool if the only source of heat is the LED phototherapy light. *Note that halogen and tungsten phototherapy lamps cannot be positioned closer to the infant than recommended by the manufacturer without incurring the risk of a burn.*

Surface Area   Increasing the surface area exposed to phototherapy is easily achieved by placing a fiber-optic/LED blanket or mattress underneath the infant, or using a system that has special blue fluorescent tubes below the baby (Table 10-2). It is not surprising that this type of "double phototherapy" is approximately twice as effective as single phototherapy in LBW infants and almost 50% better in full-term infants.[30,31] A simple way of further increasing the surface area exposed is to place some reflecting material (a white sheet or aluminum foil) around the inner surface of the bassinette or incubator. In France, the Mediprema Cradle 360 (Mediprema, Tours Cedex, France) provides 360° exposure to special blue fluorescent light and delivers highly effective phototherapy,[32] but overheating may limit the duration of phototherapy that can be used with this device.

Measuring the Dose of Phototherapy   Spectral irradiance can be measured with a spectroradiometer, a precision instrument that measures the flux of light over a series of discrete wavelengths. Clinicians and the manufacturers of phototherapy units usually use standard radiometers to measure the irradiance. These radiometers are relatively inexpensive and easy to operate but, unlike spectroradiometers, they take only a single measurement across a band of wavelengths—typically 425–475 or 400–480 nm. These wavelength bands are chosen because they represent the wavelengths at which bilirubin absorbs light maximally and will therefore undergo photochemical reactions to form excretable isomers and breakdown products. Commercial radiometers measure the irradiance in a predetermined band but display the results as the spectral irradiance (µW/cm² per nm). Examples of instruments commercially available can be found in Table 10-3.[25]

As can be seen in Table 10-3, measurement of irradiance from the same phototherapy system using different radiometers produces widely divergent results.[25] The irradiance also varies depending on where the measurement is taken. Irradiance measured below the center of the light source can be more than double that measured at the periphery of the exposed area and this drop-off at the periphery will vary with different phototherapy units. In clinical practice, average measurements are rarely used and the spectral irradiance levels provided in this chapter refer to measurements taken at the center of the exposed area of the infant or the device. Unfortunately, there is no standardized method for reporting phototherapy dosages in the clinical literature, so it is difficult to compare published studies of efficacy.

Intermittent Versus Continuous Phototherapy   Clinical studies comparing intermittent with continuous phototherapy have produced conflicting results.[33–35] In practice, trying to administer phototherapy with defined on and off times is probably more trouble than it is worth. Yet, it is rarely necessary for phototherapy to be continuous. It can, and certainly should, be interrupted during feeding or brief parental visits when eye patches are removed and normal parental bonding can occur. When TSB levels are very high, however, intensive phototherapy should be administered continuously until a satisfactory decline in the TSB has occurred.[28]

Turning the Infant   Because phototherapy acts on bilirubin that is present in the extravascular space as well as in the superficial capillaries, it has become a common practice to turn the infant at intervals supine to prone and back. Two randomized studies[36,37] and one controlled trial[38] found that turning infants every few hours did not improve the efficacy of phototherapy. For this and other reasons (back to sleep), it seems preferable for the infant to be supine during phototherapy.

Hydration and Feeding   Breastfed infants who are readmitted to the hospital with hyperbilirubinemia frequently also have excessive weight loss, largely as a result of poor caloric intake, although some of these infants are also dehydrated. In those in whom there is excessive weight loss and/or dehydration, it makes sense to provide supplemental calories and fluids using expressed breast milk, if available, or a milk-based formula and, if necessary, intravenous (IV) fluids. Because lumirubin photoisomers are excreted in the urine, maintaining adequate hydration and good urine output should help to improve the efficacy of phototherapy.[39] In a randomized controlled trial, 74 Indian infants with TSB levels >18 mg/dL and no documented hemolysis received special blue light phototherapy.[40] In the group that received supplemental IV fluids 6/37 (16%) required an exchange transfusion versus 20/37 (54%) in the group that received breastfeeding or formula only (relative risk [RR]: 0.30; 95% confidence interval [CI]: 0.14–0.66). But in a Malaysian randomized trial,[41] no difference was found in the number of infants requiring an exchange transfusion between groups that received oral or IV supplementation. The above reported incidence of exchange transfusions in an Indian population[40] is much higher than currently experienced in western countries. In Northern California Kaiser Permanente hospitals, only 1/130 (0.8%) infants with TSB levels 25–29.9 mg/dL received an exchange transfusion.[23] In our experience, if the infant is taking oral fluids and is not significantly dehydrated, IV therapy is not required and phototherapy with oral fluid supplementation is sufficient.

Guidelines for Phototherapy Use

A detailed guideline for the use of phototherapy in infants of 35 or more weeks of gestation has been published by the American Academy of Pediatrics (AAP) (Figure 10-8) and has been widely adopted in the United States and elsewhere.[46–48] Similar, consensus-based guidelines have been published recently in Canada, Israel, Norway, and the United Kingdom[7,46,49,50] and two of these guidelines include the management of infants ≤34 weeks of gestation.[7,49] Figure 10-9 shows the recommendations from Norway, which are based on birth weight. In the UK guideline,[7] graphs are provided for each gestational age. Because solid data on which to base recommendations are lacking, all of these guidelines are, of necessity, consensus based. Most recently, Maisels et al. have offered suggestions for the management of hyperbilirubinemia in the preterm infant <35 weeks gestation[51] (Table 10-4). The recommended treatment levels in this report are based on operational thresholds or therapeutic normal levels (a level beyond which a specific therapy is likely to do more good than harm).[52] It would be ideal if all of these guidelines were the product of evidence-based estimates of when the benefit of intervention exceeds the risks and costs. Such estimates should come from randomized trials or high-quality, systematic observational studies, but such studies are rare.[53,54] Treatment guidelines must, therefore, rely on relatively uncertain estimates of risks and benefits as well as the recognition that using a single TSB to predict long-term behavioral and developmental outcomes is not reliable and will lead to conflicting results.[53,54]

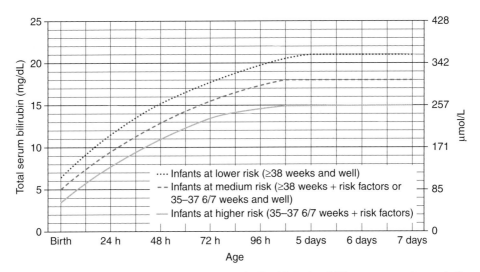

FIGURE 10-8. Guidelines for phototherapy in hospitalized infants of 35 or more weeks gestation.

- Use total bilirubin. Do not subtract direct-reacting or conjugated bilirubin.
- The lines for lower, medium, and higher risks refer to risk for neurotoxicity.
- Risk factors for neurotoxicity—isoimmune hemolytic disease, G6PD deficiency, asphyxia, significant lethargy, temperature instability, sepsis, acidosis, or albumin <3.0 g/dL (if measured).
- For well infants 35–37 6/7 weeks can adjust TSB levels for intervention around the medium risk line. It is an option to intervene at lower TSB levels for infants closer to 35 weeks and at higher TSB levels for those closer to 37 6/7 weeks.
- It is an option to provide conventional phototherapy in hospital or at home at TSB levels 2–3 mg/dL below those shown but home phototherapy should not be used in any infant with risk factors.

These guidelines refer to the use of intensive phototherapy, which should be used when the TSB exceeds the line indicated for each category. Infants are designated as "higher risk" because of the potential negative effects of the conditions listed on albumin binding of bilirubin,[42–44] the blood–brain barrier,[45] and the susceptibility of the brain cells to damage by bilirubin.[45]

Intensive phototherapy implies irradiance in the blue-green spectrum (wavelengths of approximately 430–490 nm) of at least 30 μW/cm^2 per nm (measured at the infant's skin directly below the center of the phototherapy unit) and delivered to as much of the infant's surface area as possible. Note that irradiance measured below the center of the light source is much greater than that measured at the periphery. Measurements should be made with a radiometer specified by the manufacturer of the phototherapy system.

If the total serum bilirubin does not decrease or continues to rise in an infant who is receiving intensive phototherapy, this strongly suggests the presence of hemolysis.
(Reproduced from Maisels MJ. Why use homeopathic doses of phototherapy? *Pediatrics.* 1996;98: 283–287. Copyright 1996 by the American Academy of Pediatrics.)

How Many Infants Do We Need to Treat with Phototherapy to Prevent One Exchange Transfusion?

Although it is clear that phototherapy has played an important role in the dramatic reduction in the need for exchange transfusion, it has not been clearly established how many late preterm and term infants we need to treat with phototherapy (the "number needed to treat" [NNT]) in order to prevent one infant from requiring an exchange transfusion. In the published randomized

trials,[55–57] among infants without hemolysis, 6–10 infants needed to be treated with phototherapy to prevent 1 from developing a TSB ≥20 mg/dL.[53] In those studies, however, the type of phototherapy used was much less effective than that used today,[17,28] so the NNT could be lower. As the primary function of phototherapy is to prevent the need for an exchange transfusion, Newman et al. estimated the NNT[58] among term and late preterm newborns in order to prevent one infant from reaching a TSB level

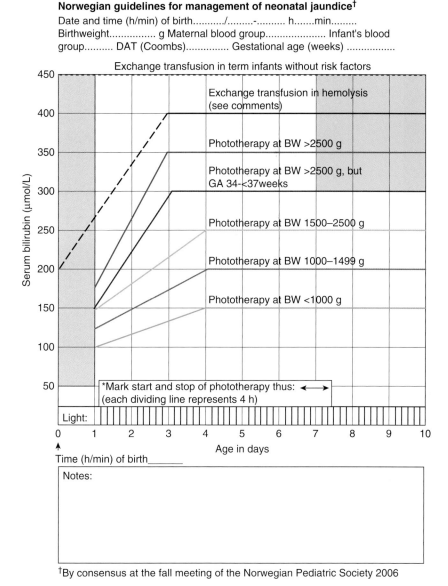

Norwegian guidelines for management of neonatal jaundice†

Date and time (h/min) of birth........../........-......... h.......min........
Birthweight............... g Maternal blood group.................... Infant's blood
group.......... DAT (Coombs)............... Gestational age (weeks) ....

Exchange transfusion in term infants without risk factors

Exchange transfusion in hemolysis (see comments)

Phototherapy at BW >2500 g

Phototherapy at BW >2500 g, but GA 34-<37weeks

Phototherapy at BW 1500–2500 g

Phototherapy at BW 1000–1499 g

Phototherapy at BW <1000 g

*Mark start and stop of phototherapy thus: ←→
(each dividing line represents 4 h)

Light:

Serum bilirubin (µmol/L)

Age in days

Time (h/min) of birth_____

Notes:

†By consensus at the fall meeting of the Norwegian Pediatric Society 2006

FIGURE 10-9. Norwegian guidelines for management of neonatal jaundice. (Reproduced from Bratlid D, Nakstad B, Hansen TWR. National guidelines for treatment of jaundice in the newborn. *Acta Paediatr.* 2011;100:499–505, with permission.)

that meets the AAP criteria for exchange transfusion.[28] There was a remarkable range in the NNT among infants who did not have a positive direct antiglobulin test (DAT, Coombs' test) (Table 10-5). For 36-week gestation boys, <24 hours old, the NNT was 10 (95% CI: 6–19) while for 41-week gestation girls who were ≥3 days old, it was 3041 (95% CI: 888–11,096). Phototherapy was less effective for infants with a positive DAT. For a 40-week gestation male infant who met criteria for phototherapy between 48 and 72 hours the NNT was 682 (95% CI: 367–1294). These numbers suggest that for infants ≥38 weeks who qualify for phototherapy between 48 and 72 hours a different

■ TABLE 10-4. Suggested Use of Phototherapy and Exchange Transfusion in Preterm Infants <35 Weeks Gestational Age

Gestational Age (Weeks)	Initiate Phototherapy (mg/dL)	Exchange Transfusion
<28 0/7 weeks	5 to 6	An exchange transfusion is recommended for infants <30 0/7 weeks if the TSB exceeds 12–13 mg/dL.
28 0/7–29 6/7 weeks	6 to 8	For those ≥30 0/7 weeks, an exchange transfusion is recommended if, in spite of intensive phototherapy,
30 0/7–31 6/7 weeks	8 to 10	TSB levels continue to rise and are 5 mg/dL above the levels listed. For all infants, an exchange
32 0/7–33 6/7 weeks	10 to 12	transfusion is recommended if the infant shows signs of acute bilirubin encephalopathy (hypertonia,
34 0/7–34 6/7 weeks	12 to 14	arching, retrocollis, opisthotonos, high-pitched cry), although it is recognized that these signs rarely occur in VLBW infants.

- This table is modified from Maisels et al,[51] and reflects the authors' recommendations for operational or therapeutic TSB thresholds—bilirubin levels at, or above which, treatment is likely to do more good than harm.[52] They are not based on good evidence.
- Use total bilirubin. Do not subtract direct-reacting or conjugated bilirubin from the total.
- For infants ≤26 weeks gestation, it is an option to use phototherapy prophylactically starting soon after birth.
- Measure irradiance at regular intervals with an appropriate spectroradiometer.
- Measure the serum albumin level in all infants who meet criteria for phototherapy.
- Use the lower range of the listed TSB levels for infants at greater risk for bilirubin toxicity, for example, those with rapidly rising TSB levels, suggesting hemolytic disease, those with serum albumin levels <2.5 g/dL and those who have one or more of the following:: (a) blood pH <7.15; (b) capillary or arterial PCO$_2$ >50 mm Hg; (c) blood culture positive sepsis; (d) apnea and bradycardia requiring bagging or intubating; (e) hypotension requiring pressor treatment; and (f) mechanical ventilation at the time of blood sampling.
- Use post-conceptional age for phototherapy, for example, when a 29 0/7 week infant is 7 days old, use the TSB level for 30 0/7 weeks.
- In the NICHD, Neonatal Research Network there was a 5% increase in mortality observed in infants <750 g who received intensive phototherapy. This observation and the evidence in neonatal rats of an increase in oxidative injury with increasing irradiance[85] suggest that it is prudent to use less intensive levels of irradiance in these infants. In VLBW infants, phototherapy is almost always prophylactic—it is used to prevent a further increase in the TSB, and TSB levels can usually be controlled by phototherapy that is less intensive. Thus, although there are no studies that show a significant increase in mortality in infants <1500 g, the trends toward a possible increase[18,95,96] suggest that it is reasonable in infants <1500 g to start phototherapy at irradiance levels of about 15 μW/cm² per nm. If the TSB continues to rise, additional phototherapy should be provided by increasing the surface area exposed (phototherapy above and below the infant, reflecting material around the incubator). If the TSB, nevertheless, continues to rise, the irradiance should be increased by switching to a higher-intensity setting on the device or by bringing the overhead light closer to the infant. Fluorescent and LED light sources can be brought closer to the infant, but this cannot be done with halogen or tungsten lamps because of the danger of a burn.

■ **TABLE 10-5.** Estimated Number Needed to Treat with Inpatient Phototherapy (95% CI) for 3.3-kg Infants Who Were Not DAT Positive, By Gender, Gestational Age, and Age at Qualifying TSB

Gestational Age (Weeks)	Age at Qualifying TSB: <24 h	Age at Qualifying TSB: 24 to <48 h	Age at Qualifying TSB: 48 to <72 h	Age at Qualifying TSB ≥72 h
Boys				
35	14 (7–40)	26 (14–57)	83 (36–190)	171 (70–426)
36	10 (6–19)	19 (12–39)	59 (31–101)	122 (68–236)
37	16 (10–28)	29 (20–58)	95 (52–168)	196 (100–407)
38	35 (14–100)	67 (31–215)	222 (107–502)	460 (196–1352)
39	74 (31–244)	142 (62–554)	476 (197–1385)	989 (373–3607)
40	106 (44–256)	204 (98–487)	682 (367–1294)	1419 (634–3755)
≥41	148 (54–428)	284 (127–780)	953 (366–3017)	1983 (676–8408)
Girls				
35	21 (12–49)	40 (21–86)	126 (50–267)	261 (105–585)
36	15 (11–26)	28 (20–51)	90 (43–146)	186 (102–347)
37	23 (16–39)	44 (31–75)	145 (73–243)	300 (146–671)
38	53 (23–134)	102 (43–236)	339 (154–730)	705 (314–2016)
39	113 (58–342)	217 (103–713)	729 (272–1730)	1516 (614–4520)
40	162 (75–400)	312 (164–704)	1046 (491–2136)	2176 (922–6107)
≥41	226 (92–702)	435 (183–1140)	1461 (510–4842)	3041 (888–11,096)

The NNT is estimated as the reciprocal of the difference between predicted probabilities of the outcome in those who did and in those who did not receive hospital phototherapy within 8 hours of their qualifying TSB level.

Reproduced from Newman TB, Kuzniewicz MW, Liljestrand P, Wi S, McCulloch C, Escobar GJ. Numbers needed to treat with phototherapy according to American Academy of Pediatrics guidelines. *Pediatrics*. 2009;123:1352–1359, with permission. Copyright 2009 by the American Academy of Pediatrics.

approach might avoid the need for phototherapy entirely. Instead of routinely admitting these infants for treatment, other options could be considered, such as improved lactation support, providing formula supplementation,[56] the use of home phototherapy (see below), or simply repeating the TSB after several hours when, in many cases, it might have decreased. If we need to treat 3000 infants with phototherapy to prevent one exchange transfusion, it is reasonable to ask whether, in many of these infants, phototherapy could have been avoided.

As noted by Newman et al., the TSB level at which phototherapy should be done "depends on the NNT one is willing to accept."[58] But to determine this number, we need much more information regarding both the costs and potential adverse effects of phototherapy as well as a better way of knowing which TSB levels (or some other measurement) represent a threat to the infant's well-being. "Unless we can quantify how bad an outcome is, it is hard to know how many people it is worth treating to prevent it."[58] In the NICHD NRN study of ELBW infants,[18] the rate of neurodevelopmental impairment (NDI) was lower with aggressive phototherapy than with conservative therapy (26% vs. 30%, RR: 0.86; 95% CI: 0.74–0.99) (see below). Based on these data, the NNT with aggressive phototherapy, on average, to prevent one case of developmental impairment in infants with birth weights <1000 g was 25.

Management of Infants <35 Weeks Gestation

Infants of <35 weeks gestation are considered to be at greater risk for the development of bilirubin-associated brain damage than term infants, although a paucity of data has made the quantification of the magnitude of this risk difficult[59] and the range of bilirubin levels used to initiate treatment in different parts of the world at different weights and gestations is remarkably wide.[49,60,61] Chronic bilirubin encephalopathy, including kernicterus at postmortem, is currently a rare event in premature neonates but it has not disappeared completely, and whether the modest elevations in TSB contribute to subtle forms of central nervous system dysfunction in premature infants remains controversial.[62–64] Some studies suggest that

■ TABLE 10-6. Criteria for Initiating Phototherapy and Exchange Transfusions in the NICHD Neonatal Research Network Trial[19]

| Birth Weight (g) | Aggressive Management | | | Conservative Management | | | |
| | Phototherapy Begins | Exchange Transfusion | | Phototherapy (mg/dL) | Begins (μmol/L) | Exchange Transfusion | |
		(mg/dL)	(μmol/L)			(mg/dL)	(μmol/L)
501–750	ASAP after enrollment	≥13.0	≥222	≥8.0	≥137	≥13.0	≥257
751–1000	ASAP after enrollment	≥15.0	≥257	≥10.0	≥171	≥15.0	≥157

Enrollment is expected within the period 12–36 hours after birth, preferably between 12 and 24 hours. Reproduced from Maisels MJ, Watchko JF. Treatment of hyperbilirubinemia. In: Buonocore G. Bracci R, Weindling M, eds. *Neonatology: A Practical Approach to Neonatal Diseases*. Milan: Springer-Verlag; 2011;629–640, with permission.

moderate hyperbilirubinemia in these infants poses no risk of neurotoxicity.[22,65] Thus, there was an urgent need for an appropriately conducted large, randomized controlled trial to attempt to provide some answers to these questions and this was undertaken by the NICHD NRN.

In this trial, "aggressive or conservative" phototherapy was instituted in 1974 ELBW infants born between 2002 and 2005, and followed to age 18–20 months of corrected age.[18] The protocol for this study is shown in Table 10-6. Compared with conservative phototherapy, aggressive phototherapy did not reduce the primary outcome of death or NDI but, in surviving infants, it did reduce the rates of NDI (RR: 0.86; 95% CI: 0.75–0.99), hearing loss (RR: 0.32; 95% CI: 0.15–0.60), mental development index score <70 (RR: 0.83; 95% CI: 0.71–0.98), and athetosis (RR: 0.20; 95% CI: 0.04–0.90). The reduction in NDI was attributable almost entirely to a decrease in infants with profound impairment in the aggressive phototherapy group (RR: 0.68; 95% CI: 0.52–0.89). The mean TSB levels were lower in the aggressive group (4.7 ± 1.1 mg/dL) than in the conservative group (6.2 ± 1.5 mg/dL) and, although these differences were statistically significant (P <.001), it is surprising that this small difference was associated with a difference in outcome. On the other hand, the mean TSB levels in the surviving impaired and unimpaired infants were identical (5.4 mg/dL), although the mean peak TSB was marginally higher (0.3 mg/dL) in the impaired cohort.

Were the improved outcomes in this study the result of lower TSB levels in the aggressive phototherapy group and were the worse outcomes in the conservative group the consequence of higher TSB levels? It is difficult to answer this question with confidence, given that the surviving impaired and unimpaired infants had identical mean TSB levels and a difference of 0.3 mg/dL in peak TSB levels. On the other hand, this was a randomized controlled trial and there were no (known) differences between the two groups prior to treatment. In term and late preterm infants, bilirubin encephalopathy is not usually associated with profound intellectual impairment, although severe motor handicap is the rule. If these outcomes are related to TSB or unbound bilirubin levels, perhaps they are the result of a combination of the effect of extreme prematurity, with its known hazards, together with the additional burden of (questionably) increased exposure to bilirubin. Perhaps aggressive phototherapy, by itself, has other, unknown benefits as well as hazards.

What should neonatologists do with this information? In many units, phototherapy is initiated in infants with birth weights <1000 g when their TSB reaches 5 mg/dL. As the TSB at the start of phototherapy in the aggressive group was 4.8 mg/dL, instituting phototherapy at a TSB of 5 mg/dL will likely have a similar effect on TSB levels as prophylactic phototherapy initiated in every infant soon after birth. If one combines these data with the previous observations from the NRN,[66] it appears that modest elevations of TSB in these tiny babies are potentially harmful and, when used in a manner similar to that employed in this study, phototherapy could help to reduce long-term NDI. The treatment levels suggested in Table 10-4 are, therefore, to some extent influenced by the NRN study.

Biological Effects and Complications

Millions of infants have been exposed to phototherapy for over 40 years and reports of significant toxicity are exceptionally rare.[6,67] Although human, animal, and in vitro studies suggest that the products of photodecomposition have no neurotoxic effects,[68,69] the data on this subject are relatively limited.

Skin

Infants with congenital erythropoietic porphyria who have been exposed to phototherapy have developed severe blistering and photosensitivity.[70] Congenital porphyria, or a family history of porphyria, is an absolute contraindication to the use of phototherapy and severe blistering and agitation during phototherapy could be a sign of this disease.[70] Rare purpuric and bullous eruptions have also been described in infants with cholestatic jaundice who are receiving phototherapy.[71,72] Tin mesoporphyrin (SnMP) is an experimental drug used to prevent and treat hyperbilirubinemia (see section "Pharmacological Therapy"). An erythematous rash has been described in infants who were treated with this drug and subsequently exposed to sunlight or daylight fluorescent bulbs.[73] The rash resolved when the light exposure was discontinued.[73]

The possibility of late dermatologic effects of phototherapy has focused on the presence of melanocytic nevi, a risk factor for malignant melanoma,[74,75] and malignant melanoma itself. The size and number of nevi have been evaluated in school-age children and adults.[75–78] Some studies have found that children who had been treated with intense blue light phototherapy had increased numbers[75,78] or an abnormal appearance of melanocytic nevi,[75] but others have not found this[79,80] and no association between phototherapy and malignant melanoma was found in the one study that has examined this.[81]

A partial-thickness burn was described on the back of a 25-week gestation 800-g infant receiving phototherapy with a fiber-optic system,[82] and the Ohmeda company reported four extremely premature infants (≤25 weeks gestation) who developed purplish-red necrotizing lesions during the use of the BiliBlanket phototherapy system. All of these infants suffered from conditions that can reduce skin integrity such as birth trauma, hypotension, poor perfusion of the skin, or bacterial contamination of the incubator or bed. The skin of these extremely premature infants is remarkable fragile and it appears unlikely that these were thermal burns. Two infants developed erythema (one was blistering) following exposure to daylight fluorescent lamps without Plexiglas shielding.[83] Children with the Crigler–Najjar syndrome receiving phototherapy for 2–3 years often develop pigmented lesions and tanning as well as skin atrophy.

The Bronze Baby Syndrome

When infants with cholestasis (direct hyperbilirubinemia) are exposed to phototherapy, they will often develop a grayish-brown discoloration of the skin, serum, and urine known as the bronze baby syndrome (BBS).[84–86] The pathogenesis of this condition is not fully understood, and, although it occurs exclusively in infants with cholestasis, not all infants with cholestatic jaundice develop this syndrome.[87–90] Infants with cholestasis accumulate porphyrins and other metabolites in the plasma, and some investigators have suggested that photosensitization of the porphyrins by bilirubin produces the color changes seen.[89,90] These conclusions have been challenged by the recent work of McDonagh,[91] who showed that bilirubin in a solution of human serum albumin (HSA) does not photosensitize the degradation of copper-porphyrins (CuP). He notes that bilirubin is a weak photosensitizer and that it is unlikely that it would photosensitize the degradation of CuP. In addition, the concentration of CuP, even in infants with cholestasis, is very small and that it is very "unlikely that CuP (which is pink in HSA solution) or CuP photoproducts are responsible for the hyperpigmentation seen in patients with the BBS."[91] He suggests that it is more likely that "the color is related to substances derived from the predominant, much more visible, and more photoreactive bilirubin pigments that are present."[84,85] There appear to be few deleterious consequences from this syndrome, although kernicterus has been described in infants who had Rh hemolytic disease and the BBS.[90,92,93] In these infants the maximum TSB level ranged from 18 to 22.8 mg/dL and the direct-reacting bilirubin from 4.1 to 8.7 mg/dL.

The effect of phototherapy on bilirubin conjugates has not been studied, but it is likely that they undergo similar photochemical reactions to bilirubin. Indeed, bleaching of jaundiced skin (photooxidation?) in adults with alcoholic cirrhosis during experimental phototherapy, with no lowering of plasma bilirubin levels, has been reported.[94] If there is a need for phototherapy, particularly in LBW, sick neonates, the presence of direct-reacting hyperbilirubinemia should not be considered a contraindication to its use. Because the products of phototherapy are excreted in the bile, the presence of cholestasis will decrease the efficacy of phototherapy. Nevertheless, in our experience, infants with direct-reacting hyperbilirubinemia often show some response to phototherapy. In those who develop the BBS, exchange transfusion should be considered if the TSB meets the threshold for exchange transfusion. In almost all circumstances, the direct-reacting serum bilirubin should not be subtracted from the TSB concentration in making decisions about exchange transfusions.[28]

Eye Damage

Because light can be toxic to the retina,[95] the eyes of infants receiving phototherapy should be protected with appropriate eye patches, but it should also be noted that eye patches can obstruct the nares and produce apnea. Commercially available eye shields, if properly applied, prevent more than 98% of light transmission.[96]

Insensible Water Loss and Thermal Regulation

Conventional phototherapy can produce an acute change in the infant's thermal environment, leading to an increase in peripheral blood flow and insensible water loss of approximately 20–25%.[97,98] LED lights produce little heat and should be much less likely to cause insensible water loss but this has not been studied. Some clinicians routinely increase maintenance fluids for LBW infants receiving phototherapy but we have not found this to be necessary. The infant's fluid status should be monitored in the usual manner—measurement of urine output, urine specific gravity, serum electrolytes, changes in body weight, and adjustments in fluid requirements made as needed.

Mortality in Very Low Birth Weight Infants

There have only been two large randomized controlled trials of phototherapy. In the first NICHD phototherapy study, conducted from 1974 to 1976, infants with birth weights of <2500 g were randomly assigned to undergo either 96 hours of phototherapy or no phototherapy.[55] For the 1063 infants with birth weights <2500 g, the RR for death with phototherapy was 1.32 (95% CI: 0.96–1.82) and among the 77 infants of ELBW (<1000 g) the RR was 1.49 (95% CI: 0.93–2.40).[99,100] In the recent NICHD NRN trial there was a 5% increase in mortality in infants with birth weights 501–750 g who received aggressive phototherapy.[18] This was not statistically significant, but a post hoc, Bayesian analysis estimated an 89% probability that aggressive phototherapy increased the rate of death in the subgroup. It is unclear why phototherapy might increase

mortality in these tiny infants but it is likely that light penetrates more deeply through the thin, gelatinous skin, reaching the subcutaneous tissues and possibly producing oxidative injury to cell membranes.[101–103] This observation and the evidence that, in neonatal rats, there is a relationship between increasing irradiance and the degree of oxidative injury as measured by dermal carbon monoxide (CO) excretion[102] suggest that it is prudent to use less intensive levels of irradiance in VLBW infants. An accepted principle of pharmacology is that we administer a drug in a dose that is adequate to provide therapeutic blood levels while minimizing the risks of toxicity. The same principles apply to phototherapy—we should provide a dose that will have the desired therapeutic effect and only resort to higher doses (with an increased possibility of toxicity) if the initial dose proves to be inadequate. In all VLBW infants, unlike term infants who are readmitted with very high TSB levels, the use of phototherapy is essentially prophylactic. TSB levels can almost always be controlled by phototherapy that is less intensive than that used in larger infants. Thus, for infants <1500 g, it is reasonable to start phototherapy at lower irradiance levels of about 15 μW/cm^2 per nm. If this does not lead to a decrease in TSB, additional phototherapy can be provided by increasing the surface area exposed (phototherapy above and below the infant, reflecting material around the incubator). If this does not prevent an increase in TSB, the irradiance can be increased.

Intravenous Alimentation

IV alimentation solutions should be protected from phototherapy lights. The exposure of amino acid solutions to light in the blue spectrum produced a significant reduction in tryptophan[104] and when a multivitamin solution was added to the amino acids, a 40% reduction in methionine and a 22% reduction in histidine occurred.[104]

Patent Ductus Arteriosus

A relationship has been described between the use of phototherapy and the risk of patent ductus arteriosus (PDA) in VLBW infants.[105–107] The mechanism for this potential effect is unclear, although it has been reported that exposure of isolated ductal rings to artificial room light resulted in photorelaxation and prevention of constriction of the rings despite stimulation with oxygen.[108] The mechanism and wavelength dependence of this curious effect have not been investigated further. There is, however, no photochemical rationale for the effect nor is it likely that phototherapy light will penetrate deeply enough to promote a significant effect on the ductus arteriosus. Two randomized controlled trials have evaluated the effect of a chest shield in infants receiving phototherapy. In the first trial[107] the incidence of PDA was significantly lower in the shielded group (30.6%) versus the exposed group (60.5%), but in a subsequent study no differences were found between the two groups.[109]

Does Intensive Phototherapy Cause Hemolysis?

There is some in vitro evidence that phototherapy can increase erythrocyte osmotic fragility[110] and produce lipid peroxidation of the red cell membrane,[111] leading to hemolysis. In one study of 24 preterm neonates,[112] standard phototherapy produced a modest, but statistically significant increase in the mean end-tidal CO concentration corrected for ambient CO (ETCOc). In contrast, in a study of 27 infants $\geq$35 weeks gestation who received intensive phototherapy (mean irradiance: $43.0 \pm 7.4\,\mu W/cm^2$ per nm at 425–475 nm), there was a steady decrease in the mean ETCOc levels over the course of phototherapy.[113] This suggests that intensive phototherapy at a high irradiance does not increase heme turnover or bilirubin production. In one study of preterm neonates,[114] 96 hours of phototherapy (irradiance not stated) produced a significant increase in blood thiobarbituric acid–reacting substances (TBARS, a measure of lipid peroxidation), suggesting that phototherapy induces oxidative stress. By contrast, Kaplan et al.[115] found no increase in TBARS or plasma protein carbonyls (representative of protein oxidation) in 41 preterm infants $\leq$35 weeks gestation during the first 24 hours of phototherapy (average irradiance 18 $\mu W/cm^2$ per nm). As phototherapy uniformly decreases TSB levels, the likelihood that it actually increases heme catabolism, even in VLBW infants, is very small.

Other Complications

Given the vast number of newborns who have been exposed to phototherapy in every corner of the globe for about four decades, it is hard to envisage some hitherto undiscovered important complication of this treatment. Nevertheless, it should be recognized that there are a number of studies of human newborns that have found some evidence of DNA damage,[116–121] alterations in cytokine levels,[122–124] and evidence of oxidative stress.[114,125,126]

The linking of disease registries with perinatal databases has suggested a possible relationship between an increased risk of childhood leukemia and phototherapy,[127] but others have not found this.[128] A Swedish study found a strong association between phototherapy and juvenile-onset diabetes,[129] but a subsequent, large, Scottish case–control study did not.[130] None of these potential late, adverse medical effects of phototherapy has been convincingly demonstrated and they need to be evaluated carefully in larger, well-designed studies. In addition, the complete absence of any abnormal neurodevelopmental outcomes including visual and auditory function, school performance, and social interactions in children with the Crigler–Najjar syndrome who have received daily phototherapy for up to 21 years is certainly reassuring.[131]

Rate of Decline in Serum Bilirubin

The effectiveness of phototherapy depends not only on the dose of light, but also on the cause and severity of the hyperbilirubinemia. During active hemolysis, the TSB may not decline or not decline as rapidly as it would in an infant without hemolysis. On the other hand, because phototherapy works on bilirubin present in the skin and superficial subcutaneous tissue, the more bilirubin present at those sites (i.e., the higher the TSB level), the more effective phototherapy will be.[132] In some infants with a TSB >30 mg/dL (513 μmol/L), intensive phototherapy can result in a decline of as much as 10 mg/dL (171 μmol/L) within a few hours.[29]

Hemolysis is more likely to be the cause of hyperbilirubinemia in infants who require phototherapy during the birth hospitalization than in those readmitted for such treatment[133–135] and phototherapy in infants treated during the birth hospitalization is almost always initiated at a lower TSB level. For both of these reasons, the level of TSB tends to fall relatively slowly in such infants.

When Should Phototherapy Be Stopped?

There is no standard for discontinuing phototherapy. The TSB level for discontinuing phototherapy depends on the age at which phototherapy is initiated and the cause of the hyperbilirubinemia. In infants who are readmitted for phototherapy following discharge after their birth hospitalization (usually for TSB levels of 18–20 mg/dL or higher), phototherapy may generally be discontinued when the TSB falls below 13–14 mg/dL. In these infants, phototherapy is usually instituted when the TSB has reached or is close to its peak and phototherapy simply assists it on its way down. In infants who receive phototherapy during the birth hospitalization, phototherapy can be discontinued when two consecutive TSB values fall below the level at which phototherapy was initiated.

Rebound

A rebound in the TSB level of 1–2 mg/dL,[134] and occasionally more,[133] can occur after phototherapy is discontinued and it is closely related to the age at which phototherapy was initiated and the cause of the hyperbilirubinemia.[133,134] Of 144 infants who first received phototherapy on readmission, only 1 (RR: 0.7%; 95% CI: 0–2.0) required repeat phototherapy, whereas of infants who received phototherapy before discharge from the nursery 13/158 (RR: 8.2%; 95% CI: 3.9–12.4) required repeat phototherapy.[134] In Israeli infants who received phototherapy prior to discharge from the hospital, 15.3% developed a rebound defined as a TSB following phototherapy of ≥15 mg/dL,[133] but in infants who only required phototherapy following readmission, 0 of 30 cases developed a rebound. Most infants who develop hyperbilirubinemia by age 48–72 hours have some degree of hemolysis[135] so that it is not surprising that infants who need phototherapy prior to discharge are much more likely to have a rebound. In these infants, after phototherapy is discontinued, it is advisable to provide a follow-up TSB measurement within 24 hours after discharge. For those who are readmitted for phototherapy, a clinical follow-up is suggested with the option of performing a TSB measurement. In these infants, once phototherapy is discontinued, discharge from the hospital should not be delayed in order to observe the infant for rebound.

Home Phototherapy

Pressures for early discharge and a desire to avoid rehospitalization have led to the widespread use of home phototherapy.[136–140] Although not recommended for infants who have severe hyperbilirubinemia (TSB >20 mg/dL),[28] when used appropriately, home phototherapy poses no obvious hazards to the infant and is certainly much cheaper than hospital treatment.[136–140] It avoids parent–child separation and there is evidence that mothers of infants who receive phototherapy at home are less likely to stop nursing their infants.[141] The recent development of LED/fiber-optic systems permits efficient phototherapy to be delivered at home and should reduce

the necessity for readmission in many cases. Figure 10-8 provides the AAP recommendations regarding TSB levels at which home phototherapy is appropriate.[28]

Sunlight Exposure

In their original description of phototherapy, Cremer et al.[4] demonstrated that sunlight lowers TSB levels. Although sunlight certainly produces sufficient irradiance in the 425- to 475-nm band to provide effective phototherapy (Table 10-3), the practical difficulties involved in safely exposing a naked newborn to the sun either inside or outside (and avoiding sunburn) generally preclude the use of sunlight as a reliable therapeutic tool. As discussed in Chapter 13, however, in low- and middle-income countries, where lack of appropriate equipment or lack of electricity often precludes the use of phototherapy, sunshine phototherapy might be the only available alternative for a severely jaundiced infant. Studies are currently being conducted using filters to protect the infant from UV exposure while utilizing the benefit of sunlight to lower the TSB.[142]

Phototherapy in Older Children and Adolescents

The definitive therapy for Crigler–Najjar syndrome is liver transplantation but, until the procedure can be performed, phototherapy is needed to prevent dangerous TSB levels from developing.[131] In the Amish population, a group in whom the Crigler–Najjar syndrome is relatively common, the cost of liver transplantation is prohibitive (and these communities do not accept any form of state or federal support). Specially designed home phototherapy devices have been created that provide adequate phototherapy to the growing child and even the adolescent.[131] In the older child, phototherapy is less effective, presumably as a consequence of thickening of the skin, an increase in skin pigmentation, and a decrease in surface area relative to body mass. In these children phototherapy is provided only during sleep to allow normal activities during the day. The most satisfactory systems provide a "tanning bed" configuration in which the child lies on a transparent surface directly above special blue fluorescent tubes. A standard mesh or high-transmission fabric stretched over an adjustable tension frame has been used.[143] This is similar to a traditional hammock and permits adequate transmission of blue light as well as patient comfort. Because LED systems generate minimal heat, they will significantly ease the discomfort experienced by the older child who requires phototherapy and, in these children, one can anticipate that the use of LED systems will become the rule.[131]

■ EXCHANGE TRANSFUSION

The use of high-intensity blue light (460–490 nm) phototherapy applied to a large surface area of the neonate, and prevention of Rh isoimmunization with Rh immunoglobulin, have greatly reduced the need for an exchange transfusion.[18,20,23,144] However, there are still circumstances, most often in the context of hemolytic disease, when exchange transfusion is necessary to prevent or correct hazardous levels of hyperbilirubinemia and reduce the risk of kernicterus. Exchange transfusion removes bilirubin-laden blood and in the treatment of immune-mediated hemolytic disease also achieves: (i) the removal of antibody-coated red blood cells (a source of "potential"

bilirubin); (ii) the correction of anemia (if present); and (iii) removal of maternal antibody.

Technique

The first report of an exchange transfusion was published in 1925 by Hart[145] and describes the technique that was implemented, in his case, for the right condition, but for the wrong, or at least speculative, reason (to remove an unknown toxin in the blood). The history of the introduction of exchange transfusion for treatment of hemolytic disease of the newborn has been described nicely elsewhere,[146] including the various ways in which exchange transfusion was achieved in those early days. Ultimately, Diamond et al.[147] described the procedure most applied now, with the typical placement of a plastic catheter into the umbilical vein, necessitating a "push–pull" method with a single syringe and a special four-way stopcock assembly for a single operator to accomplish the task (Figure 10-10). The catheter size used will vary

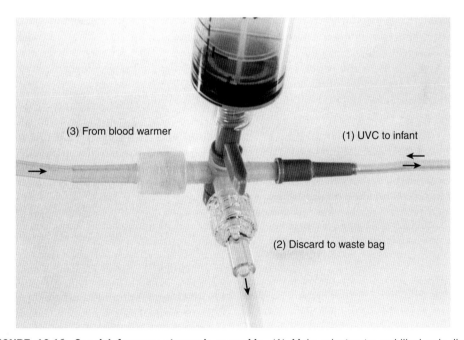

(3) From blood warmer

(1) UVC to infant

(2) Discard to waste bag

FIGURE 10-10. Special four-way stopcock assembly. (1) Male adapter to umbilical vein line; (2) female adapter to waster container; and (3) attachment to blood bag and warmer. The stopcock handle points to the port that is open to the syringe and stopcock handle is rotated in a clockwise fashion when correctly assembled (e.g., first, withdraw aliquot from infant; second, discard to waste container; third, draw fresh blood from bag; and then fourth, infuse into infant to complete one cycle). (Reproduced from Watchko JF. Exchange transfusion in the management of neonatal hyperbilirubinemia. In: Maisels MJ, Watchko JF, eds. *Neonatal Jaundice—Monographs in Clinical Pediatrics.* Amsterdam: Harwood Academic Publishers; 2000:169–176.)

with the size of the infant, usually 5 or 8 French, and inserted until there is free flow of blood, usually no more than the distance between the xiphoid process and umbilicus.[146] Alternatively, an exchange transfusion may be performed by simultaneous infusion through an umbilical venous catheter placed in the inferior vena cava and withdrawal from an umbilical arterial line.[146] When umbilical venous catheterization is unattainable, a femoral venous line[148,149] or peripheral arteries and veins may be used.[150,151]

The blood used for the procedure should be fresh (<72 hours old), citrate-phosphate-dextrose (CPD)–preserved blood, cross-matched with the infant and without any antigens that could make the transfused cells vulnerable to hemolysis. Blood for the exchange transfusion should be irradiated in order to avoid the rare occurrence of graft-versus-host disease, and should be warmed to body temperature using a blood/fluid warmer before infusion.

A "double volume" exchange refers to an exchange of twice the neonate's blood volume or ~170–200 mL/kg performed slowly in aliquots of 5–10 mL/kg body weight with each withdrawal–infusion cycle approximating 3 minutes. Using this approach a double volume exchange should take ~1.5 hours and removes ~110% of circulating bilirubin (extravascular bilirubin enters the blood during the exchange), but only 25% of total body bilirubin because at least 50% of the infant's bilirubin is typically in the extravascular compartment.[152] Many infants who require an exchange transfusion will have a high total body bilirubin load, as a result of increased production of the pigment due to hemolysis. Postexchange bilirubin levels are ~60% of preexchange values, and the reequilibration of bilirubin between extravascular and vascular compartments produces a rapid rebound (within 30 minutes) of TSB to 70–80% of preexchange levels.[152,153]

The infant's heart rate (electrocardiogram), respiratory rate, oxygen saturation, temperature, and blood pressure should be monitored continuously throughout the procedure. Citrate in CPD-preserved blood may lead to symptomatic hypocalcemia in some infants. If the infant shows signs of hypocalcemia, the procedure can be temporarily interrupted until such signs abate, as the citrate is metabolized by the liver. The routine practice of infusing calcium gluconate during an exchange transfusion is unnecessary[154] and, if done too rapidly, can lead to bradyarrhythmias and cardiac arrest. Albumin priming

to improve the efficiency of the exchange transfusion is not likely to be successful in this regard and not routinely recommended. The infusion of albumin while awaiting blood for exchange transfusion may facilitate a shift of bilirubin from the extravascular to intravascular compartment[155] and increase the efficacy of the exchange,[152,156–158] although the impact of this intervention may be modest, is difficult to predict,[159] and should not delay initiating the exchange transfusion itself.

Often not appreciated is the increased risk for paradoxical air emboli arising from a loose stopcock in the umbilical venous catheter system, with air entraining into the line in the spontaneously breathing infant. Air emboli can cross the foramen ovale and exit the left side of the heart, and potentially access the coronary arteries and cause sudden cardiac arrest, which can be refractory to resuscitation for long periods of time. Thus, checking and rechecking the integrity of all stopcock connections before, during, and after the procedure is paramount.

Once the procedure is completed, postexchange blood studies should include measurements of bilirubin, hemoglobin, platelet count, and serum glucose. The platelet count needs to be checked because the blood that has been used for the exchange transfusion is platelet-poor. Glucose should be monitored because dextrose from the CPD preservative can cause a reactive hypoglycemia induced by an insulin response.

Indications

Figure 10-11 provides the 2004 AAP guidelines for exchange transfusion in infants 35 or more weeks gestation[28] and Table 10-4 provides guidelines for infants <35 weeks gestation.

Complications

Exchange transfusion has many possible adverse effects, some of which have already been mentioned above (Table 10-7). Although mortality rates historically have been less than 1%,[21,162] it is not inconceivable that the risks might be higher when the procedure is performed by individuals who do not conduct exchange transfusions frequently (which now includes most practitioners).[64] Sick LBW infants are those at the highest risk for death or other complications[19,163] and, despite the best execution, there are always the risks associated with the administration of blood (even when appropriately screened), including infections of various kinds, mainly viral.[164]

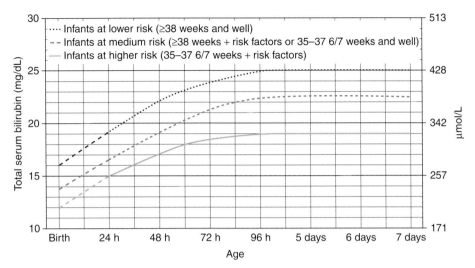

FIGURE 10-11. Guidelines for exchange transfusion in infants 35 or more weeks gestation. (Modified from American Academy of Pediatrics, Subcommittee on Hyperbilirubinemia. Clinical practice guideline: management of hyperbilirubinemia in the newborn infant 35 or more weeks of gestation. *Pediatrics*. 2004;114:297–316, with permission.)

- The dashed lines for the first 24 hours indicate uncertainty due to a wide range of clinical circumstances and a range of responses to phototherapy.
- Immediate exchange transfusion is recommended if infant shows signs of acute bilirubin encephalopathy (hypertonia, arching, retrocollis, opisthotonos, fever, high-pitched cry) or if TSB is ≥5 mg/dL (85 μmol/L) above these lines.
- The lines for lower, medium, and higher risks refer to risk for neurotoxicity.
- Risk factors for neurotoxicity—isoimmune hemolytic disease, G6PD deficiency, asphyxia, significant lethargy, temperature instability, sepsis, and acidosis.
- Measure serum albumin and calculate B/A ratio (see legend).
- Use total bilirubin. Do not subtract direct-reacting or conjugated bilirubin.
- If infant is well and 35–37 6/7 weeks (median risk), can individualize TSB levels for exchange based on actual gestational age.
- During birth hospitalization, exchange transfusion is recommended if the TSB rises to these levels despite intensive phototherapy. For readmitted infants, if the TSB level is above the exchange level, repeat TSB measurement every 2–3 hours and consider exchange if the TSB remains above the levels indicated after intensive phototherapy for 6 hours.

The following B/A ratios can be used together with but not in lieu of the TSB level as an additional factor in determining the need for exchange transfusion[160]:

Risk Category	B/A Ratio At Which Exchange Transfusion Should Be Considered	
	TSB (mg/dL)/Alb (g/dL)	TSB (μmol/L)/Alb (μmol/L)
Infants ≥38 0/7 weeks	8.0	0.94
Infants 35 0/7–36 6/7 weeks and well or ≥38 0/7 weeks if higher risk or isoimmune hemolytic disease or G6PD deficiency	7.2	0.84
Infants 35 0/7–37 6/7 weeks if higher risk or isoimmune hemolytic disease or G6PD deficiency	6.8	0.80

If the TSB is at or approaching the exchange level, send blood for immediate type and cross-match. Blood for exchange transfusion is modified whole blood (red cells and plasma) cross-matched against the mother and compatible with the infant.[161]

■ **TABLE 10-7.** Potential Complications of Exchange Transfusion

Cardiovascular	Arrhythmias
	Cardiac arrest
	Volume overload
	Embolization with air or clots
	Thrombosis
	Vasospasm
Hematologic	Sickling (donor blood)
	Thrombocytopenia
	Bleeding (overheparinization of donor blood)
	Graft-versus-host disease
	Mechanical or thermal injury to donor cells
Gastrointestinal	Necrotizing enterocolitis
	Bowel perforation
Biochemical	Hyperkalemia
	Hypernatremia
	Hypocalcemia
	Hypomagnesemia
	Acidosis
	Hypoglycemia
Infectious	Bacteremia
	Virus infection (hepatitis, CMV)
	Malaria
Miscellaneous	Hypothermia
	Perforation of the umbilical vein
	Drug loss
	Apnea

Reproduced from Watchko JF. Exchange transfusion in the management of neonatal hyperbilirubinemia. In: Maisels MJ, Watchko JF, eds. *Neonatal Jaundice—Monographs in Clinical Pediatrics*. Amsterdam: Harwood Academic Publishers; 2000: 169–176.

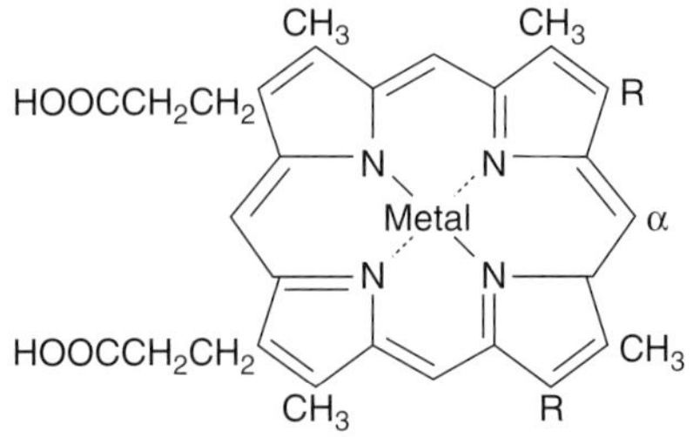

FIGURE 10-12. Metalloporphyrin structure. (Reproduced from Vreman HJ, Wong RJ, Stevenson DK. Alternative metalloporphyrins for the treatment of neonatal jaundice. *J Perinatol.* 2001;21(suppl 1):S108–S113, with permission.)

isoform of the enzyme, which is induced by conditions that result in increased availability of heme, such as hemolysis. The compounds typically affect also HO-2, the constitutive isoform. Since HO-2 is involved in important biological processes other than heme catabolism, this could potentially lead to undesirable side effects.[165] Free base porphyrins are phototoxic because they photosensitize formation of highly reactive singlet oxygen. Diamagnetic metalloporphyrins such as Sn and Zn metalloporphyrins also can photosensitize singlet oxygen formation to some degree, in marked contrast to heme. Therefore, phototoxicity is an inherent potential undesirable side effect of many metalloporphyrin drugs.

The most well studied metalloporphyrin is tin protoporphyrin (SnPP), which was the first tested in human neonates.[166] It is potent, but also has potentially serious phototoxicity. It was replaced by SnMP,[167] which has also been tested in human neonates and shows promise because of its even greater potency, allowing it to be used at much lower doses, although it still has phototoxic potential and requires intramuscular injection for administration.[73] A series of controlled clinical trials in Greece and Argentina have demonstrated that SnMP is highly effective in reducing TSB levels and the requirements for phototherapy in term and preterm infants,[168–170] including those with G6PD deficiency.[171] The only side effect reported to date has been a transient, non-dose-dependent erythema that developed in infants who received white light phototherapy after SnMP administration, but disappeared without sequelae.[73] SnMP has produced a temporary reduction in TSB levels in children with the Crigler–Najjar syndrome[172] and has prevented the need for an exchange transfusion in Jehovah's Witness newborns with Rh hemolytic

■ **PHARMACOLOGICAL THERAPY**

Drugs That Decrease Bilirubin Production

Perhaps the most promising candidate drugs for the prevention of hyperbilirubinemia are the metalloporphyrins. These compounds are synthetic analogs of heme, iron protoporphyrin (Figure 10-12), containing various metals complexed with protoporphyrin, deuteroporphyrin, mesoporphyrin, or glycol-substituted porphyrins (Table 10-8). They inhibit the first step in the two-step conversion of heme to bilirubin by competitively inhibiting HO (Figure 10-13). The target is HO-1, the inducible

■ TABLE 10-8. Porphyrin Type Based on Chelated Metal and Ring Substituent

Metal	Deuteroporphyrin (DP) (R = −H)	Mesoporphyrin (MP) (R = −CH$_2$−CH$_3$)	Protoporphyrin (PP) (R = −CH=CH$_2$)	Bis Glycol Porphyrin (BG) (R = −CHOH−CH$_2$OH)
Metal free	MfDP	MfMP	MfPP	MfBG
Iron	FeDP	FeMP	FePP (hemin)	FeBG
Zinc (Zn^{2+})	ZnDP	ZnMP	ZnPP	ZnBG
Tin (Sn^{4+})	SnDP	SnMP	SnPP	SnBG
Chromium (Cr^{2+})	CrDP	CrMP	CrPP	CrBG
Manganese (Mn^{2+})	MnDP	MnMP	MnPP	MnBG
Copper (Cu^{2+})	CuDP	CuMP	CuPP	CuBG
Nickel (Ni^{2+})	NiDP	NiMP	NiPP	NiBG

Reproduced from Vreman HJ, Wong RJ, Stevenson DK. Alternative metalloporphyrins for the treatment of neonatal jaundice. *J Perinatol.* 2001;21(suppl 1):S108–S113, with permission.

disease.[173] In a review of the published controlled trials, 129/279 (46%) infants in the control groups received phototherapy versus 13/443 (3%) in the infants who received SnMP.[168] To date over 800 infants in controlled trials have received SnMP and trials are ongoing in the United States, but this drug has not yet been approved by the FDA.

Another promising metalloporphyrin is zinc protoporphyrin (ZnPP).[174] ZnPP may be naturally present in minute amounts in normal red cells, but is most notably present in very much larger amounts in iron-deficiency anemia and lead poisoning. It has much lower potency than SnMP, but apparently no phototoxicity or other

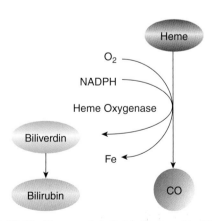

FIGURE 10-13. Heme catabolic pathway. (Modified from Stevenson DK. American Pediatric Society Presidential Address 2006: science on the edge with life in the balance. *Pediatr Res.* 2006;60:630–635. Reprinted with permission.)

adverse effects in rodents, despite being a more potent photosensitizer of singlet oxygen than protoporphyrin in vitro.[175] Zinc deuteroporphyrin IX 2,4 bis glycol (ZnBG) is more potent, with activity comparable to SnMP. It has some phototoxicity, but, like SnMP, can be used at very low doses and appears not to be photoreactive under blue phototherapy light. ZnBG is absorbed from the intestine. After oral administration it has maximum activity in liver and spleen with minimal effects in other tissues and is virtually undetectable in the brain.[176,177] It does not seem to perturb HO-1 gene expression, unlike SnMP,[178] but has not yet been tested in humans.

Hungarian investigators reported in the 1970s that IV D-penicillamine lowers bilirubin levels in newborns, including infants with ABO hemolytic disease, and can provide an alternative to exchange transfusion for Jehovah's Witness newborns.[179] The mechanism is unknown and the work has not been replicated elsewhere. In addition to metalloporphyrins, imidazole dioxolanes inhibit HO in vitro and in vivo and have high selectivity for HO-1. But they may also affect other important enzymes such as NOS and sGC, or inhibit in vivo HO activity only at high doses and induce HO-1 gene transcription, like azalanstat.[180] Biliverdin reductase inhibitors have not been developed for the purpose of treating hyperbilirubinemia.

While HO or biliverdin reductase inhibition remains a promising pharmacological approach for preventing hyperbilirubinemia and kernicterus, the permanent sequelae of bilirubin toxicity, proving that candidate drugs can prevent kernicterus, will be difficult, except in a very large population-based study, because of its low incidence. Nonetheless, any effective drug with a good safety profile is likely to replace phototherapy, and certainly exchange transfusion, as a necessity in the management of neonatal hyperbilirubinemia.

■ INTRAVENOUS IMMUNE GLOBULIN (IVIG)

Controlled trials have confirmed that the administration of IVIG to infants with Rh and ABO hemolytic disease will significantly reduce the need for exchange transfusion.[181-185] The doses usually range from 500 mg/kg given slowly over 2 hours soon after birth to 800 mg/kg given daily for 3 days. The 2004 AAP guideline recommends the use of IVIG if the TSB is rising in spite of intensive phototherapy or if the TSB is within 2–3 mg/dL of the exchange level.[28] The mechanism of action of IVIG is unknown but it is possible that it might alter the course of hemolytic disease by blocking Fc receptors and thus inhibit hemolysis. Indeed, when successful in lowering the TSB in infants with isoimmune hemolysis, IVIG treatment also reduced COHb levels (and, therefore, hemolysis), but did not lower COHb levels if the TSB was not affected.[186] Additional studies by the same investigators suggest that IVIG might be more effective in infants who have less severe hemolytic disease,[187] suggesting that the severity of the hemolysis plays a role in determining the response to IVIG.

On the other hand, after a review of published randomized controlled trials, the Cochrane Collaboration[188] concluded that the quality of these trials was not adequate to allow a recommendation for routine use of IVIG in isoimmune hemolytic disease. In addition, two recent, large randomized controlled trials of the use of IVIG in Rh hemolytic disease[189,190] found that IVIG did not reduce the need for exchange transfusion. As many clinicians are convinced that IVIG is beneficial in infants with isoimmune hemolytic disease, it will likely require additional, large randomized controlled trials before this question can be resolved.

■ DRUGS INCREASING CONJUGATION OF BILIRUBIN

Phenobarbital induces a number of hepatic enzymes, including uridine diphosphoglucuronosyltransferase (UGT),[191] and the phenobarbital response enhancer sequence of the UGT1A1 gene has been delineated.[192] Its role in reducing TSB levels in different populations has been well studied, including populations at higher risk for developing hyperbilirubinemia because of a genetic predisposition, where phenobarbital, administered to the mother antenatally, has been used successfully to lower the incidence of significant hyperbilirubinemia and exchange transfusion.[193] Nevertheless, concerns about long-term toxicity when given to pregnant women militate against the use of phenobarbital for this purpose.[194,195] The postnatal use of phenobarbital is less effective, because the TSB has often peaked prior to the clinical effectiveness of the drug. If hyperbilirubinemia were likely to be protracted, for example, in the context of ongoing increased bilirubin production, then postnatal phenobarbital administration might be useful in controlling a later-onset peak in bilirubin, as can be encountered in certain clinical conditions, such as late premature infants or an infant of a diabetic mother.

■ OTHER DRUGS FOR HYPERBILIRUBINEMIA

A few other drugs deserve mention, but are not typically used for treatment of transitional hyperbilirubinemia in the newborn. Their usage has been reviewed in detail elsewhere.[196] They include minocycline, a semisynthetic second-generation tetracycline, which may afford neuroprotection against damage caused by hyperbilirubinemia through as yet not well-defined mechanisms; clofibrate, the ethyl ester of 2-chlorophenoxy-2-methylpropionic acid, which has primarily been used as an antilipemic agent in adult patients with hyperlipoproteinemia; certain Chinese herbal remedies; and ursodeoxycholic acid (Actigall). Bilirubin oxidase has been proposed as a method to reduce the enterohepatic circulation of bilirubin and both charcoal and agar have been used to accelerate the elimination of bilirubin from the gut. The same, however, can be achieved with the establishment of good oral feeding, including breastfeeding, although formula feeding is most influential in this regard.

Of the various possible treatments besides phototherapy, the HO inhibitors are probably the most promising therapeutic agents for prevention and treatment of neonatal jaundice in order to avoid the risks of exchange transfusion. Using a targeted approach to identify high producers of the pigment would increase the therapeutic:toxic ratio favorably and maximize benefit and minimize risk for the treated infants. Until such an approach is feasible, phototherapy will remain the mainstay of treatment for neonatal jaundice.

REFERENCES

1. Dobbs RH, Cremer RJ. Phototherapy. *Arch Dis Child.* 1975;50(11):833–836.
2. Lightner DA, McDonagh AF. Molecular mechanisms of phototherapy for neonatal jaundice. *Acc Chem Res.* 1984;17:417–424.
3. Maisels MJ, McDonagh AF. Phototherapy for neonatal jaundice. *N Engl J Med.* 2008;358:920–928.
4. Cremer RJ, Perryman PW, Richards DH. Influence of light on the hyperbilirubinemia of infants. *Lancet.* 1958;1:1094–1097.
5. Lucey JF, Ferreiro M, Hewitt J. Prevention of hyperbilirubinemia of prematurity by phototherapy. *Pediatrics.* 1968;41:1047–1054.
6. Jährig K, Jährig D, Meisel P, eds. *Phototherapy: Treating Neonatal Jaundice with Visible Light.* München: Quintessenz Verlags-GmbH; 1998.
7. National Institute for Health and Clinical Excellence. *Neonatal Jaundice.* London, UK: National Institute for Health and Clinical Excellence; 2010. Available at: www.nice.org.uk/CG98.
8. McDonagh AF, Lightner DA. "Like a shrivelled blood orange"—bilirubin, jaundice and phototherapy. *Pediatrics.* 1985;75:443–455.
9. McDonagh AF. Ex uno plures: the concealed complexity of bilirubin species in neonatal blood samples. *Pediatrics.* 2006;118:1185–1187.
10. Mreihil K, McDonagh A, Nakstad B, Hansen TWR. Early isomerization of bilirubin in phototherapy of neonatal jaundice. *Pediatr Res.* 2010;67:656–659.
11. McDonagh AF. Controversies in bilirubin biochemistry and their clinical relevance. *Semin Fetal Neonatal Med.* 2010;15:141–147.
12. Myara A, Sender A, Valette V, Rostoker C, Paumier D, Capoulade C. Early changes in cutaneous bilirubin and serum bilirubin isomers during intensive phototherapy of jaundiced neonates with blue and green light. *Biol Neonate.* 1997;71:75–82.
13. Ennever JF. Blue light, green light, white light, more light: treatment of neonatal jaundice. *Clin Perinatol.* 1990;17:467–481.
14. McDonagh AF. Sunlight-induced mutation of bilirubin in a long-distance runner. *N Engl J Med.* 1986;314:121–122.
15. McDonagh AF, Maisels MJ. Photoisomerization of bilirubin in Crigler–Najjar patients. In: Kappas A, Lucey J, eds. *Treatment of Crigler–Najjar Syndrome, Conference Proceedings.* New York City: Rockefeller University; 1996.
16. Tan KL. The pattern of bilirubin response to phototherapy for neonatal hyperbilirubinemia. *Pediatr Res.* 1982;16:670–674.
17. Maisels MJ. Why use homeopathic doses of phototherapy? *Pediatrics.* 1996;98:283–287.
18. Morris BH, Oh W, Tyson JE, et al. Aggressive vs. conservative phototherapy for infants with extremely low birth weight. *N Engl J Med.* 2008;359:1885–1896.
19. Patra K, Storfer-Isser A, Siner B, Moore J, Hack M. Adverse events associated with neonatal exchange transfusion in the 1990s. *J Pediatr.* 2004;144:626–631.
20. Steiner LA, Bizzarro MJ, Ehrenkranz RA, Gallagher PG. A decline in the frequency of neonatal exchange transfusions and its effect on exchange-related morbidity and mortality. *Pediatrics.* 2007;120:27–32.
21. Keenan WJ, Novak KK, Sutherland JM, et al. Morbidity and mortality associated with exchange transfusion. *Pediatrics.* 1985;75:417–421.
22. O'Shea TM, Dillard RG, Klinepeter KL, Goldstein DJ. Serum bilirubin levels, intracranial hemorrhage, and the risk of developmental problems in very low birth weight infants. *Pediatrics.* 1992;90:888–892.
23. Newman TB, Liljestrand P, Jeremy RJ, et al. Outcomes among newborns with total serum bilirubin levels of 25 mg per deciliter or more. *N Engl J Med.* 2006;354:1889–1900.
24. Vreman HJ, Wong RJ, Murdock JR, Stevenson DK. Standardized bench method for evaluating the efficacy of phototherapy devices. *Acta Paediatr.* 2008;97:308–316.
25. Bhutani VK, Committee on Fetus and Newborn. Technical report: phototherapy to prevent severe neonatal hyperbilirubinemia in the newborn infant 35 or more weeks of gestation. *Pediatrics.* 2011;128:e1046–e1052.
26. Vreman HJ, Wong RJ, Stevenson DK. Light-emitting diodes: a novel light source for phototherapy. *Pediatr Res.* 1998;44:804–809.
27. Maisels MJ, Kring EA, DeRidder J. Randomized controlled trial of light-emitting diode phototherapy. *J Perinatol.* 2007;27:565–567.
28. American Academy of Pediatrics, Subcommittee on Hyperbilirubinemia. Clinical practice guideline: management of hyperbilirubinemia in the newborn infant 35 or more weeks of gestation. *Pediatrics.* 2004;114:297–316.
29. Hansen TWR. Acute management of extreme neonatal jaundice—the potential benefits of intensified phototherapy and interruption of enterohepatic bilirubin circulation. *Acta Paediatr.* 1997;86:843–846.
30. Holtrop PC, Ruedisueli K, Maisels MJ. Double versus single phototherapy in low birth weight newborns. *Pediatrics.* 1992;90:674–677.
31. Tan KL. Efficacy of bidirectional fiberoptic phototherapy for neonatal hyperbilirubinemia. *Pediatrics.* 1997;99:e13.
32. Corley A, Huguet-Jacquot S, Lattes F, et al. Effect of a 360 degree fluorescent tubes intensive phototherapy device on kinetics of total bilirubin (TB) and unbound

bilirubin (UBB) plasmatic levels in term neonates. *E-PAS2010*:2851.347.

33. Rubaltelli FF, Zanardo V, Granati B. Effect of various phototherapy regimens on bilirubin decrement. *Pediatrics*. 1978;61:838–841.

34. Maurer HM, Shumway CN, Draper DA, Hossaini AA. Controlled trial comparing agar, intermittent phototherapy, and continuous phototherapy for reducing neonatal hyperbilirubinemia. *J Pediatr*. 1973;82(1):73–76.

35. Lau SP, Fung KP. Serum bilirubin kinetics in intermittent phototherapy of physiological jaundice. *Arch Dis Child*. 1984;59(9):892–894.

36. Mohammadzadeh A, Bostani Z, Jafarnejad F, Mazloom R. Supine versus turning position on bilirubin level during phototherapy in healthy term jaundiced neonates. *Saudi Med J*. 2004;25:2051–2052.

37. Shinwell ES, Sciaky Y, Karplus M. Effect of position changing on bilirubin levels during phototherapy. *J Perinatol*. 2002;22:226–229.

38. Yamauchi Y, Casa N, Yamanouchi I. Is it necessary to change the babies' position during phototherapy? *Early Hum Dev*. 1989;20:221–227.

39. Wu PYK, Hodgman JE, Kirkpatrick BV, et al. Metabolic aspects of phototherapy. *Pediatrics*. 1985;75(2):427–433.

40. Mehta S, Kumar P, Narang A. A randomized controlled trial of fluid supplementation in term neonates with severe hyperbilirubinemia. *J Pediatr*. 2005;147:781–785.

41. Boo NY, Lee H-T. Randomized controlled trial of oral versus intravenous fluid supplementation on serum bilirubin level during phototherapy of term infants with severe hyperbilirubinemia. *J Paediatr Child Health*. 2002;38:151–155.

42. Cashore WJ. Free bilirubin concentrations and bilirubin-binding affinity in term and preterm infants. *J Pediatr*. 1980;96:521–527.

43. Cashore WJ, Oh W, Brodersen R. Reserve albumin and bilirubin toxicity index in infant serum. *Acta Paediatr Scand*. 1983;72:415–419.

44. Wennberg RP, Ahlfors CE, Bhutani V, Johnson LH, Shapiro SM. Toward understanding kernicterus: a challenge to improve the management of jaundiced newborns. *Pediatrics*. 2006;117:474–485.

45. Bratlid D. How bilirubin gets into the brain. *Clin Perinatol*. 1990;17:449–465.

46. Canadian Paediatric Society. Guidelines for detection, management and prevention of hyperbilirubinemia in term and late preterm newborn infants (35 or more weeks' gestation)—summary. *Paediatr Child Health*. 2007;12:401–418.

47. Fouzas S, Karatza AA, Skylogianni E, Mantagou L, Varvarigou A. Transcutaneous bilirubin levels in late preterm neonates. *J Pediatr*. 2010;157:762–766.

48. Fouzas S, Mantagou L, Skylogianni E, Mantagos S, Varvarigou A. Transcutaneous bilirubin levels for the first 120 postnatal hours in healthy neonates. *Pediatrics*. 2010;125:e52–e57.

49. Bratlid D, Nakstad B, Hansen TWR. National guidelines for treatment of jaundice in the newborn. *Acta Paediatr*. 2011;100(4):499–505.

50. Kaplan M, Merlob P, Regev R. Israel guidelines for the management of neonatal hyperbilirubinemia and prevention of kernicterus. *J Perinatol*. 2008;28:389–397.

51. Maisels MJ, Watchko JF, Bhutani VK, Stevenson DK. Clinical report: an approach to the management of hyperbilirubinemia in the preterm infant less than 35 weeks of gestation. *J Perinatol*. 2012, in press.

52. Sackett DL, Haynes RB, Guyatt GH, Tugwell P. *Clinical Epidemiology: A Basic Science for Clinical Medicine*. 2nd ed. Boston: Little, Brown and Co; 1991.

53. Ip S, Chung M, Kulig J, et al. An evidence-based review of important issues concerning neonatal hyperbilirubinemia. *Pediatrics*. 2004;114:e130–e153. Available at: www.pediatrics.org/cgi/content/full/114/1/e130:e130-e153.

54. Ip S, Glicken S, Kulig J, Obrien R, Sege R, Lau J. *Management of Neonatal Hyperbilirubinemia*. Rockville, MD: U.S. Department of Health and Human Services, Agency for Healthcare Research and Quality; 2003. AHRQ Publication 03-E011.

55. Brown AK, Kim MH, Wu PYK, et al. Efficacy of phototherapy in prevention and management of neonatal hyperbilirubinemia. *Pediatrics*. 1985;75:393–400.

56. Martinez JC, Maisels MJ, Otheguy L, et al. Hyperbilirubinemia in the breast-fed newborn: a controlled trial of four interventions. *Pediatrics*. 1993;91:470–473.

57. Maurer HM, Kirkpatrick BV, McWilliams NB, Draper DA, Bryla DA. Phototherapy for hyperbilirubinemia of hemolytic disease of the newborn. *Pediatrics*. 1985;75:407–412.

58. Newman TB, Kuzniewicz MW, Liljestrand P, Wi S, McCulloch C, Escobar GJ. Numbers needed to treat with phototherapy according to American Academy of Pediatrics guidelines. *Pediatrics*. 2009;123:1352–1359.

59. Maisels MJ, Watchko JF. Treatment of jaundice in low birthweight infants. *Arch Dis Child Neonatal Ed*. 2003;88:F459–F463.

60. Hansen TWR. Therapeutic approaches to neonatal jaundice: an international survey. *Clin Pediatr*. 1996;35:309–316.

61. Rennie JM, Sehgal A, De A, Kendall GS, Cole TJ. Range of UK practice regarding thresholds for phototherapy and exchange transfusion in neonatal hyperbilirubinaemia. *Arch Dis Child Fetal Neonatal Ed*. 2009;94: F323–F327.

62. Shapiro SM. Chronic bilirubin encephalopathy: diagnosis and outcome. *Semin Fetal Neonatal Med.* 2010;15:157–163.

63. Watchko JF, Maisels MJ. Jaundice in low birth weight infants—pathobiology and outcome. *Arch Dis Child Fetal Neonatol Ed.* 2003;88:F455–F459.

64. Watchko JF, Oski FA. Kernicterus in preterm newborns: past, present and future. *Pediatrics.* 1992;90: 707–715.

65. Yeo KL, Perlman M, Hao Y, Mullaney P. Outcomes of extremely premature infants related to their peak serum bilirubin concentrations and exposure to phototherapy. *Pediatrics.* 1998;102(6):1426–1431.

66. Oh W, Tyson JE, Fanaroff AA, et al. Association between peak serum bilirubin and neurodevelopmental outcomes in extremely low birth weight infants. *Pediatrics.* 2003;112:773–779.

67. Maisels MJ. Phototherapy. In: Maisels MJ, Watchko JF, eds. *Neonatal Jaundice.* London, UK: Harwood Academic Publishers; 2000:177–204.

68. Haddock JH, Nadler HL. Bilirubin toxicity in human cultivated fibroblasts and its modification by light treatment. *Proc Soc Exp Biol Med.* 1970;134(1):45–48.

69. Silberberg DH, Johnson L, Schutta H, Ritter L. Effects of photodegradation products of bilirubin on myelinating cerebellum cultures. *J Pediatr.* 1970;77:613.

70. Tonz O, Vogt J, Filippini L, Simmler F, Wachsmuth ED, Winterhalter KH. Severe light dermatosis following phototherapy in a newborn infant with congenital erythropoietic uroporphyria. *Helv Paediatr Acta.* 1975;30:47–56.

71. Mallon E, Wojnarowska F, Hope P, Elder G. Neonatal bullous eruption as a result of transient porphyrinemia in a premature infant with hemolytic disease of the newborn. *J Am Acad Dermatol.* 1995;33:333–336.

72. Paller AS, Eramo LR, Farrell EE, Millard DD, Honig PJ, Cunningham BB. Purpuric phototherapy-induced eruption in transfused neonates: relation to transient porphyrinemia. *Pediatrics.* 1997;100:360–364.

73. Valaes T, Petmezaki S, Henschke C, et al. Control of jaundice in preterm newborns by an inhibitor of bilirubin production: studies with tin-mesoporphyrin. *Pediatrics.* 1994;93:1–11.

74. Gandini S, Sera F, Cattaruzza MS, et al. Meta-analysis of risk factors for cutaneous melanoma: I. Common and atypical naevi. *Eur J Cancer.* 2005;41(1):28–44.

75. Csoma Z, Toth-Molnar E, Balogh K, et al. Neonatal blue light phototherapy and melanocytic nevi: a twin study. *Pediatrics.* 2011;128:e856–e864.

76. Csoma Z, Hencz P, Orvos H, et al. Neonatal blue-light phototherapy could increase the risk of dysplastic nevus development. *Pediatrics.* 2007;119:1269.

77. Csoma Z, Kemeny L, Olah J. Phototherapy for neonatal jaundice. *N Engl J Med.* 2008;358(23):2523–2524.

78. Matichard E, Le Henanff A, Sanders A, Leguyadec J, Crickx B, Descamps V. Effect of neonatal phototherapy on melanocytic nevus count in children. *Arch Dermatol.* 2006;142:1599–1604.

79. Bauer J, Buttner P, Luther H, Wiecker TS, Mohrle M, Garbe C. Blue light phototherapy of neonatal jaundice does not increase the risk for melanocytic nevus development. *Arch Dermatol.* 2004;140:493–494.

80. Mahe E, Beauchet A, Philippe A, Saiag P. Neonatal blue-light phototherapy does not increase nevus count in 9-year-old children. *Pediatrics.* 2009;123:e896–e900.

81. Berg P, Lindelof B. Is phototherapy in neonates a risk factor for malignant melanoma development? *Arch Pediatr Adolesc Med.* 1997;151:1185–1187.

82. Hussain K, Sharief N. Dermal injury following the use of fiberoptic phototherapy in an extremely premature infant. *Clin Pediatr (Phila).* 1996;35(8):421–422.

83. Siegfried EC, Stone MS, Madison KC. Ultraviolet light burn: a cutaneous complication of visible light phototherapy of neonatal jaundice. *Pediatr Dermatol.* 1992;9: 278–282.

84. Meisel P, Jahrig D, Theel L, Ordt A, Jahrig K. The bronze baby syndrome: consequence of impaired excretion of photobilirubin? *Photochem Photobiol.* 1982;3: 345–352.

85. Kopelman AE, Brown RS, Odell GB. The "bronze" baby syndrome: a complication of phototherapy. *J Pediatr.* 1972;81:466–472.

86. Tan KL, Jacob E. The bronze baby syndrome. *Acta Paediatr Scand.* 1982;71:409–414.

87. Jori G, Reddi E, Rubaetelli FF. Bronze baby syndrome: evidence for increased serum porphyrin concentration. *Lancet.* 1982;1:1072.

88. Jori G, Reddi E, Rubaltelli FF. Bronze baby syndrome: an animal model. *Pediatr Res.* 1990;27:22–25.

89. Rubaltelli FF, Da Riol R, D'Amore E, Jori G. The bronze baby syndrome: evidence of increased tissue concentration of copper porphyrins. *Acta Paediatr.* 1996;85: 381–384.

90. Rubaltelli FF, Jori G, Reddi E. Bronze baby syndrome: a new porphyrin-related disorder. *Pediatr Res.* 1983;17: 327–330.

91. McDonagh A. Bilirubin, copper-porphyrins, and the bronze-baby syndrome. *J Pediatr.* 2010;158(1):160–164.

92. Bertini G, Dani C, Fonda C, Zorzi C, Rubaltelli F. Bronze baby syndrome and the risk of kernicterus. *Acta Paediatr.* 2005;94:968–971.

93. Clark CF, Torii S, Hamamoto Y, Kaito H. The "bronze baby" syndrome: postmortem data. *J Pediatr.* 1976;88: 461–464.

94. Knodell RG, Cheney H, Ostrow JD. Effects of phototherapy on hepatic function in human alcoholic cirrhosis. *Gastroenterology.* 1976;70:1112–1116.

95. Messner KH, Maisels MJ, Leure-DuPree AE. Phototoxicity to the newborn primate retina. *Invest Ophthalmol Vis Sci.* 1978;17(2):178–182.

96. Robinson J, Moseley MJ, Fielder A, et al. Light transmission measurements in phototherapy eye patches. *Arch Dis Child.* 1991;66:59–61.

97. Dollberg S, Atherton HD, Hoath SB. Effect of different phototherapy lights on incubator characteristics and dynamics under three modes of servocontrol. *Am J Perinatol.* 1995;12(1):55–60.

98. Maayan-Metzger A, Yosipovitch G, Hadad E, Sirota L. Transepidermal water loss and skin hydration in preterm infants during phototherapy. *Am J Perinatol.* 2001;18:393–396.

99. Maisels MJ. Neonatal jaundice. In: Sinclair JC, Bracken MB, eds. *Effective Care of the Newborn Infant.* Oxford: Oxford University Press; 1992:507–561.

100. Lipsitz PJ, Gartner LM, Bryla DA. Neonatal and infant mortality in relation to phototherapy. *Pediatrics.* 1985;75:422–426.

101. Tozzi E, Tozzi-Ciancarelli MG, Di Giulio A, et al. In vitro and in vivo effects of erythrocyte phototherapy in newborns. *Biol Neonate.* 1989;56(4):204–209.

102. Vreman HJ, Knauer Y, Wong RJ, Chan M-L, Stevenson DK. Dermal carbon monoxide excretion in neonatal rats during light exposure. *Pediatr Res.* 2009;66:66–69.

103. Vreman HJ, Wong RJ, Stevenson DK. Phototherapy: current methods and future directions. *Semin Perinatol.* 2004;28:326–333.

104. Bhatia J, Mims LC, Roesel RA. The effect of phototherapy on amino acid solutions containing multivitamins. *J Pediatr.* 1980;96:284–286.

105. Barefield ES, Dwyer MD, Cassady G. Association of patent ductus arteriosus and phototherapy in infants weighing less than 1000 grams. *J Perinatol.* 1993;13(5):376–380.

106. Benders MJNL, van Bel F, van de Bor M. Cardiac output and ductal reopening during phototherapy in preterm infants. *Acta Paediatr.* 1999;88:1014–1019.

107. Rosenfeld W, Sadhev S, Brunot V, Jhavri R, Zabaleta I, Evans HE. Phototherapy effect on the incidence of patent ductus arteriosus in premature infants: prevention with chest shielding. *Pediatrics.* 1986;78:10–14.

108. Clyman RI, Rudolph AM. Patent ductus arteriosus: a new light on an old problem. *Pediatr Res.* 1978;12(2):92–94.

109. Travadi J, Simmer K, Ramsay J, Doherty D, Hagan R. Patent ductus arteriosus in extremely preterm infants receiving phototherapy: does shielding the chest make a difference? A randomized, controlled trial. *Acta Paediatr.* 2006;95:1418–1423.

110. Cuiker JO, Maglalang AC, Odell GB. Increased osmotic fragility of erythrocytes in chronically jaundiced rats after phototherapy. *Acta Paediatr Scand.* 1979;68:903–909.

111. Ostrea EJ Jr, Cepeda EE, Fleury CA. Red cell membrane lipid peroxidation and hemolysis secondary to phototherapy. *Acta Paediatr Scand.* 1985;74:378–381.

112. Aouthmany M. Phototherapy increases hemoglobin degradation and bilirubin production in preterm infants. *J Perinatol.* 1999;19:271–274.

113. Maisels MJ, Kring EA. Does intensive phototherapy produce hemolysis in newborns of 35 or more weeks gestation? *J Perinatol.* 2006;26:498–500.

114. Gathwala G, Sharma S. Phototherapy induces oxidative stress in premature neonates. *Indian J Gastroenterol.* 2002;21(4):153–154.

115. Kaplan M, Gold V, Hammerman C, et al. Phototherapy and photo-oxidation in premature neonates. *Biol Neonate.* 2005;87:44–50.

116. Aycicek A, Kocyigit A, Erel O, Senturk H. Phototherapy causes DNA damage in peripheral mononuclear leukocytes in term infants. *J Pediatr (Rio J).* 2008;84(2):141–146.

117. Galla A, Kitsiou-Tzeli S, Gourgiotis D, et al. Sister chromatid exchanges in peripheral lymphocytes in newborns treated with phototherapy and vitamin E. *Acta Paediatr.* 1992;81(10):820–823.

118. Karadag A, Yesilyurt A, Unal S, et al. A chromosomal-effect study of intensive phototherapy versus conventional phototherapy in newborns with jaundice. *Mutat Res.* 2009;676(1–2):17–20.

119. Karakukcu C, Ustdal M, Ozturk A, Baskol G, Saraymen R. Assessment of DNA damage and plasma catalase activity in healthy term hyperbilirubinemic infants receiving phototherapy. *Mutat Res.* 2009;680(1–2):12–16.

120. Tatli MM, Minnet C, Kocyigit A, Karadag A. Phototherapy increases DNA damage in lymphocytes of hyperbilirubinemic neonates. *Mutat Res.* 2008;654(1):93–95.

121. Tsai FJ, Tsai CH, Peng CT, Wang TR. Sister chromatid exchange in Chinese newborn infants treated with phototherapy for more than five days. *Zhonghua Min Guo Xiao Er Ke Yi Xue Hui Za Zhi.* 1998;39(5):327–329.

122. Kurt A, Aygun AD, Kurt AN, Godekmerdan A, Akarsu S, Yilmaz E. Use of phototherapy for neonatal hyperbilirubinemia affects cytokine production and lymphocyte subsets. *Neonatology.* 2009;95(3):262–266.

123. Procianoy RS, Silveira RC, Fonseca LT, Heidemann LA, Neto EC. The influence of phototherapy on serum cytokine concentrations in newborn infants. *Am J Perinatol.* 2010;27(5):375–379.

124. Sirota L, Staussberg R, Gurary N, Aloni D, Bessler H. Phototherapy for neonatal hyperbilirubinemia affects

cytokine production by peripheral blood mononuclear cells. *Eur J Pediatr.* 1999;158(11):910–913.

125. Aycicek A, Erel O. Total oxidant/antioxidant status in jaundiced newborns before and after phototherapy. *J Pediatr (Rio J).* 2007;83(4):319–322.

126. Gathwala G, Sharma S. Oxidative stress, phototherapy and the neonate. *Indian J Pediatr.* 2000;67(11):805–808.

127. Cnattingius S, Zack MM, Ekbom A, et al. Prenatal and neonatal risk factors for childhood lymphatic leukemia. *J Natl Cancer Inst.* 1995;87(12):908–914.

128. Roman E, Ansell P, Bull D. Leukaemia and non-Hodgkin's lymphoma in children and young adults: are prenatal and neonatal factors important determinants of disease? *Br J Cancer.* 1997;76(3):406–415.

129. Dahlquist G, Kallen B. Indications that phototherapy is a risk factor for insulin-dependent diabetes. *Diabetes Care.* 2003;26:247–248.

130. Robertson L, Harrild K. Maternal and neonatal risk factors for childhood type 1 diabetes: a matched case–control study. *BMC Public Health.* 2010;10:281.

131. Strauss KA, Robinson DL, Vreman HJ, Puffenberger EG, Hart G, Morton DH. Management of hyperbilirubinemia and prevention of kernicterus in 20 patients with Crigler–Najjar disease. *Eur J Pediatr.* 2006;165:306–319.

132. Jährig K, Jährig D, Meisel P. Dependence of the efficiency of phototherapy on plasma bilirubin concentration. *Acta Paediatr Scand.* 1982;71(2):293–299.

133. Kaplan M, Kaplan E, Hammerman C, et al. Post-phototherapy neonatal bilirubin rebound: a potential cause of significant hyperbilirubinaemia. *Arch Dis Child.* 2006;91:31–34.

134. Maisels MJ, Kring E. Rebound in serum bilirubin level following intensive phototherapy. *Arch Pediatr Adolesc Med.* 2002;156:669–672.

135. Maisels MJ, Kring E. The contribution of hemolysis to early jaundice in normal newborns. *Pediatrics.* 2006;118:276–279.

136. Meropol SB, Luberti AA, De Jong AR, Weiss JC. Home phototherapy: use and attitudes among community pediatricians. *Pediatrics.* 1993;91:97–100.

137. Plastino R, Buchner DM, Wagner EH. Impact of eligibility criteria on phototherapy program size and cost. *Pediatrics.* 1990;85(5):796–800.

138. Rogerson AG, Grossman ER, Gruber HS, Boynton RC, Cuthbertson JG. 14 years of experience with home phototherapy. *Clin Pediatr (Phila).* 1986;25(6):296–299.

139. Schuman AJ, Karush G. Fiberoptic vs conventional home phototherapy for neonatal hyperbilirubinemia. *Clin Pediatr (Phila).* 1992;31(6):345–352.

140. Slater L, Brewer MF. Home versus hospital phototherapy for term infants with hyperbilirubinemia: a comparative study. *Pediatrics.* 1984;73:515–519.

141. James J, Williams SD, Osborn LM. Home phototherapy for treatment of exaggerated neonatal jaundice enhances breast-feeding [abstract]. *Am J Dis Child.* 1990;144:431–432.

142. Slusher T, Faber K, Cline B, et al. Selectively filtered sunlight phototherapy: safe and effective for treatment of neonatal jaundice in Nigeria. *E-PAS2011*:2918.254.

143. Job H, Hart G, Lealman G. Improvements in long term phototherapy for patients with Crigler–Najjar syndrome type I. *Phys Med Biol.* 1996;41(11):2549–2556.

144. Maisels MJ. Phototherapy—traditional and nontraditional. *J Perinatol.* 2001;21:S93–S97.

145. Hart AP. Familial icterus gravis of the newborn and its treatment. *Can Med Assoc J.* 1925;15:1008–1011.

146. Watchko JF. Exchange transfusion in the management of neonatal hyperbilirubinemia. In: Maisels MJ, Watchko JF, eds. *Neonatal Jaundice.* London, UK: Harwood Academic Publishers; 2000:169–176.

147. Diamond LK, Allen FH Jr, Thomas WO Jr. Erythroblastosis fetalis. VII. Treatment with exchange transfusion. *N Engl J Med.* 1951;244:39–49.

148. Weng YH, Chiu YW. Comparison of efficacy and safety of exchange transfusion through different catheterizations: femoral vein versus umbilical vein versus umbilical artery/vein. *Pediatr Crit Care Med.* 2011;12:61–64.

149. Watchko JF. Route of exchange transfusion in neonates with hyperbilirubinemia. *Pediatr Crit Care Med.* 2011;12(110):1.

150. Sagi E, Eyal F, Armon Y, Arad I, Robinson M. Exchange transfusion in newborns via a peripheral artery and vein. *Eur J Pediatr.* 1981;137:283–284.

151. Fok TF, So LY, Leung KW, Wong W, Feng CS, Tsang SS. Use of peripheral vessels for exchange transfusion. *Arch Dis Child.* 1990;65:676–678.

152. Valaes T. Bilirubin distribution and dynamics of bilirubin removal by exchange transfusion. *Acta Paediatr.* 1963;149:1–115.

153. Brown AK, Zuelzer WW, Robinson AR. Studies in hyperbilirubinemia. II. Clearance of bilirubin from plasma and extravascular space in newborn infants during exchange transfusion. *Am J Dis Child.* 1957;93:274–286.

154. Maisels MJ, Li TK, Piechocki JT, Werthman MW. The effect of exchange transfusion on serum ionized calcium. *Pediatrics.* 1974;53:683.

155. Odell GB. The dissociation of bilirubin from albumin and its clinical implications. *J Pediatr.* 1959;55:268–279.

156. Odell GB, Cohen SN, Gordes EH. Administration of albumin in the management of hyperbilirubinemia by exchange transfusion. *Pediatrics.* 1962;30:613–621.

157. Comley A, Wood B. Albumin administration in exchange transfusion for hyperbilirubinemia. *Arch Dis Child.* 1968;43:151–154.

158. Wood B, Comley A, Sherwell J. Effect of additional albumin administration during exchange transfusion on plasma albumin-binding capacity. *Arch Dis Child.* 1970;45:59–62.

159. Ahlfors CE. Pre-exchange transfusion of albumin: an overlooked adjunct in the treatment of severe neonatal jaundice. *Indian Pediatr.* 2010;47:231–232.

160. Ahlfors CE. Criteria for exchange transfusion in jaundiced newborns. *Pediatrics.* 1994;93:488–494.

161. American Association of Blood Banks Technical Manual Committee. Perinatal issues in transfusion practice. In: Brecher M, ed. *Technical Manual.* Bethesda, MD: American Association of Blood Banks; 2002:497–515.

162. Hovi L, Siimes MA. Exchange transfusion with fresh heparinized blood is a safe procedure: experiences from 1069 newborns. *Acta Paediatr Scand.* 1985;74:360–365.

163. Jackson JC. Adverse events associated with exchange transfusion in healthy and ill newborns. *Pediatrics.* 1997;99:e7.

164. Schreiber GB, Busch MP, Kleinman SH, Korelitz JJ. The risk of transfusion-transmitted viral infections. *N Engl J Med.* 1996;334:1685–1690.

165. Loboda A, Jazwa A, Grochot-Przeczek A, et al. Heme oxygenase-1 and the vascular bed: from molecular mechanisms to therapeutic opportunities. *Antioxid Redox Signal.* 2008;10:1767–1812.

166. Drummond GS, Kappas A. Prevention of neonatal hyperbilirubinemia by tin-protoporphyrin IX, a potent competitive inhibitor of heme oxidation. *Proc Natl Acad Sci U S A.* 1981;78:6466–6470.

167. Wong RJ, Bhutani VK, Vreman HJ, Stevenson DK. Tin mesoporphyrin for the prevention of severe neonatal hyperbilirubinemia. *NeoReviews.* 2007;8:e77–e84.

168. Kappas A. A method for interdicting the development of severe jaundice in newborns by inhibiting the production of bilirubin. *Pediatrics.* 2004;113:119–123.

169. Kappas A, Drummond G, Henschke C, et al. Direct comparison of Sn-mesoporphyrin, an inhibitor of bilirubin production, and phototherapy in controlling hyperbilirubinemia in term and near-term newborns. *Pediatrics.* 1995;95:468–474.

170. Martinez JC, Garcia HO, Otheguy L, Drummond GS, Kappas A. Control of severe hyperbilirubinemia in full-term newborns with the inhibitor of bilirubin production Sn-mesoporphyrin. *Pediatrics.* 1999;103:1–5.

171. Valaes T, Drummond GS, Kappas A. Control of hyperbilirubinemia in glucose-6-phosphate dehydrogenase-deficient newborns using an inhibitor of bilirubin production, Sn-mesoporphyrin. *Pediatrics.* 1998;101(5):e1.

172. Galbraith RA, Drummond GS, Kappas A. Suppression of bilirubin production in the Crigler–Najjar type I syndrome: studies with the heme oxygenase inhibitor tin-mesoporphyrin. *Pediatrics.* 1992;89:175.

173. Kappas A, Drummond GS, Munson DP, Marshall JR. Sn-mesoporphyrin interdiction of severe hyperbilirubinemia in Jehovah's Witness newborns as an alternative to exchange transfusion. *Pediatrics.* 2001;108:1374–1377.

174. Vreman HJ, Ekstrand BC, Stevenson DK. Selection of metalloporphyrin heme oxygenase inhibitors based on potency and photoreactivity. *Pediatr Res.* 1993;33:195–200.

175. Fernandez JM, Bilgin MD, Grossweiner LI. Singlet oxygen generation by photodynamic agents. *J Photochem Photobiol B.* 1997;37:131–140.

176. Vallier HA, Rodgers PA, Stevenson DK. Oral administration of zinc deuteroporphyrin IX 2,4 bis glycol inhibits heme oxygenase in neonatal rats. *Dev Pharm Ther.* 1991;17:220–222.

177. Vreman HJ, Lee OK, Stevenson DK. In vitro and in vivo characteristics of a heme oxygenase inhibitor: ZnBG. *Am J Med Sci.* 1991;302:335–341.

178. Morioka I, Wong RJ, Abate A, Vreman HJ, Contag CH, Stevenson DK. Systemic effects of orally-administered zinc and tin (IV) metalloporphyrins on heme oxygenase expression in mice. *Pediatr Res.* 2006;59:667–672.

179. Lakatos L, Csathy L, Nemes E. "Bloodless" treatment of Jehovah's Witness infant with ABO hemolytic disease. *J Perinatol.* 1999;19(7):530–532.

180. Morisawa T, Wong RJ, Bhutani VK, Vreman HJ. Inhibition of heme oxygenase activity in newborn mice by azalanstat. *Can J Physiol Pharmacol.* 2008;86:651–659.

181. Gottstein R, Cooke R. Systematic review of intravenous immunoglobulin in haemolytic disease of the newborn. *Arch Dis Child Fetal Neonatol Ed.* 2003;88:F6–F10.

182. Miqdad AM, Abdelbasit OB, Shaheed MM, Seidahmed MZ, Abomelha AM, Arcala OP. Intravenous immunoglobulin G (IVIG) therapy for significant hyperbilirubinemia in ABO hemolytic disease of the newborn. *J Matern Fetal Neonatal Med.* 2004;16(3):163–166.

183. Rubo J, Albrecht K, Lasch P, et al. High-dose intravenous immune globulin therapy for hyperbilirubinemia caused by Rh hemolytic disease. *J Pediatr.* 1992;121:93–97.

184. Sato K, Hara T, Kondo T, Iwao H, Honda S, Ueda K. High-dose intravenous gammaglobulin therapy for neonatal immune haemolytic jaundice due to blood group incompatibility. *Acta Paediatr Scand.* 1991;80:163–166.

185. Alpay F, Sarici S, Okutan V, et al. High-dose intravenous immunoglobulin therapy in neonatal immune haemolytic jaundice. *Acta Paediatr.* 1999;88:216–219.

186. Hammerman C, Vreman HJ, Kaplan M, Stevenson DK. Intravenous immune globulin in neonatal isoimmunization: does it reduce hemolysis? *Acta Paediatr.* 1996;85:1351–1353.

187. Hammerman C, Kaplan M, Vreman HJ, Stevenson DK. Intravenous immune globulin in neonatal ABO isoimmunization: factors associated with clinical efficacy. *Biol Neonate.* 1996;70:69–74.

188. Alcock GS, Liley H. Immunoglobulin infusion for isoimmune haemolytic jaundice in neonates. *Cochrane Database Syst Rev.* 2002;(3):CD003313.

189. Smits-Wintjens VEHJ, Walther FJ, Rath MEA, et al. Intravenous immunoglobulin in neonates with rhesus hemolytic disease: a randomized controlled trial. *Pediatrics.* 2011;127:680–686.

190. Santos MC, Sa CA, Gomes SC, Camacho LA, Moreira ME. High-dose intravenous immunoglobulin therapy for hyperbilirubinemia due to Rh hemolytic disease: a randomized clinical trial. *PAS* 2010:2851.333.

191. Conney AH, Davison C, Gastel R, Burns JJ. Adaptive increases in drug-metabolizing enzymes induced by phenobarbital and other drugs. *J Pharmacol Exp Ther.* 1960;130:1–8.

192. Sugatani J, Kojima H, Ueda A, et al. The phenobarbital response enhancer module in the human bilirubin UDP-glucuronosyltransferase UGT1A1 gene and regulation by the nuclear receptor CAR. *Hepatology.* 2001;33:1232–1238.

193. Valaes T. Pharmacological approaches to the prevention and treatment of neonatal hyperbilirubinemia. In: Maisels MJ, Watchko JF, eds. *Neonatal Jaundice.* London, UK: Harwood Academic Publishers; 2000:205–214.

194. Yaffe SJ, Dorn LD. Effects of prenatal treatment with phenobarbital. *Dev Pharmacol Ther.* 1990;15:215.

195. Reinisch JM, Sanders SA, Mortensen EL, Rubin DB. In utero exposure to phenobarbital and intelligence deficits in adult men. *JAMA.* 1995;15:18–25.

196. Stevenson DK, Wong RJ, Hintz SR, Vreman HJ. Drugs for hyperbilirubinemia. In: Yaffe SJ, Aranda JV, eds. *Neonatal and Pediatric Pharmacology Therapeutic Principles in Practice.* 4th ed. Philadelphia: Wolters Kluwer/Lippincott Williams & Wilkins; 2011:221–232.

Kernicterus

Steven M. Shapiro

■ INTRODUCTION

Excessive newborn hyperbilirubinemia can cause permanent brain damage, that is, chronic bilirubin encephalopathy (BE), also known as kernicterus. The effort to understand and treat neonatal hyperbilirubinemia is for the most part an effort to prevent kernicterus and bilirubin-induced neurological dysfunction (BIND), the latter referring to subtle neurodevelopmental disabilities without classical findings of kernicterus.[1-4] Kernicterus is a matter of concern for pediatricians and neonatologists. Historically, kernicterus caused a significant number of cases of cerebral palsy (CP), particularly the athetoid or dystonic type. Kernicterus remains a significant problem in underdeveloped countries where bilirubin screening and treatment of excessive hyperbilirubinemia is not routinely available as highlighted in Chapter 13 Neonatal Jaundice in Low-Middle-Income Countries. The "classic" literature on kernicterus evolved during an era when Rh disease was the main cause and therapeutic options for treatment were limited. The resulting acute bilirubin encephalopathy (ABE) was dramatic, with prominent central nervous system (CNS) signs of lethargy, ophthalmoplegia and setting sun sign (impairment of upward gaze), high-pitched cry, opisthotonus, and seizures.[5] Both the basal ganglia, with yellow staining (icterus) of the deep nuclei or "kernel" of the brain, and brainstem auditory pathways were recognized as being particularly vulnerable.[5,6]

The association between high levels of unconjugated bilirubin in the blood and kernicterus was recognized[7] in the 1950s. In newborns with Rh hemolytic disease (gestation not provided), Mollison and Cutbush[8] described kernicterus in 1/13 or 8% of term infants with peak total serum bilirubin (TSB) levels of 19–24 mg/dL, 4/12 (33%) with TSB 25–29 mg/dL, and 8/11 (73%) with TSB 30–40 mg/dL. The authors note, however, that "in many cases only two blood samples were taken during the period of maximum jaundice…," so it is likely that the maximum TSB concentrations were actually higher. As specific therapeutic criteria were developed first to treat and then to prevent severe hyperbilirubinemia and Rh disease, the incidence of kernicterus fell dramatically. However, the level of bilirubin that is regarded as safe in human infants cannot be determined in isolation from other important risk factors, because it is bilirubin in the CNS, not bilirubin in blood bound to albumin, that is neurotoxic.

While clearly the risk of kernicterus rises as TSB rises, other risk factors, including free bilirubin, pH, albumin binding, infection, inflammation, and gestational age, may be important in combination with TSB to better predict neurotoxicity.

■ PATHOLOGY AND CLINICOPATHOLOGICAL CORRELATIONS

Pathology

Kernicterus is a pathological term originally used to describe the yellow staining (icterus) of the deep nuclei (kernel) of the brain, that is, the basal ganglia. More recently it has been used as a clinical term synonymous with chronic BE, the clinical syndrome encompassing long-term adverse neurodevelopmental sequelae corresponding to the pathological condition of kernicterus. The original pathological diagnosis included yellow staining and necrosis in the globus pallidus, subthalamic nucleus (STN), brainstem nuclei, hippocampal CA-2, and cerebellar Purkinje cells. Today, modern neuroimaging can identify characteristic, almost pathognomonic brain lesions in children with ABE and chronic BE and with clinical neurophysiology using the auditory brainstem response (ABR) we can objectively identify the characteristic findings of both ABE and chronic BE.

Clinicopathological Correlations

The clinical features of chronic BE range from deafness and severe dystonic/athetoid CP, seizures, or death (classic kernicterus) to subtle cognitive disturbances. The most extreme bilirubin-induced brain injury produces deafness and severe auditory neuropathy spectrum disorders (ANSD), extrapyramidal movement disorders and abnormal muscle tone, gaze abnormalities, and dental enamel dysplasia of the deciduous (baby) teeth.[9–11] The classic movement disorder consists of athetosis and/or dystonia, the so-called athetoid CP. These relate to pathological lesions in the basal ganglia, namely, the globus pallidus and STN, the cerebellum, and brainstem including auditory nuclei (cochlear nuclei, superior olivary complex, lateral lemniscus, trapezoid body, and inferior colliculus),[12,13] vestibular nuclei,[14] the interstitial nucleus of Cajal (upward gaze center), Dieter's nucleus (truncal tone),[13] and cerebellar Purkinje cells.

The auditory system may be affected clinically with auditory neuropathy/dyssynchrony with or without hearing loss, and, as a result, there may be difficulty understanding speech in noisy environments, even when "hearing" as measured by audiograms is normal or near-normal. The neuropathology of elevated bilirubin in the auditory system is based primarily on autopsy studies of infants with classic kernicterus,[15–17] and premature, low birth weight infants with "low-bilirubin kernicterus."[18] These studies have shown central auditory pathology, with involvement of brainstem auditory structures (e.g., the dorsal and ventral cochlear nuclei, the superior olivary complex, the nuclei of the lateral lemniscus, and the inferior colliculi), but no significant abnormalities of the inner ear structures.[19,20]

Neuroimaging

Lesions in the globus pallidus and STN can be seen on magnetic resonance imaging (MRI) scans of the brain (Figure 11-1).

In the globus pallidus, hyperintense lesions can be seen in both the external and internal portions; lesions in the STN are more difficult to visualize, but may also appear as hyperintense signals on MRI. Other lesions, such as those in auditory brainstem nuclei or cerebellum, are too small to be seen on routine MRI scans. In the context of a hyperbilirubinemic baby with a static encephalopathy, the MRI findings of bilateral hyperintensity of the globus pallidus and STN without other significant abnormalities are almost pathognomonic of BE.

Our experience is that MRIs done within a few weeks of peak bilirubin neurotoxicity in babies with ABE who go on to develop kernicterus often show striking bilateral T1 hyperintensities in the globus pallidus without significant T2 abnormalities; later, T2 and FLAIR images become hyperintense, sometimes with an intervening normal appearing MRIs. Others report a similar shift from T1 to T2 hyperintensity in the globus pallidus,[22,23] and in five preterm and three term infants followed serially, Govaert et al.[23] found that sometimes the signal changes were "subtle and easily overlooked."

Auditory Testing

Evoked potentials identify abnormalities of neuronal function with a high degree of sensitivity. These include conduction delay, desynchronization, and loss of cells, which occur in a number of pathological conditions involving brain injury, metabolic disorders, and demyelination.[24–26] ABRs, aka brainstem auditory evoked potentials (BAEPs) or responses (BAERs), are electrical potentials evoked by auditory stimulation and recorded noninvasively from the scalp. A series of characteristic waves, which arise from neural generators in the auditory nerve and brainstem fiber tracts and nuclei,[27–30] can be distinguished from the background electrical activity (electroencephalogram) by averaging the responses to many stimuli. Each ABR wave is generated by a small subpopulation of synchronously firing neural elements; thus, each component of the ABR wave reflects the activation of specific but temporally overlapping anatomical regions of the brainstem. The time between ABR waves is known as the interwave interval (IWI). This interval reflects the time it takes for nerve impulses to travel from one anatomical location to another. Dysfunction in these neural pathways causes delayed or abnormal conduction of impulses and manifests as increased IWIs, that is, the times between specific ABR waves. Desynchronization or loss of nerve cell activity also produces changes in amplitudes and morphology of the ABR waves. Thus, alterations of latencies, IWIs, and wave amplitudes indicate neuronal dysfunction.

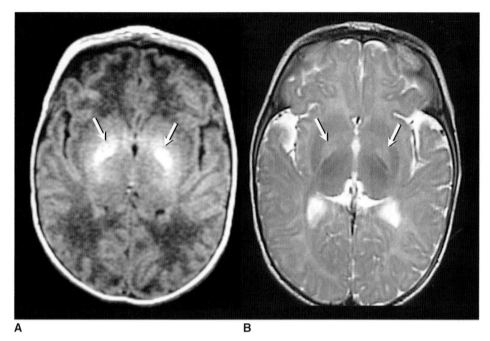

FIGURE 11-1. MRI scans illustrating hyperintensities in the globus pallidus seen in T1-weighted images early (A) and T2-weighted images later (B) after bilirubin neurotoxicity. A. T1-weighted axial MRI image obtained at 10 days of age showing bilateral hyperintense lesions in the globus pallidus (arrows) in a child born in 1995 at 37 weeks gestation with peak total bilirubin 35 mg/dL. Currently this young man is highly intelligent with moderate-to-severe dystonia and athetosis and ambulates with a walker. **B.** T2-weighted axial MRI image obtained at 2 years of age in a child born in 2002 at 38 weeks gestation with peak AO incompatibility and TSB of 46 mg/dL on day 6 of age with classic kernicterus and increased intensity of the globus pallidus bilaterally (arrows). (A: Reprinted from Shapiro SM. Bilirubin toxicity in the developing nervous system. *Pediatr Neurol.* 2003;29(5):410–421. Copyright 2003, with permisson from Elsevier. B: Reprinted from Shapiro SM, Bhutani VK, Johnson L. Hyperbilirubinemia and kernicterus. *Clin Perinatol.* 2006;33(2):387–410. Copyright 2006, with permission from Elsevier.)

ABRs were first measured in 1979 in studies of older children and adults with chronic BE[31,32] and abnormal function of the auditory nerve and the brainstem was found. In these patients, however, cochlear microphonic (CM) recordings were normal. These recordings assess the electrical output of the outer hair cells, part of the efferent auditory system in the inner ear.[31] In hyperbilirubinemic human newborns, increases in IWIs and decreases in amplitudes were found,[31,33–36] abnormalities that could be reversed when the TSB decreased spontaneously or in response to phototherapy or exchange transfusion.[35,37,38] ABR changes correlate significantly with serum levels of total and free bilirubin in the newborn period[34] and at follow-up.[39]

In 1996, patients were described with hearing impairment, normal evoked otoacoustic emissions (OAEs; a test of the mechanical integrity of the basilar membrane

of the inner ear), normal CM responses, and absent or abnormal ABRs, and the term "auditory neuropathy" was coined.[40] We and others prefer the term auditory neuropathy/dyssynchrony to better describe the condition and reflect the concern that the term "neuropathy" is inappropriate for pathologies that may only affect central auditory pathways.[41–43] Recently, the term ANSD has been applied to this condition.[44] The pathophysiology of ANSD involves inner hair cells, spiral ganglion cells, or their processes in the auditory portion of the eighth nerve or the auditory brainstem, all or any of which in theory could preserve OAEs and cochlear (CM) responses while producing severely abnormal ABRs.

Kernicterus and neonatal hyperbilirubinemia are associated with ANSD, functionally defined as absent or abnormal ABRs and normal tests of cochlear function (CMs and OAEs). Initially normal, ANSD and OAEs may become abnormal with time while CMs remain normal.

The combination of absent ABRs and normal CM responses described in 1979 in children with hearing loss due to hyperbilirubinemia[31] is thought to be the first reported case of what is now called ANSD. Notably, a history of hyperbilirubinemia and prematurity is found in over half of patients with ANSD[45] without other reported signs of kernicterus. Previously, CM responses were obtained from a transtympanic electrode; CMs are now usually obtained noninvasively from scalp recordings during the ABR, using two techniques to distinguish CM from electrical artifacts: (1) a tube from the speaker to the tympanic membrane to introduce an acoustic delay and (2) using reversing polarity of stimuli (CM responses change polarity with the stimuli, while ABR waves do not).

ANSD prevalence was found to occur in 11% of a group of children with permanent hearing deficit.[46] With the increased recognition of ANSD through neonatal programs that utilize ABR or automatic ABR screening, the incidence of diagnosed cases of ANSD is likely to increase. A recent report of universal screening found that 24% of 477 graduates from a regional perinatal center neonatal intensive care unit (NICU) fit the ANSD profile of absent ABR and present OAEs and had more hyperbilirubinemia than those infants not fitting an ANSD profile.[47] ANSD was detected by universal newborn hearing screening in 9 of 52 infants with hearing loss in 14,807 consecutively screened cases in Singapore—6/10,000 screened, and 17.3% of hearing loss.[48] Of the many possible risk factors assessed, only hyperbilirubinemia and administration of vancomycin or furosemide were more frequent in the ANSD group.

■ DEFINITIONS

Any discussions of the outcome of neonatal hyperbilirubinemia and assessment of new methods to predict outcome depend on a good, objective, and clear definition of the outcome variable, in this case kernicterus. In this section we focus on defining kernicterus and developing diagnostic criteria.

Traditional Definitions

Acute Bilirubin Encephalopathy
The Subcommittee on Hyperbilirubinemia of the American Academy of Pediatrics (AAP)[49] recommends

that the term "ABE" be used "to describe the acute manifestations of bilirubin toxicity seen in the first weeks after birth and that the term 'kernicterus' be reserved for the chronic and permanent clinical sequelae of bilirubin toxicity." Clinically, ABE has a progression of symptomatology. Initially neonates show lethargy and decreased feeding, then variable abnormal tone with both hypotonia and hypertonia, often alternating over the course of minutes, a high-pitched or shrill cry, and then truncal arching (opisthotonus) with extension of the neck (retrocollis). Neonates develop downward deviation of the eyes from impairment of vertical upward gaze, known as the setting sun sign. As they become more neurotoxic, they may develop fever, seizures, and death from cardiovascular collapse. In the acute stage, ABR changes will occur, starting with abnormalities of waves III and V from the brainstem, followed in severe cases by the loss of all ABR waves. In the acute phase MRI will show increased signal on T1-weighted images. Recently, Slusher et al. have described a characteristic "kernicterus facies," a "scared" look that combines the setting sun sign with facial dystonia and eyelid retraction, suggesting a dorsal midbrain syndrome combined with dystonia from basal ganglia dysfunction.[50]

Kernicterus or Chronic Bilirubin Encephalopathy
It is not difficult to diagnose severe chronic BE or classical kernicterus in older children and adults. Clinically there is a tetrad of (1) severe dystonia with or without athetosis, (2) severe hearing impairment or deafness due to severe auditory neuropathy/dyssynchrony, (3) impairment of the oculomotor function, especially upward gaze, and (4) dental enamel dysplasia of the deciduous (baby) teeth. Currently, laboratory studies are available to support the diagnosis. MRI scans showing abnormal signal intensity in the globus pallidus, STN (if the quality of the scan is good enough), and audiological studies show abnormalities of ABRs with normal CM responses, consistent with a diagnosis of auditory neuropathy/dyssynchrony. Other abnormalities that have been described are hypotonia and sensorimotor disturbances.

The movement disorders, athetosis (slow writhing movement) and, more commonly, dystonia (abnormal muscle tone resulting in abnormal position or postures), correspond to the lesions in the globus pallidus and subthalamic nuclei in the basal ganglia.

In classic kernicterus, there is audiometric evidence for a predominantly high-frequency hearing loss that is usually bilateral and symmetric, with recruitment and abnormal loudness growth functions.[10,51–57] Central auditory system abnormalities, either alone or in combination with sensory loss, are suggested by reports of decreased binaural fusion, auditory aphasia and imperception, word deafness, and numerous instances of patients labeled as "deaf" when objective tests show normal thresholds.[9,10,53,55–57] While deafness is a feature of classical kernicterus, studies have shown an association between moderate-to-severe hearing loss and central auditory dysfunction and elevated bilirubin levels in high-risk, low birth weight newborns in the absence of kernicterus.[58–60] Both the amount and duration of hyperbilirubinemia are risk factors.[58,59]

With current understanding and ABR and CM testing, the typical clinical auditory abnormality in chronic kernicterus is ANDS and relates to abnormalities in the brainstem auditory nuclei including the cochlear nucleus, superior olivary complex, medial nucleus of the trapezoid body, and inferior colliculus. It is also possible that bilirubin toxicity may affect the cell bodies of the auditory nerve in the spiral ganglia, or selectively affect large, heavily myelinated fibers of the auditory nerve.[61] Severe ANSD can cause a child to be deaf with absent ABRs, yet can be distinguished from the more common types of sensory deafness with ABR, CM, and other auditory testing.

The oculomotor abnormalities include impairment of upward gaze, which can be difficult to detect on physical examination in infants, and other oculomotor abnormalities including strabismus, esotropia, and exotropia. The disturbance of vertical gaze, especially upward gaze, is likely due to the selective involvement of the interstitial nucleus of Cajal in the brainstem.[14] Finally dental enamel dysplasia of the deciduous teeth may be present. An important pathological consideration is that, for the most part, bilirubin toxicity does not affect the cerebral cortex and most children with kernicterus, absent other etiologies, comorbidities, and concurrent damage (such as hypoxia–ischemia), will have normal intelligence. Learning disorders related to auditory processing problems or sensory integration or sensorimotor integration perhaps at the level of the basal ganglia may be present, and oculomotor problems may manifest as difficulties with reading and tracking visually.

Even though etiologies for hyperbilirubinemia may differ, there is still a remarkable similarity in the clinical picture of classical kernicterus from case to case. With the exception of kernicterus in extremely premature infants (see comments later regarding auditory-predominant subtype associated with prematurity), almost all cases of kernicterus have variations in tone. Many have greater or lesser amounts of truncal hypotonia. We suggest that bilirubin neurotoxicity is more likely to affect the auditory nervous system in prematurely born infants and that motor abnormalities and perhaps more cerebellar findings may be seen than with bilirubin neurotoxicity in term infants, as preterm infants may have longer but relatively lower levels of hyperbilirubinemia.

Subtle Kernicterus

Subtle neurodevelopmental disabilities related to neonatal hyperbilirubinemia, including mild neurological abnormalities and cognitive disorders, have been recognized for some time,[62–67] as have isolated hearing loss[58,68] and ANSD.[46,69–74] More recently this has been termed BIND.[2,75] Children with kernicterus generally have normal intelligence but are trapped or locked inside dysfunctional bodies, sometimes with severe disabling movement disorders, abnormal control of eye movements, and deafness.

New Definitions

Defining kernicterus is important because it can help us to understand the risk of neurological sequelae from hyperbilirubinemia and to design the appropriate research studies. No matter how carefully designed and novel prospective studies are, the validity of the results depends on the quality and objectivity of the outcome measures, that is, the dependent variables. Other authors have discussed how bilirubin (the independent variable) and other risk factors such as gestational age, infection, inflammation, and hemolysis can affect the outcome. I will focus on the dependent variable, kernicterus, that is, brain damage due to bilirubin neurotoxicity. It is important to attempt to quantify, as best one can, the definitions of kernicterus and BIND, since pairing excellent independent variables with poorly defined, imprecise, or subjective definitions of the dependent variables for outcome measures affects the quality and reliability of the studies. Thus, I have attempted to define kernicterus and BIND in at least semi-objective terms, so that outcome researchers can use similar terminology.

We lack a consistent definition of kernicterus. The absence of a single clinical sign (or combination of clinical and neurophysiological findings) that defines kernicterus makes an objective definition difficult. Perhaps for this reason, studies that attempt to relate neonatal events, including excessive neonatal hyperbilirubinemia, to an outcome of kernicterus rarely, if ever, define kernicterus. In my experience, there is a wide range of manifestations of kernicterus, varying from mild to moderate to severe, and from localized or system-specific kernicterus to classical kernicterus, including the entire triad or tetrad. The well-described differences between ABE, sub-ABE, and chronic BE (kernicterus) are also seen, as are changes that occur during the first year of life. I will attempt to define kernicterus and to establish semi-objective criteria for its diagnosis and severity. I will also describe some of the subtypes seen.

As proposed by Perlstein in 1960[10] and later by Volpe,[76] varied but distinctive patterns of sequelae following BE represent "clinical aggregates in a continuation of syndromes and the possible major predominance of one site of damage over another in the auditory or extrapyramidal category." Perlstein noted, for example, that motor involvement can range from the very severe to so mild as to be virtually unrecognizable except under the broad terms of being "awkward" or "clumsy."[10] Volpe reviewed more recent literature and suggested that impairment of auditory function is the most consistent abnormality associated with chronic postkernicteric BE, especially in premature infants, and that the auditory pathways constitute the most sensitive neural system to bilirubin injury.[76] I have seen patients with impairment of auditory function with neither athetosis nor a significant associated movement disorder and recently proposed new clinical definitions of chronic kernicterus by localization, severity, and timing, where localization was characterized as isolated, mixed, or classical and severity as mild, moderate, or severe.[2] I have suggested that kernicterus can be classified according to three dimensions of severity, location, and time. Although I had originally conceived that the time dimension would reflect time in relation to the bilirubin neurotoxic damage, that is, acute, subacute, and chronic encephalopathy, the time dimension could also represent the stage of the infant's neurodevelopment (i.e., postmenstrual age) at which the CNS is exposed to bilirubin neurotoxicity, which I believe may be an important determinant of selective susceptibility.

■ SUBTYPE CLASSIFICATION OF KERNICTERUS

Although multiple CNS locations are frequently involved in individuals with kernicterus, some appear to have their most disabling symptoms in either the auditory or motor control system. Because I have seen many children with "isolated" kernicterus, that is, predominantly auditory or motor kernicterus who also have subtle signs of involvement of the other system, I prefer to use the terms "auditory predominant" or "motor predominant" to describe children with a major disability in one system but with minimal or no involvement in the other.

Based on my examination and review of the medical records of over 100 patients with kernicterus, I have concluded that there are likely four main categories of kernicterus: (1) classical kernicterus, (2) auditory-predominant kernicterus, (3) motor-predominant kernicterus, and (4) subtle kernicterus or BIND.[2,4] All of these categories may be considered a part of a broader category of kernicterus spectrum disorders (KSDs).

Classical kernicterus refers to individuals with the classical triad or tetrad of auditory neuropathy and/or deafness or hearing loss, motor symptoms of dystonia and/or athetosis, oculomotor pareses, and dental enamel dysplasia (Table 11-1).

Motor-predominant kernicterus refers to individuals with predominantly motor symptoms of dystonia and/or athetosis with minimal auditory symptoms. Hearing loss or ANSD is absent, transient, or minimal. The motor sequelae and dystonia are probably the result of selective lesions in the globus pallidus externa (GPe), globus pallidus interna (GPi), and STN. However, abnormal coordination and hypotonia can also be caused by selective neuropathological lesions in the cerebellar Purkinje cell, which cannot currently be visualized on MRI. Similarly, brainstem lesions in the auditory, vestibular, and oculomotor nuclei and the nuclei controlling truncal tone are too small to be seen in conventional MRI scans.

Auditory-predominant kernicterus refers to individuals with predominantly auditory symptoms, that is, ANSD and/or hearing loss or deafness with relatively minimal motor symptoms. Many individuals with ANSD due to neonatal hyperbilirubinemia have been reported in the literature, although examination of tone or movements

■ TABLE 11-1. Proposed Classification of Kernicterus by Location

Kernicterus Subtype	Description
Classic kernicterus	Classic triad or tetrad of: (1) auditory neuropathy/auditory dyssynchrony ± hearing loss or deafness, (2) neuromotor symptoms, for example, dystonia, hypertonia ± athetosis, (3) oculomotor paresis of upward gaze, and (4) enamel dysplasia of the deciduous teeth. Note that the oculomotor and dental criteria may be variably present or absent
Auditory kernicterus	Predominantly auditory symptoms, that is, auditory neuropathy/auditory dyssynchrony with minimal motor symptoms
Motor kernicterus	Predominantly motor symptoms, for example, dystonia ± athetosis with minimal auditory symptoms
Subtle kernicterus or bilirubin-induced neurological dysfunction (BIND)	Subtle neurodevelopmental disabilities without classical findings of kernicterus that, after careful evaluation and consideration, appear to be due to bilirubin neurotoxicity. These may include disturbances of sensory and sensorimotor integration, central auditory processing, coordination, and muscle tone

Reprinted from Shapiro SM. Chronic bilirubin encephalopathy: diagnosis and outcome. *Seminars in Fetal and Neonatal Medicine.* 2010;15(3):157–163. Copyright 2010, with permission from Elsevier.

is rarely discussed. Virtually all patients referred to me with ANSD following neonatal hyperbilirubinemia have also had abnormalities of tone or movement, although these findings are often subtle. As discussed above, hyperbilirubinemia has recently emerged as a significant risk factor for the ANSD,[77] a nonsyndromic auditory processing problem due to dyssynchrony in the auditory nerve and/or brainstem auditory pathways causing auditory processing problems and neural, not sensory, hearing loss.[40,46,71,78–80] Hyperbilirubinemia accounts for over half of the reported cases of infants with ANSD,[45] with a predilection for premature infants.

Subtle kernicterus or BIND refers to individuals with subtle neurodevelopmental disabilities without the classical findings of kernicterus that, after careful evaluation and exclusion of other possible etiologies, appear to be due to bilirubin neurotoxicity. The findings may include auditory imperception, aphasia and central auditory processing disorders, sensory and sensorimotor integration disorders, hypotonia, ataxia, or clumsiness.

Other Possible Sequelae

It has been suggested that neonatal hyperbilirubinemia might be associated with a variety of other disorders including learning disorders, attention deficit hyperactivity disorder (ADHD), hypotonia, clumsiness and incoordination, tic disorders, central visual impairment, mental retardation, blindness, and autism,[81,82] and although a meta-analysis of 13 observations studies found an association with autism spectrum disorder overall,[83] there is no direct evidence for any of these associations and none of these findings were observed either in a study of 140 infants with TSB levels >25 mg/dL[84] or in a large case–control study.[85]

I hypothesize that an association of moderate levels of neonatal hyperbilirubinemia with disorders of language or reading could be related to central auditory processing disturbances, including mild or undiagnosed ANSD, or transient auditory abnormalities that, though resolved, might interfere with normal language development. Another hypothesis is that subtle oculomotor tracking abnormalities could lead to reading disorders (dyslexia) in some children. Finally, I hypothesize that subtle bilirubin neurotoxicity might manifest as hypotonia, incoordination, or clumsiness, given the proclivity of bilirubin neurotoxicity for the basal ganglia and cerebellum, and the clinical findings in children with classical or motor-predominant kernicterus. Finally, there is evidence to suggest that the globus pallidus may act as a sensory integrator between the somatosensory and motor systems[86]; if so, abnormal function might explain suggestions of sensory and sensorimotor integration difficulties in patients with kernicterus.

■ **TABLE 11-2.** Classification of Kernicterus by Severity and Type of Symptoms

Severity	Auditory Symptoms	Motor Symptoms
Mild	Mild (ABR abnormal but present, may normalize with time), or CAPD with no or mild hearing loss; normal or mildly delayed speech	Mild dystonia ± athetosis; mild gross motor delays, for example, walking; ambulates well, speech intelligible
Moderate	ANSD with absent or persistent abnormal ABR, mild/moderate hearing loss, may fluctuate; speech delayed or absent	Moderate hyperkinetic dystonia/"athetoid" CP; ambulates with or without assistance with athetoid/choreoathetoid gait
Severe	ANSD with absent ABR, severe-to-profound hearing loss/deafness	Severe dystonia/hyperkinetic CP; unable to ambulate, feed self, sign, speak; often with episodic severe hypertonia and muscle cramps

Abbreviations: ANSD, auditory neuropathy spectrum disorder; ABR, auditory brainstem response; CAPD, central auditory processing disorder; CP, cerebral palsy.

Reprinted and modified from Shapiro SM. Chronic bilirubin encephalopathy: diagnosis and outcome. *Seminars in Fetal and Neonatal Medicine.* 2010;15(3):157–163. Copyright 2010, with permission from Elsevier.

Classification of Kernicterus by Severity of Symptoms

The severity of kernicterus varies widely from mild to severe in children and adults. Table 11-2 provides semiobjective definitions for categorizing the range of severity of the auditory and motor sequelae of bilirubin neurotoxicity.[4] Note that the auditory symptoms may not correlate with the severity of the motor symptoms.

The severity of auditory symptoms varies from mild auditory perceptual problems (e.g., problems with hearing and understanding speech in noisy environments or on the telephone, problems localizing sounds, or problems distinguishing speech sounds such as consonants) to profound deafness. ANSD may or may not be associated with concomitant hearing loss on an audiogram. Acoustic reflex testing may be abnormal in ANSD and correlate with ABR abnormalities, and because this testing may often be done without sedation, some have used it as a screen for ANSD or in place of ABR when suspicion of ANSD is low. Children with ANSD have a severe disruption in the temporal coding of speech and an inability to cope with the dynamics of speech.[87] The low threshold of activation and high spontaneous discharge rate of large diameter axons that innervate inner hair cells in the cochlea[88] are electrophysiological properties that are ideally suited for the temporal coding of auditory information, particularly as it relates to neural synchrony and temporally dependent auditory events, such as speech comprehension.[89]

The severity of motor symptoms also varies widely, from subtle increased tone or perhaps occasional muscle cramps to severe dystonia with virtually no voluntary movements and painful muscle spasms. Spasticity, that is, velocity-sensitive hypertonia, is not a part of kernicterus, and is suggestive of other etiologies, for example, hypoxia–ischemia.

Expressive speech problems may be a significant disability, and are usually secondary to motor disability or dystonia of the speech apparatus as well as abnormal auditory function and hearing. Early treatment of severe ANSD deafness with educational programs such as Cued Speech and/or a cochlear implant may preserve language function.

Subtly to mildly affected individuals have little to no functional disability, but may have significant learning disabilities, subtle movement disorders especially under stressful conditions, and occasional muscle cramps.

Moderately affected individuals have more prominent dystonia, perhaps with athetoid movements, but eventually can talk, although they may be difficult to understand. They can feed themselves, although they may need some assistance, and they ambulate unassisted, although awkwardly and with poor stability.

Severely affected individuals have more disabling dystonia and are nonambulatory, ambulate only with assistance (e.g., a walker), or for limited periods with great difficulty. Their speech may be severely dysarthric and barely understandable.

Profoundly affected individuals are invariably wheelchair bound, do not speak, or speak only with great difficultly. They have severe to profound auditory dysfunction

■ TABLE 11-3. Proposed Research Definitions of Kernicterus at 3 Months of Age in Term and Late Preterm Infants with Total Bilirubin (TSB) ≥20 mg/dL (342 μmol/L)

Kernicterus at 3 Months	Muscle Tone[a]	ABR (nl OAE or CM)[b]	Abnormal MRI (abnl GP ± STN)[c]
Certain (three of three)	Abnormal	Abnormal	Abnormal
Probable (two of three, and one must be abnormal tone)	Abnormal	Abnormal	Normal
		Or	
	Abnormal	Normal	Abnormal
Possible (one of three)		Any one of three abnormal	

[a]Abnormal tone: hypotonia, hypertonia, and dystonia.

[b]ABR, auditory brainstem response, also known as brainstem auditory evoked potential (BAEP) or brainstem auditory evoked response (BAER); nl OAE or CM, normal otoacoustic emissions or cochlear microphonic responses (these findings are consistent with the definition of auditory neuropathy).

[c]MRI, magnetic resonance imaging; abnl GP ± STN, abnormal globus pallidus and/or subthalamic nucleus.

Reprinted and modified from Shapiro SM. Chronic bilirubin encephalopathy: diagnosis and outcome. *Seminars in Fetal and Neonatal Medicine.* 2010;15(3):157–163. Copyright 2010, with permission from Elsevier.

or deafness, and often have totally disabling dystonia with frequent or constant painful muscle cramps.

There may be some change in the degree of handicap with age, but the change is not dramatic and individuals do not usually change severity categories.

Classification by Certainty of Kernicterus

Kernicterus can further be categorized as possible, probable, and certain. This classification may be useful for research and/or medicolegal purposes. Table 11-3 provides suggested definitions of kernicterus at age 3 months and Table 11-4 at 9–18 months of age.[4] These definitions are offered as criteria that can be helpful in ongoing research in this area of clinical investigation.

■ RELATION OF KERNICTERUS SUBTYPE WITH NEURODEVELOPMENTAL AGE OF EXPOSURE

There is experimental evidence that the neurodevelopmental age of exposure at the time of peak bilirubin neurotoxicity influences the location of selective neuropathology.[90,91] We have noted an association between the subtype classification of kernicterus and the neurodevelopmental age at the time of the peak TSB and, presumably, when bilirubin neurotoxicity occurred. Isolated auditory-predominant kernicterus (ANSD) appears to be more frequently associated with hyperbilirubinemia in prematurely born babies. Preliminary data[92–94] from our population of children with kernicterus showed that

■ TABLE 11-4. Proposed Research Definitions of Kernicterus at 9–18 Months of Age in Term and Late Preterm Infants with Total Bilirubin (TSB) ≥20 mg/dL (342 μmol/L)

Kernicterus at 9–18 Months	Definition at 3 Months	Hyperkinetic Dystonia (CP)[a]	Abnormal Vertical Gaze	Dental Enamel Dysplasia
Certain	Certain or probable	Yes	Yes	Yes
Probable	Probable or Possible		Two of three abnormal	
Possible	Not kernicterus		Two of three abnormal	

[a]CP, cerebral palsy.

Reprinted from Shapiro SM. Chronic bilirubin encephalopathy: diagnosis and outcome. *Seminars in Fetal and Neonatal Medicine.* 2010;15(3):157–163. Copyright 2010, with permission from Elsevier.

those who developed isolated ANSD were more premature, at the time of the peak TSB, than those who also
developed motor symptoms.[94] Informal surveys of directors of cochlear implant centers and parents reveal that
isolated ANSD appears to be frequent in prematurely
born infants with hyperbilirubinemia. This suggests that
isolated damage to the auditory system occurs at an earlier developmental stage than damage to the basal ganglia associated with dystonic/athetoid CP. Recently, Amin
has suggested an association between apnea and ABE in
premature infants.[95] He also found ANSD as a sequelae
of severe jaundice in otherwise healthy late preterm and
term infants, who had no clinical signs of ABE.[96]

■ ARE NEURODEVELOPMENTAL PROBLEMS DUE TO HYPERBILIRUBINEMIA?

In order to determine whether hyperbilirubinemia in the
newborn period is the cause of the neurodevelopmental
disorder, one should consider the history, the physical
examination, and laboratory findings (Table 11-5).

The history should include an excessively high bilirubin
level. At a minimum the TSB should be greater than the
threshold for instituting phototherapy according to AAP
2004 guidelines,[49] and stronger evidence would be the finding of a TSB level greater than the level at which exchange
transfusion is recommended. Compounding factors,
such as sepsis, acidosis, or Rh disease, hypoalbuminemia,
extreme prematurity, or the presence of displacing agents
would be exceptions because of the possibility that bilirubin neurotoxicity could occur with significantly lower TSB
levels. In the future, measurement of free bilirubin in addition to total unconjugated bilirubin might be helpful.

A history of lethargy, decreased feeding, hypotonia,
hypertonia, retrocollis or opisthotonus, setting sun sign,
high-pitched cry, fever, or seizures occurring in the presence
of a high bilirubin level supports the diagnosis of ABE.

In an older infant or child, abnormal tone or movements, hearing loss or difficulty localizing sound or
difficulty understanding speech in noise, abnormal
eye movements such as impairment of upward gaze,
dental enamel dysplasia, or staining or flaking of the
enamel of baby teeth are consistent with the diagnosis of
kernicterus.

MRI showing bilateral abnormalities in the globus pallidus and possibly the STN, and auditory testing diagnostic
of ANSD (presence of normal CM responses, absence or

■ **TABLE 11-5.** Are Neurodevelopmental Problems Due To Hyperbilirubinemia?

History
   Excessively high bilirubin[a]
   At minimum: total bilirubin >phototherapy level
      (15–20 mg/dL)[a]
   Stronger evidence: total bilirubin >exchange level
      guidelines (20–25 mg/dL)[a]
   Neurological symptoms at time bilirubin high
      (abnormal tone, cry, posturing, eye movements)
   Other risk factors (duration, prematurity, sepsis,
      critically ill, Rh isoimmunization)
Examination
   Abnormal tone, movements
   Hearing loss (±variable), difficulty localizing sound, or
      understanding sound in noisy environments
   Abnormal eye movements, especially decreased
      upward gaze
   Dental enamel dysplasia of deciduous (baby) teeth
Laboratory-specific ABR and MRI findings
   ABR (also known as BAEP) absent or abnormal
      consistent with ANSD
   MRI abnormal globus pallidus ± subthalamic nucleus
      (hyperintensity T1 early, T2 later)

[a]In term and late-preterm infants current (2004) American
Academy of Pediatrics guidelines[49] may be tentatively used as a
guide to levels of risk.

Reprinted from Shapiro SM. Chronic bilirubin encephalopathy:
diagnosis and outcome. *Seminars in Fetal and Neonatal Medicine.*
2010;15(3):157–163. Copyright 2010, with permission from
Elsevier.

abnormality of ABR) are objective findings supporting a
diagnosis of kernicterus. Certain findings on neurological
examination suggest other etiologies. Spasticity (velocity-
dependent hypertonia) is suggestive of hypoxic–ischemic
encephalopathy or other forms of neonatal encephalopathy. Other neurological abnormalities on exam or MRI
may be suggestive of other diagnoses that may be sufficient to explain the neurological symptoms. However, kernicterus may occur concurrently with other neurological
or neurodevelopmental disorders and kernicterus may be
a comorbidity of other severe neonatal illnesses.

■ TREATMENT OF KERNICTERUS

Treatment of kernicterus is directed toward treating the
dystonia and the problems in the auditory system.

The ANSD, once defined and characterized, may be treated in several ways including Cued Speech, low amplification hearing aids, or, in more severe cases, with cochlear implantation. Reading is difficult because ANSD prevents the child from hearing the phonemic content of speech, making it difficult to decode how written letter combinations represent speech sounds. Cued Speech presents hand signals and gestures accompanying speech so that the child with ANSD can distinguish sounds and phonemes that he or she would otherwise not be able to hear. Specific educational programs such as the Wilson Reading System, which teach the phonological coding system of the English language, may help compensate for the deficit and optimize language function[97,98] (www.wilsonlanguage.com). Cochlear implantation has been used in over a dozen children with ANSD and deafness due to kernicterus. The success of cochlear implantation for ANSD is well documented in the literature,[99–101] although these cases did not always include clear examples of kernicterus. In my experience, cochlear implantation in children with hyperbilirubinemia-induced ANSD and hearing loss has usually been dramatically successful. Thus, diagnosing ANSD early in life is important because if cochlear implantation is to be considered, the earlier the implantation, the better to promote literacy and normal language function.

Treatment of dystonia includes physical, occupational, and speech therapies, medical treatments, botulinum toxin (Botox), and surgery. Benzodiazepines such as diazepam and baclofen are often beneficial. Artane, gradually building up to high doses, has been recommended by some for dystonia in children, but is usually not beneficial. Because the hypertonia disappears with sleep, fixed contractures do not occur as frequently as in CP from other causes. For this reason, orthopedic procedures, for example, tendon lengthening, are discouraged in favor of medication and Botox injections. With severe dystonia and painful muscle cramps, intrathecal baclofen, delivered by a pump, has been very successful in reducing tone and muscle spasm and improving function when oral medications have failed.

Many children with kernicterus are underweight, likely due to increased caloric requirements from their hyperkinetic movement disorder. Because they are dystonic, they also have difficulty feeding and swallowing and often require a gastrostomy to provide adequate nutrition. Other feeding difficulties include gastroesophageal reflux, emesis, and abnormal gastric motility and emptying. In my experience, many have not done well with Nissen fundoplication surgery because of persistent severe emesis and retching. These gastrointestinal problems do appear to improve with age.

Finally, deep brain stimulation (DBS) has been considered for patients who have kernicterus. This technology is promising and has been very beneficial in genetic dystonias, for example, DYT1 dystonia, but not as beneficial in secondary dystonias.[102–106] Unfortunately, the few cases of kernicterus that have been implanted have shown either no or only modest benefit.

REFERENCES

1. Johnson L, Brown AK, Bhutani VK. BIND—a clinical score for bilirubin induced neurologic dysfunction in newborns. *Pediatrics.* 1999;104(3 part 3):746–747.
2. Shapiro SM. Definition of the clinical spectrum of kernicterus and bilirubin-induced neurologic dysfunction (BIND). *J Perinatol.* 2005;25(1):54–59.
3. Smitherman H, Stark AR, Bhutan VK. Early recognition of neonatal hyperbilirubinemia and its emergent management. *Semin Fetal Neonatal Med.* 2006;11(3):214–224.
4. Shapiro SM. Chronic bilirubin encephalopathy: diagnosis and outcome. *Semin Fetal Neonatal Med.* 2010; 15(3):157–163.
5. Larroche JC. Kernicterus. In: Vinken P, Bruyn GW, eds. *Handbook of Clinical Neurology.* Vol. 6. North-Holland: Amsterdam; 1968:491–515.
6. Malamud N. Pathogenesis of kernicterus in the light of its sequelae. In: Swinyard CA, ed. *Kernicterus and Its Importance in Cerebral Palsy.* Springfield, IL: Charles C Thomas; 1961:230–246.
7. Hsia DYY, Allen FH, Gellis SS. Erthoblastosis fetalis: VIII. Studies of serum bilirubin in relation to kernicterus. *N Engl J Med.* 1952;247:668–671.
8. Mollison PL, Cutbush M. Haemolytic disease of the newborn. In: Gardner K, ed. *Recent Advances in Pediatrics.* London: J & A Churchill Ltd; 1954:110–132.
9. Byers RK, Paine RS, Crothers B. Extrapyramidal cerebral palsy with hearing loss following erythroblastosis. *Pediatrics.* 1955;15:248–254.
10. Perlstein MA. The late clinical syndrome of posticteric encephalopathy. *Pediatr Clin North Am.* 1960;7:665–687.
11. Volpe JJ. Bilirubin and brain injury. In: Volpe JJ, ed. *Neurology of the Newborn.* 2nd ed. Philadelphia: WB Saunders Co; 1987:336–356.
12. Conlee JW, Shapiro SM. Morphological changes in the cochlear nucleus and nucleus of the trapezoid body in Gunn rat pups. *Hear Res.* 1991;57(1):23–30.

13. Spencer RF, Shaia WT, Gleason AT, Sismanis A, Shapiro SM. Changes in calcium-binding protein expression in the auditory brainstem nuclei of the jaundiced Gunn rat. *Hear Res.* 2002;171(1–2):129–141.

14. Shaia WT, Shapiro SM, Heller AJ, Galiani DL, Sismanis A, Spencer RF. Immunohistochemical localization of calcium-binding proteins in the brainstem vestibular nuclei of the jaundiced Gunn rat. *Hear Res.* 2002;173(1–2):82–90.

15. Dublin W. Neurological lesions in erythroblastosis fetalis in relation to nuclear deafness. *Am J Clin Pathol.* 1951;21:935–939.

16. Dublin W. *Fundamentals of Sensorineural Auditory Pathology.* Springfield, IL: Charles C Thomas; 1976.

17. Haymaker W, Margles C, Pentschew A. Pathology of kernicterus and posticteric encephalopathy. In: Swinyard CA, ed. *Kernicterus and Its Importance in Cerebral Palsy.* Springfield, IL: Charles C Thomas; 1961:21–229.

18. Ahdab-Barmada M, Moossy J. The neuropathology of kernicterus in the premature neonate: diagnostic problems. *J Neuropath Exp Neurol.* 1984;43:45–56.

19. Gerrard J. Nuclear jaundice and deafness. *J Laryngol Otol.* 1952;66:39–46.

20. Kelemen G. Erythroblastosis fetalis. Pathologic report on the hearing organs of a newborn infant. *AMA Arch Otolaryngol.* 1956;63:392–398.

21. Shapiro SM. Bilirubin toxicity in the developing nervous system. *Pediatr Neurol.* 2003;29(5):410–421.

22. Barkovich AJ. *Diagnostic Imaging Pediatric Neuroradiology.* 1st ed. Salt Lake City, UT: Amirsys; 2007.

23. Govaert P, Lequin M, Swarte R, et al. Changes in globus pallidus with (pre)term kernicterus. *Pediatrics.* 2003;112(6 pt 1):1256–1263.

24. Hecox KE, Cone B, Blaw ME. Brainstem auditory evoked response in the diagnosis of pediatric neurologic diseases. *Neurology.* 1981;31:832–839.

25. Starr A. Sensory evoked potentials in clinical disorders of the nervous system. *Annu Rev Neurosci.* 1978;1:103–127.

26. Greenberg RP, Ducker TB. Evoked potentials in the clinical neurologies. *J Neurosurg.* 1982;56:1–18.

27. Huang C-M, Buchwald JS. Interpretation of the vertex short-latency acoustic response: a study of single neurons in the brain stem. *Brain Res.* 1977;137:291–303.

28. Jewett DL, Romano MN. Neonatal development of auditory system potentials averaged from the scalp of rat and cat. *Brain Res.* 1972;36:101–115.

29. Melcher JR, Guinan JJ Jr, Knudson IM, Kiang NY. Generators of the brainstem auditory evoked potential in cat. II. Correlating lesion sites with waveform changes. *Hear Res.* 1996;93(1–2):28–51.

30. Starr A, Hamilton AE. Correlation between confirmed sites of neurological lesions and abnormalities of far field auditory brainstem responses. *Electroencephalogr Clin Neurophysiol.* 1976;41:595–608.

31. Chisin R, Perlman M, Sohmer H. Cochlear and brain stem responses in hearing loss following neonatal hyperbilirubinemia. *Ann Otol.* 1979;88:352–357.

32. Kaga K, Kitazumi E, Kodama K. Auditory brain stem responses of kernicterus infants. *Int J Pediatr Otorhinolaryngol.* 1979;1:255–294.

33. Lenhardt ML, McArtor R, Bryant B. Effects of neonatal hyperbilirubinemia on the brainstem electrical response. *J Pediatr.* 1984;104:281–284.

34. Nakamura H, Takada S, Shimabuku R, Matsuo M, Matsuo T, Negishi H. Auditory nerve and brainstem responses in newborn infants with hyperbilirubinemia. *Pediatrics.* 1985;75:703–708.

35. Perlman M, Fainmesser P, Sohmer H, Tamari H, Wax Y, Pevsmer B. Auditory nerve–brainstem evoked responses in hyperbilirubinemic neonates. *Pediatrics.* 1983;72:658–664.

36. Kotagal S, Rudd D, Rosenberg C, Horenstein S. Brainstem auditory evoked potentials in neonatal hyperbilirubinemia. *Neurol.* 1981;31(4 Part 2):48.

37. Nwaesei CG, Van Aerde J, Boyden M, Perlman M. Changes in auditory brainstem responses in hyperbilirubinemic infants before and after exchange transfusion. *Pediatrics.* 1984;74(5):800–803.

38. Wennberg RP, Ahlfors CE, Bickers R, McMurtry CA, Shetter JL. Abnormal auditory brainstem response in a newborn infant with hyperbilirubinemia: improvement with exchange transfusion. *J Pediatr.* 1982;100(4):624–626.

39. Funato M, Tamai H, Shimada S, Nakamura H. Vigitiphobia, unbound bilirubin, and auditory brainstem responses. *Pediatrics.* 1994;93(1):50–53.

40. Starr A, Picton TW, Sininger Y, Hood LJ, Berlin CI. Auditory neuropathy. *Brain.* 1996;119(pt 3):741–753.

41. Berlin CI, Hood L, Rose K. On renaming auditory neuropathy as auditory dys-synchrony. *Auditory Today.* 2002;13(1):15–17.

42. Berlin CI, Morlet T, Hood LJ. Auditory neuropathy/dyssynchrony: its diagnosis and management. *Pediatr Clin North Am.* 2003;50(2):331–340, vii–viii.

43. Rapin I, Gravel J. "Auditory neuropathy": physiologic and pathologic evidence calls for more diagnostic specificity. *Int J Pediatr Otorhinolaryngol.* 2003;67(7):707–728.

44. Hayes D, Sininger Y. Guidelines development conference on the identification and management of infants with auditory neuropathy. Paper presented at: International Newborn Hearing Screening Conference; June 19–21, 2008; Como, Italy.

45. Madden C, Rutter M, Hilbert L, Greinwald JH Jr, Choo DI. Clinical and audiological features in auditory neuropathy. *Arch Otolaryngol Head Neck Surg.* 2002;128(9):1026–1030.

46. Rance G, Beer DE, Cone-Wesson B, et al. Clinical findings for a group of infants and young children with auditory neuropathy. *Ear Hear.* 1999;20(3):238–252.

47. Berg AL, Spitzer JB, Towers HM, Bartosiewicz C, Diamond BE. Newborn hearing screening in the NICU: profile of failed auditory brainstem response/passed otoacoustic emission. *Pediatrics.* 2005;116(4):933–938.

48. Ngo RY, Tan HK, Balakrishnan A, Lim SB, Lazaroo DT. Auditory neuropathy/auditory dys-synchrony detected by universal newborn hearing screening. *Int J Pediatr Otorhinolaryngol.* 2006;70(7):1299–1306.

49. American Academy of Pediatrics Subcommittee on Hyperbilirubinemia. Management of hyperbilirubinemia in the newborn infant 35 or more weeks of gestation. *Pediatrics.* 2004;114(1):297–316.

50. Slusher TM, Owa JA, Painter MJ, Shapiro SM. The kernicteric facies: facial features of acute bilirubin encephalopathy. *Pediatr Neurol.* 2011;44(2):153–154.

51. Crabtree N, Gerrard J. Perceptive deafness associated with severe neonatal deafness. A report of sixteen cases. *J Laryngol Otol.* 1950;64:482–506.

52. Flottorp G, Morley DE, Skatvedt M. The localization of hearing impairment in athetoids. *Acta Otolaryngol.* 1957;48:404–414.

53. Hardy WG. Auditory deficits of the kernicterus child. In: Swinyard CA, ed. *Kernicterus and Its Importance in Cerebral Palsy.* Springfield, IL: Charles C Thomas; 1961:21–228.

54. Keaster J, Hyman CB, Harris I. Hearing problems subsequent to neonatal hemolytic disease or hyperbilirubinemia. *Am J Dis Child.* 1969;117:406–410.

55. Matkin ND, Carhart R. Auditory profiles associated with Rh incompatibility. *Arch Otolaryngol.* 1966;84:502–513.

56. Rosen J. Deaf or 'aphasic'? 4. Variations in the auditory disorders of the Rh child. *J Speech Hear Dis.* 1956;21:418–422.

57. Ruben R, Lieberman A, Bordley J. Some observations on cochlear potentials and nerve action potentials in children. *Laryngoscope.* 1962;72:545–553.

58. Bergman I, Hirsch RP, Fria TJ, Shapiro SM, Holzman I, Painter MJ. Cause of hearing loss in the high-risk premature infant. *J Pediatr.* 1985;106(1):95–101.

59. de Vries LS, Lary S, Dubowitz LMS. Relationship of serum bilirubin levels to ototoxicity and deafness in high-risk, low birth-weight infants. *Pediatrics.* 1985;76(3):351–354.

60. de Vries LS, Lary S, Whitelaw AG, Dubowitz LM. Relationship of serum bilirubin levels and hearing impairment in newborn infants. *Early Hum Dev.* 1987;15(5):269–277.

61. Shaia WT, Shapiro SM, Spencer RF. The jaundiced Gunn rat model of auditory neuropathy/dyssynchrony. *Laryngoscope.* 2005;115(12):2167–2173.

62. Hyman CB, Keaster J, Hanson V, et al. CNS abnormalities after neonatal hemolytic disease or hyperbilirubinemia. A prospective study of 405 patients. *Am J Dis Child.* 1969;117:395–405.

63. Johnson L, Boggs TR. Bilirubin-dependent brain damage: incidence and indications for treatment. In: Odell GB, Schaffer R, Sionpoulous AP, eds. *Phototherapy in the Newborn: An Overview.* Washington, DC: National Academy of Sciences; 1974:122–149.

64. Naeye RL. Amniotic fluid infections, neonatal hyperbilirubinemia and psychomotor impairment. *Pediatrics.* 1978;62:497–503.

65. Odell GB, Storey GN, Rosenberg LA. Studies in kernicterus. III. The saturation of serum proteins with bilirubin during neonatal life and its relationship to brain damage at five years. *J Pediatr.* 1970;76:12–21.

66. Rubin RA, Balow B, Fisch RO. Neonatal serum bilirubin levels related to cognitive development at ages 4 through 7 years. *J Pediatr.* 1979;94(4):601–604.

67. Scheidt PC. Toxicity to bilirubin in neonates: infant development during first year in relation to maximal neonatal serum bilirubin concentration. *J Pediatr.* 1977;92:292–297.

68. Salamy A, Eldredge L, Tooley WH. Neonatal status and hearing loss in high-risk infants. *J Pediatr.* 1989;114(5):847–852.

69. Stein LK, McGee T, Kraus N, Cheatham MA. Auditory neuropathy associated with elevated bilirubin levels. Paper presented at: Abstracts of the Twentieth Midwinter Research Meeting, Association for Research in Otolaryngology; February 2–6, 1997; St. Petersburg Beach, FL.

70. Morant Ventura A, Orts Alborch M, Garcia Callejo J, Pitarch Ribas MI, Marco Algarra J. Auditory neuropathies in infants. *Acta Otorrinolaringol Esp.* 2000;51(6):530–534.

71. Simmons JL, Beauchaine KL. Auditory neuropathy: case study with hyperbilirubinemia. *J Am Acad Audiol.* 2000;11(6):337–347.

72. Tapia MC, Almenar Latorre A, Lirola M, Moro Serrano M. Auditory neuropathy. *An Esp Pediatr.* 2000;53(5):399–404.

73. Tapia MC, Lirola A, Moro M, Antoli Candela F. Auditory neuropathy in childhood. *Acta Otorrinolaringol Esp.* 2000;51(6):482–489.

74. Yilmaz Y, Degirmenci S, Akdas F, et al. Prognostic value of auditory brainstem response for neurologic outcome in patients with neonatal indirect hyperbilirubinemia. *J Child Neurol.* 2001;16(10):772–775.

75. Shapiro SM, Bhutani VK, Johnson L. Hyperbilirubinemia and kernicterus. *Clin Perinatol.* 2006;33(2):387–410.

76. Volpe JJ. Bilirubin and brain injury. In: Volpe JJ, ed. *Neurology of the Newborn.* 3rd ed. Philadelphia: WB Saunders Co; 2001:490–514.

77. Berlin CI, Hood LJ, Morlet T, et al. Multi-site diagnosis and management of 260 patients with auditory neuropathy/dys-synchrony (auditory neuropathy spectrum disorder). *Int J Audiol.* 2010;49(1):30–43.

78. Deltenre P, Mansbach AL, Bozet C, Clercx A, Hecox KE. Auditory neuropathy: a report on three cases with early onsets and major neonatal illnesses. *Electroencephalogr Clin Neurophysiol.* 1997;104(1):17–22.

79. Berlin CI, Bordelon J, St John P, et al. Reversing click polarity may uncover auditory neuropathy in infants. *Ear Hear.* 1998;19(1):37–47.

80. Stein L, Tremblay K, Pasternak J, Banerjee S, Lindemann K. Auditory brainstem neuropathy and elevated bilirubin levels. *Semin Hear.* 1996;17:197–213.

81. Maimburg RD, Vaeth M, Schendel DE, Bech BH, Olsen J, Thorsen P. Neonatal jaundice: a risk factor for infantile autism? *Paediatr Perinat Epidemiol.* 2008;22(6):562–568.

82. Maimburg RD, Bech BH, Vaeth M, Moller-Madsen B, Olsen J. Neonatal jaundice, autism, and other disorders of psychological development. *Pediatrics.* 2010;126(5):872–878.

83. Amin SB, Smith T, Wang H. Is neonatal jaundice associated with autism spectrum disorders: a systematic review. *J Autism Dev Disord.* 2011;41(11):1455–1463.

84. Newman TB, Liljestrand P, Jeremy RJ, et al. Outcomes among newborns with total serum bilirubin levels of 25 mg per deciliter or more. *N Engl J Med.* 2006;354(18):1889–1900.

85. Croen LA, Yoshida CK, Odouli R, Newman TB. Neonatal hyperbilirubinemia and risk of autism spectrum disorders. *Pediatrics.* 2005;115(2):e135–e138.

86. Boecker H, Ceballos-Baumann A, Bartenstein P, et al. Sensory processing in Parkinson's and Huntington's disease: investigations with 3D H(2)(15)O-PET. *Brain.* 1999;122(pt 9):1651–1665.

87. Rance G, Cone-Wesson B, Wunderlich J, Dowell R. Speech perception and cortical event related potentials in children with auditory neuropathy. *Ear Hear.* 2002;23(3):239–253.

88. Merchan-Perez A, Liberman MC. Ultrastructural differences among afferent synapses on cochlear hair cells: correlations with spontaneous discharge rate. *J Comp Neurol.* 1996;371(2):208–221.

89. Kraus N, Ozdamar O, Stein L, Reed N. Absent auditory brain stem response: peripheral hearing loss or brain stem dysfunction? *Laryngoscope.* 1984;94(3):400–406.

90. Keino H, Kashiwamata S. Critical period of bilirubin-induced cerebellar hypoplasia in a new Sprague–Dawley strain of jaundiced Gunn rats. *Neurosci Res.* 1989;6(3):209–215.

91. Conlee JW, Shapiro SM. Development of cerebellar hypoplasia in jaundiced Gunn rats treated with sulfadimethoxine: a quantitative light microscopic analysis. *Acta Neuropathol.* 1997;93:450–460.

92. Shapiro SM, Daymont MJ. Patterns of kernicterus related to neonatal hyperbilirubinemia and gestational age. *Pediatr Res.* 2003;53(4 part 2):398A–399A.

93. Powers KM, Miller SM, Shapiro SM. Exposure to excessive hyperbilirubinemia earlier in neurodevelopment is associated with auditory-predominant kernicterus subtype. *Ann Neurol.* 2008;64(suppl 12):S105.

94. Shapiro SM, Powers KM. Kernicterus subtypes and their association with signs of neonatal encephalopathy. *Ann Neurol.* 2010;68(suppl 14):D117–D118.

95. Amin SB. Clinical assessment of bilirubin-induced neurotoxicity in premature infants. *Semin Perinatol.* 2004;28(5):340–347.

96. Saluja S, Agarwal A, Kler N, Amin S. Auditory neuropathy spectrum disorder in late preterm and term infants with severe jaundice. *In J Pediatr Otorhinolaryngol.* 2010;74(11):1292–1297.

97. Wilson BA. *Wilson Reading System.* 3rd ed. Oxford, MA: Wilson Language Training; 1996.

98. *Wilson Reading System;* 2002. Available at: http://www.ecs.org/clearinghouse/19/01/1901.htm. Accessed November 1, 2011.

99. Shallop JK, Peterson A, Facer GW, Fabry LB, Driscoll CL. Cochlear implants in five cases of auditory neuropathy: postoperative findings and progress. *Laryngoscope.* 2001;111(4 pt 1):555–562.

100. Madden C, Hilbert L, Rutter M, Greinwald J, Choo D. Pediatric cochlear implantation in auditory neuropathy. *Otol Neurotol.* 2002;23(2):163–168.

101. Peterson A, Shallop J, Driscoll C, et al. Outcomes of cochlear implantation in children with auditory neuropathy. *J Am Acad Audiol.* 2003;14(4):188–201.

102. Cif L, El Fertit H, Vayssiere N, et al. Treatment of dystonic syndromes by chronic electrical stimulation of the internal globus pallidus. *J Neurosurg Sci.* 2003;47(1):52–55.

103. Katsakiori PF, Kefalopoulou Z, Markaki E, et al. Deep brain stimulation for secondary dystonia: results in 8 patients. *Acta Neurochir (Wien).* 2009;151(5):473–478 [discussion 478].

104. Andrews C, Aviles-Olmos I, Hariz M, Foltynie T. Which patients with dystonia benefit from deep brain stimulation? A metaregression of individual patient outcomes. *J Neurol Neurosurg Psychiatry.* 2010;81(12):1383–1389.

105. Vitek JL, Delong MR, Starr PA, Hariz MI, Metman LV. Intraoperative neurophysiology in DBS for dystonia. *Mov Disord.* 2011;26(suppl 1):S31–S36.

106. Starr PA, Turner RS, Rau G, et al. Microelectrode-guided implantation of deep brain stimulators into the globus pallidus internus for dystonia: techniques, electrode locations, and outcomes. *Neurosurg Focus.* 2004;17(1):E4.

Public Policy to Prevent Severe Neonatal Hyperbilirubinemia

Vinod K. Bhutani

■ INTRODUCTION

Newborn jaundice, regardless of its etiology, is a matter of newborn safety, and when it is unrecognized or unmonitored or progresses untreated, it can lead to severe hyperbilirubinemia.[1-5] Because kernicterus is preventable, but not treatable, public health policies need to be focused and rooted in a preventive approach.[6] Thus, neonatal hyperbilirubinemia not only is an important public health issue but also has significant clinical, societal, and economic consequences for both maternal–child health care and educational systems in the United States. Of the approximately 4 million live births each year, over 80% of term infants, and most preterm infants, manifest jaundice during the first week after birth.[6-8] Progression to severe hyperbilirubinemia is due to either increased bilirubin production or impaired bilirubin elimination.[9-11] From 1967 to 2000, about 0.14–0.16% of term infants without known Rh disease (140–160/100,000 live births) developed severe hyperbilirubinemia (total serum bilirubin [TSB] levels >20 mg/dL) that required emergency treatment, such as an exchange transfusion, and were at risk for adverse neurologic outcomes.[10,12-14] Kernicterus, the ultimate manifestation of irreversible bilirubin-induced neurologic dysfunction (BIND), is more evident among infants with concurrent hemolytic disorders, prematurity, sepsis, and glucose-6-phosphate dehydrogenase (G6PD) deficiency. In about half of the reported cases of

kernicterus in the United States, the cause is not diagnosed or investigated.[3] Estimates of the incidence of kernicterus range from 1 to 5.8 per 100,000.[15] The incidence of hazardous hyperbilirubinemia (TSB >30 mg/dL) ranges from 25 to 60 per 100,000, whereas the risk of kernicterus in this subpopulation is estimated at 1 in 4.[12] In the context of prevailing clinical practices, both the use of exchange transfusion and the occurrence of kernicterus are unusual (Figure 12-1), based on reports from health care systems that have accessible service infrastructures and the ability to respond in a timely manner.[16-18] Another public health issue is the association of the intent to breastfeed and the severity of hyperbilirubinemia that has often led to the inappropriate withholding of breast milk intake.[2,5] The societal costs of neonatal hyperbilirubinemia include the cost of predischarge risk assessment in the context of routine newborn care, interrupted breastfeeding, readmission for treatment with phototherapy and/or an urgent need for an exchange transfusion, parental–infant separation, and the onset and persistence of neurologic injury with lifelong learning and movement disorders.[19]

This chapter summarizes key and pertinent maternal–child health and other related societal issues pertaining to neonatal jaundice. It also raises key policy issues with respect to maternal–child health care practices during the first week after birth, and highlights the importance of family/societal education in order to reduce the risk of permanent neurologic sequelae caused by hyperbilirubinemia.

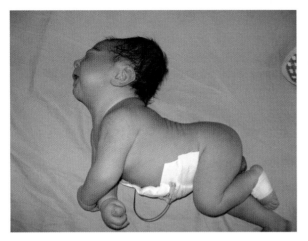

FIGURE 12-1. Infant with acute advanced bilirubin encephalopathy (post-exchange transfusion). Note the classic facies, hypertonia with retrocollis, opisthotonus, and cephalohematoma. (Photograph contributed by Dr Numan Alhamdani, Children's Hospital, Baghdad, Iraq, 2010.)

■ TABLE 12-1. Standard Definitions for Severity of Neonatal Hyperbilirubinemia at Age >72 Hours[3]

Adjective	TSB Level (At Age >72 Hours)	TSB Percentile
Low risk (mild)	<14 mg/dL (239 µmol/L)	<40th percentile
Significant (moderate)	>17 to ≤20 mg/dL (292–342 µmol/L)	>95th percentile
Severe	>20 to ≤25 mg/dL (343–427 µmol/L)	>98th percentile
Extreme (excessive)	>25 to ≤30 mg/dL (428–513 µmol/L)	>99.9th percentile
Hazardous (fulminant)	>30 mg/dL (>513 µmol/L)	>99.99th percentile

■ BACKGROUND

Statement of the Problem

Over 3 million live births in the United States occur after 35 weeks gestation and should have benign outcomes with little or no threat of neurologic compromise from medical conditions during the first year after birth. Proven preventive health measures provided in well baby nurseries have been effective in reducing infant mortality and morbidity in this group of infants. Among the leading causes of neurologic injuries during infancy, kernicterus is one of those conditions that might be prevented. Whether preventive measures are implemented through best clinical practice models or mandated through patient safety strategies has been a matter of recent debate.[2,19–24]

Standard definitions for the severity of neonatal hyperbilirubinemia at age >72 hours are listed in Table 12-1.[3] Confirmation of the diagnosis is made by a transcutaneous bilirubin (TcB) and/or a TSB measurement. Progression of newborn jaundice to severe hyperbilirubinemia and suggested clinical actions are shown in Table 12-2. A range of TSB levels, rather than a singular threshold level, actually represents a range of risk for developing BIND in otherwise healthy term infants.[2,6,25–27] A spectrum of BIND further defines more subtle neurologic manifestations in vulnerable infants who have experienced an exposure to bilirubin of lesser degree than generally described in previous publications.[28] Such neurologic manifestations (kernicterus spectrum disorders) include various neurologic processing problems, with disturbances of visual motor, auditory, speech, language, and cognition among infants with a prior history of moderate to severe hyperbilirubinemia of variable duration.[29] It is in this context that predischarge screening combined with assessment of gestational age is most predictive of subsequent development of severe hyperbilirubinemia at age >72 hours and can direct timely interventions to prevent an infant from progressing to kernicterus.[2,21,24,30–34]

Traditional epidemiological investigations have failed to track accurately the national incidence of kernicterus.[3,17,19,24] Strategies to prevent its surrogate, severe hyperbilirubinemia, are amenable to setting an "aviation safety standard" for newborn care services during the first week after birth. Now, a better understanding of system failures[2,5] has led to considerable progress in quality improvement and should encourage the development of a national strategy to prevent kernicterus.[5,19,21,24] The cause of kernicterus could be considered as largely a system failure in neonatal care in the first week after birth, probably related to the fact that multiple providers deliver health care services at many different sites to the same infant. A contributing root cause might also be an insufficient understanding of the potential for BIND in the professional community of physicians, nurses, maternal and child health care providers, child health advocates, lactation consultants, as well

■ **TABLE 12-2.** Progression of Newborn Jaundice to Severe Hyperbilirubinemia and Suggested Clinical Action

Clinical Event	Incidence[a] (Range)	Action	Analogy
Newborn jaundice	About 84%	Bilirubin screening	"Use of a seat belt"
Bilirubin >75th percentile for age (hours)	25–30%	Evaluate and treat	"Safety precaution"
Bilirubin >15 mg/dL	8–12%	Consider use of phototherapy	"Effective prevention"
Use of intensive phototherapy	4–8%	For bilirubin rate of rise >5 mg/dL per 24 hours	"Crash-cart approach"
Use of exchange transfusion	Rare event	Emergency procedure for any neurologic signs	"Crash landing"
Bilirubin level >30 mg/dL[b]	Avoidable event	Intensive monitoring for lifesaving interventions	"Sentinel event"

[a]Estimated range, based on cumulative review of literature.

[b]At facilities with limited access to intensive newborn care, this threshold for referrals may be lowered to 20–25 mg/dL, based on local experiences.

as third-party payors and the lay society in general. Thus, compounding factors could have contributed to the following: (a) early hospital discharge at age <72 hours (before the risk of severe hyperbilirubinemia is appreciated); (b) insufficient evidence to identify risks of severe jaundice in healthy term and late preterm newborns; (c) an increase in breastfeeding but without counseling and sufficient support to ensure optimal lactation; (d) perceived medical cost constraints complicating reimbursement for follow-up at age 3–5 days; (e) a paucity of educational materials to help families learn about the problem; and (f) a failure of the health care system to provide predischarge screening and identify infants at increased risk for severe hyperbilirubinemia and ensure postdischarge follow-up.[19] In response to such deficiencies, the American Academy of Pediatrics (AAP) guideline for the management of newborn jaundice now recommends updated approaches and practices to prevent severe neonatal hyperbilirubinemia as well as avoid the development of acute bilirubin encephalopathy (ABE) and kernicterus.[21]

A public health question is whether the AAP guideline might be implemented as a national "aviation safety" measure of quality and safety. Using occurrence of defect per critical encounters of adverse icteric experiences (based on critical to quality [CTQ] characteristics), we calculated the defect rate per encounter as the CTQ index, converted to defect rate per million well baby discharges, and determined specific sigma values. Successful implementation of "aviation" safety and quality standards could allow a

defect-free experience of 99.99966% to achieve a 6 sigma level of care. For comparison, a sigma level of 4–4.5 represents safety standards prevalent in the US steel industry in the 1960s. Using a TSB level >25 mg/dL as a surrogate, we have previously calculated a 4.5 sigma level in the pre-phototherapy era of the 1960s and a sigma level of 4.45 in the 1990s.[3,4,19] Rates for readmission (1988–1998) show a 4 sigma level performance. In a Danish population-based report of kernicterus,[35] 6 cases over a 5-year period (estimated at 3 per 100,000 well babies) suggest a 5.5 sigma level. An unproven hypothesis is whether the coordination of current multiorganizational strategies would limit nationwide adverse experiences of TSB >30 mg/dL to 3–4 well babies per million live births and achievement of a 6 sigma level of care.

Currently, the national incidence of kernicterus is not known, but is likely to be low, and the incidence of other more subtle posticteric sequelae is unknown. The US Preventive Services Task Force (USPSTF) has recognized efforts made by clinicians to eliminate this rare, but devastating, condition by instituting system-level measures to screen for hyperbilirubinemia and aggressively manage infants with high bilirubin levels.[24] The USPSTF also has noted that there is adequate evidence to support screening using risk factors and/or hour-specific bilirubin measurements for the identification of infants at risk for developing severe hyperbilirubinemia. Because of the remote relationship between a history of hyperbilirubinemia and the subsequent (often delayed) diagnosis of kernicterus

■ TABLE 12-3. A Community-Based Toolkit To Track Progression of Jaundice (May Be Complemented With a Selective Use of a Transcutaneous or Objective Measure of Skin Color)

Assessment of Jaundice (At Well Baby Visits)	Date and Time (Age) (Suggested Timed Visits)	Jaundice Location	Jaundice Intensity			TcB at Sternum	Risk Status (Percentile)[a]
			Zone	Lemon (Mild)	Orange (Deep)		
1	<24 hours						b
2	24–48 hours					X	
3	3–5 days					X	
4	7–14 days						c
5	2–4 weeks						d

[a]Obtain (X) and plot TcB on hour-specific bilirubin nomogram to assess risk of subsequent severe hyperbilirubinemia.

[b]Obtain TcB for any jaundice.

[c]Obtain TcB/TSB for deep jaundice or if in zone 4 or 5.

[d]Persistence of jaundice after age 2 weeks should trigger screening for hypothyroidism, inborn errors of metabolism, biliary atresia, etc.

later in childhood, it remains unproven whether or not a neonatal screening test will reliably identify all infants who will develop the condition.

■ RECENT CHANGES IN PREVENTIVE APPROACHES

Significant advances to prevent severe hyperbilirubinemia during the first week after birth can be attributed to system-based approaches to the management of neonatal jaundice. Clinicians are now less likely to rely on visual assessment of jaundice alone to predict bilirubin levels. They also recognize that there is little evidence to support reliance on clinical judgment alone. They know that bilirubin concentrations should be interpreted in the context of postnatal age in hours. Moreover, there have been technical advances in TcB measurements.[7,36–41] A community-based toolkit to track progression of jaundice complemented by the selective use of a TcB monitor or other objective measure of skin color is presented in Table 12-3. This toolkit has been adapted by several state and national professional organizations, as well as health care networks and birthing facilities. Such advances are likely to balance the risk of early discharge after birth (age <72 hours) and the absence of direct medical supervision for the infant cared for at home.

An analysis of existing literature on testing TSB levels in the first 24 hours of life indicates that a TSB ≥17 mg/dL (range 2.9–12.0% of all risk levels) can be predicted with a sensitivity of 94% (95% confidence interval [CI]: 88–97%).[36–38,40] On the other hand, the specificity of prediction is 62% (95% CI: 59–65%). These data also indicate that a TSB ≥6 mg/dL at about 24 hours of age is a sensitive predictor of later severe hyperbilirubinemia. In another study, combining a TSB >5 mg/dL at <24 hours with clinical variables (maternal blood group O, maternal age, intent for exclusive breastfeeding, and maternal education) was also predictive.[42] This evidence confirms a long-standing clinical "pearl" that visible jaundice in the first 24 hours of life is a risk factor for the later development of severe hyperbilirubinemia.[43] Thus, any visible or suspected jaundice in the first 24 hours requires urgent medical attention (within a couple of hours), which must include TSB measurement and an investigation of potential underlying causes.[1,2,7,40] Current evidence also suggests that it is possible to identify babies who are likely to develop significant hyperbilirubinemia using a predischarge TSB (age 24 to <60 hours) plotted on an hour-specific nomogram.[2,41] The evidence for this recommendation is listed in Table 12-4.

■ PROGRESS IN REDUCING RISK OF ADVERSE OUTCOMES

The AAP has published a guideline for the management of hyperbilirubinemia in the newborn infant ≥35 weeks gestation in 2004[2] that followed a Joint Commission on

■ TABLE 12-4. Summary of Studies That Used Predischarge Risk Assessment To Predict High Late Bilirubin Measurements

Author	Study Design	Number Enrolled	High Bilirubin Predicted	Predischarge Risk Assessment	AUC (95% Confidence Interval)
Keren et al.[8]	PC (SC)	522	>95th percentile (by age <7 days)	Visual assessment of jaundice	0.65 (0.50–0.80)
Sarici (2004)[37]	PC (SC)	366	>95th percentile (by age <7 days)	Early TSB, plotted on nomogram	–
Keren et al.[31]	RC (SC)	993	>95th percentile (by age <7 days)	Clinical risk factors	0.71 (0.66–0.76)
Newman et al.[34]	RC (MC)	5706	>20 mg/dL (by 48 h)	Clinical risk factors	0.69 (–)
Newman et al.[34]	NCC (MC)	275	>25 mg/dL (by 30 days)	Clinical risk factors	0.83 (0.77–0.89)
Newman et al.[14]	NCC (MC)	496	>25 mg/dL (by 48 h)	Clinical risk factors	0.84 (0.79–0.89)
Keren et al.[32]	PC (SC)	823	>95th percentile (by age <7 days)	Clinical risk factors	0.91 (0.86–0.96)
Bhutani[61]	PC (MC)	982	Use of phototherapy	Gestational age	0.76 (0.68–0.84)
Bhutani[61]	PC (MC)	982	Use of phototherapy	Select clinical risk factors	0.86 (0.79–0.93)
Bhutani et al.[30]	PC (SC)	2840	>95th percentile (by age <7 days)	TSB, plotted on nomogram	0.83 (0.79–0.90)
Keren et al.[31]	RC (SC)	996	>95th percentile (by age <7 days)	Early TSB, plotted on nomogram	0.83 (0.80–0.86)
Newman et al.[34]	RC	5706	>20 mg/dL	Early TSB, plotted on nomogram	0.83 (0.80–0.85)
Keren et al.[32]	PC (SC)	823	>95th percentile (by age <7 days)	Early TcB, plotted on nomogram	0.92 (0.89–0.95)
Bhutani[61]	PC (MC)	982	Use of phototherapy	TcB/TSB, plotted on nomogram (hours)	0.87 (0.82–0.93)
Keren et al.[32]	PC (SC)	823	>95th percentile (by age <7 days)	Combined clinical and bilirubin risk	0.96 (0.93–0.98)
Bhutani[61]	PC (MC)	982	Use of phototherapy	Combined clinical and TcB/TSB (hours)	0.95 (0.92–0.98)

PC, prospective cohort; RC, retrospective cohort; SC, single center; MC, multicenter; NCC, nested case control.

Accreditation of Healthcare Organizations (JCAHO) Sentinel Alert[20] and the Centers for Disease Control and Prevention (CDC) *Morbidity and Mortality Weekly Report* (*MMWR*).[44] Subsequently, similar consensus-based guidelines were developed and implemented in Denmark,[45,46] Canada,[47] Israel,[43,48] Brazil,[42] Europe,[49] Norway,[50] and the United Kingdom.[51] Over the past several years, the AAP guideline has been widely implemented in the United States. Recent publications have also reported the beneficial effect of this guideline in reducing the acute adverse events attributed to severe hyperbilirubinemia, including reduced rates of readmission, TSB levels >25 and >30 mg/dL, and the need for exchange transfusion.[16–18,52] Some concerns have been raised about a marginal increase in the use of phototherapy.[16,17,52] This may be due to an improved early recognition of severe hyperbilirubinemia when TSB levels are actually measured rather than relying on the visual assessment of jaundice alone.

■ RECENT MULTINATIONAL REVIEWS

Promotion of Breastfeeding

Suboptimal breastfeeding among preterm infants is a public health problem. Increasing the rates of breast-feeding initiation, duration, and exclusivity is a national health objective and one of the goals of Healthy People 2010 and 2020. The Department of Health and Human Services,[53] AAP,[54] and the American College of Obstetrics and Gynecology (ACOG)[55] have supported vigorously this initiative. The rates of intent to breastfeed are routinely reported to the CDC.[56] More recently, much evidence has focused on the prenatal and intrapartum period as critical for the success of exclusive (or any) breastfeeding.[57] Many states, including California, also report the use of breastfeeding at the hospital level.[58] Exclusive breastfeeding rates during birth hospital stay have been recorded by the California Department of Public Health using the framework of newborn genetic disease screening program. These birth hospitalization breastfeeding data range from 8% to over 90%. Prevalence of the initiation of breastfeeding and continued breastfeeding at 6 months of age among mothers of term infants in the United States have reached their highest levels recorded to date, 73.8% and 41.5%, respectively; exclusive breastfeeding through 3 months was 30.5%. The AAP recommends that, as a primary mode of prevention for severe hyperbilirubinemia, clinicians should advise mothers to nurse their infants at least 8–12 times per day for the first several days. Poor caloric intake and/or dehydration associated with inadequate breastfeeding may contribute to the development of hyperbilirubinemia. Providing appropriate support and advice to breastfeeding mothers increases the likelihood that breastfeeding will be successful. Clinicians also need to assess the adequacy of intake in breast-feeding infants during the entire neonatal period. Data from a number of studies indicate that unsupplemented breastfed infants experience their maximum weight loss by day 3 and, on average, lose 6.1 ± 2.5% of their birth weight. It is estimated that 5–10% of exclusively breast-fed infants lose 10% or more of their birth weight by day 3, suggesting that adequacy of intake should be followed closely. Evidence of adequate intake in breastfed infants includes four to six thoroughly wet diapers in 24 hours and the passage of three to four stools per day by the fourth day. By the third to fourth day, the stools in adequately breastfed infants should have changed from meconium to a mustard yellow, mushy stool. Nationwide policies for newborn jaundice should promote successful breastfeeding and provide toolkits to identify breast-fed infants who are at risk for dehydration because of inadequate intake.

Predischarge Risk Assessment

The bilirubin load for an infant represents the net accumulated bilirubin in circulation—the balance of bilirubin production, conjugation, elimination, and enterohepatic circulation. The hour-specific bilirubin nomogram has been recommended as one approach for predicting severe neonatal hyperbilirubinemia and was developed based on the hypothesis that TSB levels measured early in the postnatal course, expressed as a percentile with respect to the infant's age in hours, are predictive of an infant's later TSB levels.[30]

The Agency for Healthcare Research and Quality (AHRQ) sponsored the development of Evidence Syntheses through its Evidence-Based Practice Centers. With guidance from the USPSTF, evidence for clinical preventive services in the primary care setting was reviewed. Such review serves as the foundation for the recommendations of the USPSTF, which provides age- and risk-factor-specific recommendations for the delivery of these services in the primary care setting. The evidence regarding the benefits, limitations, and cost-effectiveness of a broad range of clinical preventive services would help further awareness, delivery, and coverage of preventive care as an integral part of quality primary health care. In a recent systematic review for evidence[21,41] of the effectiveness of strategies to prevent kernicterus, there was no study that addressed directly the effectiveness of using risk factor assessment and/or bilirubin testing to reduce the incidence of the condition. The reviewed studies used different threshold values and definitions of hyperbilirubinemia. In one study, two consecutive TSB readings plotted on the nomogram had greater predictive accuracy than a single TSB measurement. Another study indicated that predischarge TcB plotted on an hour-specific nomogram of bilirubin levels derived from healthy babies could predict hyper-bilirubinemia with 100% sensitivity and 88% specificity. The threshold values for defining severe hyperbilirubinemia were different for the TcB (≥75th percentile) and TSB (≥95th percentile) levels. Current data suggest comparable predictability of the risk score (newborn and familial jaundice history and clinical characteristics) and the modified risk index (i.e., the risk score without family history of jaundice in a newborn) in predicting later severe hyperbilirubinemia (TSB >95th percentile for age in hours) or use of phototherapy. Studies also suggest that the combination of using the modified risk index with early TSB levels significantly enhanced prediction when compared with using either one of the strategies alone. None of the studies in this review assessed potential harms of screening. Ip et al.[4] have previously reported that one needs to treat 6–10 otherwise healthy jaundiced neonates with TSB ≥15 mg/dL by phototherapy in order to prevent the TSB in one infant from rising above 20 mg/dL. However, no substantive harm could be attributed to phototherapy by either of the systematic reviews reported by AHRQ in 2004 and 2009.[4,41] Based on these reviews, the USPSTF concluded that a study to evaluate directly the effectiveness of different strategies to reduce the incidence of kernicterus would not be feasible given the rare occurrence of the condition. For practical reasons, studies on the effectiveness of different strategies to reduce the incidence of BIND could only rely on a surrogate outcome such as the TSB level. Outcomes of multiple recent international reviews described above and the most recent AHRQ review[41] also confirm the earlier report[30] that predischarge TSB plotted on hour-specific bilirubin nomograms show good accuracy in predicting subsequent hyperbilirubinemia (Figure 12-2).

Effective Use of Phototherapy

Clinical trials have validated the efficacy of phototherapy in reducing excessive unconjugated hyperbilirubinemia,

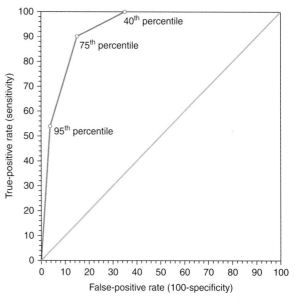

FIGURE 12-2. Receiver operating characteristic (ROC) curve of hour-specific bilirubin levels (18–60 hours) to predict significant hyperbilirubinemia.[30]

and the use of phototherapy has drastically curtailed the use of exchange transfusions.[1,2,59–61] The initiation and duration of phototherapy is defined by a specific range of TSB levels on the basis of an infant's postnatal age and the potential risk for developing BIND (Table 12-5). Aggressive implementation of phototherapy for excessive hyperbilirubinemia, sometimes referred to as the "crash-cart" approach, has been reported to reduce the need for exchange transfusions, and, possibly, reduce the severity of BIND. Barriers to effective use of phototherapy are

---

■ **TABLE 12-5.** Guidelines To Initiate Effective Phototherapy[a] Based on Clinical Risk of Neurotoxicity

Risk of Bilirubin Neurotoxicity	Clinical Risk Factors[b]	Bilirubin Level at Age 48 hours	Bilirubin Level at Age >96 hours
High risk	Risk factors + late term	11 mg/dL (188 µmol/L)	15 mg/dL (257 µmol/L)
Moderate risk	Late preterm + no risk factors	13 mg/dL (222 µmol/L)	18 mg/dL (308 µmol/L)
	Risk factors + term infants		
Low risk	Term infants + no risk factors	15 mg/dL (257 µmol/L)	21 mg/dL (359 µmol/L)

[a]In absence of access to effective phototherapy devices, the infant should be treated with devices at a lower irradiance (see text) at TSB levels 2–3 mg/dL (35–50 µmol/L) lower than those recommended above or considered a higher risk category.

[b]Clinical risk factors: isoimmune hemolysis, G6PD deficiency, sepsis, acidosis, hypoalbuminemia (albumin ≤3.0 g/dL), and lethargy.[3]

■ **TABLE 12-6.** Barriers To Effective Phototherapy

Light source

Phototherapy devices in resource-constrained settings often contain light sources that deliver suboptimal light emission spectrum and irradiance level. Such light sources, including white fluorescent tube lamps, are often used because of their low cost and ready availability, but provide negligible treatment. Light sources with a proper light emission spectrum and irradiance level are often of markedly higher cost and less readily available

Maintenance

Maintenance of medical devices is often a challenge in resource-constrained settings. Effective maintenance is particularly important for phototherapy devices because of the need to check for optimal irradiance levels at regular intervals. Due to maintenance constraints in resource-constrained settings, phototherapy devices in use on patients often contain burned out or missing light bulbs as well as devices that have been in use longer than manufacturer's recommendations. Often, light bulbs may be replaced with suboptimal selections. Furthermore, devices receiving infrequent maintenance may accumulate dust between the light sources and protective clear plastic, further reducing the irradiance delivered to the patient

Environment

The lack of consistent electricity poses a significant barrier to administration of phototherapy in many resource-constrained settings. Power may not be available from the electrical grid for hours or days at a time. Additionally, when grid electricity is available, it may be subject to voltage surges that can damage phototherapy devices, especially fluorescent tube lamps

Operational

Lack of awareness of requirements for effective phototherapy treatment among medical staff administering phototherapy can hamper the delivery of effective treatment. In resource-constrained settings with severe staffing shortages, nurses are often delegated the administration of phototherapy. Such nurses, as well as some pediatricians, may not have a clear understanding of how phototherapy works or the requirements for effective treatment. Additionally, few nurseries in resource-constrained settings can afford a flux meter. Without this important verification tool, medical staff is unable to accurately assess the efficacy of their seemingly functioning phototherapy devices or make necessary adjustments for effective treatment

Reported in literature, as anecdotes or as direct observations. Please review hour-specific bilirubin guidelines for phototherapy.[2]

---

described in Table 12-6. Affordable access to effective phototherapy devices (see checklist in Table 12-7) is an urgent global public health need.

Reducing the Need for Exchange Transfusion

Neonatal exchange transfusion was introduced in the late 1940s to decrease the mortality due to rhesus hemolytic disease of the newborn and to prevent kernicterus in surviving infants.[62] Development and widespread use of Rh immunoglobulin (RhoGAM), improvements in diagnostic prenatal ultrasound, intensive phototherapy, and an AAP guideline for management of hyperbilirubinemia have resulted in worldwide declining needs for neonatal exchange transfusion over the last two to three decades. Technological breakthroughs and simulation training

have emerged to improve the safety of this lifesaving procedure that often needs to be conducted at Level II regional centers in the developing world. Among many nations and regions with poorly developed health care infrastructures, an exchange transfusion still remains a frequent, but unsafe, rescue procedure because of absent or suboptimal community-based use of phototherapy, ineffective phototherapy devices, late referrals, delayed recognition of excessive TSB levels, and the higher prevalence of G6PD deficiency. Currently, the estimated use of exchange transfusions in the United States (for infants with TSB >30 mg/dL) is at about 3/100,000 live births. However, based on the adverse events encountered in an era of declining technical skills, preventive solutions are needed for safer interventions and less reliance on neonatal exchange transfusion as a rescue intervention.

■ **TABLE 12-7.** Checklist for Technical Specifications for Effective Phototherapy Devices

Checklist	Technical Requirements	Recommended Specifications
1	Regulatory approval	FDA 510K clearance or CE mark
2	Light emission spectrum	Blue light (400–520 nm) with a peak wavelength of 450 ± 20 nm
3	Light spectral irradiance	≥30 μW/cm²/nm at the level of the baby (as measured with device-specific irradiance meter)
4	Light source	Light emitting diodes (LEDs) with lifetime of at least 20,000 h (irradiance must be ≥30 μW/cm²/nm at 20,000 h)
5	Illuminated surface area (footprint)	Assure uniformity over the light footprint area: uniformity of spectral irradiance over a 30 × 50 cm rectangular footprint such that ratio of minimum and maximum irradiance values over this area exceeds 0.4
6	Device energy requirements	(i) Device is compatible with 90–240 V and 48–60 Hz power input (ii) Device has a circuit breaker for overload protection
7	Device structural requirements (all devices)	(i) Height adjustable from approximately 1.20 to 1.60 m (measured from bottom surface of enclosure to ground) (ii) Lights are protected by clear plastic cover (iii) Light source enclosure must be tiltable from horizontal to >30° upwards (iv) Device is topple resistant and will not fall on a 10° incline (v) Device is easily portable
8	Device structural requirements (all devices with stands)	(i) Stand is sturdy and stable (ii) Stand has castors (at least two castors with brakes) (iii) Height of stand's base is less than 8 cm, in order for base of phototherapy stand to fit under the stands of radiant warmers

Devices should have a 5-year warranty (including provisions for rapid repair or replacement, a spare set of fuses, a pictorial guide and operating instructions for use by all health care providers, as well as contact information for direct access to manufacturers).

Assessing Neonatal G6PD Deficiency Through Public Policy Initiatives

G6PD deficiency, a commonly occurring genetic enzyme deficiency, is the most easily identified inherited disorder that causes newborn jaundice, severe hyperbilirubinemia, and ABE.[63–67] Chinevere et al.[68] reported the overall US incidence of G6PD deficiency in US military recruits of diverse races and ethnicities. The gender-categorized incidences ranged from 0% to 12.4% (Table 12-8). The African American male is at the highest risk, an observation substantiated by multiple observational studies.[69–71] Newborn screening for G6PD deficiency has led to identification of at-risk infants and has led to public health educational programs to prevent or recognize "favism" crises following hemolytic triggers.[72–77] This may not be unexpected in countries in which there is a high background incidence of G6PD deficiency, and therefore it is not surprising that in recent reports it is a major etiological factor for kernicterus in countries such as Turkey, Nigeria, Oman, Malaysia, Taiwan, China, Philippines, Philippines, India, and Mediterranean nations. However, an association between G6PD deficiency and severe hyperbilirubinemia and/or ABE is now being noted in other countries because of changing demographics, including the United States, in which the overall incidence of G6PD deficiency is low, and in which G6PD deficiency is not yet recognized as being a health hazard to warrant universal newborn screening.[78] The most striking of these reports is that of the Pilot Kernicterus Registry, in which G6PD deficiency affected 26 of the 125 (20.8%) newborns reported,[6] compared with the overall incidence of the condition in the United States (0.5–2.9%) as reported by Beutler.[63]

Significant research gaps exist in our understanding of the lifelong population burden of G6PD deficiency.

■ **TABLE 12-8.** Frequency of G6PD Deficiency Among UD Military Recruits

Ethnicity of Recruits Tested for G6PD Deficiency	Total Recruits Tested	Gender Differences of G6PD Deficiency		
		Male Recruits Tested	Males with G6PD Deficiency (%)	Females with G6PD Deficiency (%)
African American	11,276	8513	12.2	4.1
Asian	2123	1658	4.3	0.9
Hispanic	5304	4462	2.0	1.2
Caucasian	42,126	38,108	0.3	0.0
American Indian/Alaskan	604	492	0.8	0.9
Other	1869	1643	3.0	1.8
Total	63,302	54,876	2.5	1.6

Data from Chinevere TD, Murray CK, Grant E Jr, Johnson GA, Duelm F, Hospenthal DR. Prevalence of glucose-6-phosphate dehydrogenase deficiency in U.S. Army personnel. *Mil Med.* 2006;171:905–907.

However, the acute and reported life-threatening neonatal manifestations of G6PD deficiency syndrome and the need to educate families and society of known preventive measures warrant an urgent inquiry to define a national neonatal G6PD screening strategy. US population-based studies to determine the optimal and risk-based strategies for targeted routine newborn screening have not been conducted. Screening tests are available based on enzyme assay, but point-of-care application has yet to be developed. Whether neonatal G6PD screening can lead to a reduction in the incidence of severe neonatal hyperbilirubinemia has not been tested prospectively in the ethnically diverse US population.

Economic Consequences of Public Policy Initiatives

Newman and coworkers, in their recent commentary, observed that in the absence of universal screening, detection and management of clinically significant hyperbilirubinemia during the birth hospitalization relies on several imperfect steps.[18] These include: (1) reliance on nurses and physicians to remember to examine the infant for onset of jaundice; (2) the need to distinguish visually between jaundice that is and jaundice that is not clinically significant for the infant's age in hours; and (3) the need to combine information from this visual assessment of jaundice and/or a TSB level with the knowledge of the newborn's other risk factors to determine the need for

and timing of repeat bilirubin measurements, follow-up visits, and treatments.[21] It is well known that newborn nurseries are busy places where multiple individuals care for families in a time-constrained environment that is often not suitable for parental education. These potentially suboptimal environments limit the ability to assess jaundice in the dim light found in many hospital rooms, to define an undistracted time for parental coaching, and to integrate the multiple and often conflicting instructions that demand unrestricted parental attention. An imperfect system places an onerous burden on the bedside nurse whose total responsibility for the clinical care and education of both mother and infant is complemented by one or two assessments by a physician. Based on these experiences, the Expert AAP Panel[18] and Newman[22] compared the devastating effects of kernicterus with the costs and risks of screening and supported the benefit of routine bilirubin screening. Recently, Suresh and Clark[79] conducted a theoretical incremental cost-effectiveness analysis using a decision analysis model and a spreadsheet to estimate the direct costs and outcomes, including the savings resulting from prevented kernicterus, for an estimated annual cohort of 2.8 million healthy term newborns who are eligible for early discharge. For an incidence of kernicterus 1:100,000 and a relative risk reduction (RRR) of 0.7, the cost estimate to prevent 1 case of kernicterus was $5,743,905, if routine predischarge TcB measurements with selective follow-up and laboratory testing were used. As expected, sensitivity analyses for cost per case are highly dependent on the population incidence of kernicterus. In their model, annual cost savings were best estimated if the incidence of kernicterus were high (1:10,000 births or higher) and the RRR were high (>0.7). However, sensitivity analyses were not conducted for varying incidences of a kernicterus surrogate, such as hazardous hyperbilirubinemia (TSB >30 mg/dL), or an RRR >0.95 (to approach higher sigma thresholds). In addition, because resource utilization is not likely to be generalizable, the cost per case of kernicterus, quality-adjusted life years, and the benefit of averting other adverse outcomes due to hyperbilirubinemia also should be considered.

Many health care providers and institutions have adopted bilirubin screening policies independent of their potential economic consequences, such as increased phototherapy use, in order to prevent severe neonatal hyperbilirubinemia since excessive TSB levels have been recommended as surrogate indices for kernicterus. In a study of 101,272 neonates at the Intermountain Healthcare hospitals,[16] the practice of routine predischarge screening resulted in a decrease in the incidence of TSB levels >25 mg/dL per 100,000 from 66 to 25 per 100,000 (RRR = 0.62). In a separate study at Hospital Corporation of America hospitals,[17] out of 1,028,817 infants, 129,345 were delivered before implementation of a routine predischarge bilirubin screening program in their individual hospitals compared with 899,472 infants delivered after implementation of this program; the incidence of infants with TSB ≥30.0 mg/dL dropped from 9 to 3 per 100,000 (RRR = 0.67). This change was associated with a small, but statistically significant, increase in phototherapy use. In summary, the cost of routine predischarge screening for all healthy newborns is only marginally more than that for a bilirubin test for infants at low clinical risk for severe hyperbilirubinemia: the formula-fed, white, Anglo-Saxon female infant with no bruising at birth with blood type O and whose mother's blood type is type A, B, or Rh positive and who has a negative Coomb's test. This cohort represents <10% of the population.

■ THE SOCIETAL ROLE

Randomized controlled trials to prevent kernicterus are not likely to be done and such studies are probably not ethically feasible because of easy access to effective treatment options for severe hyperbilirubinemia in most countries.[24] Thus, the only available way to delineate strategies to improve access to effective prevention or treatment is through a detailed root cause analysis of infants who develop kernicterus in prevailing health care systems. We have previously reported the outcome of a root cause analysis for a convenience sample of cases that were reported to the Pilot US Kernicterus Registry from 1992 to 2004, prior to the updated 2004 AAP guideline.[6] The underlying hypothesis for this analysis was that we would identify additional clinical observations and commonly occurring lapses in management that might be useful for the identification of safer and more effective ways to manage newborn jaundice. All cases were found to have multiple root causes or lapses in the care provided by multiple providers at multiple sites. Delays in intervention were often related to a pervasive lack of awareness of impending irreversible BIND. The most common root causes are shown in Table 12-9 and were based on the Institute of Medicine patient safety matrix.

The antecedent clinical and health services lapses reported to the Pilot US Kernicterus Registry revealed deficiencies in the clinical and public health management of newborn jaundice that may not be recognizable easily by traditional epidemiological investigation or surveillance. The following observations were made:

1. Kernicterus cases are continuing to be reported in the United States.
2. Over 95% of the kernicterus cases were attributed to a multifactorial failure of the postpartum and newborn health care delivery system.
3. These cases represent the minimum number of infants diagnosed with kernicterus and are likely to be a "tip of the iceberg."
4. Virtually all cases of kernicterus in the Registry could have been prevented with early identification of potentially severe hyperbilirubinemia (TSB > 40th percentile), recognition (before discharge or at early follow-up) of TSB increase at >0.2 mg/(dL h) and initiation of timely medical care and intensive phototherapy and exchange transfusions.
5. Kernicterus is a low-frequency condition with current interventions, but an unacceptable outcome in prevailing health practices.
6. For nearly all cases with ABE, responses to parental and family concerns and involvement were inadequate.

| ■ **TABLE 12-9.** Example of a Patient Safety Analysis for an Infant With ABE[6] |

Patient Centeredness	Safety	Effective Care	Timeliness
No teaching of jaundice recognition or its progression. No warning that untreated jaundice could be a risk for brain damage	Failed to recognize severity of jaundice or severity of hyperbilirubinemia or risk factors for hemolysis	Did not recognize clinical risk factors for subsequent hyperbilirubinemia or signs of suboptimal lactation	Did not determine infant's hyperbilirubinemia. Did not increase enteral milk intake. Did not arrange for an early and timely follow-up
Poor communication of the need for jaundice follow-up or to track its regulation	Inadequate record or documentation of enteral milk intake or urine/stool output	Did not intervene by checking TSB or TcB for early onset of jaundice (age <30 hours) or at progression of jaundice	Failed to follow up bilirubin levels either prior to discharge or at follow-up. Failed to initiate rapid and appropriate bilirubin reduction treatments
Lack of MD response to repeated calls by parents to progressive clinical signs	No lactation support or guidance for assessment of milk production or milk transfer. Did not recognize signs of progressive ABE	No lactation support services or counseling. Did not institute phototherapy and arrange for an exchange transfusion	Limited transfer of health care information from birthing hospital to follow-up service site (no discharge plan). Referral to emergency room with scant resources to manage severe hyperbilirubinemia

7. Data from this Registry validate the consensus opinion that there is no evidence of a specific TSB level linked to the onset of ABE.
8. Successful implementation of a systems-based approach to manage newborn jaundice could serve as an index for the integrity of the postpartum health delivery system.
9. Effective implementation of the 2004 AAP guideline is an urgent matter.
10. National awareness and partnerships with new and expectant parents are important.

The optimization of clinical practice has been a driving force in the educational efforts initiated by the AAP, CDC, the Association of Women's Health, Obstetric and Neonatal Nurses (AWHONN), and JCAHO. These educational efforts include standardized guidelines for the management of neonatal jaundice for pediatricians and emergency room physicians. Most of the patient education materials (brochures, videos, resource links, posters, and transcripts) are currently available online for public access and can be viewed at www.aap.org/jaundice, www.cdc.gov/jaundice, www.jcaho.org/kernicterus, and

www.pickonline.org. The California Perinatal Quality Care Collaborative (CPQCC) has developed and implemented a "Severe Neonatal Hyperbilirubinemia Toolkit" (http://www.cpqcc.org/quality_improvement.htm). Statewide or regional initiatives to report severe neonatal hyperbilirubinemia (TSB levels >25 mg/dL) along with outcomes for newborn screening for other inherited disorders may be feasible through a partnership of providers and society to implement a state-driven or national program: (1) apply an aviation safety standard approach to address gaps in newborn health care delivery using health care information technology solutions; (2) implement statewide (regional) and national surveillance for severe neonatal hyperbilirubinemia; and (3) provide national and global education and empowerment aids for new and expectant parents.

A description of a health care professional and societal partnership was reported in two recent articles and partially described here.[23,80] In an effort to build "Health and Society" partnerships, a group of parents consented to have video clips and case histories of their children compiled into the "BIND video documentary" prepared by Dr Lois Johnson. One of the mothers, Sue Sheridan, had been invited to testify at the President's Summit Meeting on Medical Errors in September 2000. Joined by other families, these parents were invited to the first screening of the documentary at an AAP satellite meeting in Chicago in October 2000. Sheridan stated that "a confluence of events and far-sighted visions occurred when the parents met as a group and with concerned physicians for the first time. The families decided to form a support and advocacy group (Parents of Infants and Children with Kernicterus [PICK]). Along with the physicians (who subsequently constituted their advisory board), they chose to build a foundation for our partnerships." The proposed revision of the 1994 AAP practice parameters for newborn jaundice galvanized the medical advisory board and PICK to conceive and conduct a unique gathering of parents, medical experts on neonatal jaundice and kernicterus, representatives of health care regulatory agencies, and pediatric and nursing professional organizations at the Historic Library at Pennsylvania Hospital, Philadelphia, Pennsylvania, in February 2001. The objective for this full-day meeting on "Strategies for a System-Wide Approach in the Management of Hyperbilirubinemia to Prevent Kernicterus" was to develop a framework for a systemwide change in the predischarge and postdischarge management of neonatal jaundice.[23] At the conclusion of the workshop, the meeting participants generally agreed that systemwide awareness and application of strategies would advance the goal of prevention of BIND. Together with their Medical Advisory Board (V. K. Bhutani, A. K. Brown, W. J. Cashore, L. H. Johnson, S. A. Shapiro, M. J. Maisels, D. K. Stevenson), this informed, articulate, and dedicated parents' group developed a comprehensive syllabus, which contained statements by the parents, a representative body of pertinent medical literature, and an estimated incidence of hyperbilirubinemia in excess of the 95th percentile. Sheridan arranged for the participation in the meeting of representatives of AHRQ, CDC, Healthcare Financing Administration (HCFA), JCAHO, Maternal Child Health Bureau (MCH), National Institutes of Health (NIH), and the Office of Science Planning. In collaboration with their medical advisory board, PICK also sent invitations to representatives of the AAP (represented by M. J. Maisels), AWOHNN (represented by S. Gennaro), Making Advances Against Jaundice in Infant Care (MAJIC, a joint project of Harvard School of Public Health and the AAP,

represented by M. H. Palmer), National Association of Neonatal Nurses (NANN, represented by A. Schwoebel), and the Harvard Life Bridge Program (Boston Children's Hospital, represented by J. J. Volpe and A. Duplesis), all of whom agreed to attend.[23] As a follow-up to this meeting, JCAHO, AHRQ, AAP, AWHONN, and CDC reviewed their roles in the prevention of severe hyperbilirubinemia and kernicterus, publishing their results and suggestions for action (see section "Useful Web Sites"). The National Quality Forum (AHRQ) declared kernicterus as one of the "never events," the only pediatric condition in this list. PICK observed that the stumbling blocks for a measurable change in practice have been: (1) a lack of "greatest strength of evidence" that a specific TSB level causes brain damage; (2) the inability to conduct a prospective randomized controlled trial for ethical considerations; (3) the lack of institutional will to implement universal bilirubin screening (which is system based and would identify babies at risk and allow for early, prophylactic, and aggressive intervention based on their risk status while reassure a much larger segment of parents of well baby of a benign outcome) until it is deemed "cost-efficient"; and (4) an inordinate delay in response to this "epidemic" as reports of new cases of neonatal kernicteric death and delayed interventions occur. Just as their children's treatment for hyperbilirubinemia was ineffective, signs of opisthotonus and hypertonicity were not recognized and the final diagnosis of kernicterus delayed and disputed; annually scores of newborns and children continue to journey through similar yet completely preventable adversities.

PICK's "call for action" noted that timeliness of effective and efficient practices requires urgent implementation of the safest practices and overcome the breakdowns in health systems while evidence for newborn jaundice management identified in infants who developed kernicterus (Table 12-10); alternative practices are prospectively studied with mandatory follow-up and outcome validation.[19] It is in this context that parents and prospective parents have a responsibility to the community to achieve as well as maintain (through effective oversight) safer birthing, a safer first week, a safer first month, and a healthy childhood for our children. The parent–physician partnership has continued to advocate universal bilirubin screening prior to discharge and implementation of a system-based approach to prevent kernicterus. They also embarked on a Safety and Family Education (SAFE) program for management of newborn jaundice to define

■ **TABLE 12-10.** Breakdowns in Health Systems for Newborn Jaundice Management Identified in Infants Who Developed Kernicterus (Reported in 1992–2002[5,6])

1. Failure to recognize the clinical significance of jaundice within the first 24 h after birth
2. Failure of clinicians to recognize the limitations of visual recognition of jaundice
3. Failure of clinicians to recognize the onset and progression of clinical jaundice and document its severity by bilirubin measurement before discharge from the hospital
4. Failure to ensure post-discharge follow-up based on the severity of predischarge hyperbilirubinemia
5. Failure to respond to parental concerns of newborn jaundice, poor feeding, lactation difficulties, and change in newborn behavior and activity in a timely manner
6. Failure to provide ongoing effective lactation support in breastfeeding babies to ensure adequacy of intake
7. Failure to recognize the impact of skin color, race, ethnicity, and family history on severity of newborn jaundice and risk of brain damage
8. Failure to diagnose the cause of hyperbilirubinemia prior to onset of ABE
9. Failure to institute interventional strategies to prevent severe hyperbilirubinemia when bilirubin is rising more rapidly than expected
10. Failure to aggressively treat severe hyperbilirubinemia with intensive phototherapy or exchange transfusion for "hazardous" bilirubin levels
11. Failure to communicate with parents and educate them about the potential irreversible risks of jaundice during newborn period and infancy
12. Failure to provide developmental follow-up after exposure to severe hyperbilirubinemia

Data from Johnson LH, Bhutani VK, Brown AK. System-based approach to management of neonatal jaundice and prevention of kernicterus. *J Pediatr.* 2002;140:396–403; and Johnson L, Bhutani VK, Karp K, Sivieri EM, Shapiro SM. Clinical report from the pilot USA Kernicterus Registry (1992 to 2004). *J Perinatol.* 2009;29 Suppl 1:S25–S45.

presentinel trigger events that place a newborn at risk for kernicterus, to expand the Pilot Kernicterus Registry to a formal, ongoing national surveillance system, and to prepare a national outreach campaign to achieve a "zero tolerance of kernicterus."

■ MATERNAL CHILD HEALTH CARE INFRASTRUCTURE AND PUBLIC POLICY

Kernicterus due to Rh blood group incompatibility used to be a major cause of cerebral palsy prior to introduction of RhoGAM prophylaxis, legislation to test the Rh-negative status of women of childbearing age, universal access to phototherapy, and rescue use of exchange transfusion to treat excessive hyperbilirubinemia.[80] By the mid-1990s, however, cases of kernicterus not due to Rh disease were reported, including cases in apparently healthy term newborns. Guidelines from the AAP emphasized timely and efficient management of severe neonatal hyperbilirubinemia.[1,2] Primary prevention is usually conducted at a birthing facility with medical supervision and surveillance. It includes ensuring a structured and practical approach to the identification

and care of infants with jaundice and adequate breastfeeding of infants. Secondary prevention is through vigilant monitoring, usually daily, of neonatal jaundice during the first week after birth. The intent of the education and screening is to identify infants at risk for severe hyperbilirubinemia to ensure timely outpatient follow-up within 24–72 hours of discharge from the birthing facility. Palmer et al. recognized that the wider "ecosystem" of care constrains local health care providers and parents in ways that limit their ability to prevent kernicterus. For instance, cumbersome reimbursement policies for obtaining TSB in the ambulatory setting delay urgently needed test results, and lack of standardization across clinical laboratories makes the results difficult to interpret.[81] Also, parents have difficulty arranging for a clinician to check their child after discharge given the vulnerability and interdependence of a recently delivered mother and her breastfeeding newborn and the resistance of clinicians to changing patterns of care. Flawed interactions between many different parties perpetuate the problems. The whole "ecosystem" has been undergoing a change in the United States to ensure a safe first week of life for all newborns.[82]

The absence of or fractured existence of maternal–child health care systems is evident in nations with underdeveloped health care planning or those disrupted by war or civil strife. In a 4-month study during 2007–2008 in Baghdad, Hameed et al. reported bilirubin encephalopathy in 88 of 162 infants admitted for severe hyperbilirubinemia, which represented an estimated incidence of 1749 (95% CI: 1649–1849) per 100,000 live births. Of the 88 infants with BIND, 53 (over 60%) sustained posticteric sequelae consistent with kernicterus or death.[83] There were difficulties in reaching the hospital because of road blockages and dangers during travel, as well as personal constraints that prevented families from seeking timely medical attention. More importantly, subsequent questioning of the families also highlighted the poor knowledge about newborn jaundice, its course, and treatment as well as the lack of understanding about the necessity for urgent intervention. Clinician–community partnerships are needed to prevent adverse newborn outcomes (Table 12-11). Appropriate and affordable technologies are also needed. These include tools to promote and enhance visual assessment of the degree of jaundice, such as simpler TcB measurements and readily available TSB measurements that could be incorporated into routine treatment and follow-up. Widespread screening for G6PD deficiency is needed, as this is often a major cause of neonatal jaundice and kernicterus worldwide. Moreover, recognition and treatment of Rh hemolytic disease, another known preventable cause of kernicterus, should not be forgotten in developing countries. Additionally, effective phototherapy is crucial if kernicterus is to be a "never event." Finally it is essential to conduct appropriate population-based studies to accurately elucidate the magnitude of the problem. However, knowledge alone will not be sufficient. To relegate severe neonatal jaundice and its sequelae to the history books, screening and interventions must be low cost, technologically appropriate, and easily accessible for low- and middle-income nations.[84,85]

■ RESEARCH NEEDS

There is a need to better understand the natural history of BIND. Population-based surveillance for BIND or kernicterus is necessary for an understanding of the incidence of the condition and of its risk factors. There is a need to assess whether current efforts to screen neonates to prevent severe hyperbilirubinemia are associated with a reduction in kernicterus. The unintended consequences of the institution of universal bilirubin screening will also need further study, such as interruption of breastfeeding, abuse of phototherapy, prolonged hospitalization, or inadvertent maternal–infant separation.

■ POLICY ISSUES TO PREVENT SEVERE NEONATAL HYPERBILIRUBINEMIA

Based on multiple systematic reviews of best available evidence and explicit consideration of cost-effectiveness, the policies given in the next subsections need consideration for implementation as "best practices" to reduce adverse consequences related to neonatal hyperbilirubinemia.

Birthing Facility Care

A. Identify and assess for following clinical risk factors for significant hyperbilirubinemia:
 1. Visible jaundice in the first 24 hours of life
 2. A gestational age of <39 weeks
 3. A mother who intends to breastfeed exclusively
 4. Signs of bruising or cephalohematoma
 5. Risk of blood group incompatibility
 6. Risk of inherited hemolytic disorders such as G6PD deficiency
B. At-risk infants are monitored for onset and progression of jaundice:
 1. Examine all babies for jaundice with assessment of vital signs.
 2. Do not rely on visual inspection to estimate the bilirubin concentration.

■ **TABLE 12-11.** Clinician–Community Partnership to Prevent Adverse Newborn Outcomes

1. Aviation safety standard for newborn postpartum newborn health delivery
2. Statewide (regional) surveillance for severe neonatal hyperbilirubinemia
3. National surveillance program for severe neonatal hyperbilirubinemia
4. Health care information technology solution to bridge postpartum gaps between the birthing institution and the postnatal medical home for the infant
5. National and global education and empowerment of new and expectant parents

C. Measure bilirubin concentration based on clinical judgment and routinely before discharge:
   1. Use a TcB (for age in hours) as a noninvasive screening test.
   2. Measure TSB for age in hours: if a TcB device is not available or for TcB levels >15 mg/dL or prior to use of phototherapy.
   3. Always measure TSB for infants with jaundice <24 hours of age and those receiving phototherapy.
D. Management of hyperbilirubinemia with phototherapy:
   1. Use TSB concentration and determine risk of BIND to decide thresholds for use of effective phototherapy.
   2. Encourage breaks for breastfeeding and parental handling and allow for continual treatment with phototherapy.
   3. Continue breast milk intake and breastfeeding support.
   4. There is no need to routinely give additional fluids or feeds.
   5. Provide protection for retina and diaper hygiene.
   6. Monitor effectiveness of phototherapy and its use by testing irradiance, light wavelength, and exposure of body surface area and its duration.
   7. Consider "crash-cart" for infants at risk for rescue intervention with exchange transfusion.

Home Care

Providing safe and effective care requires coordination among the multiple levels of the health care system. These levels comprise the newborn (patient, family, and community), nursery or primary care practice (microsystem), hospital or managed care organization (macrosystem), and policy, payment, or regulatory issues (environmental system). Contemporary care practices associated with childbirth and the newborn often reflect disruptions in coordination of these processes and place newborns at risk for poor outcomes. Parental education and assistance for the first few days at home include lactation support, assessment for onset and progression of jaundice, need for a follow-up visit with 2 days of discharge, and an understanding that newborn jaundice is usually benign, but can have serious irreversible neurologic consequences in the absence of timely intervention. The AAP Safe and Healthy Beginnings Initiative, a quality improvement project, targets newborn nurseries, primary care practices, and coordination between

these sites using a system-based approach to facilitate implementation of the 2004 guideline for management of hyperbilirubinemia.

Follow-Up Office-Based Care

A checklist for the front office staff that handles follow-up visits should contain the medical requirements for a first office visit for a newborn. Designation as a "well baby" visit may have an unintended consequence of a low-risk visit, when, in fact, the first office visit deals with a multitude of unresolved issues that relate to newborn transition. These include an assessment of breastfeeding (adequacy of milk intake, lactation support, intake and output evaluation), assessment for progression of jaundice, evaluation for heart murmurs, sepsis and hygiene assessment, examination of the umbilical cord, skin assessment, as well as an evaluation of parental coping. The ability to handle phone calls from parents of newborn infants requires an ability to ask probing questions, to triage health care concerns, and to offer reassurance. Having an algorithm for office personnel to follow would be helpful in this regard. In addition, office staff should be in a position to coordinate multidisciplinary interactions for the families, such as meetings with nurses, nurse practitioners, lactation experts, or physicians. Each office should also maintain a standard operating procedure for laboratory tests. Clinicians should review emergency procedures for rapid transfer of a jaundiced infant to a neonatal intensive care facility and a communication plan for direct contact with a neonatologist or pediatric intensivist. Generally, referral to an emergency room should be avoided unless requested to do so by the contacted neonatal–pediatric facility.

Emergency Readmission Care

An infant admitted with severe hyperbilirubinemia or with levels that exceed the thresholds for intensive phototherapy requires urgent and expert attention. The evaluation and interventions need to be implemented in a matter of a couple of hours. If the TSB level is approaching or is at hazardous levels or onset of ABE is recognized, the goal of therapy is to dramatically reduce the bilirubin load promptly, safely, and expeditiously.

Triage for a Jaundiced Newborn Arriving at the Emergency Room

The triage process should be guided by ongoing staff education, as well as development and sharing of a predetermined local protocol and action plan. This plan should include the following:

1. *Technology supplies*: There must be ready access to phototherapy devices, monitoring equipment, and a transport isolette.
2. *Clinical assessment*: Identification of risk factors is paramount, including a neurologic examination.
3. *Testing*: There should be access to TcB testing and other immediate laboratory studies (such as bilirubin, albumin, blood type, electrolytes).
4. *Informed consent*: The parents should be informed about the medical emergency and the need for action.
5. *Treatment*: There should be the capability to initiate immediate intensive phototherapy (or transfer to another facility for therapy) within about an hour of arrival.

■ CONCLUSIONS

The prevention and treatment of neonatal hyperbilirubinemia have been improved over the past four decades but still face significant clinical and societal challenges. New, affordable technologies could alter the economic paradigms and help us implement not only local but also global approaches. To achieve both the highest standards for patient safety (as enunciated by the Institute of Medicine) and evidence-based disease reduction, maternal–child health care infrastructure during the first week after birth needs to be urgently reengineered. These standards should be worldwide and emphasize medical–societal partnerships that are transparent, evidence-based practice, mandatory, and actively promoted to meet professional and family expectations.

■ USEFUL WEB SITES

AHRQ, http://www.ahrq.gov/clinic/epcsums/neonatalsum.htm

Joint Commission, http://www.jointcommission.org/SentinelEvents/SentinelEventAlert/sea_31.htm

CDC, http://www.cdc.gov/ncbddd/dd/kernichome.htm

AAP: Professional, http://aappolicy.aappublications.org/cgi/content/full/pediatrics;114/1/297

Committee of Fetus and Newborn

Family, http://www.aap.org/family/healthychildren/07school/HC-07School-Jaundice.pdf

Association of Women's Health, Obstetric Nursing and Neonatal Nursing, http://www.awhonn.org/awhonn/product.detail.do?productCode 1/4PA8–2ND, http://www.awhonn.org/awhonn/content.do?name1/402_PracticeResources/2C2_Fo us_Hyperbili.htm

BiliTool, http://www.bilitool.org/

Parent support, http://www.pickonline.org/

■ USEFUL POLICIES AND THEIR ACCESS

These are available at the AAP, CDC, AWOHNN, NAAN, and JCAHO web sites and include:

- Joint Committee on Infant Hearing, American Academy of Audiology, American Academy of Pediatrics, American Speech-Language-Hearing Association, Directors of Speech and Hearing Programs in State Health and Welfare Agencies. Year 2000 position statement: principles and guidelines for early hearing detection and intervention programs. *Pediatrics.* 2000;106:798–817.
- Committee on Hospital Care. Family-centered care and the pediatrician's role. *Pediatrics.* 2003;112:691–696.
- American Academy of Pediatrics Committee on Fetus and Newborn. Hospital stay for healthy term newborns. *Pediatrics.* 2004;113(5):1434–1436. This policy is a revision of the policy posted on October 1, 1995.
- Ip S, Chung M, Kulig J, et al. American Academy of Pediatrics Subcommittee on Hyperbilirubinemia. An evidence-based review of important issues concerning neonatal hyperbilirubinemia. *Pediatrics.* 2004;114:e130–e153.
- Subcommittee on Hyperbilirubinemia. Management of hyperbilirubinemia in the newborn infant 35 or more weeks of gestation. *Pediatrics.* 2004;114:297–316.
- Gartner LM, Morton J, Lawrence RA, et al.; American Academy of Pediatrics Section on breastfeeding. Breastfeeding and the use of human milk. *Pediatrics.* 2005;115:496–506.
- Markenson D, Reynolds S. American Academy of Pediatrics Committee on Pediatric Emergency Medicine, Task Force on Terrorism. The pediatrician and disaster preparedness. *Pediatrics.* 2006;117:E340–E362.
- Kaye C. Committee on Genetics. Newborn screening fact sheets. *Pediatrics.* 2006;118:E934–E963.
- Engle WA, Tomashek KM, Wallan C. American Academy of Pediatrics Committee on Fetus and Newborn. "Late-preterm" infants: a population risk. *Pediatrics.* 2007;120:1390–1401.

- Joint Committee on Infant Hearing. Year 2007 position statement: principles and guidelines for early hearing detection and intervention programs. *Pediatrics.* 2007;120:898–921.
- Newborn Screening Authoring Committee. Newborn screening expands: recommendations for pediatricians and medical homes—implications for the system. *Pediatrics.* 2008;121:192–217.

■ ACKNOWLEDGMENT

Supported in part by HRSA/MCHB U21MC04403.

REFERENCES

1. American Academy of Pediatrics. Practice parameter: management of hyperbilirubinemia in the healthy term newborn. Provisional Committee for Quality Improvement and Subcommittee on Hyperbilirubinemia. *Pediatrics.* 1994;94:558–565.
2. American Academy of Pediatrics. Management of hyperbilirubinemia in the newborn infant 35 or more weeks of gestation. *Pediatrics.* 2004;114:297–316.
3. Bhutani VK, Johnson LH, Jeffrey Maisels M, et al. Kernicterus: epidemiological strategies for its prevention through systems-based approaches. *J Perinatol.* 2004;24:650–662.
4. Ip S, Chung M, Kulig J, et al. American Academy of Pediatrics Subcommittee on Hyperbilirubinemia. An evidence-based review of important issues concerning neonatal hyperbilirubinemia. *Pediatrics.* 2004;114:e130–e153.
5. Johnson LH, Bhutani VK, Brown AK. System-based approach to management of neonatal jaundice and prevention of kernicterus. *J Pediatr.* 2002;140:396–403.
6. Johnson L, Bhutani VK, Karp K, Sivieri EM, Shapiro SM. Clinical report from the pilot USA Kernicterus Registry (1992 to 2004). *J Perinatol.* 2009;29(suppl 1):S25–S45.
7. Bhutani VK, Vilms RJ, Hamerman-Johnson L. Universal bilirubin screening for severe neonatal hyperbilirubinemia. *J Perinatol.* 2010;30(suppl):S6–S15.
8. Keren R, Tremont K, Luan X, Cnaan A. Visual assessment of jaundice in term and late preterm infants. *Arch Dis Child Fetal Neonatal Ed.* 2009;94:F317–F322.
9. Dennery PA, Seidman DS, Stevenson DK. Neonatal hyperbilirubinemia. *N Engl J Med.* 2001;344:581–590.
10. Johnson L, Bhutani VK. Guidelines for management of the jaundiced term and near-term infant. *Clin Perinatol.* 1998;25:555–574, viii.
11. Maisels MJ. Jaundice. In: MacDonald M, Seshia M, Mullett M, eds. *Avery's Neonatology: Pathophysiology and Management of the Newborn.* Philadelphia: Lippincott Williams and Wilkins; 2005:768–846.
12. Bhutani VK, Johnson L. Kernicterus in the 21st century: frequently asked questions. *J Perinatol.* 2009;29 (suppl 1):S20–S24.
13. Newman TB, Klebanoff MA. Neonatal hyperbilirubinemia and long-term outcome: another look at the Collaborative Perinatal Project. *Pediatrics.* 1993;92:651–657.
14. Newman TB, Xiong B, Gonzales VM, Escobar GJ. Prediction and prevention of extreme neonatal hyperbilirubinemia in a mature health maintenance organization. *Arch Pediatr Adolesc Med.* 2000;154:1140–1147.
15. Ip S, Chung M, Trikalinos T, DeVine D, Lau J. *Screening for Bilirubin Encephalopathy.* Rockville, MD: Agency for Healthcare Research and Quality; 2009.
16. Eggert LD, Wiedmeier SE, Wilson J, Christensen RD. The effect of instituting a prehospital-discharge newborn bilirubin screening program in an 18-hospital health system. *Pediatrics.* 2006;117:e855–e862.
17. Mah MP, Clark SL, Akhigbe E, et al. Reduction of severe hyperbilirubinemia after institution of predischarge bilirubin screening. *Pediatrics.* 2010;125:e1143–e1148.
18. Usatin D, Liljestrand P, Kuzniewicz MW, Escobar GJ, Newman TB. Effect of neonatal jaundice and phototherapy on the frequency of first-year outpatient visits. *Pediatrics.* 2010;125:729–734.
19. Bhutani VK, Johnson L. A proposal to prevent severe neonatal hyperbilirubinemia and kernicterus. *J Perinatol.* 2009;29(suppl 1):S61–S67.
20. Joint Commission on Accreditation of Healthcare Organizations. Kernicterus threatens healthy newborns. *Sentinel Event Alert.* 2001;(18):1–4.
21. Maisels MJ, Bhutani VK, Bogen D, Newman TB, Stark AR, Watchko JF. Hyperbilirubinemia in the newborn infant ≥35 weeks' gestation: an update with clarifications. *Pediatrics.* 2009;124:1193–1198.
22. Newman TB. Universal bilirubin screening, guidelines, and evidence. *Pediatrics.* 2009;124:1199–1202.
23. Sheridan SE. Parents of infants and children with kernicterus. *J Perinatol.* 2005;25:227–228.
24. US Preventive Services Task Force. Screening of infants for hyperbilirubinemia to prevent chronic bilirubin encephalopathy: US Preventive Services Task Force recommendation statement. *Pediatrics.* 2009;124:1172–1177.
25. Hanko E, Lindemann R, Hansen TW. Spectrum of outcome in infants with extreme neonatal jaundice. *Acta Paediatr.* 2001;90:782–785.
26. Shapiro SM, Bhutani VK, Johnson L. Hyperbilirubinemia and kernicterus. *Clin Perinatol.* 2006;33:387–410.
27. Van Praagh R. Diagnosis of kernicterus in the neonatal period. *Pediatrics.* 1961;28:870–876.

28. Ahlfors CE. Criteria for exchange transfusion in jaundiced newborns. *Pediatrics.* 1994;93:488–494.

29. Soorani-Lunsing I, Woltil HA, Hadders-Algra M. Are moderate degrees of hyperbilirubinemia in healthy term neonates really safe for the brain? *Pediatr Res.* 2001;50:701–705.

30. Bhutani VK, Johnson L, Sivieri EM. Predictive ability of a predischarge hour-specific serum bilirubin for subsequent significant hyperbilirubinemia in healthy term and near-term newborns. *Pediatrics.* 1999;103:6–14.

31. Keren R, Bhutani VK, Luan X, Nihtianova S, Cnaan A, Schwartz JS. Identifying newborns at risk of significant hyperbilirubinaemia: a comparison of two recommended approaches. *Arch Dis Child.* 2005;90:415–421.

32. Keren R, Luan X, Friedman S, Saddlemire S, Cnaan A, Bhutani VK. A comparison of alternative risk-assessment strategies for predicting significant neonatal hyperbilirubinemia in term and near-term infants. *Pediatrics.* 2008;121:e170–e179.

33. Newman TB, Liljestrand P, Escobar GJ. Infants with bilirubin levels of 30 mg/dL or more in a large managed care organization. *Pediatrics.* 2003;111:1303–1311.

34. Newman TB, Liljestrand P, Escobar GJ. Combining clinical risk factors with serum bilirubin levels to predict hyperbilirubinemia in newborns. *Arch Pediatr Adolesc Med.* 2005;159:113–119.

35. Ebbesen F. Recurrence of kernicterus in term and near-term infants in Denmark. *Acta Paediatr.* 2000;89:1213–1217.

36. Agarwal R, Kaushal M, Aggarwal R, Paul VK, Deorari AK. Early neonatal hyperbilirubinemia using first day serum bilirubin level. *Indian Pediatr.* 2002;39:724–730.

37. Sarici SU, Serdar MA, Korkmaz A, Erdem G, Oran O, Tekinalp G, Yurdakök M, Yigit S. Incidence, course, and prediction of hyperbilirubinemia in near-term and term newborns. *Pediatrics.* 2004;113(4):775–780.

38. Carbonell X, Botet F, Figueras J, Riu-Godo A. Prediction of hyperbilirubinaemia in the healthy term newborn. *Acta Paediatr.* 2001;90:166–170.

39. Lo SF, Jendrzejczak B, Doumas BT. Laboratory performance in neonatal bilirubin testing using commutable specimens: a progress report on a College of American Pathologists study. *Arch Pathol Lab Med.* 2008;132:1781–1785.

40. Rennie J, Burman-Roy S, Murphy MS. Neonatal jaundice: summary of NICE guidance. *BMJ.* 2010;340:c2409.

41. Chung M, Ip S, Yu W, et al. *Interventions in Primary Care to Promote Breastfeeding: A Systematic Review.* Rockville, MD: Agency for Healthcare Research and Quality; 2008.

42. Facchini FP, Mezzacappa MA, Rosa IR, Mezzacappa Filho F, Aranha-Netto A, Marba ST. Follow-up of neonatal jaundice in term and late premature newborns. *J Pediatr (Rio J).* 2007;83:313–322.

43. Seidman DS, Ergaz Z, Paz I, et al. Predicting the risk of jaundice in full-term healthy newborns: a prospective population-based study. *J Perinatol.* 1999;19:564–567.

44. Centers for Disease Control and Prevention. Kernicterus in full-term infants—United States, 1994–1998. *MMWR Morb Mortal Wkly Rep.* 2001;50:491–494.

45. Ebbesen F, Andersson C, Verder H, et al. Extreme hyperbilirubinaemia in term and near-term infants in Denmark. *Acta Paediatr.* 2005;94:59–64.

46. Bjerre JV, Petersen JR, Ebbesen F. Surveillance of extreme hyperbilirubinaemia in Denmark. a method to identify the newborn infants. *Acta Paediatr.* 2008;97:1030–1034.

47. Canadian Pediatric Society. Guidelines for detection, management and prevention of hyperbilirubinemia in term and late preterm newborn infants (35 or more weeks' gestation)—summary. *Paediatr Child Health.* 2007;12:401–418.

48. Kaplan M, Bromiker R, Schimmel MS, Algur N, Hammerman C. Evaluation of discharge management in the prediction of hyperbilirubinemia: the Jerusalem experience. *J Pediatr.* 2007;150:412–417.

49. Bhutani VK, Maisels MJ, Stark AR, Buonocore G. Management of jaundice and prevention of severe neonatal hyperbilirubinemia in infants ≥35 weeks gestation. *Neonatology.* 2008;94:63–67.

50. Bratlid D, Nakstad B, Hansen TW. National guidelines for treatment of jaundice in the newborn. *Acta Paediatr.* 2011;100:499–505.

51. National Institute for Health and Clinical Excellence. *Neonatal Jaundice.* London: National Institute for Health and Clinical Excellence; 2010. Available at: www.nice.org.uk/CG98.

52. Bhutani VK, Johnson LH, Schwoebel A, Gennaro S. A systems approach for neonatal hyperbilirubinemia in term and near-term newborns. *J Obstet Gynecol Neonatal Nurs.* 2006;35:444–455.

53. Department of Health and Human Services, Office on Women's Health. *HHS Blueprint for Action on Breastfeeding.* Washington, DC: Department of Health and Human Services Office on Women's Health; 2000:1–33.

54. American Academy of Pediatrics. Breastfeeding and the use of human milk. *Pediatrics.* 2005;115:496–506.

55. Committee on Health Care for Underserved Women, American College of Obstetricians and Gynecologists. ACOG Committee Opinion No. 361: breastfeeding: maternal and infant aspects. *Obstet Gynecol.* 2007;109:479–480.

56. Centers for Disease Control and Prevention. *Breastfeeding Report Card, United States—2007: Outcome Indicators.* Atlanta, GA: Centers for Disease Control and Prevention; 2007.

57. Ip S, Chung M, Raman G, et al. Breastfeeding and maternal and infant health outcomes in developed countries. *Evid Rep Technol Assess (Full Rep).* 2007;(153):1–186.

58. California Department of Public Health GDB. *California In-Hospital Breastfeeding as Indicated on the Newborn Screening Test Form, Statewide, County and Hospital of Occurrence.* 2006.

59. Maisels MJ, McDonagh AF. Phototherapy for neonatal jaundice. *N Engl J Med.* 2008;358:920–928.

60. Vreman HJ, Wong RJ, Stevenson DK. Phototherapy: current methods and future directions. *Semin Perinatol.* 2004;28:326–333.

61. Bhutani VK, Stark AR, Lazzeroni LA, et al. (ICTERUS Study Group). Pre-discharge assessment predicts significant hyperbilirubinemia risk in a diverse cohort of US newborns. E-PAS 2008:6130.11.

62. Bhutani VK, Cline BK, Donaldson KM, Vreman HJ. The need to implement effective phototherapy in resource-constrained settings. *Semin Perinatol.* 2011;35: 192–197.

63. Beutler E. G6PD deficiency. *Blood.* 1994;84:3613–3636.

64. Bowman JM. RhD hemolytic disease of the newborn. *N Engl J Med.* 1998;339:1775–1777.

65. Kaplan M, Beutler E, Vreman HJ, et al. Neonatal hyperbilirubinemia in glucose-6-phosphate dehydrogenase-deficient heterozygotes. *Pediatrics.* 1999;104:68–74.

66. Kaplan M, Muraca M, Hammerman C, et al. Imbalance between production and conjugation of bilirubin: a fundamental concept in the mechanism of neonatal jaundice. *Pediatrics.* 2002;110:e47.

67. Kaplan M, Renbaum P, Levy-Lahad E, Hammerman C, Lahad A, Beutler E. Gilbert syndrome and glucose-6-phosphate dehydrogenase deficiency: a dose-dependent genetic interaction crucial to neonatal hyperbilirubinemia. *Proc Natl Acad Sci U S A.* 1997;94:12128–12132.

68. Chinevere TD, Murray CK, Grant E Jr, Johnson GA, Duelm F, Hospenthal DR. Prevalence of glucose-6-phosphate dehydrogenase deficiency in U.S. Army personnel. *Mil Med.* 2006;171:905–907.

69. Beal AC, Chou SC, Palmer RH, Testa MA, Newman C, Ezhuthachan S. The changing face of race: risk factors for neonatal hyperbilirubinemia. *Pediatrics.* 2006;117: 1618–1625.

70. Herschel M, Beutler E. Low glucose-6-phosphate dehydrogenase enzyme activity level at the time of hemolysis in a male neonate with the African type of deficiency. *Blood Cells Mol Dis.* 2001;27:918–923.

71. Nock ML, Walsh MC. Newborn screening program for glucose-6-phosphate-dehydrogenase deficiency (G6PD):

creation, implementation, and early results. *E-PAS2008:* 635848.2.

72. Al Otaibi SF, Blaser S, MacGregor DL. Neurological complications of kernicterus. *Can J Neurol Sci.* 2005;32: 311–315.

73. Joseph R, Ho LY, Gomez JM, Rajdurai VS, Sivasankaran S, Yip YY. Mass newborn screening for glucose-6-phosphate dehydrogenase deficiency in Singapore. *Southeast Asian J Trop Med Public Health.* 1999;30(suppl 2):70–71.

74. Meloni T, Forteleoni G, Meloni GF. Marked decline of favism after neonatal glucose-6-phosphate dehydrogenase screening and health education: the northern Sardinian experience. *Acta Haematol.* 1992;87:29–31.

75. Missiou-Tsagaraki S. Screening for glucose-6-phosphate dehydrogenase deficiency as a preventive measure: prevalence among 1,286,000 Greek newborn infants. *J Pediatr.* 1991;119:293–299.

76. Nkhoma ET, Poole C, Vannappagari V, Hall SA, Beutler E. The global prevalence of glucose-6-phosphate dehydrogenase deficiency: a systematic review and meta-analysis. *Blood Cells Mol Dis.* 2009;42:267–278.

77. Padilla CD, Therrell BL. Newborn screening in the Asia Pacific region. *J Inherit Metab Dis.* 2007;30:490–506.

78. Centers for Disease Control and Prevention. Impact of expanded newborn screening—United States, 2006. *MMWR Morb Mortal Wkly Rep.* 2008;57:1012–1015.

79. Suresh GK, Clark RE. Cost-effectiveness of strategies that are intended to prevent kernicterus in newborn infants. *Pediatrics.* 2004;114:917–924.

80. Bhutani VK, Johnson L. Kernicterus: lessons for the future from a current tragedy. *NeoReviews.* 2003;4:30.

81. Palmer RH, Keren R, Maisels MJ, Yeargin-Allsopp M. National Institute of Child Health and Human Development (NICHD) conference on kernicterus: a population perspective on prevention of kernicterus. *J Perinatol.* 2004;24:723–725.

82. Lannon C, Stark AR. Closing the gap between guidelines and practice: ensuring safe and healthy beginnings. *Pediatrics.* 2004;114:494–496.

83. Hameed NN, Na' Ma AM, Vilms R, Bhutani VK. Severe neonatal hyperbilirubinemia and adverse short-term consequences in Baghdad, Iraq. *Neonatology.* 2011;100: 57–63.

84. Bhutani VK, Stevenson DK. The need for technologies to prevent bilirubin-induced neurologic dysfunction syndrome. *Semin Perinatol.* 2011;35:97–100.

85. Slusher TM, Zipursky A, Bhutani VK. A global need for affordable neonatal jaundice technologies. *Semin Perinatol.* 2011;35:185–191.

Neonatal Jaundice in Low- and Middle-Income Countries

Tina M. Slusher and Bolajoko O. Olusanya

■ GLOBAL SCOPE OF NEONATAL JAUNDICE AND ASSOCIATED DISABILITIES

For the most part, in the developed world, neonatal jaundice occurs without significant morbidity and/or mortality due to early diagnosis and treatment.[1] However, most literature from low-middle-income countries (LMICs) suggests that it accounts for significant morbidity and mortality in contrast to that in the United States and developed world (Table 13-1).[2–18] For example, based on limited population-based data available worldwide, severe neonatal jaundice is about 100-fold greater in Nigeria than in the developed world. In one of the few population-based studies from the developed world, Ebbesen et al.[17] from Denmark reported that 24/100,000 neonates met exchange blood transfusion (exchange transfusion [ET]) criteria, while 9/100,000 developed acute bilirubin encephalopathy (ABE), in comparison to results from the only population-based study in Nigeria, in which Olusanya et al. reported 1860/100,000 infants had an EBT.[19] Based on the limited data available, ABE is at least as common as tetanus as a cause of neonatal deaths in Nigeria, Kenya, and Pakistan,[11,13,20–23] and likely in most LMICs often ranking as one of the top five causes of neonatal death.[8,11,13,24]

The available literature indicates that, in LMICs, a significant proportion of survivors of severe neonatal hyperbilirubinemia have signs of chronic bilirubin encephalopathy or kernicterus[1] (e.g., cerebral palsy, deafness, and language processing disorders (Table 13-2).[25–34] Children with disabilities are a tremendous burden on families in

LMICs, where resources are already stretched thin; such children are often left with few or no options for improved quality of life[35,36] and experience greater maltreatment than do those without disabilities. Notably, children with communication problems have a greater preponderance of first incidents of maltreatment by their mothers/caretakers from birth to 5 years than any other group of disabled children.[37–40] Such adverse childhood experiences are associated with significant short- and long-term medical, mental, psychosocial, and economic problems.[41–45] Overall, children suffering from the effects of neonatal hyperbilirubinemia readily fit into UNICEF's category of "excluded and invisible"[46] children. Unfortunately, current global efforts are doing little to highlight the burden of neonatal hyperbilirubinemia; *these children are excluded from the global burden of disease measurement.*[47]

■ NEED FOR POPULATION-BASED ABE CASE ASCERTAINMENT

Efforts to reduce or eliminate the sequelae of severe neonatal hyperbilirubinemia are hampered by a lack of adequate tools to objectively quantify the problem's magnitude.[48] One glaring gap is the paucity of population-based studies in the developing world; only two of the five countries represented in the literature are from the LMICs.[14,19,49–51] According to Lawn et al., population-based data on severe acute neonatal morbidities including jaundice are limited and only two cohort hospital-based follow-up studies on neonatal encephalopathy exist.[48,52] Studies by the World Health Organization (WHO) and

■ **TABLE 13-1.** Morbidity and Mortality Associated With Neonatal Jaundice

Country	No. of Infants, Definition	Year(s)	No. of ET/No. of ABE
Bolivia[2]	1167, 428 TSB ≥25 mg/dL	2000–2004	362/15
China[3]	41,535 admissions, 17,582 NNJ	2005–2006	NR/357
Egypt[4]	281 without TSB >25 mg/dL	2005–2006	229/29
Egypt[5]	408 without TSB >95% for age	2006–2008	112/16
India[6]	3791 births, 551 needing treatment	1994–1995	141/NR
Iran[7]	346 without NNJ	2004–2006	50/NR
Kenya[8]	432 ≤ 7 days, 75 NNJ (1080 <90 days)	1999–2001	30/10 plus/24% death
Nigeria[9]	4198 admitted, 722 TSB >19.9 mg/dL	2001–2005	87/42
Nigeria[10]	1686 admitted	2001–2003	90/27
Nigeria[11]	206 admissions, 44 NNJ	2002	36/6
Nigeria[12]	55 infants	1991–1992	NR/9
Nigeria[13]	7225 admissions	1981–1990	13% death
Pakistan[14]	1690 live births, 466 NNJ	2004–2006	1.8/1000 LB/NR
Thailand[15]	No denominator	1994–2003	165/NR
Turkey[16]	774 with NNJ, 93 with TSB ≥25 mg/dL	2000–2004	NR/6
Denmark[17]	12,334 births/32 with extreme hyperbilirubinemia	2000–2001	32 infants with TSB > ET limit/12 without CNS involvement
USA[18]	125 with kernicterus	1992–2004	91/125

ABE: acute bilirubin encephalopathy; ET: exchange transfusion; LB: live births; NNJ: neonatal jaundice; NR: not recorded; TSB: total serum bilirubin; CNS: central nervous system.

others have been limited by the lack of an appropriate survey instrument to accurately determine the percentage of infants with ABE in the community.[53] WHO published *A Standard Verbal Autopsy Method for Investigating Causes of Death in Infants and Children*[54] to provide a tool for health care workers to arrive at a reasonable cause of death in countries where systems for recording deaths are not well developed or where most deaths occur outside of medical facilities. This tool employs a structured interview with the next of kin (or significant other) to conduct mortality investigations. Specific questions for ABE and kernicterus are absent from this questionnaire, except to ask about whether the infant "was yellow," and about postneonatal deaths, which excluded neonatal jaundice as a preexisting condition, and posed only general questions about tone and eye movements. Large-scale efforts to prevent ABE are crucial, but are unlikely to happen until the actual burden of disease from severe hyperbilirubinemia is appreciated including appropriate population-based studies.

Available data suggest that the detection and treatment of severe neonatal hyperbilirubinemia is not rated high on the list of priorities in LMICs. However, recently the multinational Global Prevention of Kernicterus Network has been formed with the express purpose of both bringing the problem to the world's attention and developing affordable, sustainable solutions.

■ **NEED FOR EARLY DETECTION OF NEONATAL JAUNDICE**

Efforts to both define the magnitude of the problem and treat the problem effectively are also limited by lack of a screening tool. Neither visual assessment for jaundice nor any kind of quantitative measure of bilirubin is available in most locations in many LMICs. Recognition of jaundice and appropriate referral to and treatment at the community level is often lacking with delayed referral hampering timely recommended treatment.[10,55]

■ **NEED FOR DIAGNOSIS OF DEGREE OF JAUNDICE AND COMMON ETIOLOGIES**

As the first step, mothers, traditional birth attendants, community health workers, as well as more advanced health care providers should be taught to visually assess

■ **TABLE 13-2.** Disabilities Associated with Neonatal Jaundice

Country	Sequelae	Frequency due to NNJ
Brazil[25]	Hearing loss	6% of hearing loss from NNJ
Kenya[26]	Eye movement disorder, dyskinesia movement disorder	12/23 with NNJ seen in FU 11/23 with NNJ seen in FU
India[27]	CP, DD, or abnormal ABR	12/15 FU post-ET with ABE
India[28]	CP	16.7% of <19 years old with CP had ABE
Malaysia[29]	Hearing loss	28/128 with NNJ
Nigeria[30]	Communication disorder	4.3% of communication disorders
Nigeria[31]	Hearing loss	13.5% of DHI children
Nigeria[32]	Hearing loss	19.7% of infants with HL
Turkey[33]	CP	Post-NNJ common
Zimbabwe[34]	CP, DD	5/43 FU, 11/43 FU

ABE: acute bilirubin encephalopathy; ABR: auditory-evoked brainstem response; CP: cerebral palsy; DD: developmental disabilities; DHI: deaf and hearing impaired; ET: exchange transfusion; FU: follow-up; NNJ: neonatal jaundice.

perform jaundice evaluations in some locations including Pakistan[14,57] and Bangladesh.[58] If possible, every infant should be reevaluated on days 2–4 of life. One logical solution in many locations may be to set up the BCG (tuberculosis vaccine) clinic appointment during this time interval. In addition to assessing feeding problems, cord care, and general issues with the newborn, the infant should be assessed visually for jaundice. If there is jaundice present, the infant should be reevaluated the following day and at least daily if jaundice appears to be progressing. In many locals trained traditional birth attendants and other trained community health workers will be essential in this process as transport and other obstacles will make it impossible for these babies to be brought to higher-level health care facilities for screening. If any infant is noted to be jaundiced in the first day of life or have jaundice involving the hands and feet at any point, the infant should be referred urgently for further evaluation in a center capable of performing TSB measurements and phototherapy at a minimum.

Measuring TSB levels is a challenge facing many health care facilities in LMICs. Many facilities have no way of measuring TSB, and those that do often lack resources such as reagents, blood collection tubes, centrifuges, and a consistent supply of electricity to run the machines. In addition, many machines require large volumes of blood from infants from whom the sample is difficult to obtain, discouraging frequent rechecks even when clinically indicated. Finally, the cost of supplies and limited trained lab personnel also preclude appropriate bilirubin rechecks in many facilities. Each of these obstacles needs to be addressed in health care facilities and every effort should be made to provide TSB levels at admission and as needed around the clock. In the event that there is a delay in obtaining

jaundice after birth and at least for the following week. Recognizing its limitation, the modified Kramer scale[56] (Figure 13-1) can still be used to improve visual assessment. Community health workers have been taught to

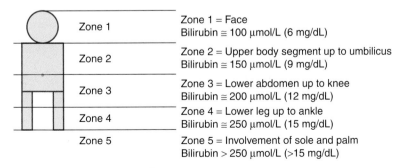

Zone 1 = Face
Bilirubin ≅ 100 µmol/L (6 mg/dL)

Zone 2 = Upper body segment up to umbilicus
Bilirubin ≅ 150 µmol/L (9 mg/dL)

Zone 3 = Lower abdomen up to knee
Bilirubin ≅ 200 µmol/L (12 mg/dL)

Zone 4 = Lower leg up to ankle
Bilirubin ≅ 250 µmol/L (15 mg/dL)

Zone 5 = Involvement of sole and palm
Bilirubin > 250 µmol/L (>15 mg/dL)

FIGURE 13-1. Modified Kramer scale.[56]

■ TABLE 13-3. Agents That May Provoke Hemolysis in Neonates with G6PD Deficiency[59-61]

Naphthalene
Mentholated products such as mentholated rub/dusting
  powder
Vitamin K analogs (K3)
Henna
Triple dye
Sulfanilamide powder
Maternal ingestion of aflatoxins
Maternal ingestion of fava beans

TSB levels in an infant deemed to have significant jaundice, phototherapy should be initiated and a TSB level measured as soon as possible. If this is not possible, the serum should be separated from the cells and the sample stored in the dark.

In many parts of the world, glucose-6-phosphate dehydrogenase (G6PD) deficiency is an important cause of severe neonatal hyperbilirubinemia. Efforts to provide low-cost, easy-to-perform G6PD testing are urgently needed to help identify at-risk infants. Health care providers and parents should be told to avoid products commonly used in normal newborn care such as mentholated rub, mentholated dusting powder, naphthalene balls, and other agents (e.g., certain foods such as fava beans) that might trigger hemolysis in a G6PD-deficient infant (Table 13-3).[59-61] Harmful practices such as applying mentholated rub on the fontanel should be avoided; instead, alternatives such as petroleum jelly in cultures should be suggested.

Routine blood typing of pregnant women and, when indicated, the use of $Rh_o(D)$ immune globulin are standard practices in the developed world but, in many settings, especially in rural areas, blood typing is not available. Rh immune globulin is usually unavailable and, when available, is often cost prohibitive. Although the incidence of Rh hemolytic disease is substantially lower in many LMICs compared with the United States and Europe before the use of Rh immune globulin, tens of thousands of mothers in India, Pakistan, and Kenya are nevertheless sensitized to the D antigen.[62] Routine blood typing should be done for all women of childbearing age either during or before pregnancy. One practical approach to blood typing could involve the routine screening of young women in secondary schools together with tetanus immunization. Blood

typing could also be done on all students on school entry and become part of their personal health records. Mothers at risk for ABO or Rh incompatibility should be counseled to observe their infants for jaundice and seek treatment early. It is important to plan ahead to have Rh immune globulin available and affordable, perhaps through international subsidies to those women who need it.

■ NEED FOR ACCURATE DIAGNOSIS OF ACUTE BILIRUBIN ENCEPHALOPATHY/ KERNICTERUS

Generally ABE/kernicterus is a clinical diagnosis made easily by an experienced clinician using established physical signs and symptoms (Table 13-4).[63] These signs and symptoms may be scored using the bilirubin-induced neurologic dysfunction (BIND) II score (Table 13-5).

Johnson et al.[64] developed a scoring system to categorize the severity of ABE. We have modified this score for use in LMICs where it might help to better differentiate ABE from other illnesses such as tetanus, since confirmatory testing such as auditory-evoked responses and magnetic resonance imaging (MRI) are usually unavailable. Reporting a BIND II score (Table 13-5) may also be useful in communicating with other clinicians and investigators regarding the severity of ABE and the change in the score in response to treatment. One group of physical findings,

■ TABLE 13-4. Major Clinical Features of Acute Bilirubin Encephalopathy (ABE)

Initial phase
Slight stupor ("lethargic," "sleepy")
Slight hypotonia, paucity of movement
Poor sucking, slightly high-pitched cry

Intermediate phase
Moderate stupor—irritability
Tone variable—usually increased, some with retrocollis/
  opisthotonos
Minimal feeding, high-pitched cry

Advanced phase
Deep stupor to coma
Tone usually increased, pronounced retrocollis/
  opisthotonos
No feeding, shrill cry

Reprinted with permission from Volpe J. *Neurology of the Newborn.* 5th ed. Philadelphia: Saunders Elsevier. Copyright © Elsevier 2008.

■ **TABLE 13-5.** Bilirubin-Induced Neurologic Dysfunction (BIND) II Score

Clinical Sign (Score Most Severe Sign)	Score	Severity
Mental status		
☐ Normal	0	None
☐ Sleepy but arousable	1	Mild
☐ Decreased feeding		
☐ Lethargy		
☐ Poor suck and/or	2	Moderate
☐ Irritable/jittery with short-term strong suck		
☐ Semi-coma		
☐ Apnea	3	Severe
☐ Seizures		
☐ Coma		
Muscle tone		
☐ Normal	0	None
☐ Persistent mild hypotonia	1	Mild
☐ Moderate hypotonia		
☐ Moderate hypertonia		
☐ Increasing arching of neck and trunk on stimulation without spasms of arms and legs and without trismus	2	Moderate
☐ Persistent retrocolis		
☐ Opisthotonos	3	Severe
☐ Crossing or scissoring of arms or legs but without spasms of arms and legs and without trismus		
Cry pattern		
☐ Normal	0	None
☐ High-pitched	1	Mild
☐ Shrill	2	Moderate
☐ Inconsolable crying or		
☐ Cry weak or absent in child with previous history of high pitched or shrill cry	3	Severe
Oculomotor/eye movements/facies		
☐ Normal	0	None, mild
☐ Sun-setting		
☐ Paralysis of upward gaze		
☐ Disconjugate eye movements	3	Severe
☐ Blank stare		
☐ Aimless eye movements		
Total BIND II (ABE score)	_____	

Scores of 1–4 are consistent with mild ABE but cannot be differentiated from sepsis or other neonatal illnesses without ancillary testing, such as ABR and/or MRI. Scores 5–8 are consistent with moderate ABE. Scores ≥9 are consistent with severe ABE. The BIND score may include different stages for different categories, for example, scores of 4 or 5 might represent the sum of one for cry and two for muscle tone and/or arousal state. Modified with permission from Dr. Lois Johnson.

which may be particularly helpful in making the diagnosis, is the "kernicteric facies" (Figure 13-2). It is described under the oculomotor/facial findings of the BIND II and recently reported in the literature.[65]

The infant with ABE/kernicterus should be evaluated for other illnesses such as birth asphyxia, meningitis, and other causes of encephalitis. These and other neonatal illnesses increase the risk of ABE/kernicterus in an infant

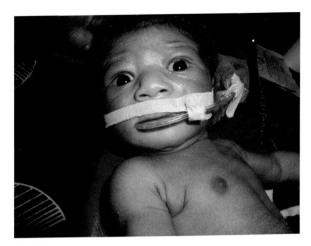

FIGURE 13-2. Kernicteric facies.

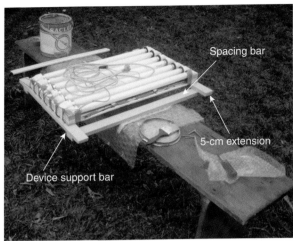

FIGURE 13-3. Assembling the locally made phototherapy device.

with significant hyperbilirubinemia. They can occur alone or in combination with ABE/kernicterus and will need additional treatment.

■ TREATMENT

Implementing phototherapy can be difficult to achieve in LMICs because the appropriate light sources as well as electricity are often not available. ETs carry a higher risk due to the limited ability to screen the blood, intermittent availability of blood, limited monitoring available to the infants during an ET, and higher risk of transmission of infectious diseases such as HIV due to the higher risk in the general population. In addition, the number of institutions that can perform ETs is limited. Because of these limitations, health care providers often elect to begin phototherapy when TSB levels are about 2–3 mg/dL below that suggested by the 2004 American Academy of Pediatrics (AAP) recommendations,[1] and continue phototherapy until the bilirubin drops below 12 mg/dL.

"Intensive phototherapy" (defined in the AAP guideline[1] as delivering an irradiance ≥30 µW/cm²/nm) is rarely available in LMICs. Nevertheless, more effective phototherapy can be achieved using simple, locally available supplies. These devices can usually be made and maintained for a fraction of the cost of the commercial devices used in high-income countries (Figures 13-3 to 13-5). Double phototherapy can be provided by building a fixed unit for the side of incubators/isolettes or beside the bed (meaning bed, bassinette, cot, or wherever the infant sleeps) of the

term infant or below the bed of the infant using a Plexiglas surface for the infant to lie on.

Even with locally made devices, more effective phototherapy can be provided with white sheets placed around the infant's bed, and by decreasing the distance between the phototherapy device and the infant to 10–15 cm.[66] Depending on the light source, caution must be exercised, to avoid overheating or causing a burn. Overheating can be prevented by placing term infants in beds or bassinettes and by treating them in well-ventilated areas. Infant temperatures should be monitored regularly even in the

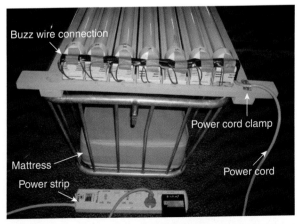

FIGURE 13-4. Locally made phototherapy device inverted over a cradle to display fully assembled device.

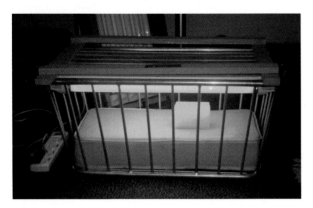

FIGURE 13-5. Phototherapy in use with a cradle.

larger term infants as hypothermia may be a problem at night or in cooler seasons even in the tropics.

Special blue bulbs are more efficient[1] but almost never available in many locations. Bulbs should be kept clean and replaced when they burn out or at 2000 hours[67] (whichever comes first) or flicker or begin to look visibly dim. The use of irradiance meters should be encouraged, as measuring the irradiance of the units is the only way to ensure that effective phototherapy is being provided. Irradiance meters can also be used to educate health care providers that simply having light does not equate with "having effective phototherapy."[66] Low-cost, reliable irradiance meters are urgently needed.

Although unfiltered sunlight phototherapy should never be the recommended treatment for neonatal jaundice, even in LMICs, at times it is the only option available, at least emergently, in very remote rural areas without readily available transportation. Its use is not ideal for many reasons including potential for sunburn, temperature instability, and harm from prolonged exposure to UV/IR light. The use of sunlight phototherapy filters and battery- and solar-powered units is currently being investigated.[68,69] Until such units are readily available, unfiltered sunlight phototherapy may be the only option for some infants. While seeking a more appropriate option, mothers can be advised to place their unclothed infant (with eyes covered) in the sun every 1–2 hours for about 15–30 minutes while monitoring the infant closely for sunburn and overheating and seeking to refer the infant to a center for phototherapy. Nonetheless, unfiltered sunlight should be viewed as an emergency, suboptimal treatment and not standard of care even in LMICs.

ETs should be available for infants with any neurologic symptoms consistent with ABE or those meeting ET criteria. Unless both intensive phototherapy and frequent TSB testing are readily available, blood should be sent for typing and cross-matching as soon as a severely jaundice infant is admitted or when signs of ABE are present. Blood should be screened for both HIV and hepatitis B and, whenever possible, obtained from volunteer rather than paid donors. Since blood components are rarely available, whole blood is generally used for ETs. If possible, blood that is less than 2–3 days old should be used.

Complications of ETs are listed in Chapter 9.[7,70–72] Because of difficulties in administering intravenous (IV) fluids, feedings are not usually withheld in infants following an ET.

■ FOLLOW-UP OF INFANTS AND CHILDREN WITH ELEVATED TSB LEVELS/ABE/ KERNICTERUS

See Chapter 10.

■ FOLLOW-UP AND TREATMENT IN SUBSEQUENT PREGNANCIES

Depending on the etiology of the jaundice, mothers who have one significantly jaundiced infant are at risk of having subsequent affected infants.[1] During the admission of any infant with significant neonatal jaundice, especially in those infants needing an ET or having ABE, a mother should be counseled regarding future pregnancies. She should be reminded that ABE is generally preventable and she should be encouraged to have regular prenatal care and to deliver at a facility capable of providing frequent TSB levels, quality phototherapy, and ETs if needed. Depending on G6PD risk, she should be counseled to avoid practices known to increase hemolysis in these infants. Even if she delivers at home or in a health care facility not able to provide the recommended evaluations or treatment, she should be encouraged to have each subsequent infant screened for jaundice immediately on recognition of jaundice and again at days 2–3 and 4–5 of life.

Although controversial and not conclusively proven,[73] it may be appropriate to consider prenatal phenobarbital for the mother, especially if her previous infants' jaundice was known or suspected to be hemolytic in origin.[74]

Phenobarbital may be especially important if the mother is going to deliver far from facilities capable of doing bilirubin measurements and providing phototherapy and ETs if needed. A recent review of the literature by Chawla and Parmar[75] suggested that phenobarbital given to low birth weight infants reduced their need for phototherapy, duration of phototherapy, and need for an ET. While not likely applicable in areas with an ample supply of intense phototherapy, this may prove very helpful in limited resource settings subject to additional validation studies.

■ MOVING FORWARD IN LMICS

Goals for the future, as we move to eliminate ABE/kernicterus worldwide, include improving the availability and quality of diagnostic and treatment modalities. Recognizing that severe jaundice is common and can progress to death or lifelong problems is the critical first step. Developing appropriate tools to determine the magnitude of severe neonatal jaundice is paramount and an important next step. These tools need to be used to screen large populations to determine the incidence of ABE/kernicterus as a cause of both morbidity and mortality. Meeting these goals requires mass screening of neonates for jaundice. This will require a change in health care policy for many LMICs. Part of the policy change should include putting in place an *expectation* that every infant be screened, and then developing a *system* for screening of every infant, including those born at home or in small health care facilities. As previously noted, screening may be easiest if added to already existing follow-up such as the BCG (tuberculosis vaccine) clinics where neonates routinely receive this vaccine. Importantly, neonates would need to come to this clinic or any other screening facility early enough to allow effective treatment of jaundiced infants. Screening requires widely available, low-tech, durable, low-cost methods to objectively measure TSB levels, including reagents, supplies, and equipment.

Treatment challenges exist as well. Many of these can potentially be met with low-tech, low-cost devices currently being developed and tested, including innovative phototherapy methods such as sunlight filters, solar-powered devices, and battery-operated devices. More affordable and accessible irradiance meters to monitor phototherapy devices are needed and being developed. Studies of effective and affordable pharmacologic agents are needed. Heme oxygenase inhibitors are ideal[76] if they can be provided safely and at low cost (see Chapter 10).

Women of reproductive age must be trained during antenatal clinics to recognize jaundice and seek evaluation and care for their jaundiced infants before it progresses to ABE. All health care workers must likewise be trained in early recognition and referral and/or treatment as appropriate. Policy makers must be made aware of the necessity of screening and essential treatment. Education is mandatory at all levels from the mother and her village health care worker to professionals and policy makers. Only then will we move toward a world without ABE/kernicterus.

■ ACKNOWLEDGMENTS

We would like to thank Hendrik J. Vreman, PhD, for designing and constructing the locally made phototherapy devices. Full details of their construction can be found in Kamat DM, Fischer PR, eds. *American Academy of Pediatrics Textbook of Global Child Health.* Elk Grove Village, IL: American Academy of Pediatrics; 2011. In press.

REFERENCES

1. American Academy of Pediatrics Subcommittee on Hyperbilirubinemia. Management of hyperbilirubinemia in the newborn infant 35 or more weeks of gestation. *Pediatrics.* 2004;114:297–316.
2. Salas AA, Mazzi E. Exchange transfusion in infants with extreme hyperbilirubinemia: an experience from a developing country. *Acta Paediatr.* 2008;97:754–758.
3. Subspecialty Group of Neonatology, Pediatric Society, Chinese Medical Association. Epidemiologic survey for hospitalized neonates in China. *Zhongguo Dang Dai Er Ke Za Zhi.* 2009;11:15–20.
4. Seoud I, Iskander I, Gamaleldin R, Khairy D, Khairy M, Wennberg RP. How well does serum bilirubin concentration identify babies at high risk for developing kernicterus. E-PAS2009. 2009;2842.395.
5. Seoud I, Khairy MA, Khairy DA. Neonatal jaundice in Cairo University Pediatric Hospital. *J Arab Child.* 2007;18:177–187.
6. Narang A, Gathwala G, Kumar P. Neonatal jaundice: an analysis of 551 cases. *Indian Pediatr.* 1997;34:429–432.
7. Behjati S, Sagheb S, Aryasepehr S, Yaghmai B. Adverse events associated with neonatal exchange transfusion for hyperbilirubinemia. *Indian J Pediatr.* 2009;76:83–85.
8. English M, Ngama M, Musumba C, et al. Causes and outcome of young infant admissions to a Kenyan district hospital. *Arch Dis Child.* 2003;88:438–443.

9. Ogunlesi T, Dedeke I, Adekanmbi A, Fetuga M, Ogunfowora O. The incidence and outcome of bilirubin encephalopathy in Nigeria. *Niger J Med.* 2007;4: 354–359.

10. Owa JA, Ogunlesi TA. Why we are still doing so many exchange blood transfusion for neonatal jaundice in Nigeria. *World J Pediatr.* 2009;5:51–55.

11. Eneh AU, Oruamabo RS. Neonatal jaundice in a special care baby unit (SCBU) in Port Harcourt, Nigeria: a prospective study. *Port Harcourt Med J.* 2008;2:110–117.

12. Slusher TM, Vreman HJ, McLaren DW, Lewison LJ, Brown AK, Stevenson DK. Glucose-6-phosphate dehydrogenase deficiency and carboxyhemoglobin concentrations associated with bilirubin-related morbidity and death in Nigerian infants. *J Pediatr.* 1995;126:102–108.

13. Owa JA, Osinaike AI. Neonatal morbidity and mortality in Nigeria. *Indian J Pediatr.* 1998;65:441–449.

14. Tikmani S, Warraich H, Abbasi F, Rizvi A, Darmstadt G, Zaidi A. Incidence of neonatal hyperbilirubinemia: a population based prospective study in Pakistan. *Trop Med Int Health.* 2010;5:502–507.

15. Sanpavat S. Exchange transfusion and its morbidity in ten-year period at King Chulalongkorn Hospital. *J Med Assoc Thai.* 2005;88:588–592.

16. Tiker F, Gulcan H, Kilicdag H, Tarcan A, Gurakan B. Extreme hyperbilirubinemia in newborn infants. *Clin Pediatr (Phila).* 2006;45:257–261.

17. Ebbesen F, Andersson C, Verder H, et al. Extreme hyperbilirubinaemia in term and near-term infants in Denmark. *Acta Paediatr.* 2005;1:59–64.

18. Johnson L, Bhutani VK, Karp K, Sivieri EM, Shapiro SM. Clinical report from the pilot USA Kernicterus Registry (1992 to 2004). *J Perinatol.* 2009;29(suppl 1): S25–S45.

19. Olusanya B, Akande A, Emokpae A, Olowe S. Infants with severe neonatal jaundice in Lagos, Nigeria: incidence, correlates and hearing screening outcomes. *Trop Med Int Health.* 2009;3:301–310.

20. Okechukwu A, Achonwa A. Morbidity and mortality patterns of admissions into the special care baby unit of University of Abuja Teaching Hospital. *Niger J Clin Pract.* 2009;4:389–394.

21. Ugwu R, Eneh A, Oruamabo R. Mortality in the special care baby unit of the University of Port Harcourt Teaching Hospital (UPTH). Why and when do newborns die? *Niger J Paediatr.* 2006;3:133–134.

22. Simiyu DE. Morbidity and mortality of neonates admitted in general paediatric wards at Kenyatta National Hospital. *East Afr Med J.* 2003;80:611–616.

23. Rahim F. Pattern and outcome of admissions to neonatal unit of Khyber Teaching Hospital, Peshawar. *Pak J Med Sci.* 2007;23:249–253.

24. Islam M. Morbidity pattern and mortality of neonates admitted in a tertiary level teaching hospital in Bangladesh. *Mymensingh Med J.* 2010;19:159–162.

25. da Silva LP, Queiros F, Lima I. Etiology of hearing impairment in children and adolescents of a reference center APADA in the city of Salvador, state of Bahia. *Braz J Otorhinolaryngol.* 2006;72:33–36.

26. Gordon AL, English M, Tumaini Dzombo J, Karisa M, Newton CR. Neurological and developmental outcome of neonatal jaundice and sepsis in rural Kenya. *Trop Med Int Health.* 2005;10:1114–1120.

27. Mukhopadhyay K, Chowdhary G, Singh P, Kumar P, Narang A. Neurodevelopmental outcome of acute bilirubin encephalopathy. *J Trop Pediatr.* 2010;56:333–336.

28. Banerjee TK, Hazra A, Biswas A, et al. Neurological disorders in children and adolescents. *Indian J Pediatr.* 2009;76:139–146.

29. Boo NY, Oakes M, Lye MS, Said H. Risk factors associated with hearing loss in term neonates with hyperbilirubinaemia. *J Trop Pediatr.* 1994;40:194–197.

30. Somefun OA, Lesi FE, Danfulani MA, Olusanya BO. Communication disorders in Nigerian children. *Int J Pediatr Otorhinolaryngol.* 2006;70:697–702.

31. Olusanya BO, Somefun AO. Sensorineural hearing loss in infants with neonatal jaundice in Lagos: a community-based study. *Ann Trop Paediatr.* 2009;29:119–128.

32. Olusanya BO, Okolo AA. Adverse perinatal conditions in hearing-impaired children in a developing country. *Paediatr Perinat Epidemiol.* 2006;20:366–371.

33. Ozturk A, Demirci F, Yavuz T, et al. Antenatal and delivery risk factors and prevalence of cerebral palsy in Duzce (Turkey). *Brain Dev.* 2007;29:39–42.

34. Wolf MJ, Wolf B, Beunen G, Casaer P. Neurodevelopmental outcome at 1 year in Zimbabwean neonates with extreme hyperbilirubinaemia. *Eur J Pediatr.* 1999; 158:111–114.

35. Green SE. "What do you mean what's wrong with her?": stigma and the lives of families of children with disabilities. *Soc Sci Med.* 2003;57:1361–1374.

36. Hibbard RA, Desch LW; American Academy of Pediatrics Committee on Child Abuse and Neglect, American Academy of Pediatrics Council on Children with Disabilities. Maltreatment of children with disabilities. *Pediatrics.* 2007;119:1018–1025.

37. Knutson JF, Johnson CR, Sullivan PM. Disciplinary choices of mothers of deaf children and mothers of normally hearing children. *Child Abuse Negl.* 2004;28: 925–937.

38. Kvam MH. Sexual abuse of deaf children. A retrospective analysis of the prevalence and characteristics of childhood sexual abuse among deaf adults in Norway. *Child Abuse Negl.* 2004;28:241–251.

39. Sullivan PM, Knutson JF. Maltreatment and disabilities: a population-based epidemiological study. *Child Abuse Negl.* 2000;24:1257–1273.

40. Togonu-Bickersteth F, Odebiyi AI. Influence of Yoruba beliefs about abnormality on the socialization of deaf children: a research note. *J Child Psychol Psychiatry.* 1985;26:639–652.

41. Dubowitz H, Bennett S. Physical abuse and neglect of children. *Lancet.* 2007;369:1891–1899.

42. Dube SR, Felitti VJ, Dong M, Giles WH, Anda RF. The impact of adverse childhood experiences on health problems: evidence from four birth cohorts dating back to 1900. *Prev Med.* 2003;37:268–277.

43. Hildyard KL, Wolfe DA. Child neglect: developmental issues and outcomes. *Child Abuse Negl.* 2002;26:679–695.

44. Glaser D. Child abuse and neglect and the brain—a review. *J Child Psychol Psychiatry.* 2000;41:97–116.

45. Olusanya BO, Ruben RJ, Parving A. Reducing the burden of communication disorders in the developing world: an opportunity for the millennium development project. *JAMA.* 2006;296:441–444.

46. UNICEF. *State of the World's Children 2006.* New York: UNICEF, UNICEF House; 2005.

47. Jamison DT. *World Bank. Disease Control Priorities in Developing Countries.* New York: Oxford University Press; 1993.

48. Lawn JE, Osrin D, Adler A, Cousens S. Four million neonatal deaths: counting and attribution of cause of death. *Paediatr Perinat Epidemiol.* 2008;22:410–416.

49. Bjerre JV, Petersen JR, Ebbesen F. Surveillance of extreme hyperbilirubinaemia in Denmark. A method to identify the newborn infants. *Acta Paediatr.* 2008;97:1030–1034.

50. Manning D, Todd P, Maxwell M, Jane Platt M. Prospective surveillance study of severe hyperbilirubinaemia in the newborn in the UK and Ireland. *Arch Dis Child Fetal Neonatal Ed.* 2007;92:F342–F346.

51. Sgro M, Campbell D, Shah V. Incidence and causes of severe neonatal hyperbilirubinemia in Canada. *CMAJ.* 2006;175:587–590.

52. Lawn RE, Rudan I, Rubens C. Four million newborn deaths: is the global research agenda evidence-based? *Early Hum Dev.* 2008;84:809–814.

53. Bryce J, Boschi-Pinto C, Shibuya K, Black RE. WHO estimates of the causes of death in children. *Lancet.* 2005;365:1147–1152.

54. Anker M, Black RE, Coldham C, et al. *A Standard Verbal Autopsy Method for Investigating Causes of Death in Infants and Children.* Geneva: World Health Organization; 1999.

55. Ogunfowora OB, Daniel OJ. Neonatal jaundice and its management: knowledge, attitude and practice of community health workers in Nigeria. *BMC Public Health.* 2006;6:19.

56. Manzar S. Cephalo-caudal progression of jaundice: a reliable, non-invasive clinical method to assess the degree of neonatal hyperbilirubinaemia. *J Trop Pediatr.* 1999;45:312–313.

57. Hatzenbuehler L, Zaidi AK, Sundar S, et al. Validity of neonatal jaundice evaluation by primary health-care workers and physicians in Karachi, Pakistan. *J Perinatol.* 2010;30:616–621.

58. Darmstadt GL, Baqui AH, Choi Y, et al. Validation of community health workers' assessment of neonatal illness in rural Bangladesh. *Bull World Health Organ.* 2009;87:12–19.

59. Kaplan M, Hammerman C. Understanding and preventing severe neonatal hyperbilirubinemia: is bilirubin neurotoxicity really a concern in the developed world? *Clin Perinatol.* 2004;31:555–575, x.

60. Sodeinde O, Chan MC, Maxwell SM, Familusi JB, Hendrickse RG. Neonatal jaundice, aflatoxins and naphthols: report of a study in Ibadan, Nigeria. *Ann Trop Paediatr.* 1995;15:107–113.

61. Valaes T. Severe neonatal jaundice associated with glucose-6-phosphate dehydrogenase deficiency: pathogenesis and global epidemiology. *Acta Paediatr Suppl.* 1994;394:58–76.

62. Zipursky A, Paul VK. The global burden of Rh disease. *Arch Dis Child Fetal Neonatal Ed.* 2011;96:F84–F85.

63. Volpe J. Bilirubin and brain injury. In: *Neurology of the Newborn.* 5th ed. Philadelphia: Saunders Elsevier; 2008:635–637.

64. Johnson L, Brown AK, Bhutani VK. BIND—a clinical score for bilirubin induced neurologic dysfunction in newborns. *Pediatr Suppl.* 1999;104:746–747.

65. Slusher T, Owa JA, Painter M, Shapiro S. The kernicteric facies: facial features of acute bilirubin encephalopathy. *Pediatr Neurol.* 2011;44:153–154.

66. Cline BK, Vreman HJ, Faber KL, et al. Phototherapy device effectiveness in Nigeria: current irradiance levels and simple strategies for improvement. E-PAS2011. 2011;1450.540.

67. Tan K. Phototherapy for neonatal jaundice. *Clin Perinatol.* 1991;18:423–439.

68. Slusher T, Faber K, Cline BK, et al. Selectively filtered sunlight phototherapy: safe and effective for treatment of neonatal jaundice in Nigeria. E-PAS2011. 2011;2918.254.

69. Malkin R, Anand V. A novel phototherapy device: the design community approach for the developing world. *IEEE Eng Med Biol Mag.* 2010;29:37–43.

70. Gomella TL, Cunningham MD, Eyal FG, Zenk KE. *Neonatology: Management, Procedures, On-Call Problems, Diseases, and Drugs.* New York: McGraw-Hill; 2004.

71. Hosseinpour Sakha S, Gharehbaghi MM. Exchange transfusion in severe hyperbilirubinemia: an experience in northwest Iran. *Turk J Pediatr.* 2010;52:367–371.

72. Badiee Z. Exchange transfusion in neonatal hyperbilirubinaemia: experience in Isfahan, Iran. *Singapore Med J.* 2007;48:421–423.

73. Thomas JT, Muller P, Wilkinson C. Antenatal phenobarbital for reducing neonatal jaundice after red cell isoimmunization. *Cochrane Database Syst Rev.* 2007:CD005541.

74. Trevett TN Jr, Dorman K, Lamvu G, Moise KJ Jr. Antenatal maternal administration of phenobarbital for the prevention of exchange transfusion in neonates with hemolytic disease of the fetus and newborn. *Am J Obstet Gynecol.* 2005;192:478–482.

75. Chawla D, Parmar V. Phenobarbitone for prevention and treatment of unconjugated hyperbilirubinemia in preterm neonates: a systematic review and meta-analysis. *Indian Pediatr.* 2010;47:401–407.

76. Stevenson DK, Wong RJ. Metalloporphyrins in the management of neonatal hyperbilirubinemia. *Semin Fetal Neonatal Med.* 2010;15:164–168.

Index

Page references followed by *f* indicate figures; those followed by *t* indicate tables.